Contents

a Lange medical book

CURRENT
Diagnosis &
Treatment
of Pain

Edited by

Jamie H. Von Roenn, MD
Professor of Medicine
Department of Medicine
Division of Hematology/Oncology
Feinberg School of Medicine
Robert H. Lurie Comprehensive
Cancer Center
Northwestern University
Chicago, Illinois

Judith A. Paice, PhD, RN
Director, Cancer Pain Program
Department of Medicine
Division of Hematology/Oncology
Feinberg School of Medicine
Robert H. Lurie Comprehensive
Cancer Center
Northwestern University
Chicago, Illinois

Michael E. Preodor, MD
Instructor in Medicine
Department of Medicine
Division of Hematology/Oncology
Feinberg School of Medicine
Robert H. Lurie Comprehensive
Cancer Center
Northwestern University
Chicago, Illinois

Lange Medical Books/McGraw-Hill
Medical Publishing Division

New York   Chicago   San Francisco   Lisbon   London   Madrid
Mexico City   Milan   New Delhi   San Juan   Seoul   Singapore   Sydney   Toronto

Current Diagnosis & Treatment of Pain

1 2 3 4 5 6 7 8 9 0 DOC/DOC 0 9 8 7 6

ISBN: 0-07-144478-5

Notice

Medicine is an ever-changing science. As new research and clinical experience broaden our knowledge, changes in treatment and drug therapy are required. The authors and the publisher of this work have checked with sources believed to be reliable in their efforts to provide information that is complete and generally in accord with the standards accepted at the time of publication. However, in view of the possibility of human error or changes in medical sciences, neither the authors nor the publisher nor any other party who has been involved in the preparation or publication of this work warrants that the information contained herein is in every respect accurate or complete, and they disclaim all responsibility for any errors or omissions or for the results obtained from use of the information contained in this work. Readers are encouraged to confirm the information contained herein with other sources. For example and in particular, readers are advised to check the product information sheet included in the package of each drug they plan to administer to be certain that the information contained in this work is accurate and that changes have not been made in the recommended dose or in the contraindications for administration. This recommendation is of particular importance in connection with new or infrequently used drugs.

This book was set in Adobe Garamond by TechBooks.
The Editors were Joe Rusko, Harriet Lebowitz, and Regina Y. Brown.
The Production Supervisor was Sherri Souffrance.
The Cover Designer was Mary McKeon.
The Indexer was Robert Swanson.
RR Donnelly was the Printer and Binder.

This book is printed on acid-free paper.

International Edition ISBN 0-07-110460-7

Authors

Tasha Burwinkle, PsyD, PhD
Senior Fellow, Department of Psychology,
    University of Washington, Seattle, Washington
tburwinkle@aol.com
Psychological Interventions

Edwin L. Capulong, MD
Spine Medicine Fellow, The Cleveland Spine
    Institute, Cleveland, Ohio
capuloe@ccf.org
Osteoarthritis & Rheumatoid Arthritis

Kelly J. Cooke, DO
Associate Medical Director, Palliative Care Center &
    Hospice of the North Shore, Rush North Shore
    Medical Center, Skokie, Illinois
kcooke@carecenter.org
Assessment of Pain & Common Pain Syndromes

Russell C. DeMicco, DO
Associate Staff, The Cleveland Clinic Spine Institute,
    Cleveland, Ohio
demiccr@ccf.org
Osteoarthritis & Rheumatoid Arthritis

Elizabeth Ely, PhD, RN
Research Assistant Professor of Pediatrics, Drexel
University College of Medicine; St. Christopher's
    Hospital for Children, Philadelphia, Pennsylvania
eely@drexelmed.edu
Sickle Cell Disease

Perry G. Fine, MD
Professor of Anesthesiology, University of Utah,
    Salt Lake City, Utah
fine@aros.net
Legal & Regulatory Issues in Pain Management

Scott Fishman, MD
Chief, Division of Pain Medicine,
    Department of Anesthesiology and Pain Medicine;
    Associate Professor of Anesthesiology,
    University of California, Davis
smfishman@ucdavis.edu
Legal & Regulatory Issues in Pain Management

James Fricton, DDS, MS
Diagnostic and Biological Sciences, University of
    Minnesota, Minneapolis, Minnesota
frict001@umn.edu
Temporomandibular Disorders & Orofacial Pain

Michel Volcy Gomez, MD
Professor of Neurology, Department of Neurology,
    School of Medicine, University of Antioguia,
    Medellin, Colombia, South America;
    Neurologist Headache Specialist,
    Clinica medellin El Poblado
    and the Neurological Institute
    of Antioquia, medellin, Colombia
Medvol98@yahoo.com
Headaches

R. Norman Harden, MD
Associate Professor, Department of Physical Medicine
    and Rehabilitation, Feinberg School of Medicine,
    Northwestern University, Chicago, Illinois
nharden@ric.org
Neuropathic Pain

Joshua M. Hauser, MD
Director of Education, Beuhler Center on Aging,
    Palliative Care and Home Hospice Program, Division
    of General Internal Medicine, Department of
    Medicine, Feinberg School of Medicine,
    Northwestern University Medical School, Chicago,
    Illinois
j-hauser@northwestern.edu
Pain in the Elderly

Salim Hayek, MD, PhD
Staff, Department of Pain Management, Cleveland
    Clinic Foundation, Cleveland, Ohio
hayeks@ccf.org
Interventional Procedures for Pain Control

Fred M. Howard, MS, MD
Professor of Obstetrics and Gynecology,
   University of Rochester School of Medicine and
   Dentistry; Director of Gynecology, Department of
   Obstetrics and Gynecology, Strong Memorial
   Hospital, Rochester, New York
fred_howard@urmc@rochester.edu
Chronic Pelvic Pain

Euphemia Jacob, PhD, RN
Research Fellow in Pediatric Oncology,
   Texas Children's Hospital, Houston, Texas
exjab@texaschildrenshospital.org
Sickle Cell Disease

Kenneth L. Kirsh, PhD
Pharmacy Practice, Science,
   College of Pharmacy, University of Kentucky,
   Lexington, Kentucky
klkirsh@uky.edu
Pain & Addictive Disease

John D. Loeser, MD
Professor of Neurological Surgery and Anesthesiology,
   University of Washington, Seattle, Washington
jdloeser@u.washington.edu
The Current Issues in Pain Management

Gaurav Mathur, MD
Fellow, Palliative Medicine, Department of Pain
   Medicine and Palliative Care, Beth Israel
   Medical Center, New York, New York
gmathur@myrealbox.com
Pain in HIV & AIDS

Daniel J. Mazanec, MD
Associate Professor of Medicine, Cleveland Clinic
   Lerner College of Medicine, Case Western Reserve
   University; Vice Chairman, The Cleveland Clinic
   Spine Institute; Head, Section of Medical Spine,
   Cleveland Clinic, Cleveland, Ohio
mazaned@ccf.org
Osteoarthritis & Rheumatoid Arthritis

Timothy J. Ness, MD, PhD
Department of Anesthesiology, University of Alabama
   at Birmingham; University of Alabama Hospital,
   Birmingham, Alabama
loch@uab.edu
Visceral Pain

Judith A. Paice, PhD, RN
Director, Cancer Pain Program, Department of
   Medicine, Division of Hematology/Oncology,
   Feinberg School of Medicine, Northwestern
   University, Robert H. Lurie Comprehensive Cancer
   Center, Chicago, Illinois
j-paice@northwestern.edu
Cancer Pain
Pain Management in Palliative Care

Steven D. Passik, PhD
Associate Attending Psychologist, Memorial Sloan
   Kettering Cancer Center; Associate Professor of
   Psychiatry, CUMC
passiks@mskcc.org
Pain & Addictive Disease

Russell K. Portenoy, MD
Chairman, Department of Pain Medicine and Palliative
   Care, Beth Israel Medical Center, New York,
   New York
Pain & Addictive Disease

Michael E. Preodor, MD
Instructor in Medicine, Department of Medicine,
   Division of Hematology/Oncology, Feinberg School
   of Medicine, Northwestern University, Robert H.
   Lurie Comprehensive Cancer Center, Chicago,
   Illinois
m-preodor@northwestern.edu
Pain Management in Palliative Care

Edgar Ross, MD
Assistant Professor of Anesthesia, Harvard Medical
   School; Director, Pain Management Center, Brigham
   and Women's Hospital, Chestnut Hill, Massachusetts
edross@partners.org
Back Pain

Samuel Samuel, MD
Associate Staff, Department of Pain Management,
   Cleveland Clinic Foundation, Cleveland, Ohio
Interventional Procedures for Pain Control

Peter A. Selwyn, MD, MPH
Professor of Family and Social Medicine, Internal
Medicine Chair, Department of Family and Social
Medicine, Albert Einstein College of Medicine,
Montefiore Medical Center, Bronx, New York
pselwyn@montefiore.org
Pain in HIV & AIDS

Steven P. Stanos, DO
Medical Director, Chronic Pain Center, Rehabilitation
Institute of Chicago, Department of Physical
Medicine and Rehabilitation, Feinberg School of
Medicine, Albert Einstein College of Medicine,
Northwestern University, Chicago, Illinois
sstanos@rehabchicago.org
Rehabilitation Issues: Pain Control

Michael Stanton-Hicks, MB, BS
Vice Chairman, Division of Anesthesia, Department of
Pain Management, Cleveland Clinic Foundation,
Cleveland, Ohio
Stanton@ccf.org
Interventional Procedures for Pain Control

Roland Staud, MD
Associate Professor of Medicine, Division of
Rheumatology, University of Florida, Gainesville,
Florida
staudr@ufl.edu
Fibromyalgia

Brad Stuart, MD
Senior Medical Director, Sutter VNA & Hospice,
Emeryville, California
stuartb@sutterhealth.org
Chest Pain

Stewart J. Tepper, MD
Assistant Clinical Professor of Neurology,
Yale University School of Medicine, New Haven,
Connecticut; Director, The New England Center for
Headache, Stanford, Connecticut
sjtepper@aol.com
Headaches

Kati Thieme, PhD
Behavioral and Pain Therapist, University of
Heidelberg, Central Institute of Mental Health,
Mannheim, Germany
Psychological Interventions

Jay Thomas, MD, PhD
Associate Clinical Professor of Medicine, Department
of Medicine, University of California, San Diego,
Clinical Medical Director, San Diego Hospice and
Palliative Care, San Diego, California
jthomas@sdhospice.org
Pharmacologic Therapies for Pain

Dennis C. Turk, PhD
John and Emma Bonica Professor of Anesthesiology &
Pain Research, Department of Psychology,
University of Washington, Seattle, Washington
turkdc@u.washington.edu
Psychological Interventions

Martha L. Twaddle, MD
Assistant Professor of Medicine, NUSM, Chicago,
Illinois; Assistant Professor, ENH-Corp Hospital;
Assistant Professor, Rush North Shore Hospital,
Skokie, Illinois
mtwaddle@carecenter.org
Assessment of Pain & Common Pain Syndromes

Mark D. Tyburski, MD
Department of Physical Medicine and Rehabilitation,
Northwestern University; Rehabilitation Institute of
Chicago, Chicago, Illinois
tyburski@physical-medicine.org
Rehabilitation Issues: Pain Control

Charles F. von Gunten, MD, PhD
Associate Clinical Professor of Medicine, Department
of Medicine, University of California, San Diego;
Director, Center for Palliative Studies, San Diego
Hospice & Palliative Care, San Diego, California
cvongunten@sdhospice.org
Pharmacologic Therapies for Pain

Jamie H. Von Roenn, MD
Professor of Medicine, Department of Medicine,
Division of Hematology/Oncology, Feinberg School
of Medicine, Robert H. Lurie Comprehensive Cancer
Center, Northwestern University, Chicago, Illinois
j-vonroenn@northwestern.edu
Pain Management in Palliative Care

Preface

Although the world is full of suffering, it is full also of the overcoming of it.

Helen Keller, 1880–1968

Suffering is a universal phenomenon. Yet one symptom that contributes greatly to the suffering seen in people with acute and chronic illnesses—pain—can usually be effectively managed. Pain is the most common reason patients seek assistance from their healthcare provider. Pain also is a major contributor of impaired quality of life. As a result, all physicians must be skilled in the accurate diagnosis and comprehensive management of pain. *Current Diagnosis and Treatment of Pain* presents the information necessary for the practicing physician to provide skilled pain treatment. This concise, yet authoritative, text also increases awareness of the role of other disciplines in pain control and indicates when referral to a specialist may be appropriate.

Distinguishing Features

- Consistent format that facilitates rapid access to clinically useful information
- Pain assessment principles
- Pharmacologic and interventional approaches to pain control
- Rehabilitation in pain management
- Chapters devoted to specific pain syndromes commonly seen in medicine, including arthritis, headache, back pain, neuropathy, painful visceral syndromes, sickle cell pain
- Attention to regulatory concerns relevant to pain management
- Practical guide to the management of pain in persons with addictive disease
- End-of-life issues
- Evidence-based recommendations

Intended Audience

Primary care physicians, residents, and nursing trainees will find this text a useful, reliable, and up-to-date resource for the assessment and management of common pain syndromes. Fellows, house officers, and medical students will appreciate this quick, yet comprehensive introduction to the field of pain. Advanced practice nurses and physician's assistants also will find the approach provided here to be practical and clinically relevant.

Jamie H. Von Roenn, MD
Judith Paice, PhD, RN
Michael E. Preodor, MD

To all of those patients who suffered in pain, touched our lives,
and taught us so much

The Current Issues in Pain Management

John D. Loeser, MD

HISTORY

The present status of pain control is understandable only by looking backward at the developments of the past 45 years. In the 1960s and 1970s, John J. Bonica, MD, called attention to the inadequate treatment of pain as well as the absence of scientific information about the physiologic and psychological mechanisms of pain. Almost single-handedly, Bonica stimulated interest in physicians and scientists, raised funds from the National Institutes of Health and pharmaceutical companies, and attracted a motivated group of followers who carried his message all over the world. Before the efforts of Bonica, pain was always the by-product of a disease, and physicians who treated the diseases were expected to manage their patients' pains. Unfortunately, this often did not happen. Patients suffered needlessly, scientists did not recognize the need for basic and clinical studies on pain, and no one was willing to fund the necessary research.

By 1980, Bonica had changed the scene dramatically. The International Association for the Study of Pain and many of its national chapters had been founded, journals were being published, granting agencies recognized the need for funding of pain research, and clinical care was improving. Training programs and educational activities at all levels and in all the health professions expanded dramatically. Professional organizations were founded to provide a forum as well as educational activities about pain.

The treatment of pain has always been part of the physician's duties; only in the past 25 years have we seen the development of specialists in this new area of medicine. New concepts and new technologies have led to the development of the field of pain medicine.

In spite of major improvements in the understanding of the anatomy, physiology, and psychology of pain, and the application of many new treatments, chronic pain continues to be undertreated. Patients' complaints of pain remain second only to the common cold as a reason to see a primary care practitioner in the United States. Treatment of postoperative pain and cancer pain has im-proved significantly as has the management of pediatric and geriatric pain problems.

KEY DEVELOPMENTS

The improvements in pain management have been based primarily upon new concepts and paradigm shifts. Technologic advances in drugs, drug delivery systems, stimulation systems, and strategies of psychological interventions have all been significant.

Paradigm Shifts

A critical leap forward was the Melzack-Wall gate hypothesis, published in *Science* in 1965. This hypothesis focused attention upon modulation of afferent information, both at the dorsal horn and at suprasegmental levels. Line labeling was wrong; the nervous system was capable of controlling the upstream flow of information to the brain by modulating afferent activity through downstream circuits. This theory led directly to the attempt to reduce pain by non-noxious afferent input, such as transcutaneous electrical nerve stimulation and spinal cord stimulation with implanted electrical devices. It also paved the way for research on peripheral nociceptive mechanisms and dorsal horn synaptic mechanisms that could be influenced by medications. Drugs were studied, developed, and marketed that could alter the downstream modulation of dorsal horn information processing. The gate hypothesis also led to the realization that pain behaviors were influenced by affective and environmental events and that psychological strategies could be used to help reduce the impact of noxious stimulation on a person's cognitive and affective processes. This key theory led to the realization that a biopsychosocial approach to pain was far more effective than the traditional biomedical concept of pain being a genetically determined response of the brain to a noxious event.

A second paradigm shift was the recognition that tissue damage was not synonymous with pain and not directly linked to suffering or to pain behaviors. In 1982, the terms "nociception," "pain," "suffering," and "pain behavior" were defined and helped channel thinking, research, and patient care into different components that could be addressed by specific pharmacologic, psychological, or surgical techniques. There are only loose linkages between tissue damage, pain, suffering, pain behaviors, and disability. Suffering and the behaviors it can generate are not always due to tissue damage (nociception) or to pain. Pain behaviors can be perpetuated by environmental factors and anticipated consequences—influences that cannot be evaluated.

The importance of listening to the patient's story and placing it within the context of his or her thoughts, beliefs, and culture, cannot be overemphasized; without listening to the patient, the symptom presentation and the responses (or lack thereof) to treatment cannot be understood. Just listening to the patient's narrative can have a therapeutic effect.

In some ways, the biggest conceptual change was promulgated by Wilbert Fordyce at the University of Washington; he demonstrated that the environment strongly influenced pain behaviors, and factors outside the patient were often responsible for the perpetuation of chronic pain behaviors. In addition, how people think and what they fear and anticipate are also strong determinants of suffering and pain behavior. Good pain management programs are now built upon a cognitive-behavioral approach and incorporate physical, pharmacologic, and psychological treatment strategies. Indeed, the best outcomes data that we have for the treatment of chronic pain comes from such programs. No isolated surgical, pharmacologic, physical, or psychological treatment has been shown to be as good as multidisciplinary pain management for refractory chronic pain. Unfortunately, this form of treatment is thought to be expensive and is poorly funded by most insurance programs.

Role of Opioids

Another conceptual change relates to the use of opioids in the treatment of both acute and chronic pain. Fear of opioids discouraged the rational use of these drugs except in the setting of trauma or postsurgical pain. Eventually, the lessons learned from the management of cancer pain reduced some of the fear of opioids. By the 1990s, much more aggressive use of opioids in the treatment of cancer pain was becoming standard. Although opioids are used more frequently, efficacy data for opioid therapy in noncancer pain conditions are scarce. Other forms of treatment for chronic pain may be more effective than opioids. Finally, the discovery of opiate receptors in the dorsal horn of the spinal cord led to the spinal administration of opioids. For properly selected patients, this has offered a dramatic improvement in pain relief.

CONCEPTS OF PAIN

Physician-Patient Communication

The individual and his society can only understand the relationships between tissue damage, a person's report of pain, and the behaviors manifested by the patient if there is a meaningful conceptualization of the phenomena of pain and shared definitions of the terms that are used in a discussion of pain. Discussions of pain and suffering often fail because of disagreement about the meanings of the words used. Understanding their pain and suffering requires listening to the patients' stories.

Mechanisms of Pain & Suffering

The aspect of pain and suffering has long been overlooked by pain researchers. Reflex responses to noxious stimuli can occur without consciousness, but the presence of a nociceptive reflex is not a proxy for pain. A patient with a spinal cord transection due to injury may feel no pain when his toe is squeezed, but this noxious stimulus may generate a set of somatic and autonomic reflex responses.

The development of brain imaging by positron emission tomography (PET) or functional magnetic resonance imaging (fMRI) has opened new windows for understanding the mechanisms by which pain, suffering, and their narratives are generated in the human brain. To make full use of this technology, we need concepts and terms that are reflective of the events within the nervous system that lead to the phenomena we wish to investigate.

Components of Pain

Four components comprise the complex phenomenon of pain: nociception, pain, suffering, and pain behavior (Figure 1–1). These components can help generate useful models that are compatible with what we are learning from brain imaging and psychological studies. This model allows us to construct a scientific vocabulary that will aid in research and clinical management.

A. NOCICEPTION

Nociception is the detection of tissue damage by specialized transducers attached to the A delta and C fibers that transmit signals to the dorsal horn. Peripheral transducers may be biased by inflammatory and neural changes in their immediate environments and thereby alter their response characteristics. The nociceptive transducers, in their basal state, turn on at a level of mechanical, thermal, or chemical energy that is just sufficient to damage cells. Nociception can be blocked by local or regional anesthesia, usually accomplished by sodium channel blockers since they prevent axonal depolarization. Nociception can also be blocked by downstream modulation from

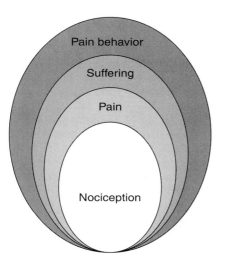

Figure 1–1. Nociception, pain, suffering and pain behavior are the four components that are necessary and sufficient to describe the phenomenon of pain. They have been drawn in an onion-skin pattern to emphasize that all *except* pain behavior are personal, private, internal events that cannot be measured objectively. (Reproduced, with permission, from Loeser JD. Concepts of Pain. In: Stanton-Hicks M, Boas RA, editors. *Chronic Low Back Pain.* New York: Raven Press, 1982:145–148.)

the brain to the dorsal horn, as originally proposed in the Melzack-Wall gate hypothesis, for example, by hypnosis or distraction. Modulation is a feature of the human brain and is just as worthy of study as are afferent projection systems.

B. PAIN

The response to nociception is properly labeled pain. Pain is generated in the spinal cord and brain by nociceptive input (in the intact animal). Injuries to the peripheral nervous system, spinal cord, or brain can lead to the report of pain even in the absence of a noxious stimulus; for example, patients who have had a limb amputated may report pain in the missing limb (phantom limb pain). Some well-known clinical examples of pain without nociception include the following:

1. Thalamic syndrome.
2. Tic douloureux.
3. Phantom limb pain.
4. Complex regional pain syndrome.
5. Atypical facial pain.
6. Postparaplegic pain.
7. Postherpetic neuralgia.
8. Nerve root avulsion pain.

9. Arachnoiditis.
10. Postthoracotomy pain.

C. SUFFERING

Suffering is a negative affective response generated in the brain by pain, fear, anxiety, stress, loss of loved objects, and other psychological states. What we do not know is whether this negative affective response to pain originates within the brain when information saying "pain" is received, or whether nociceptive information reaching the dorsal horn of the spinal cord leads to the activation of circuits leading to the production of both pain and suffering at the spinal and brainstem levels. That is, is suffering added onto pain in the brain or does it have an anatomic underpinning that starts in specific spinal projection systems? Very little research has been done on suffering, either from the physiologic perspective or from the behavioral viewpoint, although recent functional imaging studies have elucidated brain regions that play a role in suffering.

Suffering should be important to health care providers. Along with pain, it is what drives patients to seek medical care. However, to understand suffering, clinicians must listen to the patient, and listening takes time. Because of the demands on physicians' time, few patients have adequate access to their physicians to allow for an understanding of their suffering.

D. PAIN BEHAVIORS

Suffering usually leads to pain behaviors. Grimacing, moaning, limping, lying down, continuous seeking of medical care, and failing to work are common pain behaviors that often occur when someone is suffering. All pain behaviors are real. The proper question for the health care provider is not the validity of the patient's complaints, but which of the four components is contributing to the complaint and what can be done to alleviate the symptoms.

Pain behaviors are always influenced by environmental prequels and consequences, either actual or anticipated. Pain behaviors that are chronic and expressed over time reveal with special clarity the influence of the environment: behavior, in this sense, is the result of learning. The role of anticipated consequences is nicely demonstrated in the 1993 work of Waddell and colleagues, who showed that fears about back injury were a major determinant of disability status and health care consumption.

Only pain behaviors, the things a person says and does, or avoids doing, can be measured. They are truly objective—in the sense of constituting recordable events—but they do not quantify the events within the patient. They have qualities that can be described: onset, duration, intensity, frequency, periodicity, type. Pain behaviors can be measured also in terms of the amount of disability they produce, the consumption of health care, or their impact upon quality of life.

How societies deal with suffering differs widely at different points in history. To some degree this difference is due to variations in the resources available to a society, but more is involved than resources. A society must be able to define and identify suffering before it can effectively respond.

Chapman CR et al. A passion of the soul: an introduction to pain for consciousness researchers. *Conscious Cogn.* 1999;8:391. [PMID: 10600241]

Loeser JD et al. A taxonomy of pain. *Pain.* 1975;1:81. [PMID: 1235978]

Melzack R et al. Pain mechanisms: a new theory. *Science.* 1965;150:971. [PMID: 5320816]

Waddell G et al. A Fear-Avoidance Beliefs Questionnaire (FABQ) and the role of fear-avoidance beliefs in chronic low back pain and disability. *Pain.* 1993;52:157. [PMID: 8455963]

TYPES OF PAIN

There are four types of pain that are important to distinguish in the clinical setting: transient pain, acute pain, chronic pain due to cancer, and chronic pain due to nonmalignant diseases.

There is no evidence that the neurophysiologic mechanisms underlying these four types of pain are different or that different neural circuits are involved, but in clinical medicine, the principles of management of each type are so different that it is important to discuss them independently. The future will tell us if these diverse types of pain have different neural substrates.

Transient Pain

Transient pain is elicited by the activation of nociceptors in the absence of tissue damage, such as with a needle stick. It occurs frequently in everyday life and is rarely a reason to seek health care. Relevant only to procedural pain, this is not a major issue in clinical medicine, although it is important in pediatric health care and in the performance of certain procedures such as venipuncture, lumbar puncture, and bone marrow aspiration. It has, however, been the subject of most experimental pain paradigms in humans and animals until the past 20 years. The failure to look at animal models of pain associated with tissue damage was one of the reasons why so little useful information was gleaned from such studies.

Acute Pain

Acute pain is elicited by injury to the body and the activation of nociceptive transducers at the site of damage. The local injury alters the response characteristics of the regional nociceptors, their central connections, and the autonomic nervous system in the region. Nociceptor activity is processed in the dorsal horn and leads to the report of pain when upstream projection systems reach the brain. Healing of damaged tissue occurs and the restoration of normal nociceptor function is even more rapid than the entire healing process. Acute pain is a common medical problem, seen after surgery and trauma. The role of the health care provider is to treat the injury (eg, immobilization, suture of the skin) and to provide analgesia until the nociceptor function returns to baseline. After the acute injury has healed, the pain abates and the person can resume normal activities.

Chronic Pain due to Cancer

Chronic pain due to cancer is almost always associated with continuing tissue damage due to the disease process or the treatments (ie, surgery, radiation, chemotherapy). Although there is always a role for environmental factors and affective disturbances in the genesis of pain behaviors, these are not usually the predominant etiologic factors in patients with cancer pain. Furthermore, many patients with severe pain associated with cancer are nearing the end of their lives and palliative therapies are required. Issues such as social stigma of using opioids, work and functional status, and health care consumption are not likely to be important in the overall case management. Hence, the typical strategy for cancer pain management is to get the patient as comfortable as possible using opioids and other medications, surgery, and physical measures.

Chronic Pain due to Nonmalignant Diseases

Chronic pain due to nonmalignant diseases is an entirely different management problem. Typically, the pain complaints have been triggered by injury or disease in the past. Healing from such an injury should have occurred long ago. The pain is likely being perpetuated by factors other than those that were present at the time of the injury. The body is unable to heal because of a nerve injury, the loss of a body part, or changes in the central nervous system that persist after healing. Reorganization of spinal and brain modulatory systems may have occurred after the original traumatic events in the periphery, or the injury was directly to the nervous system and there is disruption of normal pathways; compensatory mechanisms may be perpetuating the pain. Because the pain is present over time, stress, affective, and environmental factors are likely to play a large role. When dealing with chronic pain, clinicians should not just focus upon the patient's symptoms but must also evaluate the roles of affective and environmental factors. Treatment must incorporate not only symptom relief but also restoration of well behaviors, including work. This means that chronic pain is not well managed by the utilization of Cartesian or Aristotelian concepts of the separation of mind and body. Instead, it requires a biopsychosocial model. Since the altered nervous system may not be amenable to standard pain-relieving therapies, control of pain through the activation of modulatory circuits may be the best available treatment. Hence, psychological strategies built upon cognitive and behavioral principles are useful.

Chronic pain, especially low back pain, is common, affecting 80% of persons at some point in their life. Most episodes of back pain are self-limiting, regardless of the health care delivered. The introduction of Western health care to Oman led to a surge of disability ascribed to low back pain without a change in the prevalence of pain. Health care and its many meanings and cultural links altered the way people thought about their symptoms and what actions they took because of their complaints.

Waddell G. 1987 Volvo award in clinical sciences. A new clinical model for the treatment of low-back pain. *Spine.* 1987;12:632. [PMID: 2961080]

PATIENT ISSUES

Issues that patients with acute and chronic pain face include the following:

1. There is wide variability in the resources allocated to pain management.
2. There are many subspecialties among pain specialists, making it difficult for patients to find the physician who might be most helpful.
3. There are very few commonly agreed upon treatment algorithms and almost no evidence-based treatment plans.

Acute Pain

Inadequate management of acute pain is still common in the United States due to the lack of resources. Efforts by the community of pain specialists have succeeded in making pain "the fifth vital sign." The Joint Commission on Accreditation of Hospitals has mandated that hospitals assess and treat pain in every inpatient and outpatient.

Nursing has played a leadership role in this change in procedures and policies. However, postoperative and posttrauma pain is very variably treated. Techniques of drug administration beyond oral medications or the intramuscular injection are not readily available in smaller hospitals. To some degree this is due to the lack of funding for pain management services. Furthermore, not all

institutions have the equipment or staff to offer patient-controlled analgesia, intravenous infusions, or neuraxial opioids. Advanced pain management techniques are expensive and potentially hazardous, so there are often arguments against their use. Nurses need extensive training and physicians need very detailed education to provide the full gamut of acute pain management services. There remains a tendency to say "It is only pain" and "just wait until nature solves the problem in a few days." In addition, often there is a belief that pain is somehow good for the patient when, in fact, there are plenty of data to show that pain delays recovery from surgery and raises the likelihood of many complications.

Acute pain management can be improved without the development of new drugs or techniques of administration, although both of these will happen and lead to better patient care in selected cases. In the interim, physicians, nurses, and pharmacists need to be better educated about the available options. We must work to change the reimbursement systems prevalent in hospitals so that the provision of good pain management services is financially rewarded. Some HMOs have solved this problem by determining that they will have trained physicians and nurses on staff to provide the best possible pain management services. Other prepaid health care plans virtually exclude pain management services for their members. Hospitals as well as physicians need to be rewarded for providing optimal treatment for acute pain. Of course, we can anticipate that there will be new, useful drugs and treatments. However, we cannot wait for these to appear and must do a better job with what is available.

Chronic Pain due to Cancer

Tremendous progress has been made in the past 25 years in the management of cancer pain. Some interventional techniques, such as regional anesthesia and implantation of intrathecal catheters, have advanced the care of patients with chronic pain due to cancer. However, the progress in cancer pain management is mainly due to the more aggressive use of opioids and adjunctive medications.

Social stigmata are fewer, and the federal and state agencies do not scrutinize prescriptions for cancer pain nearly as much as they do for patients with chronic pain of nonmalignant origin. The treatment ladder for cancer pain established by the World Health Organization (WHO) has been widely accepted throughout the world and has set a reasonable initial approach into every physician's repertoire. Some patients with cancer pain require immediate implementation of strong opioids and rigid interpretation of the WHO ladder can be an impediment to their adequate treatment. It is commonly accepted that patients with cancer should not have to suffer with pain and that they are entitled to every possible effort to reduce their pain, no matter what the dose of medication or the magnitude of the intervention to control pain. This is not to say that there is not a large amount of variability in the quality of pain relief services that are offered to cancer patients. There have been successful lawsuits claiming inadequate attempts at pain relief by physicians and nursing homes, and certainly there will be more litigation on this issue. Clearly, both better tools for the treatment of pain due to cancer and more universal application of the medications and delivery strategies than we have available today are needed. Moreover, the desires of patients to obtain pain relief seem to be congruent with the interests of health care providers to make this possible. This is clearly not the case in patients with chronic pain due to nonmalignant disease.

Chronic Pain due to Nonmalignant Disease

Patients with chronic pain due to nonmalignant diseases often do not get adequate treatment. There are many factors that contribute to this unhappy state of affairs. First, accurate diagnosis of the causes of the pain may not be possible. Second, adequate treatments for the pain, even when the cause is thought to be known, may not be available. Third, we do not understand the mechanisms underlying chronic pain, and therefore, all of the treatments are empiric and lack a rational basis. Fourth, apparently identical injuries do not predictably lead to pain, so the link between tissue damage and the complaint of pain is not strong. This suggests, of course, that in addition to the tissue damage that might start a chronic pain process, there are changes in the nervous system in response to injury that long outlast the inciting cause of pain. Also, environmental and affective factors may contribute to chronic pain and may not be discernable by examination of the patient or the imaging studies.

Treatment of Nonmalignant Pain

The treatments for chronic pain due to a nonmalignant disease are often inadequate. Anticonvulsants, antidepressants, antiarrhythmics, nonsteroidal anti-inflammatory drugs, and opioids sometimes work but often do not. If the data on efficacy of opioids in the treatment of this type of chronic pain is carefully examined, a 30% reduction in Visual Analogue Scale pain levels seems to be standard. Now, reducing a pain from a 9 to a 6 is certainly helpful, but a level 6 pain is by no means a cure of the problem of pain.

Determining peripheral mechanisms of pain has become a focus of drug companies, so that they can develop drugs aimed at treating all pain syndromes that have a similar mechanism. Thus far, we have not succeeded in identifying mechanisms underlying any pain syndrome. Hypotheses based upon animal experimentation are plentiful but unproven in humans. The role of

genetic differences in response to injury has been studied in rodents, but human studies are few and far between. It may be that specific genes determine how a person's spinal cord responds to an injury or it may be that genes determine the behaviors produced in the brain in response to an injury. Hopefully, fMRI and PET scanning will provide insights into how the brain functions in response to injury and what parts of the brain are involved in generating a behavioral and affective response.

Finally, the roles of affect and environment in the generation and perpetuation of chronic pain are largely unexplored. Clearly, environmental factors play a role; however, how and why they impinge on those parts of the brain that generate pain behaviors is not understood. Again, genetic factors may be in play. Past experiences and anticipated consequences are also relevant factors in many patients with chronic pain. For many patients, these factors may be more important than the precipitating injury, but health care providers often ignore them. Curing chronic pain is a very rare event.

Variations in the Treatment of Pain

Patients with chronic pain are subjected to wide variations in the type of care they receive. There is no commonly agreed upon diagnostic or therapeutic algorithm for most chronic pain states. In addition to all the alternative care options, within allopathic medicine the treatment that the patient receives is more a reflection of the type of physician that is consulted than the patient's diagnosis. Csordas and Clark illustrated this problem by studying the 25 available pain treatment facilities in a single urban community in the United States. They reported that 27 different treatment modalities were used, with no two treatment facilities offering identical programs. Patient selection criteria, intensity and duration of treatment, the components of treatment, costs, and follow-up plans all differed. In addition, what treatment options exist for any particular patient are determined not only by the physician's wishes but also by the type of health insurance program that the patient is enrolled within; benefits for pain management vary widely and the payers often participate too much in the treatment decision-making process.

Measuring Outcomes

Determining outcomes for pain management and ascertaining the effects of treatment upon those outcomes is not the least of the problems. Whoever gets to determine the relevant outcomes will strongly influence what treatments are offered to patients with chronic pain. Almost everyone agrees that one aspect of outcome is the patient's self-rating of his or her pain, often obtained with a Visual Analogue Scale, although other validated measures exist. Most experts agree that this is only a portion of the information needed to determine the effects of a treatment. A patient's report of pain is certainly an important communication, but the meaning of this behavior needs to be determined by acquiring more information. Such things as functional status, health care consumption, and work status are also highly relevant in the assessment of the effects of treatment.

Functional status may be ascertained on validated questionnaires, such as the Oswestry, SF-36, or other objective measures of the patient's behavior. Health care consumption can include such markers as visits to the emergency department, office visits, hospitalizations, and medication consumption. Working, either in the home or at outside employment, is a helpful measure of outcome. Finally, there are numerous quality-of-life measures that can be used to assess overall well-being.

Once criteria for the measurement of outcome has been established, it is possible to determine costs of achieving that outcome and develop comparative measures of cost-effectiveness for different treatment strategies. Such measures do not take into account the risks to the patient nor do they consider patient preference as a determinant of outcome. This has been shown in several studies to make an important contribution to a successful outcome.

In the United States, far more resources are devoted to the transplantation of hearts than to management of chronic pain, even though the economic and social burden of chronic pain dwarfs that of end-stage heart disease.

New Developments

There are many new drugs that have been developed that are used for pain management. Ironically, few, if any, were actually developed as pain-relieving substances; most have been marketed initially as anticonvulsants or antidepressants, blood pressure control agents, or anti-spasticity drugs. One area that has seen great activity is the treatment of neuropathic pain. Opioids are often not as useful for this type of pain; anticonvulsants have long been known to help some patients. New anticonvulsants, such as gabapentin, are now used more often to treat pain than they are to treat epilepsy, which was its original indication. Similar sodium channel blockers are being evaluated as pain relieving drugs. There has been a surge of interest in neuropathic pains in the past decade. It has at last become widely recognized that neuropathic pain often does not respond to standard analgesics, opioids, or other medications. The pharmaceutical industry has targeted the development of neuropathic pain treatment. Systemic and topical agents that are now available have significantly increased the treatment options and improved overall treatment results.

Modern brain imaging techniques, such as PET scanning and fMRI scanning, have improved the understanding of brain function. This is likely to lead to new drug treatments as well as an explosion of electrical stimulation techniques to treat pain. Motor cortex stimulation for neuropathic pain is likely to be the next major step forward, but associated conditions (such as depression, obsessive-compulsive disorder, and panic disorder) may soon have treatment opportunities through implanted stimulation or drug delivery systems. Functional imaging of the brain is a new area of endeavor, and it is not clear how far this area will develop into new treatment modalities.

Intrathecal drug delivery systems have been used clinically for the past 15 years to treat both spasticity and pain. The technology is reasonably effective, but better hardware is on the horizon. In addition, there is the opportunity to develop an entirely new set of pharmacologic agents that will work at the dorsal horn level to alter spinal cord function. Other methods of delivering drugs that do not require a pump or fluid delivery system are also under development.

New medications that target specific molecular complexes or membrane channels are being studied. Coupling a toxic agent to a protein that is incorporated at specific sites in the cell membrane or cytoplasm offers a new way of selectively damaging specific axons or synapses and sparing other classes of cells. Making use of axon transport systems permits the delivery of a drug to sites remote from the injection point in a highly selective fashion. Similarly, targeting specific genes within neural and glial cells to alter their function can become a new therapeutic modality.

Ablative neurosurgical procedures have become much less common in pain management, in part because of the development of aggressive oral and intrathecal opioid therapy, but also because long-term results were found to be not as good as the early proponents had claimed. Widespread use of opioid therapy seems to be meeting a similar fate; opioid use is becoming more limited. Behavioral and cognitive techniques are not being used as much as the evidence suggests they should. Funding issues may be at play in this area as well as an unawareness of the potential benefits of biobehavioral medicine. Many of the alternative health care pain treatment strategies are going to fall by the wayside as outcomes-based medicine studies the efficacy for such modalities as chiropractic manipulation, acupuncture, dietary regimens, food supplements, and magnets.

There are some patients who respond well to opioids with reduced pain behaviors and increased functional abilities. Then, there are others who manifest rapid tolerance and never get pain relief. Other patients have intractable side effects that cannot be adequately controlled. Yet, most patients have both some benefits and some problems with opioids. No one yet knows how to predict who will have a good response and who will not. The percentage of good results with opioid therapy is not known.

Csordas TJ et al. Ends of the line: diversity among chronic pain centers. *Soc Sci Med*. 1992;34:383. [PMID: 1566120]

Kalauokalani D et al. Lessons from a trial of acupuncture and massage for low back pain: patient expectations and treatment effects. *Spine*. 2001;26:1418. [PMID: 11458142]

Mondloch MV et al. Does how you do depend on how you think you'll do? A systematic review of the evidence for a relation between patients' recovery expectations and health outcomes. *CMAJ*. 2001;165:174. [PMID: 11501456]

SOCIETAL ISSUES

Costs of Chronic Pain

The treatment of patients with chronic pain due to non-malignant diseases is an issue for society as well as the individual patient. Health care resources are finite and what is consumed in one area is not available in another. Furthermore, the costs of the social support systems provided to those who are unable to work because of pain are three to four times the costs of the health care they consume. Not only are there direct costs of wage replacement systems and the administration of such programs, but there are indirect costs such as loss of taxes on income and expenditures, loss of skilled workers necessitating training of new workers, and the huge psychological and economic burden placed on those who do not work and their families.

The magnitude of the chronic pain problem in industrialized societies is enormous. Population surveys, utilization of resources such as hospitalization data, operations performed, outpatient visits, prescriptions, over-the-counter medications, physical treatments all indicate the widespread prevalence of chronic pain. We have very little data on the use and costs of complementary and alternative medicine, but we do know that they are heavily used. By far, the most important type of chronic pain from the viewpoint of the patient, health care providers, and society is low back pain. The point prevalence for low back pain in the United States and European countries ranges from 14 to 42%, and the lifetime prevalence ranges from 51 to 81%. Surprisingly, the 5% of back pain patients who do not respond to therapy are responsible for 90% of all costs for back pain. We know that the correlations between pain, suffering, pain behaviors, and work disability are generally low and explain less than 25% of the variance.

In addition, the disability ascribed to chronic pain has become a major cost for developed societies. The total

costs are thought to be $100 billion in the United States and $9 billion in the United Kingdom. Estimates suggest that 1 to 5% of the gross domestic product is expended on low back pain in Western societies. Disability costs far exceed health care costs. One way of looking at the costs of chronic pain is from survey data such as that published by Stewart et al. In the American workforce, 53% of workers report having had a pain problem in the past two weeks, 13% have lost productive time averaging 4.6 hours per week. This loss of productive time is estimated to cost $61 billion per year and accounts for about 25% of all costs related to pain in the workplace. Chronic pain costs American businesses $240 billion each year, and these costs are rapidly increasing.

Headache is the most common form of pain recalled in most surveys. Over 75% of the adult population report having headaches, and 5% report headaches more than 100 days per year. Although headaches are responsible for many sickness days and much absenteeism, they are not a major cause of health care costs and wage replacement. Other types of pain are also relatively common: menstrual pains, abdominal pain, extremity pain, neck pain, arthritis pain, and dental pain. Added together, these do not equal the impact of low back pain on health care or disability systems.

Disability Ascribed to Chronic Pain

Disability ascribed to chronic pain is a major concern for society because over 75% of the costs are related to the inability to work and not the symptom of pain. We know that addressing only the symptom of pain behavior fails to restore most patients with chronic pain to gainful employment. This is a major problem for medicine in the United States, since physicians are mandated to determine on the basis of a history, physical examination, and diagnostic studies whether or not a patient is capable of employment. There are serious ethical issues hidden in this mandate because the doctor-patient relationship is violated by providing information about the patient to a governmental agency or insurance company without the patient's consent or with the coercion that the insurance company will only pay for care if it has full access to the patient's medical records.

Rating Disability

Determining the amount of disability that is ascribed to a complaint of pain is a problem. The American Medical Association Guide for the Assessment of Impairment, now in its fifth edition, is the commonly used system; the idea behind this guide is that loss of a body part or the function of this part can be given a percentage of total disability. However, there has never been any validation of the methods promulgated in this volume, and pain is largely ignored by those rating disability. Yet, disability ascribed to pain is the major cause of disability in the federal programs in the United States.

Managing Disability

Yet another issue is the management of disability ascribed to pain. The systems that are in place in the United States today seem to have been designed to use behavioral principles to increase and prolong disability, rather than the reverse as most would desire. Being enmeshed in a compensation system is a type of comorbidity that adversely affects outcomes for any condition, including pain. Financial incentives, such as a high wage-replacement ratio, tend to perpetuate disability. The systems tend to have dehumanizing influence that contributes to the failures of the health care system to rehabilitate vast numbers of patients.

Cultural Differences & Aging Populations

As our population ages, chronic diseases including chronic pain associated with arthritis and neuropathy become more prevalent. More health care resources will be required to adequately manage the complaints of the elderly. Outcomes-based diagnostic and therapeutic algorithms are essential. Preventive programs would, of course be most effective, but insurance companies are generally not interested in such because the average beneficiary changes insurance carriers every three years. We cannot wait for such data to be produced, for patients want their symptoms alleviated now, with whatever resources may be available and with whatever treatment strategies their provider has to offer.

Quo Vadis?

Despite the widespread use of opiates for chronic, nonmalignant pain, there are no data on long-term efficacy or complications. Furthermore, there is no head-to-head testing of one type of treatment versus another. Prodigious numbers of nerve blocks and corticosteroid injections are performed for back pain with little, if any, evidence for long-term outcomes. The cost for these injection therapies was over $250 million to Medicare, which funds a minority of health care costs in the United States. Major increases in the rate of surgery for low back pain have not resulted in improved function or pain relief in most patients. Chiropractic and naturopathic practitioners are treating more and more pain sufferers but results are unclear. The role of nonspecific treatment factors in clinical outcomes needs much more exploration.

Vast sums are spent by individuals and society in the treatment of chronic pain and support of those who do not work because of pain. Patients suffer without adequate treatments and now 15% of the gross national product goes to health care in the United States. The costs, both to the patient and society are large. We need a new conceptualization of the meaning of the complaint of pain and its management.

Loeser JD et al. Doctors, diagnosis, and disability: a disastrous diversion. *Clin Orthop Relat Res.* 1997;(336):61. [PMID: 9060487]

Loeser JD et al. Incentive effects of workers' compensation benefits: a literature synthesis. *Med Care Res Rev.* 1995;52:59. [PMID: 10143575]

Luo X et al. Estimates and patterns of direct health care expenditures among individuals with back pain in the United States. *Spine.* 2004;29:79. [PMID: 14699281]

Merrill DG. Hoffman's glasses: evidence-based medicine and the search for quality in the literature of interventional pain medicine. *Reg Anesth Pain Med.* 2003;28:547. [PMID: 14634948]

Stewart WF et al. Lost productive time and cost due to common pain conditions in the US workforce. *JAMA.* 2003;290:2443. [PMID: 14612481]

van Tulder M et al. Low back pain. *Best Pract Res Clin Rheumatol.* 2002;16:761. [PMID: 12473272]

Assessment of Pain & Common Pain Syndromes

Martha L. Twaddle, MD & Kelly J. Cooke, DO

ESSENTIALS OF DIAGNOSIS

- *The diagnosis of pain is based on the patient's complaint and his or her description of the experience of the symptom.*
- *Because there is currently no objective means to quantify pain, it is essential to believe and accept the patient's report of pain.*
- *In cases of chronic or persistent pain, physical signs and diagnostic evidence may be absent or confusing.*
- *A pain inventory form including an anatomic figure can be useful in substantiating, documenting, and tracking a patient's pain as well as evaluating the patient's response to interventions.*

GENERAL CONSIDERATIONS

The International Association for the Study of Pain (IASP) defines pain in terms of the stimulus and response: "Pain is an unpleasant sensory and emotional experience associated with actual and potential tissue damage, or described in terms of such damage."

"Pain is whatever the experiencing person says it is existing whenever he says it does." McCaffrey

Differences Between Acute & Chronic Pain

Pain is typically described as acute or chronic. Many specialists use the term "persistent" in place of chronic or combine the two. The designation between these types of pain has to do with the duration of the symptom as well as the physiologic response of the person (Table 2–1).

A. ACUTE PAIN

Typically, acute pain is associated with immediate tissue injury and is of limited duration. The pain initiates a warning response to the person to avoid further injury by activating the sympathetic nervous system. Thus, the patient would experience vasoconstriction, rapid pulse,

and "fight or flight" physiology. In addition, the patient is often agitated and may groan and show signs of heightened awareness and activity.

In severe acute pain, such as labor or myocardial infarction, patients may be immobilized as well as demonstrate dissociation and decreased responsiveness to their environment. Acute pain usually responds to treatment. The ideal therapy is prompt and sufficient administration of analgesic medication along with reassurance and support.

B. CHRONIC OR PERSISTENT PAIN

Typically, chronic or persistent pain perpetuates long after the tissue injury has resolved or healed, so the reason for the pain is not obvious. In patients with chronic pain, physiologic adaptation to the persistent pain stimulus may be accompanied by the following signs and symptoms: depressive symptoms, withdrawal, anorexia, fatigue, hypersomnolence or insomnia, irritability or mood lability, lack of initiative and inactivity. These signs and symptoms may be subtle and require observation over time and input from family, friends, and caregivers about any behavioral changes.

Patients may not necessarily look like they are experiencing pain; their pulse and facial expressions would not reflect the stimulus of pain. Patients in persistent pain can interact and even laugh, but distraction cannot sustain a pain-free state.

Chronic or persistent pain tends to respond poorly to treatment because it is deeply embedded within the physiology and psychology of the patient. The ideal management requires a multidisciplinary, whole-person approach and long-term care.

Pain Descriptors

Patients should be allowed to describe their pain in their own words. The clinician can then ask specific questions to elicit the adjectives that will help identify the cause, facilitate the diagnosis as well as determine possible approaches to alleviate the pain.

Table 2–1. Characteristics That Differentiate Acute from Chronic Pain.

Acute pain	Chronic pain
Elicited by immediate tissue injury	Perpetuates after tissue injury has resolved or healed
Serves as a "warning" of tissue damage or injury; protective of further injury	Serves no useful function
Activates nociceptors	Involves central sensitization and permanent structural abnormalities of the central nervous system
Activates sympathetic nervous system	Physiologic adaptation
Limited duration	Prolonged duration
Remits with resolution and healing of injury	Persists long after resolution and healing of injury
Directly associated with injury, postoperative conditions, and disease processes	Remotely associated with injury, surgical procedures, and disease processes
Responsive to treatment	Recalcitrant to treatment

The clinical terms that will help describe the quality and character of pain include acute or chronic; diffuse or localized; throbbing or achy; dull or cramping; burning, tingling, stabbing, or shooting; sharp or tender; constant or intermittent; and breakthrough or incident.

Describing the pain as **acute** or **chronic** establishes the timing and duration of the pain (see Table 2–1) and thus the mechanisms involved. The term **"diffuse"** suggests a central process or an inflammatory condition. **Localized** pain is associated with a discrete injury, a peripheral nerve lesion, or the immediate postoperative state.

Throbbing aching pain is suggestive of bone disease, such as bone metastases or muscle strain and soft tissue injury. The terms **"dull"** and **"cramping"** are often associated with visceral pain states, such as irritation or inflammation of the viscera (as in organs) or functional pain syndromes involving the intestines.

The descriptors **burning** and **tingling** or **stabbing** and **shooting** are often associated with nerve injury or pathologic changes involving nerves and the transmission of the pain stimulus.

When the terms **"sharp"** or **"tender"** are used, clarification is necessary. Sharp can indicate sudden and acute or may be used as part of the description for nerve-related pain. Tender may reflect a lower level of pain or be used to describe aching, dull pain.

Constant or **intermittent** refers to the timing of the pain. Constant pain means that it is always present. This type of pain is best treated with scheduled medication around the clock. Intermittent pain, however, is unpredictable. Therefore, it is best treated with medication as needed.

The terms **"breakthrough"** or **"incident"** pain are not synonymous. Breakthrough pain describes an unexpected pain exacerbation that suddenly surpasses the analgesia provided by a previously effective therapy or scheduled medication. It requires prompt response to rescue the patient from pain. Incident pain occurs with a specific activity, such as coughing, lifting, or walking; it is therefore predictable and often reproducible. In order to prevent the pain from occurring, it is best treated with therapies or medication before the specific activity.

Classification

By convention, pain is typically classified in terms of pathophysiology and is referred to as nociceptive, inflammatory, or neuropathic pain syndromes (Table 2–2). Additional pain syndromes usually involve combinations of these classifications or are described in terms of pain due to an overarching diagnosis, such as cancer pain (see Pain Syndromes section).

A. NOCICEPTIVE PAIN

This type of pain involves stimuli ascending via normal nerves traveling along sensory neurons and ascending via the spinothalamic pathways of the spinal cord. It includes both somatic and visceral pain.

Somatic pain is typically well localized in the superficial cutaneous or deeper musculoskeletal structures (eg, immediate postoperative wounds, bone metastases, muscle sprain). Visceral pain is usually poorly localized and often referred from deeper structures, such as the intestines (eg, constipation, early appendicitis).

B. INFLAMMATORY PAIN

Inflammatory pain is transmitted via normal nerves and pathways such as in nociceptive pain. However, the degree of tissue damage leads to the activation of acute and chronic inflammatory mediators that potentiate pain, lower thresholds for conduction, and sensitize the central nervous system to the incoming stimulus.

Table 2–2. Pathophysiologic Classifications of Pain.

	Classification		
	Nociceptive	***Inflammatory***	***Neuropathic***
Transduction	Peripheral receptors transduce mechanical, thermal, and chemical stimuli into action potentials	Significant tissue damage results in physiologic changes in the nervous system that potentiate pain Proinflammatory mediators lower the threshold for transduction	Results from a lesion in the peripheral or central nervous system
Transmission	Via intact nerves to the spinal cord	Changes the properties and function of neurons peripherally and centrally	Abnormal since the nerves themselves are altered Changes perpetuate in the properties and function of neurons peripherally and centrally
Electrical activity	Processed and interpreted as pain	Processed and interpreted as pain	Processed and interpreted as pain
Pain response	Adaptive, protective pain phenomena	Exaggerated	Exaggerated and abnormal
Examples	Minor surgery Vaccinations	Postoperative rheumatoid arthritis	Postherpetic neuralgia Lumbar radiculopathy AIDS Polyneuropathy

Examples include chronic inflammatory conditions, such as arthropathies and arthritis, ischemic vasculopathies, later postoperative wounds, and burns.

C. NEUROPATHIC PAIN

This type of pain arises in an area that is neurologically abnormal and is caused by a lesion of the peripheral or central nervous system. Most mechanisms of injury are poorly understood but may include incisional or crush damage of nerve tissue and nutritional, chemical, ischemic, metabolic, neoplastic or paraneoplastic insults to the peripheral or central nervous system.

Pain is typically perceived or described as being electrical in quality (ie, burning, shooting, stabbing, buzzing, tingling) or associated with numbness or abnormal temperatures. The sensation in the area affected and involved in the pain is usually abnormal. For example, nonnoxious stimuli (such as touch, light pressure, or temperature) are often either amplified hyperalgesic or numbed. The sensation created by the stimuli may be unassociated with the stimulus itself (ie, light feather touch can hurt, cold may feel hot, sharp prick stimuli may be numbed). Examples of neuropathic pain include postherpetic neuralgia, phantom limb pain, postthoracotomy chest pain, and diabetic neuropathy.

Carr D, Novak G, Rathmell JP, et al. *The Spectrum of Pain: Case-Based Medicine Teaching Series.* New York, McMahon Publishing Group, 2005.

McCaffery M. The patient's report of pain. *Am J Nurs.* 2001;101:73. [PMID: 12585068]

Woolf CJ. Pain: Moving from symptom control toward mechanism-specific pharmacologic management. *Ann Intern Med.* 2004;140:441. [PMID: 15023710]

ASSESSMENT OF PAIN

History

The **history taking** uses questions that are open-ended and directed toward understanding the pain syndrome and ideally finding a reversible cause to the pain (Table 2–3). Important information to gather includes the following: onset and duration, location, severity or intensity rated using a measurement tool, quality or character, aggravating factors, alleviating factors, and any previous treatments and their effect.

Additional questions should address how the pain impacts the patient's functional status, specifically activities of daily living (ADLs), instrumental activities of daily living (IADLs), and advanced activities of daily living (AADLs) (Tables 2–4 to 2–6). This functional assessment and documentation is particularly important in

Table 2–3. Suggested Open-Ended Questions to Ask during the Patient Interview.

Tell me about your pain.
Where do you feel the pain?
Does it travel or shoot?
What does it feel like?
What other words might describe your pain?
What makes your pain feel better?
What makes the pain worse?
What medications help your pain?
Can you make yourself hurt?
Can you reproduce the pain?

follow-up since the restoration of function can attest to the impact of pain relief therapies.

The use of an **anatomic figure** to indicate areas of pain can aid in history taking. Having the patient label areas of pain on a drawing can be compared with a similar schematic generated during the physical examination. This may present a visual of pain that gives insight into cause.

Clinical Findings

A. PHYSICAL EXAMINATION

The physical examination includes assessment of the presence of signs and symptoms that might reflect the pathophysiology of the underlying pain. The vital signs may be elevated in patients with acute pain or normal in patients with persistent pain. The appearance of the patient may reflect discomfort or may reveal a flattened affect. Patients often put forth great effort to obscure the level of their distress. Examining the pain area should include looking for distortions in anatomy, changes in color or consistency of the skin, and spasms or fasciculation of the underlying muscle. Palpation should be gentle initially, building gradually to assess for deeper pathology.

Table 2–4. Additional Questions to Assess How Pain Impacts Functional Status.

What does your pain mean to you?

How does your pain impact
    your role in your family?
    your ability to work?
    your role at work?
    your role in your community?

What does it mean to you to suffer?
Do you feel that you are suffering?

Table 2–5. Numeric Scale to Describe Pain and Affect on ADLs.

Number	Description
0	No pain
1–2	Mild pain or discomfort No interference with ADLs or instrumental or advanced ADLs
3	Mild to moderate pain More distracting Instrumental ADLs may be impacted
4	Moderate pain Limiting activity (instrumental and advanced ADLs)
5–6	Moderate pain Increasing severity
7	Moderate to severe pain ADLs affected
8–9	Severe
10	Worse pain possible Immobilized or overwhelmed by pain

ADLs, activities of daily living.

Palpating the same area with different approaches gives insight into the reproducibility of the pain. Distracting the patient during palpation can sometimes quiet anticipatory pain and guarding.

The physical examination can reflect the pathophysiology causing pain. For example, **nociceptive somatic pain** typically intensifies with palpation of a specific area (ie, pressure on a rib eliciting focal pain might reflect fracture or metastatic disease). Pain that intensifies with activity may reflect bone or muscle abnormalities or injuries. An example of **nociceptive visceral pain** includes sudden onset of retrosternal chest pain radiating to the jaw caused by myocardial ischemia. Physical palpation does not exacerbate or increase the pain. Another example of nociceptive visceral pain is generalized discomfort of the abdomen, many times associated with nausea. Palpation only worsens pain once inflammation has begun.

Rapid distention of the renal collecting system associated with blockage causes severe pain. The distention of the kidney can cascade into splinting and spasm of the lateral abdominal muscles. Depending on where in the renal pelvis and ureter the obstruction exists, the pain will be referred to varying locations:

1. Distention of the renal pelvis causes pain in the costovertebral angle

2. Distention of the ureteropelvic segment produces pain adjacent to the anterior superior iliac crest

Table 2–6. Assessing Functional Status by Evaluating Activities of Daily Living.

Activities of Daily Living
Eating/feeding
Personal hygiene
Toileting (bowel and bladder continence)
Bathing
Dressing
Walking
Instrumental Activities of Daily Living[a]
Opening containers
Writing
Dialing a phone
Home chores
Doing laundry
Reaching into low cupboards
Doing yardwork
Vacuuming
Advanced Activities of Daily Living[b]
Writing checks, balancing checkbook, keeping financial records
Handling business affairs, papers, and taxes
Shopping alone for clothes, groceries, or supplies
Playing games of skill such as bridge, chess, or crossword puzzles
Participating in creative hobbies such as sewing, stamp collecting, painting
Preparing a meal
Traveling independently out of the neighborhood

[a]Tasks require a finer level of motor coordination than the basic activities.
[b]Assess patient's independence.

3. Distention of the midureter manifests in pain in the lower mid-inguinal area

4. Distention of the ureterovesical portion causes suprapubic pain.

Palpation of the site of pain will not increase the pain complaint.

Inflammatory pain is aggravated by deep breathing; rebound of the abdomen would likely reflect inflammatory pain. Pain that is intensified with a full inspiration and associated with abnormal lung sounds or rubs indicates pleuritic inflammation. Pain associ-ated with reddened, swollen joints suggests inflammatory arthropathies.

Neuropathic pain is characterized by the following: allodynia, a condition in which ordinarily nonpainful stimuli evoke pain; hyperalgesia, an exaggerated response to nonpainful or mildly painful stimulus; causalgia, abnormalities of skin temperature and color compared with surrounding areas; atrophy and loss of hair in affected area; weakness of a muscle group associated with pain; and numbness to stimuli in the painful area.

B. THE INTERDISCIPLINARY ASSESSMENT

The expansion of the history and physical to include the input of a multidisciplinary or interdisciplinary team is the ideal approach in the assessment and management of pain. This approach incorporates not only the physical aspects of pain but also explores and documents the psychological/psychiatric, social, spiritual/religious, and cultural aspects of pain that would augment and complicate the patient's suffering.

1. Psychological and psychiatric assessments— Questions are directed toward manifestations of stress, mechanisms of coping, signs and symptoms of depression and anxiety, and behavior patterns that may help or hinder rehabilitation.

Examples of behaviors that may reflect pain include changes in appetite, such as anorexia; sleep disturbances, such as restlessness and frequent awakenings; agitation or aggressiveness; the above prompted by physical touch or changes in position; and decreased socialization and withdrawal.

When using behavioral cues for assessment, a patient's behavior will need to be reassessed after treatment with analgesic drugs. There may not be a clearcut response. Thus, a defined trial of a medication with ongoing observation will be necessary.

Remember, if pain has been uncontrolled for a period of time and thus associated with sleep disturbances and sleep deprivation, relief of pain may initially be associated with somnolence. Thus, it is critically important to allow several days (more than 72 hours) or more of the medication trial to truly assess its impact on behavior and function.

2. Social assessments—The impact of pain may have significant financial and social repercussions. These can magnify the experience of pain and aggravate feelings of helplessness, hopelessness, and despair. The social assessment could also involve how a family system is affected by the patient's pain and an assessment of possible equipment or home environment needs.

3. Spiritual and religious assessments—These assessments include elucidation of faith traditions, rituals, or lack thereof. For some, the exploration of this dimension of self serves as a keyhole into unspoken hopes and fears.

Patients may articulate how faith or religious rituals help them cope with the impact of pain or how they perceive their pain is a form of punishment for prior deeds.

4. Cultural assessments—A cultural assessment represents more than documentation of heritage; it includes ethnicity, language, family/community hierarchy and rituals as well as dietary practices. This facet of whole-person care may give insight into cultural preferences regarding disclosure of medical information and decision making.

It is key to remember that spiritual/religious and cultural aspects of a patient often impact his or her choice of descriptors, tolerance of pain, or acceptance of medications or other treatment modalities.

C. IMAGING STUDIES AND SPECIAL TESTS

Though there is no single test or series of tests that can definitely demonstrate the nature of the pain complaint, diagnostic testing can give insight into possible causes.

1. Radiographic imaging—Plain films can help elucidate structural changes in bone or soft tissue that correlate with the area involved in pain. These films may show bone damage from fractures or neoplastic disease, or the loss of bone integrity impinging on neighboring nerve or soft tissue. In the case of spinal films, abnormal findings can exist in people who have no sensation of pain, and relatively normal-appearing tissue or bone can be the source of significant pain stimuli since inflammation is not evident on radiographic films.

2. Electrodiagnostic evaluations—Electromyography and electroneuromyography may give evidence of nerve and muscle injury. However, these studies are highly individualized and the electrodiagnostician must thoughtfully plan the approach and scope of testing to narrow or clarify the possible areas of injury and associated pathology.

Pain Rating Scales

The severity or intensity of pain can be assessed using pain scales. It is important to choose a developmentally appropriate scale based on the age and cognitive status of the patient. The most extensively tested multidimensional scale for assessment is the McGill Pain Questionnaire. It takes 5 to 15 minutes to complete and is more thorough than other scales. The most commonly used scale is the Numeric Pain Intensity Scale (0 to 10). With this scale, 0 corresponds to no pain and 10 the worst imaginable pain.

For patients who have difficulty choosing a number between 0 and 10, using a schematic similar to a ruler

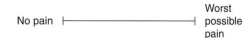

Figure 2–2. Visual Analogue Scale.

might be easier because the patient can point to a number along a continuum (Figure 2–1). Alternatively, some patients find it is easier to rate their pain by merely using the words mild, moderate, or severe. For others, the Visual Analogue Scale (VAS) is beneficial. Here the patient has the opportunity to shade in the amount of pain that exists along a continuum from no pain to worst possible pain (Figure 2–2). A final common pain scale is the Wong Baker FACES Scale (Figure 2–3). This scale shows six faces that depict a range of anguish secondary to pain. Figure 2–4 shows a comprehensive pain assessment tool.

Pain distress can be tied to functional status. Asking how pain affects activity or rating pain along with its functional impact allows a means to track improvement in a multidimensional outcome (see Table 2–6).

Moskowitz E, McCann CB. (1957). Functional disability and handicap. *J Clin Oncol.* 1995;9:2149-2151.

Memorial Sloan-Kettering Pain Assessment Card. www.mskcc.org/mskcc/html/5855.cfm; April 8, 2005.

PAIN ASSESSMENT IN THE COGNITIVELY IMPAIRED

In several studies, particularly targeting nursing home patients, the results demonstrate that there is no evidence of the masking of pain complaints by cognitive impairment. Although many older patients and cognitively impaired patients may underreport their experience of pain, their self-reports are found to be no less valid than other individuals who are cognitively intact. The challenge of assessing pain in the cognitively impaired has to do with the tools that are used to glean the results.

Assessing pain, however, in elderly patients who cannot respond verbally will negate the value of using any type of verbal descriptive tools, such as the Numeric Pain Scale described earlier. Functional status tools may be influenced by cognitive decline or morbidities such as hemiplegia, which may not necessarily involve pain.

In assessing the severely cognitively impaired patient, referring to the tools used by pediatricians may be helpful. For example, the Wong Baker FACES Scale was developed for children and could be helpful in assessing pain in the cognitively impaired patient (Table 2–7).

| 0 | 1 | 2 | 3 | 4 | 5 | 6 | 7 | 8 | 9 | 10 |

None ➔ Mild pain ➔ Moderate ➔ Severe pain

Figure 2–1. The Numeric Pain Intensity scale.

Pain assessment scales.

A. Numeric Scale

No pain   Worst pain

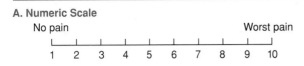

    1   2   3   4   5   6   7   8   9   10

B. Numeric Scale Translated into Word and Behavior Scales[1]

Pain intensity	Word scale	Nonverbal behaviors
0	No pain	Relaxed, calm expression
1–2	Least pain	Stressed, tense expression
3–4	Mild pain	Guarded movement, grimacing
5–6	Moderate pain	Moaning, restless
7–8	Severe pain	Crying out
9–10	Excruciating pain	Increased intensity of above

C. Wong-Baker FACES Pain Rating Scale [1]

0	1	2	3	4	5
No Hurt	Hurts Little Bit	Hurts Little More	Hurts Even More	Hurts Whole Lot	Hurts Worst

[1]Especially useful for patients who cannot read English and for pediatric patients.

Figure 2–3. Wong Baker FACES Scale. (Wong DL, Hockenberry-Eaton M, Wilson D, Winkelstein ML, Ahmann E, DeVito-Thomas PA. *Whaley and Wong's Nursing Care of Infants and Children*, ed. 6. St. Louis, 1999, Mosby, p 1153. Copyrighted by Mosby-Year Book, Inc. Reprinted by permission.)

Pain & Delirium in the Cognitively Impaired Patients

There is frequently an expressed concern that the use of analgesics can contribute to delirium in older patients. Studies of patients who have had hip fractures demonstrated that it is the undertreatment of pain that is a significant contributing factor to delirium. In fact, insufficient doses of opioids after the fracture or its repair are associated with an increased risk of delirium in both cognitively intact and cognitively impaired patients.

In hospital, it is common to write a prescription for pain medications to be given on an as-needed basis. However, the cognitively impaired patient may not be capable of interpreting their discomfort and translating this into a request for analgesics.

Closs SJ et al. A comparison of five pain assessment scales for nursing home residents with varying degrees of cognitive impairment. *J Pain Symptom Manage.* 2004;27:196. [PMID: 15010098]

Kovach CR et al. The assessment of discomfort in dementia protocol. *Pain Manag Nurs.* 2002;3:16. [PMID: 11893998]

Krulewitch H et al. Assessment of pain in cognitively impaired older adults: a comparison of pain assessment tools and their use by non-professional caregivers. *J Am Geriatr Soc.* 2000;48:1607. [PMID: 11129750]

Litaker D et al. Preoperative risk factors for postoperative delirium. *Gen Hosp Psychiatry.* 2001;23:84. [PMID: 11313076]

Manz BD et al. Pain assessment in the cognitively impaired and unimpaired elderly. *Pain Manag Nurs.* 20001:106. [PMID: 11709864]

Morrison RS et al. A comparison of pain and its treatment in advanced dementia and cognitively intact patients with hip fracture. *J Pain Symptom Manage.* 2000;19:240. [PMID: 10799790]

Morrison RS et al. Relationship between pain and opioid analgesics on the development of delirium following hip fracture. *J Gerontol A Biol Sci Med Sci.* 2003;58:76. [PMID: 12560416]

Proctor WR et al. Pain and cognitive status among nursing home residents in Canada. *Pain Res Manag.* 2001;6:119. [PMID: 11854774]

Taylor LJ et al. Pain intensity assessment: a comparison of selected pain intensity scales for use in cognitively intact and cognitively impaired African American older adults. *Pain Manag Nurs.* 2003;4:87. [PMID: 12836153]

PAIN ASSESSMENT TOOL

Patient _____ Date _____ Time _____

Medical Record Number _____ **Hospice Diagnosis:** _____

Level of consciousness (all that apply):
☐ ☐ ☐ Drowsy ☐ Unable to respond
Full Confusion

Do you have pain in any new places?
☐ Yes, new pain site ☐ No new pain site

Have you experienced pain, discomfort, or soreness at rest or with movement now or in the PAST WEEK?
☐ Yes ☐ No pain now ☐ No pain since last visit ☐ No pain behaviors observed

What pain medication(s) has the patient taken/been given in the past 24 hours? ☐ None
☐ See Medication Record
Meds: _____
Effective? ☐ Yes ☐ No

Pain Intensity Information	Number on 0-10 Scale
At rest for a minimum of 3 min	
With activity as you are able to do	
Worst over past 24 hours	
Least over past 24 hours	
Number you would **like your PAIN to be**	
Number you **could tolerate or live with**	

What does your pain keep you from doing? _____
_____
_____

How does your pain change with time?
☐ Brief ☐ Intermittent ☐ Rhythmic ☐ Unable to answer
☐ Constant ☐ Momentary ☐ Steady
☐ Continuous ☐ Periodic ☐ Transient

Does your pain affect your life in other ways? ☐ Unable to answer
☐ Agitation ☐ Hives ☐ Physical activity ☐ Pt denies
☐ Anger ☐ Hopelessness ☐ Rash
☐ Anxiety ☐ Insomnia ☐ Relationships
☐ Appetite ☐ Itching ☐ Restlessness
☐ Concentration ☐ Life enjoyment ☐ Suicidal thoughts
☐ Constipation ☐ Medication side effects ☐ Vomiting
☐ Depression ☐ Mood changes
☐ Diarrhea ☐ Nausea

What kind of things increase you pain?
☐ Nothing ☐ Sitting ☐ Unable to answer
☐ Bathing ☐ Standing
☐ Dressing ☐ Walking
☐ Eating ☐ Speaking/ Conversation
☐ Grooming ☐ Stress
☐ Toileting ☐ Time-of-day
☐ Position change/transfers ☐ Weather
☐ Reclining/lying

What kind of things relieve your pain? ☐ Unable to answer
☐ Breathing exercises ☐ Massage ☐ Nothing
☐ Cold ☐ Medications ☐ Social support
☐ Distraction ☐ Music ☐ Stockings
☐ Heat ☐ Position-change ☐ TENS
☐ Immobility ☐ Relaxation ☐ Visualization
☐ Walking

BEHAVIORAL OBSERVATION

Observe the patient – Check boxes for behavior observed

	At Rest	With Activity*	CG/Family Observation
☐ **No pain behaviors observed (Do not complete table.)**			
1. **Vocal complaints-Nonverbal:** (Expression of pain not in words: moans, groans, grunts, cries, gasps, sighs)			
2. **Facial Grimaces/Winces:** (Furrowed brow, narrowed eyes, tightened lips, dropped jaw, clenched teeth, distorted expressions)			
3. **Bracing:** (Clutching or holding onto side rails, furniture, or affected area during movement)			
4. **Restlessness:** (Constant or intermittent shifting of position, rocking, intermittent or constant hand motions, inability to keep still)			
5. **Rubbing:** (Massaging affected area)			
6. **Vocal complaints –Verbal:** (Words expressing discomfort or pain – "ouch," "that hurts," cursing during movement, or exclamations of protest – "stop," "that's enough")			

Activity Observed: ☐ Standing ☐ Walking ☐ Position Changes/Transfers ☐ Speaking ☐ Eating ☐ Other:

CLINICAL PERCEPTION, INTERVENTIONS, EDUCATION

Clinician Perception: What factors do you perceive interfere with quality pain management?
☐ None –Pain managed ☐ Patient not taking prescribed medication ☐ Family/caregiver not giving prescribed meds
☐ Psychosocial/spiritual reasons ☐ Current medication ineffective ☐ Non-pharmacological interventions not used
☐ Need prescription refill ☐ Side effects ☐ Other_____
☐ Teaching done ☐ **Continued**

_____ _____
RN Signature Date

Figure 2–4. Comprehensive pain assessment tool. *Continued*

CLINICAL PROGRESS NOTES

Patient Name _____ Medical Record Number _____ Page _____ of _____

DATE	TIME	☐ ON CALL	TC	DT	TT	V

"What does your pain feel like? I will read some words describing the nature of your pain. When I say any word that feels like your pain, stop me so I can mark it." If the patient mentions a word that describes a specific site, mark the letter for that site (A, B, C, E, etc.). After saying all the words, ask which site feels like each word the patient selects and write the letter of the site in the box next to the word.

☐ Flickering ☐   ☐ Sharp ☐   ☐ Tingling ☐   ☐ Fearful ☐   ☐ Penetrating ☐
☐ Quivering ☐   ☐ Cutting ☐   ☐ Itchy ☐   ☐ Frightening ☐   ☐ Piercing ☐
☐ Pulsing ☐   ☐ Lacerating ☐   ☐ Smarting ☐   ☐ Terrifying ☐   ☐ Tight ☐
☐ Throbbing ☐   (If no selection,   ☐ Stinging ☐   ☐ Punishing ☐   ☐ Drawing ☐
☐ Beating ☐   clarify instructions)   ☐ Dull ☐   ☐ Grunting ☐   ☐ Squeezing ☐
☐ Pounding ☐   ☐ Pinching ☐   ☐ Sore ☐   ☐ Cruel ☐   ☐ Tearing ☐
☐ Jumping ☐   ☐ Pressing ☐   ☐ Hurting ☐   ☐ Vicious ☐   ☐ Cool ☐
☐ Flashing ☐   ☐ Gnawing ☐   ☐ Aching ☐   ☐ Killing ☐   ☐ Cold ☐
☐ Shooting ☐   ☐ Cramping ☐   ☐ Heavy ☐   ☐ Wretching ☐   ☐ Freezing ☐
☐ Pricking ☐   ☐ Crushing ☐   ☐ Tender ☐   ☐ Blinding ☐   ☐ Nagging ☐
☐ Boring ☐   ☐ Tugging ☐   ☐ Taut ☐   ☐ Annoying ☐   ☐ Nauseating ☐
☐ Drilling ☐   ☐ Pulling ☐   ☐ Rasping ☐   ☐ Troublesome ☐   ☐ Agonizing ☐
☐ Stabbing ☐   ☐ Wrenching ☐   ☐ Splitting ☐   ☐ Miserable ☐   ☐ Dreadful ☐
☐ Lancinating ☐   ☐ Hot ☐   ☐ Tiring ☐   ☐ Intense ☐   ☐ Torturing ☐
☐ Shock-like ☐   ☐ Burning ☐   ☐ Exhausting ☐   ☐ Unbearable ☐   ☐ Other Words:
                 ☐ Scalding ☐   ☐ Sickening ☐   ☐ Spreading ☐
                 ☐ Searing ☐   ☐ Suffocating ☐   ☐ Radiating ☐   ☐ Unable to answer

_____

_____

_____

_____

_____

_____

_____

_____

_____

_____

_____

_____

_____

_____

_____

_____

_____

_____

_____

_____

_____

Signature _____

Figure 2–4. (Continued)

Table 2–7. Comparison of Pain Scales.

Population	Numeric scale	Visual analogue scale	Wong baker faces scale	McGill pain inventory
	Generally well-accepted and understood Can be written or oral	Generally easily understood Requires a tool for the tester to give the patient Numeric rating can be extracted from color level	Easily understood, although may reflect emotional response to pain rather than severity of symptom	Most extensively tested pain inventory available More time intensive for tester and patient Requires more interpretation
Children	Younger children may not be able to do	Color code intensity effective means for measurement	Developed for children	Younger children cannot complete
Adults	Effective	Advantageous with language barriers About 10% of adults are confused by test	Helpful for individuals not familiar with scaling their experiences	Effective and reproducible
Cognitively impaired	Effectiveness varies with degree of cognitive dysfunction	Effectiveness varies with degree of cognitive dysfunction	Effectiveness varies with degree of cognitive dysfunction	Effectiveness varies with degree of cognitive dysfunction

PAIN SYNDROMES

Grouping pain complaints based on physical findings or underlying diagnoses gives rise to many types of pain syndromes. As the understanding of pain pathophysiology expands, syndromes are better understood in terms of their defined pathology and mechanisms of pain transmission.

Cancer Pain

The pain associated with cancer may be caused by the disease or may result from some of the therapies used in treating the disease. The pain may also result from a comorbidity that is activated or aggravated in the diagnosis or treatment of the primary neoplastic process, such as arthritis or migraine.

Cancer pain is not unique in its pathophysiology; it is both acute and chronic and nociceptive, inflammatory, and neuropathic in its physiology.

Unremitted cancer pain may have significant impact on the patient's well-being and ability to undergo and tolerate treatments such as chemotherapy and radiation. Unrelieved cancer pain may have such a negative impact on the functional status of the patient that it can influence the actual prognosis in the course of disease.

Functional Pain

Functional pain lacks a recognizable cause; it has no clear peripheral or central pathophysiology, and yet is associated with persistent pain. The mechanisms are not yet well-defined and remain an area of active research.

Complaints of functional pain include irritable bowel syndrome, tension and migraine headache, as well as myofascial pain syndromes.

Complex Regional Pain Syndrome

The pathophysiology of this syndrome is complex and poorly understood. Complex regional pain syndrome (CRPS) is difficult to treat. It is believed to be neuropathic with dysautonomic signs. CRPS typically involves a constant burning sensation with intermittent paroxysms and includes two subtypes.

CRPS type I (previously known as reflex sympathetic dystrophy) is defined as continuing pain, allodynia, or hyperalgesia in which the pain is disproportionate to the inciting event and shows evidence of edema, changes in blood flow, and or abnormal motor function in the area of pain.

CRPS type II (previously known as causalgia) is similar to type I, but the presence of pain, allodynia, or hyperalgesia is not necessarily limited to the distribution of the injured nerve.

Phantom Pain

Phantom limb sensations are common after the loss of a limb but not always associated with pain. Phantom limb pain is a chronic pain condition associated with perceived pain in the absent limb. Phantom limb pain can be severe and debilitating, usually involving neuropathic pain and central sensitization from peripheral nerve damage.

Bone Pain

Bone pain is typically described as dull, aching, and constant; it is generally localized to the area of pathology with limited radiation. The pain can be aggravated by movement such as flexion or extension and sometimes by percussion.

Metastatic disease involving the long bones can be referred to the knee from lesions in the hip. Any patient with a malignancy who complains of dull, achy back pain should be assessed for an impending cord compression.

Pleural Pain

Typically, pleural pain is localized to the involved area; however, given the distribution of the pleura, it may involve the entire chest. The pain is described as sharp and shooting and is reproducible with a deep inhalation or cough. Pleural pain usually involves inflammation and nociceptive pathways. It may be associated with distinct physical findings such as a pleural rub with inhalation.

Plexopathies

The term "plexopathies" refers to pain syndromes associated with an anatomically described peripheral nerve plexus. The neurologic abnormalities involve several nerves in the plexus. In the case of a brachial plexopathy, pain is aggravated by a deep breath or movement of the neck and shoulder. Deep palpation of the shoulder may reproduce pain or suggest fullness. The pain in brachial plexopathy may be related to neoplastic encroachment into the nerves, adhesions and impingement after infection, surgery, or radiation treatment.

Bladder Pain

Bladder pain is most commonly associated with inflammation and manifests with urgency, frequency, and loss of control. It is associated with painful spasms of the bladder itself, especially as it distends with urine.

Rectal Pain

Abnormalities of the rectum can often be painless until inflammatory changes occur or obstruction results. Complaints are usually associated with burning, bloody or mucoid discharge, and rectal urgency. Tenesmus is the sensation of incomplete emptying of the rectum and is usually associated with inflammation.

Galer BS et al. IASP diagnostic criteria for complex regional pain syndrome: a preliminary empirical validation study. International Association for the Study of Pain. *Clin J Pain.* 1998;14:48. [PMID: 9535313]

ASSESSMENT & REASSESSMENT

The frequency of formal reassessment and redocumentation of pain depends on pain severity and the intensity of treatment. In severe pain states, when the titration of therapies is occurring frequently, pain levels should be reassessed and documented every 30 to 60 minutes using an effective tool. If pain is less intense and is perhaps being addressed with an oral pharmacologic regimen, reassessment and documentation of pain should initially be done in correlation with the half-life or pharmacodynamics of the medication being prescribed. For example, with a long-acting opioid with an 8-hour half-life, pain might be reassessed every 6 to 8 hours and dosing adjustments made every 24 hours. In a more stable pain state, reassessment and reaffirmation of pain management is individualized to the patients. Some patients need monthly follow-ups and reassessments, others can go quarterly or biannually with stability in their pain management approach.

Pharmacologic Therapies for Pain 3

Jay Thomas, MD, PhD & Charles F. von Gunten, MD, PhD

ESSENTIAL CRITERIA

- *Pain is subjective; the only measure of pain is a patient's report.*
- *Optimal treatment of pain requires addressing the physical, psychological, social, and spiritual/existential dimensions of the person experiencing the pain.*
- *Pharmacologic treatment of pain requires an understanding of the underlying pathophysiology of the pain (ie, whether pain is nociceptive, neuropathic, or mixed).*
- *Opioids are the foundation of the pharmacologic treatment of severe pain independent of cause, but adjunctive medications and their combinations are often required for optimal control of severe neuropathic pain.*

General Considerations

Optimal treatment of pain requires an understanding of the pathophysiology underlying the pain (ie, whether the pain is nociceptive, neuropathic, or mixed). Moreover, since pain is subjective, clinicians need to have an understanding of what the patient is experiencing emotionally. One important part of a multifaceted treatment program is pharmacologic intervention. The World Health Organization (WHO) has developed a useful three-step ladder that helps organize the pharmacologic approach to pain management (Figure 3–1):

1. Medications in Step 1 are used for mild pain, typically rated as 1 to 3 on an 11-point scale where 0 is no pain and 10 is the worst pain possible.
2. Medications in Step 2 are used for moderate pain, typically rated as 4 to 6.
3. Medications in Step 3 are used for severe pain, rated 7 to 10.

Using clinical judgment, the ladder can be entered at any step. For example, if a patient has a broken bone, the clinician need not start at Step 1 and wait until pain control fails before moving on to the next step. It is also important to remember that even if pain is sufficiently severe to require medications from a higher step, combination therapy with medications from lower steps may still be used synergistically. Finally, clinicians may use adjunctive medications to optimize pain control at each step.

STEP 1: TREATING MILD PAIN

Nonsteroidal Anti-inflammatory Drugs

A. PHARMACODYNAMICS

The predominant action of nonsteroidal anti-inflammatory drugs (NSAIDs) is to inhibit the enzyme cyclooxygenase (COX), which mediates the conversion of arachidonic acid to prostaglandins and thromboxanes. Isozymes of this enzyme exist. COX-1 is expressed constitutively in many tissues and regulates gastric cytoprotection, renal autoregulation of blood flow, platelet aggregation, and vascular homeostasis. COX-2 is constitutively expressed in a few tissues, such as the central nervous system (CNS), bone, and kidney, but predominantly is induced in inflammatory states. A third isozyme, COX-3 is an RNA splice variant of COX-1 and appears to be localized predominantly in the CNS but is also present in the heart. Its clinical significance remains unclear.

NSAIDs impact pain processing in two known ways. First, peripheral nociceptors (afferent sensory nerve fibers that signal pain) are sensitized by inflammation and in turn augment inflammation. For example, in the presence of inflammation, a normally silent peripheral C-fiber may start firing in response to a mild stimulus, and its response to a normal noxious stimulus is enhanced. In addition, the activated nociceptor may release inflammatory mediators that maintain or strengthen the inflammatory milieu. By reducing inflammation, NSAIDs decrease this peripheral sensitization and neurally mediated augmentation of inflammation. Second, COX is present in the spinal cord and has been implicated in CNS events that lead to central sensitization. In an experimental example of this central sensitization known as "wind up," a repetitive peripheral noxious stimulus can lead to central spinal changes that in turn lead to peripheral

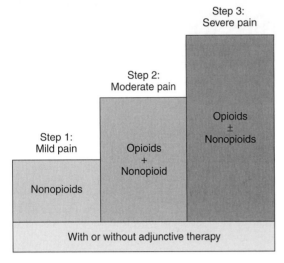

Figure 3–1. A 3-step ladder developed by The World Health Organization to help organize the pharmacologic approach to pain management. On a numeric scale, mild pain is rated between 1 and 3; moderate pain, between 4 and 6; and severe pain, between 7 and 10. Adjunctive medications may be added to any step.

hyperalgesia and allodynia. Hyperalgesia is a state where a noxious stimulus is perceived as more intense than it normally would. Allodynia is a state where a non-noxious stimulus, such as light touch, is perceived as painful. NSAIDs have experimentally been shown to prevent this central sensitization and enhancement of pain.

NSAIDs include nonselective COX inhibitors (eg, aspirin, ibuprofen, naproxen) and COX-2 selective inhibitors (eg, celecoxib, rofecoxib, valdecoxib), which have a 200- to 300-fold greater inhibitory effect on COX-2 than COX-1. Rofecoxib and valdecoxib are no longer available in the United States due to cardiac side effect concerns.

There may also be nonprostaglandin-mediated effects of NSAIDs. Studies indicate that NSAIDs may decrease neutrophil-endothelial cell interaction and may also decrease the production of nitric oxide. However, the clinical significance of these effects is unknown.

There are multiple classes of NSAIDs listed in Table 3–1. They include acetic acids, fenamates, naphthylalkanones, oxicams, propionic acids, and the COX-2 selective inhibitor. All agents inhibit COX but there may be differences in other pharmacodynamic properties that may help explain the variability in individual response.

B. Pharmacokinetics

NSAIDs in general are well absorbed and have high oral bioavailability. Oral forms typically reach peak effect for analgesia in 1 to 3 hours. NSAIDs are metabolized by the liver. Half-lives are variable. They all have a ceiling effect for efficacy but the risk of side effects continues to escalate with increasing dose.

Some NSAIDs are formulated as an elixir or suppository. These formulations can facilitate dosing when patients, especially those receiving palliative care, have difficulty swallowing pills. When formulations are not available commercially, pharmacists often compound an alternate formulation. In some circumstances, palliative care physicians have taken advantage of the fact that the oral and rectal routes of administration for many medications have similar pharmacokinetics. Often, oral pills can be used rectally with good effect. In fact, some oral time-release formulations retain their long-acting properties when used rectally, eg, morphine sulfate.

C. Prescribing Guidelines

The authors recommend the use of nonselective NSAIDs as first-line agents for several reasons. First, there is no clear analgesic benefit of COX-2 selective NSAIDs over nonselective agents. Second, COX-2 selective agents may increase the risk of cardiovascular events, and even low-dose aspirin negates the gastroprotective advantage of COX-2 selective agents. If gastric protection is needed with nonselective NSAIDs, a proton pump inhibitor or misoprostol is effective prophylaxis. Whether nonselective NSAIDs significantly increase the risk of cardiovascular events requires further study. Individual risk-benefit analysis must guide prescribing practice.

Typically, doses are started low. When steady state is reached after 3 to 5 doses, doses can be titrated up to maximum recommended doses limited by either achieving an effect or side effect. NSAIDs, independent of class, appear to be equally efficacious as analgesics but an individual patient may respond variable to them. If one NSAID fails at maximal doses, it is reasonable to try another agent in a different class. Typical dosing of NSAIDs is shown in Table 3–1.

Especially when used long term, frequency of dosing may affect patient compliance; therefore, once or twice a day dosing may be advantageous. Renal function should be monitored after initiating an NSAID as well as intermittently thereafter if the NSAID is to be given long term.

D. Common Side Effects

1. Gastrointestinal effects—COX-1 is involved in gastric protection. Therefore, COX-1 inhibition by nonselective COX inhibitors increases the risk of peptic ulcer, and COX-2 selective NSAIDs have less risk of gastrointestinal tract toxicity. However, studies have shown that concurrent use of even low-dose aspirin obviates the COX-2 selective gastrointestinal advantage. Furthermore, studies have shown that the use of either a proton pump inhibitor or misoprostol, a synthetic

Table 3-1. Prescribing Guidelines for Nonsteroidal Anti-Inflammatory Drugs.

Drug	Trade name	Dosing	Maximum daily dose
Acetic Acids			
Diclofenac	Cataflam/Voltaren	50 mg PO bid–tid	200 mg
	Voltaren XR	100 mg PO qd–bid	200 mg
Etodolac	Lodine	200–400 mg PO q6–8h	1200 mg
	Lodine XL	400–1000 mg PO qd	1200 mg
Indomethacin	Indocin	25–50 mg PO/per rectum tid	200 mg
		(Also available as 5 mg/mL suspension or 50 mg suppository)	
	Indocin SR	75 mg PO qd–bid	150 mg
Ketorolac	Toradol	10 mg PO q4–6h	40 mg
	Toradol parenteral	30 mg IM/IV q6h, (15 mg if patient > 65 years)	120 mg; NTE 5 days
Sulindac	Clinoril	150–200 mg PO bid	400 mg
Tolmetin	Tolectin	200–600 mg PO tid	1800 mg
	Tolectin DS	400 mg PO tid	1600 mg
COX-2 Inhibitor			
Celecoxib	Celebrex	100–200 mg PO bid	400 mg
Fenamates			
Meclofenamate		50–100 mg PO q4–6h	400 mg
Mefenamic acid		50–100 mg PO tid–qid	400 mg
	Ponstel	250 mg PO q6h prn	750 mg
Naphthylalkanones			
Nabumetone	Relafen	1 g PO qd–bid	2 g
Oxicams			
Meloxicam	Mobic	7.5–15 mg PO qd	15 mg
		(Also available as 7.5 mg/ 5 mL elixir)	
Piroxicam	Feldene	10–20 mg PO qd	20 mg

Continued

Table 3–1. Prescribing Guidelines for Nonsteroidal Anti-Inflammatory Drugs. (*Continued*)

Drug	Trade name	Dosing	Maximum daily dose
Propionic Acids			
Fenoprofen	Nalfon Nalfon 200	200–600 mg PO tid–qid	3200 mg
Flurbiprofen	Ansaid	50–100 mg PO bid–tid	300 mg
Ibuprofen	Motrin	200–800 mg PO q4–6h	3200 mg
Ketoprofen	Actron Orudis Oruvail	25–75 mg PO q6–8h	300 mg
Ketoprofen SR		200 mg PO qd	200 mg
Naproxen	Aleve	200–400 mg PO q8–12h	1200 mg
	Anaprox	275–550 mg PO bid	1100 mg
	Anaprox DS	550 mg PO bid	1100 mg
	Naprelan	375–1000 mg PO qd	1500 mg
	Naprosyn	250–500 mg PO bid	1500 mg
Oxaprozin	Daypro	600–1800 mg PO qd	1800 mg
Salicylates, Acetylated			
Aspirin		325–650 mg PO q4h	4000 mg
		300–600 mg per rectum q4h	
Salicylates, Nonacetylated			
Diflunisal	Dolobid	250–500 mg PO q8–12h	1500 mg
Salsalate	Disalcid	500–1000 mg PO tid	3000 mg
	Salflex	500–1000 mg PO tid	3000 mg

NTE, not to exceed.

analogue of prostaglandin E_1, in conjunction with a nonselective NSAID can significantly protect against ulcer formation.

2. Hematologic effects—Platelet COX-1 is responsible for thromboxane A_2 generation. Thromboxane A_2 mediates platelet activation and aggregation. Thus, in general, nonselective NSAIDs (nonacetylated NSAIDs, such as salsalate, are exceptions) increase the risk of bleeding, while COX-2 selective inhibitors have no antiplatelet activity and no effect on bleeding risk. However, recent clinical trials have implicated some of the COX-2 selective inhibitors in increased risk of cardiovascular events. A plausible explanation for this phenomenon is that COX-2 selective inhibitors reduce endothelial cell prostaglandin I_2 (prostacyclin) production but leave platelet prothrombotic thromboxane A_2 production unaffected.

A nonselective COX inhibitor, naproxen, has also recently been implicated in increased risk of cardiovascular events, although the strength of this association is unclear. The National Institutes of Health (NIH) stopped a large trial designed to determine whether celecoxib or naproxen versus placebo decreased the risk of developing Alzheimer's disease. Without releasing exact numbers, the NIH stated naproxen increased the risk of cardiovascular events 50% over placebo.

To clearly resolve the cardiovascular effects of both nonselective and COX-2 selective inhibitors, further studies are required.

3. Renal and hemodynamic effects—In normal circumstances, glomerular perfusion is not dependent on prostaglandins. However, in cases of chronic renal insufficiency and prerenal conditions, such as volume depletion, liver failure, and congestive heart failure, glomerular perfusion is dependent on prostaglandin-mediated vasodilation. NSAIDs, by inhibiting this vasodilation, can decrease glomerular filtration rate and worsen renal function. Systemically, NSAID inhibition of vasodilation leads to increased vascular tone. This effect elevates blood pressure and can worsen preexisting heart failure. Both nonselective and COX-2 selective NSAIDs can adversely affect renal and systemic hemodynamics.

Acetaminophen

A. PHARMACODYNAMICS

Acetaminophen's mechanism of action remains controversial. It has no peripheral anti-inflammatory effects. Its analgesic and antipyretic effects are believed to be centrally mediated. As mentioned previously, a COX-1 RNA splice variant termed "COX-3" has been identified in the brain. Acetaminophen is active as an inhibitor of this enzyme. Mouse studies have shown acetaminophen to reduce brain prostaglandin levels in a parallel with analgesia. Mice altered to lack either COX-1 or COX-2 showed this effect to be dependent on the COX-1 gene, which is needed to produce COX-3.

B. PHARMACOKINETICS

Acetaminophen is 60 to 90% orally bioavailable. Its onset of action is 15 to 30 minutes and peak serum levels (C_{max}) are reached in 40 to 60 minutes. The half-life is about 2 to 4 hours. Acetaminophen is extensively metabolized in the liver. Importantly, about 10% of it is converted to a highly reactive toxic metabolite that is normally inactivated by glutathione. When glutathione stores are depleted, the toxic metabolite can cause severe hepatotoxicity. Given this dose-dependent toxicity, acetaminophen also has a ceiling effect.

C. PRESCRIBING GUIDELINES

Typical dosing is 500 to 1000 mg orally every 4 to 6 hours. However, maximal dosing should not exceed 4 g/d due to the risk of hepatotoxicity. This maximal amount should be further reduced for those with underlying liver disease or who consume three or more alcoholic drinks per day. Acetaminophen is available in tablet, capsule, elixir, and suppository forms.

D. COMMON SIDE EFFECTS

Other than dose to dependent hepatotoxicity as described above, acetaminophen is generally well tolerated. Long-term therapy at high doses can lead to nephrotoxicity.

Chandrasekharan NV et al. COX-3, a cyclooxygenase-1 variant inhibited by acetaminophen and other analgesic/antipyretic drugs: cloning, structure, and expression. *Proc Natl Acad Sci U S A.* 2002;99:13926. [PMID: 12242329]

Ghilardi JR et al. Constitutive spinal cyclooxygenase-2 participates in the initiation of tissue injury-induced hyperalgesia. *J Neurosci.* 2004;24:2727. [PMID: 15028765]

Silverstein FE et al. Gastrointestinal toxicity with celecoxib vs nonsteroidal anti-inflammatory drugs for osteoarthritis and rheumatoid arthritis: the CLASS study: a randomized controlled trial. Celecoxib Long-term Arthritis Safety Study. *JAMA.* 2000;284:1247. [PMID: 10979111]

STEP 2: TREATING MODERATE PAIN

On this step of the ladder, Step 1 medications (NSAIDs and acetaminophen) are commonly combined with opioids. Table 3–2 lists these agents as well as their prescribing categories.

Opioids themselves have no theoretical ceiling effect. However, by virtue of their formulation, these combined agents have a ceiling effect imposed by their Step 1 component.

The opioids used in combination with NSAIDs and acetaminophen include tramadol, codeine, hydrocodone, and oxycodone. The less potent opioids codeine and tramadol are discussed in this section and the more potent opioids will be addressed below in Step 3: Treating Severe Pain.

Codeine

A. PHARMACODYNAMICS

Codeine, as all clinically useful opioid analgesics, eventually acts at μ opioid receptors, which are located in the brain and in the spinal cord. (See the Pharmacodynamics section under Step 3: Treating Severe Pain for a more detailed discussion of the action of μ-receptors.)

B. PHARMACOKINETICS

Codeine is predominantly a prodrug of morphine. Liver metabolism via the cytochrome P450 system enzyme CYP2D6 leads to activation. Patients who lack this enzyme (approximately 5 to 10% of whites) or who have concomitant inhibitors of it (such as fluoxetine or paroxetine) derive little analgesia from codeine. Orally, it is 40% bioavailable and reaches peak effect in about 1 hour. Half-life is 2.5 to 3.5 hours.

C. PRESCRIBING GUIDELINES

The usual dose of codeine alone, a schedule II drug, is 30 to 60 mg orally every 4 hours. Fixed combinations of codeine (15, 30, or 60 mg) with acetaminophen (300 mg) are available and are schedule III. Because some patients cannot activate codeine and there are drug interactions that weaken its efficacy, codeine preparations are not front-line Step 2 agents.

Other Step 2 opioid combinations contain hydrocodone or oxycodone, which are roughly equipotent. The authors consider these medications equally

Table 3–2. Medications Used in Step 2: Treating Moderate Pain.

Generic name	Trade name	Formulation (mg)	FDA schedule	Max dose
Acetaminophen/Codeine	Tylenol #2	(300/15)	III	
	Tylenol #3	(300/30)	III	
	Tylenol #4	(300/60)	III	
Acetaminophen/Hydrocodone	Hycopap	(500/5)	III	
	Lorcet HD	(500/5)	III	
	Lorcet Plus	(650/7.5)	III	
	Lorcet	(650/10)	III	
	Lortab	(500/2.5) (500/5) (500/7.5) (500/10)	III	
	Lortab Elixir	(500/7.5 per 15 mL)	III	
	Maxidone	(750/10)	III	
	Norco	(325/5) (325/7.5) (325/10)	III	
	Vicodin	(500/5)	III	
	Vicodin ES	(750/7.5)	III	
	Vicodin HP	(660/10)	III	
	Zydone	(400/5) (400/7.5) (400/10)	III	
Acetaminophen/Oxycodone	Endocet	(325/5) (325/7.5) (325/10) (500/7.5) (650/10)	II	
	Percocet	(325/2.5) (325/5) (325/7.5) (325/10) (500/7.5) (650/10)	II	
	Roxicet	(325/5) (500/5)	II	
	Roxicet Elixir	(325/5 per 5 ml)	II	
	Tylox	(500/5)	II	
Acetaminophen/Tramadol	Ultracet	(325/37.5)	Uncontrolled	
Ibuprofen/Hydrocodone	Vicoprofen	(200/7.5)	III	
Ibuprofen/Oxycodone	Combunox	(400/5)	II	
Tramadol	Ultram	(50)	Uncontrolled	400 mg

The above tablets can be dosed 1–2 PO every 4–6 hours as needed.
*Denotes maximal dose limited by Step 1 component.

efficacious, but since hydrocodone preparations are schedule III and oxycodone preparations are schedule II, hydrocodone preparations are more commonly prescribed. The choice of prescribing an agent containing acetaminophen or ibuprofen depends on whether inflammation is present, in which case an NSAID would be preferred, or depends on the side effects that each agent can cause.

Because the acetaminophen amount varies in different formulations, the prescriber must ensure that the total acetaminophen content does not exceed a toxic level, taking into account not only the Step 2 agent but also any other acetaminophen preparations a patient may be taking.

D. COMMON SIDE EFFECTS

Codeine and other opioids share the same set of side effects. For a full discussion of these effects, please refer to the section Common Side Effects in the following section Step 3: Treating Severe Pain.

Tramadol

A. PHARMACODYNAMICS

Tramadol is a weak μ-receptor agonist. It has several orders of weaker magnitude affinity for the μ-receptor than morphine. However, in addition, neuronal serotonin release is enhanced while also inhibiting serotonin and norepinephrine reuptake. This reuptake inhibition is similar mechanistically to the tricyclic antidepressants. Quantitatively, reuptake inhibition is also 1 to 2 orders less in magnitude than tricyclic antidepressants. Tramadol has also been cited to have anti-inflammatory activity that is independent of COX inhibition. It is hypothesized that tramadol's weak effects synergize to make it a clinically useful analgesic. By virtue of its multiple mechanisms of action, tramadol may be useful for mild to moderate nociceptive and neuropathic pain. A clinical trial demonstrated its efficacy in treating diabetic neuropathy.

B. PHARMACOKINETICS

Tramadol is 75% orally bioavailable. The liver metabolizes it to an active metabolite, O-desmethyltramadol, which has increased activity over its parent compound. Time to peak plasma tramadol concentration is about 2 hours and its half-life is 6 hours.

C. PRESCRIBING GUIDELINES

The typical dose for tramadol is 50 to 100 mg orally every 4 to 6 hours. The maximum recommended dose is 400 mg/d. Although the risk of addiction may be lower than with opioids, there is still some risk. However, in general, the risk of addiction to opioids when used for pain is overstated. Physical dependence does occur and withdrawal may occur with rapid cessation.

Since tramadol is an opioid with its own inherent adjunctive properties, it could be considered a first-line Step 2 agent when mild to moderate pain has a neuropathic component. Because of its multiple, synergistic properties, tramadol may be effective with fewer opioid side effects than a pure μ-receptor agonist titrated to equal efficacy. For example, tramadol may cause less constipation than an equally analgesic dose of an oxycodone-containing product.

D. COMMON SIDE EFFECTS

CNS effects, such as dizziness and somnolence, and gastrointestinal effects, such as constipation and nausea, are the most commonly cited side effects. Maximal dosing is limited due to concerns for lowering seizure thresholds.

Harati Y et al. Double-blind randomized trial of tramadol for the treatment of the pain of diabetic neuropathy. *Neurology.* 1998;50:1842. [PMID: 9633738]

STEP 3: TREATING SEVERE PAIN

Opioids

A. PHARMACODYNAMICS

Clinically used opioid analgesics are agonists at μ-receptors. They include morphine, oxycodone, hydromorphone, fentanyl, and methadone. In the brain, these μ-receptors are located in areas such as the periaqueductal gray, known to be involved in mediating pain. In the spinal cord, they are located in the dorsal horn where small fiber pain afferents synapse.

Mu receptors are transmembrane proteins that are coupled to G-proteins. Presynaptically, opioid binding can lead to blockage of calcium channels and thus a decrease in the release of neurotransmitters thus damping pain signaling. Postsynaptically, opioid binding can lead to increased potassium conductance that hyperpolarizes the neuron and makes it less likely to fire to transmit a pain signal.

In addition to μ-receptor agonism, methadone uniquely has two other pharmacodynamic effects. First, it is an *N*-methyl-D-aspartate (NMDA) receptor antagonist. At the spinal cord level, the NMDA receptor is involved in central facilitation in "wind up" and neuropathic pain. In this state, pain may be refractory to even high-dose opioids. Inhibition of the NMDA receptor can block this "wind up" and increase the efficacy of opioids at the μ receptor. Second, methadone can block presynaptic serotonin reuptake.

Older equianalgesic tables indicated methadone was roughly equianalgesic with morphine. However, empirically, when patients who are taking high-dose opioids are rotated to methadone, it is observed that a much lower dose of methadone is effective than the dose calculated from traditional equianalgesic tables. This increased efficacy is attributed to the synergism of methadone's multiple pharmacodynamic properties.

The concept that the dose of a medication must be increased over time to maintain the same pharmacodynamic effect is called tolerance. Opioid tolerance at the cellular and molecular level overall remains an enigma. To explain tolerance, researchers have invoked processes such as receptor downregulation, receptor desensitization, NMDA receptor upregulation, as well as others. Tolerance to opioid effects varies. For example, tolerance never seems to develop to the constipating effects of opioids whereas tolerance rapidly develops to respiratory depression. Tolerance to analgesia develops in animals, but empirically in humans, chronic stable pain is often well treated with stable doses of opioids.

Among opioids, tolerance also varies. If a patient who is tolerant to one opioid is switched to another opioid, it is observed that there is incomplete cross-tolerance (Table 3–3). The second opioid is more effective than would be expected from equianalgesic conversion calculations. There is some tolerance due to the effects of the first opioid but it is incomplete. The practical effect of incomplete cross-tolerance is that when rotating to a new opioid the calculated equianalgesic dose must be reduced by 25 to 50% to have a similar pharmacodynamic effect. When patients remain in pain or are having intolerable opioid side effects, this phenomenon can be used in a process called **opioid rotation.** By switching to an alternative opioid, analgesia may be enhanced and side effects may be reduced due to incomplete cross-tolerance.

B. PHARMACOKINETICS

It is important to divide opioids into two types—hydrophilic and lipophilic—when discussing the pharmacokinetics of opioids. The major differences between hydrophilic and lipophilic opioids are their pharmacokinetic and metabolite profiles.

1. Hydrophilic opioids—Morphine, codeine, hydrocodone, oxycodone, and hydromorphone are examples of clinically useful hydrophilic opioids. The hydrophilic opioids share a similar pharmacokinetic profile.

Table 3–3. Opioid Rotation and Incomplete Cross-Tolerance.

When changing from one opioid to another:
- Due to incomplete cross tolerance
  - Start with 50–75% of the calculated equianalgesic dose
  - Use more, if pain is uncontrolled
  - Use less, if adverse effects are present
- If converting to methadone, use the conversion factors listed in Table 3–5.

Hydrophilic opioid oral bioavailability ranges from 35 to 70%. There is an extensive hepatic first-pass effect. Because of this effect, conversion from oral to parenteral dosing requires reduction by approximately a factor of three. For example, 30 mg of oral morphine would be converted to 10 mg of IV morphine.

Morphine has an active metabolite, morphine-6-glucouronide (M6G) that is even more potent than morphine itself. M6G must be cleared renally. When creatinine clearance is compromised, M6G may accumulate and cause opioid neurotoxicity (eg, myoclonus, delirium, seizure). It is believed the other hydrophilic opioids may also have renally cleared metabolites that can cause toxicity with accumulation.

For the short-acting hydrophilic opioids, the time to maximal serum concentration (C_{max}) depends on the dosing route: orally, C_{max} is 60 minutes; subcutaneously, C_{max} is about 30 minutes; intravenously, C_{max} is about 6 minutes. The half-life of the hydrophilic opioids is approximately 4 hours. Steady-state levels are reached after 4 to 5 half-lives; thus, steady-state levels will be reached in 16 to 20 hours.

These short-acting opioids may be subject to the bolus effect. Patients may experience side effects when serum levels are maximal yet later experience recurrent pain as trough levels are approached before the next scheduled dose. Either continuous infusion or long-acting opioids are needed to avoid this bolus effect.

Examples of long-acting forms of the hydrophilic opioids include morphine (eg, MS Contin, Kadian), oxycodone (eg, Oxycontin), and hydromorphone exist. Depending on the formulation, the half-life is 12 to 24 hours. At steady state, peak and trough effects are blunted thus avoiding the bolus effect. Long-acting formulations also improve patient compliance by reducing dosing frequency, reducing pill burden, and reducing sleep interruptions from pain or dosing.

2. Lipophilic opioids—Examples of the major lipophilic opioids are fentanyl and methadone. Because of their affinity for lipids, fentanyl and methadone have high bioavailability, and they rapidly cross the blood-brain barrier. The liver metabolizes fentanyl and methadone, but there are no known active or toxic metabolites (unlike the hydrophilic opioids).

The noninvasive forms of fentanyl include a transdermal patch and a transmucosal lozenge. The transdermal delivery system establishes equilibrium with the subcutaneous tissue and systemically delivers a defined amount per hour. Its bioavailability approaches 100%. Available patches deliver 12.5, 25, 50, 75, and 100 mcg/h. After placement of a patch, 12 to 16 hours are needed to reach clinically significant levels. During this time, other short-acting opioids are needed to maintain analgesia. The patch is typically replaced every

3 days, although some patients may require a change every 2 days.

The lozenge contains fentanyl in a candy matrix that is applied by twirling against the buccal mucosa until it is consumed. It is available in 200, 400, 600, 800, 1200, and 1600 mcg doses. It must be uniquely titrated for each patient's pain. The effective dose has no correlation with the oral morphine equivalent dose a patient is currently receiving. The typical starting dose for fentanyl lozenge is 200 mcg. If pain is not relieved in 15 minutes, a second 200-mcg lozenge is consumed. If this controls the pain, the appropriate dose is 400 mcg. If this does not control the pain, titration is resumed at the next episode of pain starting with 400 mcg and repeating the above procedure. Approximately half of the bioavailable amount is absorbed transmucosally and has kinetics of action similar to the intravenous route. Onset of action is within 5 to 10 minutes. The other bioavailable half is swallowed and has the kinetics of the oral route. Overall, peak serum levels are achieved in 20 to 40 minutes. In addition to its rapid onset of action, it also has a relatively rapid offset of 1 to 3 hours. Given this kinetic profile, it is advantageous for short-lived breakthrough pain. Other short-acting opioids with longer half-lives may still have significant serum levels even after the short-lived breakthrough pain has diminished. In this situation, a patient has a relative opioid excess and attendant opioid side effects, eg, lethargy.

Methadone has a long and variable half-life that can range from 8 to 72 hours. Thus, it may take from 1 to 15 days for steady state to be reached. Careful individual titration is necessary to avoid accumulation over time. Methadone is typically taken every 8 hours, but some patients may only need to take it once or twice daily. Methadone has some drug interactions. Carbamazepine, phenobarbital, phenytoin, and rifampin can increase methadone metabolism; whereas, amitriptyline and cimetidine can decrease its metabolism. Methadone may also increase zidovudine levels.

C. Prescribing Guidelines

Table 3–4 outlines prescribing guidelines for opioids. When rapidly titrating opioids to treat uncontrolled pain, it is best to use short-acting agents on an as-needed basis until the pain is controlled and daily requirements have been established. This method also works best when clinically significant renal insufficiency is present. Renally cleared active opioid metabolites may accumulate, but patients will integrate this fact in their dosing as needed. The time to C_{max} of the route the opioid is being administered determines how often titration can be performed. For example, the time to C_{max} for an oral hydrophilic opioid is about 1 hour. Therefore, if a patient still has significant pain 1 hour after an oral dose of a hydrophilic opioid, there should be no expectation of

Table 3–4. Opioid Titration Guidelines.

- Titrate with short-acting hydrophilic opioid; can be given at intervals based on the time to peak serum levels (C_{max}) as needed; oral, ~1 hour; subcutaneous, ~30 minutes; intravenous ~10 minutes)
- Calculate 24-hour requirements and convert to long-acting opioid; if pain persists at steady state, adjust as follows:
  For mild to moderate pain, increase daily dose 25–50%
  For moderate to severe pain, increase daily dose 50–100%
- For breakthrough pain, give 5–15% of the total daily dose at intervals based on the time to C_{max} as needed as above with short-acting opioid

better analgesia by waiting because serum levels will only fall with the passage of time. Thus, it is rational and safe to give an appropriate amount of a hydrophilic opioid orally on the hour until pain is adequately controlled.

If the route is intravenous, C_{max} is approximately 6 to 10 minutes. Thus, doses could be repeated every 10 minutes until pain is tolerable. If pain is still severe at the C_{max}, the short-acting opioid could be safely doubled without fear of respiratory depression. Similarly, if pain is still severe at steady state, the total daily opioid dose can also be safely doubled. For example, if a patient takes 30 mg of immediate-release morphine orally, yet remains in severe pain 1 hour later at C_{max}, doubling the oral morphine dose to 60 mg would be clinically safe as titration to tolerable pain control is pursued. Once patients are no longer opioid naïve, it is the relative change in dose that matters, not the absolute values.

Once 24-hour opioid requirements are established, the dosing is converted to a long-acting regimen. This conversion enhances compliance by reducing the burden of taking pills frequently, by eliminating the bolus effect of short-acting agents, and by allowing for sleep that is uninterrupted by pain or dosing. If at steady state, pain remains at a mild to moderate level, the 24-hour dose can be increased 25 to 50%. If pain remains at a moderate to severe level, the 24-hour dose can be increased 50 to 100%. A 100% increase represents a doubling of the 24-hour dose and is safe in the context of continued pain.

When titrated as above, long-acting hydrophilic opioids are still safe and most cost-effective for treating patients with clinically significant renal insufficiency. When renal function is changing, there may be a role for opioids without active or toxic metabolites that must be renally cleared, such as methadone or fentanyl. However, hydrophilic opioids may still be useful if dose or frequency of dosing is decreased. Sometimes, returning to "as-needed" dosing is effective for analgesia and avoiding opioid side effects as renal function is declining and patients are approaching death.

When the oral route cannot be used for long-acting agents, there are still several options that can be used before resorting to continuous parenteral administration. First, the fentanyl transdermal patch can be used. Next, some long-acting hydrophilic opioid preparations are capsules containing small time-release granules. The capsules can be opened and the granules can be put down an enteral feeding tube (eg, Kadian). Finally, as mentioned previously, some oral long-acting formulations can be used rectally (eg, MS Contin).

For pain that breaks through a basal opioid regimen, clinicians can give 5 to 15% of the 24-hour requirement as a breakthrough dose. Again, since hydrophilic opioids have a C_{max} of about 1 hour, this breakthrough dosing is safely given up to every hour if pain persists. If pain is persistent, requiring multiple breakthrough doses per day, the total opioid use (basal plus breakthrough) per day can be totaled and divided into dosing of a long-acting agent. For example, if a patient is taking 60 mg of oral morphine sulfate every 12 hours and needs 12 extra 10-mg doses of immediate-release morphine sulfate in a day, the basal regimen can be adjusted to long-acting morphine sulfate 120 mg orally every 12 hours.

This kind of persistent breakthrough pain must be distinguished from incident breakthrough pain that is incited by a particular event. For example, for a patient with an acute vertebral compression fracture, there may be little pain when lying at rest but there may be severe pain on weight bearing to go to the bathroom. Although multiple doses of breakthrough medication may be required per day, these doses would not be rolled into the basal opioid regimen. Doing so would give a relative excess of opioid when the patient is pain free when lying and not enough opioid for the acute pain exacerbation when standing.

When converting from one opioid to another, equianalgesic conversion tables guide dosing (Table 3–5). It is important to note that these conversions are only guidelines and clinical judgment is needed to individualize dosing for patients. Moreover, because of the phenomenon of incomplete cross-tolerance (see Table 3–3), calculated equianalgesic doses must be reduced by 25 to 50% for equal effect. Sometimes, when pain is not well controlled and opioids are being rotated, clinicians purposely do not take into account incomplete cross-tolerance in order to have a net increase in opioid effect. It is comforting to know that for opioid tolerant patients, even two-fold differences in dosing of an opioid will not cause life-threatening complications.

Conversion from other opioids to methadone requires special consideration (see Table 3–5). Methadone, as discussed previously, has multiple pharmacodynamic actions, making it more potent than predicted from traditional equianalgesic tables. In cases of neuropathic or opioid-resistant pain, methadone needs to be uniquely titrated based on the total oral morphine equivalent dose a patient is currently receiving. The higher the oral morphine equivalent dose, the more potent methadone may be and the conversion must be adjusted accordingly. For example, at an oral morphine equivalent dose of

Table 3–5. Equianalgesic Dosing Guidelines for Chronic Pain.

Changing opioids		
Oral/rectal dose (mg)	**Analgesic**	**Parenteral IV/SC/M dose (mg)**
150	Meperidine	50
150	Tramadol	—
150	Codeine	50
15	Hydrocodone	—
15	Morphine	5
10	Oxycodone	
3	Hydromorphone	1
2	Levorphanol	1
—	Fentanyl	0.050

Transdermal fentanyl
Morphine 50 mg $\approx$ Fentanyl 25 mcg/h PO in 24 hours   transdermal patch

Methadone		
	Conversion ratio	
Daily morphine dose (mg/24 hr PO)	**Morphine PO**	**Methadone PO**
<100	3 :	1
101–300	5 :	1
301–600	10 :	1
601–800	12 :	1
801–1000	15 :	1
>1000	20 :	1

Adjusting for incomplete cross-tolerance based on pain control	
Poor	100%
Moderate	75%
Excellent	50%

(Reprinted From San Diego Hospice & Palliative Care.)

300 mg/d, a conversion factor of 5 would be used, yielding a methadone dose of 60 mg/d. At an oral morphine equivalent dose of 1000 mg/d, a conversion factor of 15 would be used, yielding a similar methadone dose of ~ 67 mg/d.

Given methadone's long and variable half-life, it is not typically used to titrate acutely for severe pain. Therefore, patients are often taking high doses of other opioids before being converted to methadone. This conversion requires careful attention. If methadone potently relieves pain, a patient may be left with a relative excess of the original opioid. In theory, this excess could suppress respirations since pain is no longer present as an antidote.

There are many conversion protocols in use. Bruera et al have published a conservative conversion to methadone over 3 days. First, the targeted methadone dose per day is calculated as above. Then,

1. On day 1, the current opioid is decreased by one-third, and methadone is initiated at one-third of the final targeted dose.
2. On day 2, the original opioid is decreased by another third, and the methadone is titrated up to two-thirds of the final targeted dose.
3. On day 3, the original opioid is discontinued, and the methadone dose is titrated up to the full, targeted dose.

During this conversion, the authors recommend using the original opioid for breakthrough pain at the original breakthrough dose. If patients have significant pain relief early in the conversion, the original opioid can continue to be tapered, but the methadone dose can be maintained without further up-titration. Again, due to methadone's long and variable half-life, patients must be carefully monitored for lethargy as an early sign of accumulation. Typically, this occurs within 3 to 5 days of initiating long-term therapy, but may occur later. If it is noted, the methadone should be held and then restarted at a lower or less frequent dose. Due to the complexity of methadone dosing, expert consultation may be indicated.

Methadone may also be started as the initial opioid, particularly when neuropathic pain is present. In opioid naïve patients with moderate pain, 5 mg of oral methadone 2 or 3 times daily is a reasonable starting dose. Doses can be titrated up every 3 to 5 days as indicated, again monitoring for signs of accumulation. The authors use a short-acting hydrophilic opioid for breakthrough pain during titration.

D. COMMON SIDE EFFECTS

All the opioids share similar side effects (Table 3–6); the common include nausea, constipation, and altered cognition (eg, sedation, mental clouding). Although respiratory depression is much feared, it is not common when opioids are dosed appropriately. This statement is

Table 3–6 Opioid Side Effects.

Common
Constipation
Nausea/vomiting
Sedation
Dry mouth
Sweats
Uncommon
Dysphoria/delirium
Myoclonus/seizures
Pruritus/urticaria
Urinary retention
Respiratory depression

especially true when opioids are titrated in the presence of pain, which is a powerful antagonist to respiratory depression. The other less common side effects include dysphoria, delirium, myoclonus, seizures, pruritus and urticaria, and urinary retention.

Side effects typically occur at the time of opioid initiation and at times of dose increments. At any given opioid dose, tolerance to the side effect may develop but is variable. Tolerance to respiratory depression happens quickly. Tolerance to nausea and cognitive changes typically occurs within a few days to 1 week. Unfortunately, tolerance to constipation never develops.

To avoid having to discontinue opioid therapy, side effects can be treated. Nausea is usually well controlled with an antidopaminergic antiemetic. Since gastric motility is slowed by opioids, a particularly effective agent is metoclopramide, which has promotility effects in addition to antidopaminergic effects. Sedation and mental clouding may respond to stimulants such as methylphenidate or modafinil. Since tolerance to constipation never develops, a bowel regimen should be instituted at the same time opioids are initially prescribed. Typically, a stimulant laxative, such as senna, is combined with a stool softener, such as docusate, to treat opioid-induced constipation. New agents to treat opioid-induced constipation are in clinical trials and may be available in the near future. These agents are peripherally acting opioid antagonists that do not cross the blood-brain barrier. Therefore, they do not negate the opioids' central analgesia but can reverse the peripheral constipating effects.

Dysphoria and delirium may be managed by opioid rotation, reducing the opioid dose by adding an adjunctive agent, or adding a psychoactive agent to treat symptoms (eg, an antipsychotic to treat delirium). Opioids can directly cause mast cell degranulation independently of IgE, resulting in pruritus and urticaria. Opioid rotation and antihistamines can be useful. Myoclonus and seizures indicate neurotoxicity and opioids should be rotated, potentially to opioids lacking active or toxic metabolites that need to be renally cleared. Urinary retention can be treated with a catheter, and opioid rotation can be attempted.

Morley JS et al. Low-dose methadone has an analgesic effect in neuropathic pain: a double-blind randomized controlled crossover trial. *Palliat Med.* 2003;17:576. [PMID: 14594148]

Thwaites D et al. Hydromorphone neuroexcitation. *J Palliat Med.* 2004;7:545. [PMID: 15353098]

Waldhoer M et al. Opioid receptors. *Annu Rev Biochem.* 2004;73:953. [PMID: 15189164]

ADJUNCTIVE MEDICATIONS

Table 3–7 lists the typical dosing for adjunctive medications, including antidepressants, anticonvulsants, sodium channel blockers, NMDA receptor antagonists, α_2-agonists, and corticosteroids.

Antidepressants

A. Pharmacodynamics

Tricyclic antidepressants were the first antidepressants found to be effective for neuropathic pain. The analgesic effect has been separated from the antidepressant effect. Consistent with this observation is that doses effective for analgesia are typically lower than doses required for depression. Amitriptyline is the best studied of the tricyclic antidepressants. It blocks both serotonin and norepinephrine reuptake. There is also evidence that it can act as an NMDA receptor antagonist.

The tricyclic antidepressants vary in their anticholinergic effects. Amitriptyline is the most potent anticholinergic, while nortriptyline and desipramine have the least effect.

Serotonin-norepinephrine reuptake inhibitors (SNRIs) are also effective for neuropathic pain. The US Food and Drug Administration (FDA) has approved duloxetine for diabetic neuropathy. Studies on venlafaxine indicate efficacy for neuropathic pain as well.

Selective serotonin reuptake inhibitors (SSRIs) that block presynaptic reuptake have had varied success in neuropathic pain. In randomized controlled trials, fluoxetine was no better than placebo, but citalopram and paroxetine showed some efficacy.

B. Pharmacokinetics

In general, acute pharmacokinetics are not as important for this class since acute analgesia is not expected. Doses are titrated up over time as tolerated and to efficacy. Typically, analgesia occurs within 1 week once an effective dose has been reached, but it may take weeks to titrate to this level. Tricyclic antidepressants have long half-lives and can be taken once per day, often at bedtime. Duloxetine also has a long half-life and can be taken once per day. Venlafaxine is typically taken 2 to 3 times a day, but once an effective dose is found, there is a long-acting form that can be dosed daily.

C. Prescribing Guidelines

Overall, tricyclic antidepressants and the newer SNRIs appear more effective than SSRIs. There have been no head-to-head comparisons of tricyclic antidepressants with SNRIs. Tricyclic antidepressants are more cost effective, but because they have more side effects, they may be less well tolerated than SNRIs.

Tricyclic antidepressants are prescribed using the adage, "Start low and go slow." Amitriptyline, nortriptyline, and desipramine are started at 10 to 25 mg orally at bedtime and titrated up to about 100 mg/d. Titration occurs every few days to 1 week as tolerated until efficacy or side effects limit dosing. Analgesia ensues within 1 week of attaining an effective dose.

The dose of duloxetine approved by the FDA for treating diabetic neuropathy is 60 mg orally once a day. If side effects are experienced, the dose can be reduced and titrated up as tolerated. Venlafaxine can be started at 75 mg/d orally in two or three divided doses. The dose can be titrated up by 75 mg about every 4 days until efficacy or a side effect is reached. Typically, effective analgesic doses range from 75 to 225 mg/d. There is an extended-release once-a-day formulation that can reduce the burden of pills.

D. Common Side Effects

The anticholinergic properties of tricyclic antidepressants induce dry mouth, constipation, urinary retention, and sedation. Many of the side effects wane over time. The sedating properties can be advantageous when insomnia is present. Tricyclic antidepressants should not be used in patients with narrow-angle glaucoma. At the lower doses that are effective for analgesia, levels need not be monitored and cardiovascular side effects are uncommon. However, especially for geriatric patients and patients with known cardiac problems, orthostatic hypotension and cardiac conduction abnormalities should be monitored. Overdose of tricyclic antidepressants can be lethal, so prescribers must remain vigilant for signs of suicidal ideation.

The SNRIs and the SSRIs are well tolerated overall. Headaches, gastrointestinal upset, and sexual dysfunction are the most common side effects reported.

Anticonvulsants

A. Pharmacodynamics

Anticonvulsants are effective neuropathic pain medications most likely by virtue of their membrane stabilizing

Table 3–7 Prescribing Guidelines for Adjunctive Medications.

Drug	Trade name	Dosing	Maximum daily dose
Tricyclic Antidepressants			
Amitriptyline	Elavil	10–150 mg PO qhs	150 mg
Nortriptyline	Aventyl HCl	10–150 mg PO qhs	150 mg
	Pamelor	10–150 mg PO qhs	150 mg
Desipramine	Norpramin	10–150 mg PO qhs	150 mg
SNRIs			
Duloxetine	Cymbalta	60 mg/d PO	60 mg
Venlafaxine	Effexor	37.5–75 mg PO bid–tid	375 mg
	Effexor XR	37.5–225 mg/d PO	225 mg
Anticonvulsants			
Gabapentin	Neurontin	100–1200 mg PO tid (Also available as 50 mg/mL elixir)	3600 mg
Pregabalin	Lyrica	25–200 mg PO tid	600 mg
Carbamazepine	Carbatrol Equetro Tegretol	200–800 mg PO bid (Also available as 100 mg/5 mL elixir)	1600 mg
Oxcarbazepine	Trileptal	150–600 mg PO bid	2400 mg
		(Also available as 300 mg/5 mL elixir)	
Lamotrigine	Lamictal	25–200 mg PO bid	400 mg
Valproic acid	Depakene	10–15 mg/kg/d	60 mg/kg/d
		(Also available as 250 mg/5 mL elixir)	
Topiramate	Topamax	25–200 mg PO bid	400 mg
Sodium Channel Blockers			
Lidocaine parenterally	Xylocaine	~1 mg/kg/h infusion	Must monitor serum levels; Target 3–5 mg/L
Lidocaine 5% patch	Lidoderm	1–3 patches q12–24h	NA
Mexiletine	Mexitil	150–250 mg PO qd to tid	10 mg/kg/day
NMDA Receptor Antagonists			
Dextromethorphan	Delsym Silphen DM	20–90 mg PO tid (Available as 30 mg/5 mL or 10 mg/5 mL elixir)	120 mg
Ketamine	Ketalar	Start with 0.1 mg/kg/h parenterally	Titrate to effect or side effect
Methadone		See Table 3–4 for dosing (Available as 5, 10, 40 mg tablets or	
	Methadose	1 mg/mL or 10 mg/mL elixir)	
	Dolophine	See Table 3–4 for dosing	

Continued

Table 3–7 Prescribing Guidelines for Adjunctive Medications. (*Continued*)

Drug	Trade name	Dosing	Maximum daily dose
α_2-**Agonists**			
Clonidine	Catapres	0.1–0.3 mg PO tid	2.4 mg
	Catapres–TTS	0.1–0.3 mg/24 h patch every wk	
Corticosteroids			
Dexamethasone	Decadron	2–20 mg/d PO/SC/IV	Variable
		(Also available as 4 mg/mL elixir)	
Prednisone		5–60 mg/d PO	Variable

NA, not applicable; NMDA, *N*-methyl-D-aspartate.

properties. Although not definitively known, gabapentin and pregabalin (recently FDA approved) probably act by binding to a calcium channel subunit that appears to be upregulated in nerves in certain neuropathic pain states. Carbamazepine, oxcarbazepine, and lamotrigine appear to inhibit sodium channels. Valproic acid, in addition to inhibiting sodium channels, may also enhance levels of the inhibitory neurotransmitter GABA. Topiramate, in addition to inhibiting sodium channels, may also enhance GABA activity and inhibit an NMDA receptor.

B. PHARMACOKINETICS

Acute analgesic effects are not expected from this class of drugs. Gabapentin has variable absorption that decreases as the dose increases. For example, 300 mg of oral gabapentin three times daily is about 60% bioavailable; whereas, 1200 mg orally three times daily is only about 33% bioavailable. Pregabalin has an oral bioavailability of about 90%. Of note, both gabapentin and pregabalin are primarily excreted unchanged renally. Therefore, in renal insufficiency, their dosage must be modified. Carbamazepine has many potential drug interactions that must be monitored. The newer anticonvulsants, especially gabapentin and pregabalin, tend to have fewer interactions than the older anticonvulsants.

C. PRESCRIBING GUIDELINES

Gabapentin is commonly considered the first-line anticonvulsant. It is well tolerated, does not require that serum levels be monitored, and has few drug interactions. It is usually started at low dose and titrated to effect. The minimal effective dose is 900 mg/d, but doses have been titrated up to 4500 mg/d. A common mistake is discontinuing gabapentin for lack of efficacy before titrating up to clinically effective levels. The disadvantages of gabapentin include its variable absorption and time needed to titrate to effect.

Pregabalin shares gabapentin's advantages, but also is more potent and has predictable bioavailability. These characteristics make it easier and faster to titrate to effect. In clinical studies, pregabalin was titrated to effect in about 1 week, whereas gabapentin titration required about 4 weeks. The typical dosage for pregabalin starts at 25 to 50 mg orally three times daily and can be titrated up to 200 mg orally three times daily.

Table 3–7 lists the typical dosages for the other anticonvulsants.

D. COMMON SIDE EFFECTS

Headache, dizziness, ataxia, and nausea are common side effects seen among anticonvulsants. Somnolence and dizziness are the most common side effects associated with gabapentin and pregabalin therapy. These effects can usually be controlled by titrating up slowly and by habituation over time.

In addition, carbamazepine can also cause the syndrome of inappropriate antidiuretic hormone (SIADH), hepatitis, and bone marrow suppression, so appropriate laboratory tests should be performed. Oxcarbazepine, a metabolite of carbamazepine, is better tolerated overall than carbamazepine but can still cause hyponatremia. In addition to the above common side effects, valproic acid can induce thrombocytopenia. Topiramate can block carbonic anhydrase lowering serum bicarbonate levels, which should be monitored.

Sodium Channel Blockers

A. PHARMACODYNAMICS

Lidocaine, a nonselective sodium channel blocker, is effective in neuropathic pain syndromes such as diabetic neuropathy and postherpetic neuralgia, and there are case reports of effectiveness in cancer pain. Researchers have identified sodium channels on damaged nerves and dorsal root ganglion cells that fire spontaneously after damage.

Systemic lidocaine can suppress this ectopic, spontaneous firing at a concentration that does not affect normal nerve and cardiac conduction. This suppressive ability may at least partially explain nonselective sodium channel blockers' utility in neuropathic pain. An oral congener of lidocaine, mexiletine, is presumed to operate similarly. Systemic lidocaine has been used as a predictor of response to oral mexiletine but the usefulness of this practice has not been well substantiated.

B. Pharmacokinetics

Lidocaine can be given parenterally; a topical 5% patch is also available. Lidocaine 5% patches do not have significant systemic absorption in usual clinical applications. It is metabolized by the liver and has a half-life of ~100 minutes.

Mexiletine has oral bioavailability approaching 90%. It is metabolized by the liver and has peak serum levels in 2 to 3 hours. Half-life is about 10 to 14 hours.

C. Prescribing Guidelines

Parenteral lidocaine has been used to treat diabetic neuropathy and postherpetic neuralgia in small trials. Based on preliminary observations, parenteral lidocaine may quickly control neuropathic or opioid-refractory cancer pain and provide a window of opportunity for other agents to be titrated to effective levels. The authors challenge opioid-refractory patients with a lidocaine dose of 1 to 2 mg/kg given intravenously over 20 minutes. As soon as 30 minutes after administration, pain relief is measured. If pain is improved, a continuous lidocaine infusion is started at 1 mg/kg/h. Steady-state levels are checked 8 to 9 hours later; the infusion is adjusted based on efficacy and side effects to a level between 2 mg/L and 5 mg/L. The authors do not use cardiac monitoring in a hospice population. Moreover, there is a good safety record in published small trials. However, larger trials are needed to substantiate the efficacy and safety of parenteral lidocaine. Currently, parenteral lidocaine is best used in consultation with a specialist.

Lidocaine patches are applied over the painful area and left in place for 12 hours. Studies have used up to 3 patches left in place for 24 hours with good efficacy and no increase in side effects.

Mexiletine is usually started at 150 mg/d orally for 3 days, titrated to 300 mg/d orally for another 3 days, and then titrated to a dose of 10 mg/kg.

D. Common Side Effects

Systemic lidocaine at therapeutic levels (2 to 5 mg/L) is well tolerated with the most frequent complaints being somnolence and dizziness. However, it does have a relatively narrow therapeutic window. Therefore, serum levels should be monitored. Above 8 mg/L, myoclonus may occur, and at higher levels the risk of seizure (>10 mg/L) and cardiovascular collapse (>25 mg/L) increases. Topical lidocaine patches are well tolerated. In typical usage, clinically significant serum levels are not a concern. Mexiletine can cause gastrointestinal upset in up to 40% of patients, limiting its clinical usefulness.

NMDA Receptor Antagonists

A. Pharmacodynamics

As discussed previously, the NMDA receptor is involved in the spinal process of "wind up" and is believed to be involved in the generation of neuropathic pain and opioid tolerance. Inhibition of the NMDA receptor can have potent analgesic effects. Clinically available NMDA receptor antagonists that have been reasonably studied include methadone, dextromethorphan, and the dissociative anesthetic, ketamine. They all have approximately the same affinity for the NMDA receptor. For best efficacy, it is likely that NMDA receptor antagonists should be used in conjunction with opioids.

B. Pharmacokinetics

As discussed earlier, methadone has a long and variable half-life, requiring slow titration. Dextromethorphan is available orally in short- and long-acting forms. In the short-acting form, it has an onset of action of 15 to 30 minutes. Ketamine is available as a parenteral solution that has also been used orally. There is a significant first-pass effect when taken orally. The liver metabolizes ketamine to norketamine. Norketamine is equipotent with ketamine as an analgesic but only one-third as potent as an anesthetic. Orally, ketamine has an onset of action of 30 minutes.

C. Prescribing Guidelines

In chronic severe pain, when there is time for titration, the authors recommend methadone. It provides both μ receptor agonism and NMDA receptor antagonism. Dosing based on previous opioid levels is shown in Table 3–5.

In crescendo pain where there is no time to titrate medications slowly, ketamine has a kinetic advantage. In palliative care populations, ketamine has been used parenterally at low dose with good effect. Dosing is usually started at 0.1 to 0.2 mg/kg/h parenterally and titrated to effect. At low dose, the risk of psychotomimetic effects is reduced. If they appear, low-dose benzodiazepines are usually able to control the negative effects.

Dextromethorphan has had mixed success in the literature, and its dose has been limited by side effects. Typical dosing in the literature ranges from 20 mg orally three times daily to 90 mg orally three times per day.

D. COMMON SIDE EFFECTS

Methadone shares the opioid side effects already discussed. Dextromethorphan and ketamine can cause dysphoria, hallucinations, somnolence, and dizziness.

α_2-Agonists

A. PHARMACODYNAMICS

Clonidine and dexmedetomidine are α_2-agonists that are effective for both nociceptive and neuropathic pain. Tizanidine is another α_2-agonist used in spasticity but has not been well studied otherwise as an analgesic. They have CNS and peripheral nervous system effects. In the spinal cord, α_2-agonists have effects similar to the opioids but act through a different receptor, thus potentially providing additive effects. Specifically, they alter calcium and potassium conductance. Presynaptically, they decrease neurotransmitter release; and postsynaptically, they hyperpolarize the neuron making it less likely to fire. α_2-agonists also have a sympatholytic effect that may be mediated both spinally and at postganglionic nerve terminals with the net effect of decreasing catecholamine release. This decreased sympathetic outflow may help in certain forms of sympathetically driven neuropathic pain, such as complex regional pain syndromes.

B. PHARMACOKINETICS

Clonidine is available as an oral agent and a transdermal patch. Orally, it is 75 to 100% bioavailable, and the patch is 60% bioavailable. Dexmedetomidine is available as a parenteral solution, but the buccal and oral routes of administration have also been studied.

C. PRESCRIBING GUIDELINES

Dexmedetomidine needs further study to be useful routinely. Clonidine is typically started at 0.1 mg/d orally and titrated to efficacy or intolerable side effects. To limit systemic effects, α_2-agonists are often used intraspinally, but this technique requires specialist assistance and is beyond the scope of this chapter.

D. COMMON SIDE EFFECTS

Clonidine and dexmedetomidine share hypotension and bradycardia as potential side effects. Clonidine tends to cause more dry mouth and somnolence.

Corticosteroids

A. PHARMACODYNAMICS

Corticosteroids are potent anti-inflammatory drugs. They include hydrocortisone, prednisone, methylprednisolone, and dexamethasone. They bind a cytosolic receptor that translocates to the nucleus and alters transcriptional regulation. One subsequent effect is to suppress the action of nuclear factor κ B, which induces many inflammatory cytokines. Corticosteroids are often used at supraphysiologic doses, above what should be needed for receptor-mediated effects. Researchers hypothesize that there may be a direct effect of corticosteroids dissolved in membranes.

Corticosteroids reduce pain in several ways. As stated previously, inflammation sensitizes some nociceptors. Corticosteroids, by reducing inflammation, can reduce pain. Second, neural compression causes pain. By decreasing inflammation and edema, such as peritumoral edema, corticosteroids relieve nerve compression and pain. Finally, studies have shown that corticosteroids can decrease the spontaneous firing of sodium channels in neuromas. This suppression may be an example of a direct membrane effect.

The corticosteroids differ in their mineralocorticoid effect, which affects salt retention. Dexamethasone has the least mineralocorticoid effect, and therefore is often used when patients are hypoalbuminemic with fluid third spacing.

B. PHARMACOKINETICS

Corticosteroids have high oral bioavailability and can also be administered parenterally. Their plasma half-lives are short, but with the exception of hydrocortisone, their duration of action is long, allowing for once a day dosing.

C. PRESCRIBING GUIDELINES

Especially in patients with advanced medical illness potentially facing the end of life, dexamethasone is often the first-line corticosteroid due to its minimal mineralocorticoid effect and its long duration of action that supports once a day dosing. As a pain adjunct, doses range from 4 mg/d to 20 mg/d. Dexamethasone can be given orally, rectally, intravenously, and subcutaneously. Typically, doses are started at high levels to determine whether there is an effect. If there is no clinical benefit in 1 to 2 days, the corticosteroid can simply be discontinued without fear of adrenal suppression. If there is a clinical benefit, the dose can be tapered down to the minimally effective dose. In this population, long-term sequelae are typically not relevant.

In other inflammatory pain syndromes, corticosteroids may have a role, but due to long-term sequelae, this role is usually time-limited.

D. COMMON SIDE EFFECTS

Patients who have been taking the equivalent of 20 mg/d of prednisone for more than 3 weeks should be assumed to have suppression of the hypothalamic-pituitary-adrenal axis. Hyperglycemia and corticosteroid-induced psychosis can occur early after starting corticosteroids.

Longer-term sequelae include osteoporosis, Cushing syndrome, cataracts, peptic ulcer, and myopathy.

Overall Prescribing Recommendations for Adjunctive Medications & Their Combinations

The literature provides little guidance on the optimal use of adjunctive medications and their combinations (see Table 3–7). However, a recent randomized, double-blind, active placebo-controlled, crossover trial of neuropathic pain demonstrated that the combination of morphine and gabapentin provided better analgesia with fewer side effects at lower doses than either agent alone. This study indicated opioids were effective treatment for neuropathic pain but highlighted the fact that combination therapy can be synergistic for analgesia and a reduction in side effects. Further studies are needed to quantitatively assess other adjunctive combinations.

For moderate to severe neuropathic pain, the authors recommend methadone for consideration as a first-line therapy. Its multiple pharmacodynamic properties make it an effective analgesic. It is an opioid with its own adjunctive properties. In addition to efficacy, major advantages of methadone are decreased pill burden, long-lasting effects, and cost effectiveness. Its major disadvantages include its slow titration, complicated opioid conversion calculation, and potential for accumulation due to its long and variable half-life. Prescribers should consider expert consultation until they are knowledgeable in the use of methadone.

Gabapentin and pregabalin are also recommended for consideration as first-line adjunctive medications. The above-cited study provides evidence of its useful combination with opioids. Their major advantages include a good side effect profile, little drug interaction, and no need to monitor serum levels. The major disadvantage of gabapentin is its variable absorption that worsens with increased dosage.

Although it has been poorly studied in the literature, the authors recommend further combinatorial therapy for resistant pain syndromes. Anecdotally, in severe cancer pain syndromes, the authors have effectively combined μ-receptor agonists, NMDA receptor antagonists, neuron-specific calcium-channel blockers, sodium channel blockers, tricyclic antidepressants, and anti-inflammatory drugs for optimal pain control. Clearly, there is a need for more evidence to guide clinical practice. However, in its absence, the principal of combining analgesics that may work through different pathways to produce synergism is rational.

Arnold LM et al. A double-blind, multicenter trial comparing duloxetine with placebo in the treatment of fibromyalgia patients with or without major depressive disorder. *Arthritis Rheum.* 2004;50:2974. [PMID: 15457467]

Devor M et al. Corticosteroids suppress ectopic neural discharge originating in experimental neuromas. *Pain.* 1985;22:127. [PMID: 4047699]

Galer BS et al. The lidocaine patch 5% effectively treats all neuropathic pain qualities: results of a randomized, double-blind, vehicle-controlled, 3-week efficacy study with use of the neuropathic pain scale. *Clin J Pain.* 2002;18:297. [PMID: 12218500]

Gilron I et al. Morphine, gabapentin, or their combination for neuropathic pain. *N Engl J Med.* 2005;352:1324. [PMID: 15800228]

Rosenstock J et al. Pregabalin for the treatment of painful diabetic peripheral neuropathy: a double-blind, placebo-controlled trial. *Pain.* 2004;110:628. [PMID: 15288403]

Schulte H et al. The synergistic effect of combined treatment with systemic ketamine and morphine on experimentally induced windup-like pain in humans. *Anesth Analg.* 2004;98:1574. [PMID: 15155308]

Thomas J et al. Intravenous lidocaine relieves severe pain: results of an inpatient hospice chart review. *J Palliat Med.* 2004;7:660. [PMID: 15588357]

Interventional Procedures for Pain Control

4

Samuel Samuel, MD, Salim Hayek, MD, PhD, & Michael Stanton-Hicks, MB, BS

Interventional nerve blocks remain the mainstay treatment of chronic pain despite advances in pharmacologic and nonpharmacologic modalities. However, multiple factors (including social, emotional, financial, and legal issues) further compound the complexity of chronic pain, necessitating a multidisciplinary approach to its management. Such a discussion is beyond the scope of this chapter, which will primarily focus on interventional nerve blocks for chronic pain conditions and when the primary care physician should refer patients for these procedures. Some aspects of the techniques are described to assist the internist in determining whether a patient might tolerate the procedure. Although the internist is unlikely to be performing these techniques, it is important to understand the goals of the procedures, the potential benefits, and the possible complications.

While diagnostic regional anesthetic procedures have been applied to practically every peripheral and cranial nerve, in the interest of demonstrating that by its interruption either somatosensory, visceromotor, or sudomotor efferents abolish or change the described pain, it is probably the systematic blocking of the axial spine and sympathetic blocks that have the greatest usefulness in clinical diagnosis of chronic pain conditions.

Interventional nerve blocks can be broadly classified into three types: diagnostic blocks, prognostic blocks, and therapeutic blocks. Prognostic blocks are conducted to predict the efficacy of a neurodestructive procedure (to prevent a potentially unnecessary operation). Prognostic blocks also temporarily provide patients the sensations of a more definitive procedure, thereby allowing them to determine whether the resulting numbness might be tolerable to them.

The use of blocks for diagnosis and prognosis depends on an assumption of anatomic consistency. Nerve structures are expected to be found in predictable places and to have predictable connections, but there are important limitations to these assumptions, with most anatomic parameters showing normal variance. There is 50% accuracy in guessing vertebral level for needle placement without fluoroscopy and for this reason most nerve block techniques have no validity unless conducted under flu-

oroscopic guidance. The use of a high-resolution C-arm image intensifier with associated computerized image generation is considered to be essential if the results are to contribute to both diagnosis and definitive therapeutic maneuvers.

Nerve blocks are used for diagnosis and treatment of multiple pain syndromes, including low back pain, headache, abdominal pain, failed back surgery syndrome, post- thoracotomy pain syndrome, postherpetic neuralgia, myofascial pain syndrome, pain secondary to malignancy, compression fractures, complex regional pain syndrome (CRPS) type I and type II, whiplash injuries, pain originating from vascular insufficiency, diabetic neuropathy, and the diagnosis of central pain syndrome.

■ DIAGNOSTIC BLOCKS

SELECTIVE NERVE ROOT SHEATH INJECTION

 ESSENTIAL CRITERIA

- *Useful diagnostically and therapeutically.*
- *Diagnostically, symptomatic nerve roots causing radiculopathic symptoms can be identified and the source of pain for subsequent surgical interventions can be pinpointed.*
- *Therapeutically, nerve root irritation resulting from lateral recess spinal stenosis, disk herniations, or dynamic nerve root irritation from instability or spondylolysis can be treated.*

General Considerations

Chronic back pain, radiculopathies, and their associated disabilities represent a significant health problem. At some time in life, 70 to 85% of all people have back pain, with an annual prevalence ranging from 15 to 45%. Symptoms are most common in middle-aged adults, with back pain equally common in men and women. Back pain is the most frequent reason for activity limitation in persons younger than 45 years of age, the second leading reason for doctor visits and absenteeism from work, and the third common cause for surgical interventions.

The primary site of back pain is the lower back in 85% of back pain sufferers. Annually, about 2% of the work force has back injuries covered by the Bureau of Workers Compensation. The total annual direct cost of treating this subgroup of patients rose from $4.6 billion in 1977 to $11.4 billion in 1994. From 1979 to 1990, rates of back surgery in the United States increased dramatically; the increase in surgical rates was especially marked for spinal fusions.

Patient Selection

Back pain associated with radiculopathy is the main indication for selective nerve sheath injection, since the contribution of root inflammation to pain may not be certain or the level of the lesion may be unclear.

Imaging

Computed tomography (CT) or magnetic resonance imaging (MRI) and electrophysiologic evaluation by electromyography may be inconsistent or may be inconclusive. Abnormal imaging findings in asymptomatic persons (prevalence as high as 40%) demonstrates the inability of abnormal anatomy to indicate a pain source. A further cause of confusion is the presence of disease at multiple levels, because the origin of pain may be any one site or a combination of sites. Finally, evaluation is especially difficult after laminectomy because imaging is impeded by the presence of hardware or the presence of scar tissue in the epidural space.

Duration of Benefit

In diagnostic blocks, the duration of the block essentially reflects the duration of action of the local anesthetic used (short, intermediate, or long-acting). Therapeutic benefit from the block is variable, with multiple confounding variables involved; however, the average success rate after 12 months of follow-up is approximately 75–80% in patients with disk abnormality.

Technique

When used therapeutically, a mixture of local anesthetic and corticosteroid is used. Corticosteroids decrease pain due to inflammation and sensitization of nerve fibers through their anti-inflammatory action and the release of phospholipase A_2 inhibitor. Corticosteroids also block

nociceptive input, block the transmission in C fibers but not in Aβ fibers and inhibit the formation of adhesion and fibrosis.

Complications

The following are possible complications due to selective nerve root sheath injection:

1. Damage to the nerve root.
2. Intrathecal injection.
3. Intravascular injection (in case of corticosteroid injection, anterior spinal artery syndrome may result from intravascular injection and embolization of the artery of Adamkiewicz).
4. Bleeding.
5. Pneumothorax.

Stanton-Hicks M. Nerve blocks in chronic pain therapy—are there any indications left? *Acta Anaesthesiol Scand.* 2001;45:1100. [PMID: 11683660]

DIFFERENTIAL EPIDURAL BLOCK

 ESSENTIAL CRITERIA

- *Valuable in diagnosing chronic abdominal pain, chronic pelvic pain, and thoracic pain of unknown origin.*

General Considerations

When the location of pain makes diagnosis difficult (as in abdominal pain), differential nerve blocks can be valuable in providing the information necessary to verify a certain diagnosis and delineate a treatment plan. The test relies on the selective differential blockade of one structure, without blocking others, using specific concentration of local anesthetic and saline. The three classes of nerve fibers are as follows:

1. A fibers (which are further subdivided into Aa [motor function and proprioception], Ab [touch and pressure], Ag [muscle spindle tone], and Ad [pain and temperature sensation]).
2. B fibers (thin myelinated preganglionic autonomic nerves).
3. C fibers (unmyelinated fibers mediating pain and temperature impulses).

Technique

The test can be carried out using epidural, spinal anesthesia, or peripheral nerve plexus blocks and interpreted in an antegrade or retrograde fashion. In the antegrade approach, the clinician observes the gradual onset of analgesia with increasing doses of local anesthetics injected, whereas in the retrograde approach, after analgesia is achieved with a large bolus, the clinician observes the relationship between the block wearing off and the gradual return of pain. For instance, in cases of visceral abdominal pain, pain is abolished first in the antegrade approach and its relief outlasts the duration of local anesthesia in the retrograde approach. Musculoskeletal pain, on the other hand, returns as soon as dermatomal anesthesia is resolved.

Two shortcomings of this technique are that (1) the differential nerve blocks can be very time consuming and (2) occasionally, no clear-cut end points are obtained, with overlap of results making interpretation of the test difficult.

Complications

The following are possible complications of a differential epidural block:

1. Postdural puncture headache with an incidence ranging from 1 to 7% after neuraxial blocks.
2. Bleeding (including epidural hematoma).
3. Infection (abscess formation, meningitis).
4. Inadvertent intrathecal injection with resultant spinal anesthesia.
5. Local anesthetic toxicity.

ZYGAPOPHYSEAL JOINT INJECTION (FACET JOINT INJECTION)

1. Lumbar Facet Syndrome

 ESSENTIAL CRITERIA

Indications

- *Low back pain with radiation to the hip and buttock.*
- *Cramping lower extremity pain (usually not lower than the knee).*
- *Low back stiffness (especially in the morning) and pain that is commonly aggravated by prolonged sitting or standing.*
- *Patients with axial low back pain who have not responded to conservative therapy (nonsteroidal anti-inflammatory drugs, rest, and physical therapy).*

- *Absence of radiologic evidence of disk herniation, lumbar stenosis, or foraminal stenosis with resultant nerve root impingement.*

Signs

- *Paraspinal tenderness, worse over the affected joint.*
- *Positive facet loading (hyperextension, rotation, and side bending).*
- *Absence of signs of nerve root irritation as well as hip, buttock, and back pain on straight leg rising.*

General Considerations

The zygapophyseal (facet) joints are paired diarthrodial joints between the posterior elements of the adjacent vertebrae that can contribute drastically to the problem of low back pain. The percentage of all patients with low back pain who have a significant proportion of their pain attributable to the facet joint varies from 15 to 50% in published series.

Injection of a small amount of local anesthetic into the facet joint (0.5 mL, 0.75% bupivacaine) or interruption of the median branch nerves to the facet joints are standardized techniques for the diagnosis of zygapophyseal joint-symptoms. Because each joint is innervated by at least two medial branches, two adjacent levels should always be blocked.

Patient Selection

Table 4–1 shows a scoring system that was developed to determine which patients will benefit from facet joint injection. Patients with a score of 60 points or higher had 100% prolonged response from a facet joint injection. A score of 40 points or higher predicted 78% prolonged response.

Table 4–1. Scorecard for Probability of Pain Relief with Facet Joint Injection.

Back pain associated with groin or thigh pain	+30 points
Reproduction of pain with extension-rotation	+30 points
Well-localized paraspinal tenderness	+20 points
Significant radiographic changes	+20 points
Pain below the knee	−10 points

Helbig T, Lee CK. The lumbar facet syndrome. *Spine.* 1988;13:61.

Duration of Benefit

The duration of pain relief in diagnostic blocks probably reflects the duration of the local anesthetic used. Patients with consistent pain relief with such a block but of short duration may benefit from radiofrequency ablation of the median branch block with reported duration of up to 1 year. Another alternative to radiofrequency lesioning is pulsed radiofrequency, with reported duration of 4 months and decreased incidence of complications compared with radiofrequency ablation.

Technique

Unless there are localizing signs, the L4–5, L5–S1 are the most affected joints. The block is performed under fluoroscopy with the patient in the prone position and a pillow placed under the lower abdomen. After the back is prepared and draped, the facet joint or the junction of the transverse process with the facet joint (in case of median branch block) is identified. Using a 22-gauge spinal needle, the needle is introduced and a mixture of 0.5 mL of 0.75% bupivacaine and 20 mg of triamcinolone is injected into each of the designated joint or median branch.

Complications

Although rare, complications may include infection, transient radicular pain, subarachnoid injection, backache, muscle spasm, allergic reaction, joint rupture and necrosis in case of intra-articular injection, and neuritis in the case of radiofrequency ablation.

Dreyfuss PH et al. Lumbar zygapophysial (facet) joint injections. *Spine J.* 2003;3:50S. [PMID: 14589218]

Saal JS. General principles of diagnostic testing as related to painful lumbar spine disorders: a critical appraisal of current diagnostic techniques. *Spine.* 2002;27:2538. [PMID: 12435989]

2. Cervical Facet Syndrome

ESSENTIAL CRITERIA

- *Neck pain and stiffness.*
- *Shoulder, suprascapular, scapular, and upper arm pain.*
- *Headaches, mostly occipital.*
- *Decreased range of motion of the neck.*
- *Pain on lateral flexion on the affected side.*
- *Decreased discomfort with forward flexion.*
- *Tenderness over the affected joints.*

General Considerations

Cervical facet joint has been shown to be the most commonly involved structure following neck injury, especially in whiplash injury. This injury represents 1 of the major causes of neck pain with an estimated incidence of 4 per 1000 population. An estimated 42% of whiplash injuries become chronic, with pain persisting in about 10% of the cases; it may also result from twisted neck and poor sleep postures.

Chronic neck pain represents about 30% of the chronic pain conditions, with a staggering impact on US society; an estimated annual cost of about $90 billion is split between treatment and work losses. This economic impact reflects the importance of recognizing and promptly treating conditions that lead to chronic neck pain.

Cervical facet joints and its innervations are slightly different than the lumbar facet joints. The atlanto-occipital (C0–1) and the atlantoaxial (C1–2) are innervated by C1 and C2 ventral rami and not the dorsal primary ramus; hence, the intra-articular injection is the only way to block these joints. Cervical facet joints from C3–T1 are supplied by medial branches of the dorsal rami above and at the same level as the joint, so either intra-articular or median branch block could be used for diagnostic or therapeutic purposes. Table 4–2 describes the distribution of pain of cervical facet joint origin.

Patient Selection

Patients with cervicogenic headaches may benefit from facet joint medial branch block since the third occipital nerve (dorsal ramus C3) has a close anatomic proximity to and innervates the C2–3 zygapophyseal joint. This joint and the third occipital nerve appear most vulnerable to trauma from acceleration-deceleration ("whiplash")

Table 4–2. Distribution of Pain of Cervical Facet Joint Origin.

Joint	Distribution
C2–3	Occiput and cervical
C3–4	Neck
C4–5	Lateral aspect of the nape of the neck and shoulder
C5–6	Arm
C6–7	Shoulder or upper dorsum as far down as the scapula

Adapted from Benzon et al: *Essentials of Pain Medicine and Regional Anesthesia.* Elsevier, 1999.

injuries of the neck. Pain from the C2–C3 zygapophyseal joint is referred to the occipital region but is also referred to the frontotemporal and periorbital regions.

Duration of Benefit

Despite the wide variability in the duration of pain relief with cervical facet injection, some reports cite pain relief and improved range of motion for up to 12 months. In conjunction with the facet injection, other adjuvant treatment includes traction, local heat, manipulation with correction of facet subluxation, and medical treatment with nonsteroidal anti-inflammatory drugs (NSAIDs).

Technique

With the patient lying prone (some clinicians advocate a lateral or even a supine position with easier accessibility to the airway), the posterior neck is prepared and draped. Under fluoroscopic guidance, a 22-gauge spinal needle is inserted at the desired levels to be blocked; the importance of slow advancement of the needle with serial anteroposterior and lateral fluoroscopic imaging for correct needle placement and direction must be emphasized. After negative aspiration (close proximity of the vertebral artery), 0.5 mL of 0.75% bupivacaine and 20 mg of triamcinolone is injected.

Complications

In addition to the complications of the lumbar facet blocks, complications related to the cervical facet injection include epidural and intrathecal injection progressing to total spinal anesthesia, intravascular injection, and seizures.

Bogduk N et al. Biomechanics of the cervical spine Part 3: minor injuries. *Clin Biomech (Bristol, Avon).* 2001;16:267. [PMID: 11358613]

Freeman MD et al. A review and methodologic critique of the literature refuting whiplash syndrome. *Spine.* 1999;24:86. [PMID: 9921598]

Kwan O et al. A review and methodologic critique of the literature supporting 'chronic whiplash injury': part I–research articles. *Med Sci Monit.* 2003;9:RA203. [PMID: 12942047]

Peloso P et al; Cervical Overview Group. Medicinal and injection therapies for mechanical neck disorders. *Cochrane Database System Rev.* 2005;(2):CD000319. [PMID: 15846603]

Siegmund GP et al. Mechanical evidence of cervical facet capsule injury during whiplash: a cadaveric study using combined shear, compression, and extension loading. *Spine.* 2001;26:2095. [PMID: 11698885]

DISCOGRAPHY

 ESSENTIAL CRITERIA

- *Axial back pain that is the predominant feature of discogenic pain in the lower back.*
- *Gluteal extension is not uncommon; however, there is an absence of radicular symptoms, with no weakness affecting the lower extremity and the pain rarely follows dermatomal or myotomal patterns.*
- *The pain is worse with positions that increase the intradiscal pressure, including standing for a long time, prolonged sitting due to back flexion, and intolerance to cumulative axial loading.*

General Considerations

Discography can be considered as a purely diagnostic modality for the diagnosis of back pain. Discography is only indicated to rule out or to rule in discogenic pain with concordant or nonconcordant pain in the suspected degenerated disk.

For diagnostic purposes, MRI is sensitive in detecting disk abnormalities, yet MRI is capable of detecting degenerated, desiccated disks. Therefore, discography is considered the gold standard and an invaluable adjunct for the diagnosis of discogenic pain.

Patient Selection

Indications for discography include, but are not limited to, the following:

1. Further evaluation of demonstrably abnormal disks to help assess the extent of the abnormality or correlation of the abnormality with the clinical symptoms. Such symptoms may include recurrent pain from a previously operated disk and lateral disk herniation.
2. Patients with persistent, severe symptoms in whom other diagnostic tests have failed to reveal clear confirmation of a suspected disk as the source of pain.
3. Assessment of patients who have not responded to surgical intervention to determine whether there is painful pseudoarthrosis or a symptomatic disk in a posteriorly fused segment and to help evaluate possible recurrent disk herniation.
4. Assessment of disks before fusion to determine whether the disks within the proposed fusion segment are symptomatic and to determine whether disks adjacent to this segment are normal.

While the specificity may range from 20 to 90% depending on patient selection, discography results should be carefully validated and the procedure should be performed by an experienced clinician. Most clinicians will perform discography on two consecutive disks.

Technique

After placing the patient in a prone position, a posterolateral extraspinal approach with fluoroscopic guidance to the desired disks is used. The skin is prepared and draped. The C-arm is then obliquely rotated until the facet joint "shadow" projects to about the middle of the vertebral body. A 22- or 25-gauge 6-inch needle with introducer is inserted, until it reaches the inner third of the disk. Upon confirmation of needle position using a true anteroposterior and lateral pictures, 0.5–1.5 mL of water-soluble radio-opaque contrast material is injected. The patient's response, the distribution of the dye, resistance, and volume injected are all noted and recorded.

A normal disk accommodates between 0.5 mL and 1.5 mL of contrast material; in the case of a fissured disk, there will be a path of least resistance with an increase in the capacitance of the disk and apparent abnormal spread of the contrast. However, these findings should be accompanied by concordant pain to label this study as a positive provocative discography.

Complications

Discitis represents one of the most devastating complications of discography. Thus, discography requires a surgically sterile environment with extreme caution when entering the disk, and despite lack of data to support the use of prophylactic antibiotics, most clinicians do provide a dose of antibiotics prior to the procedure.

Nausea, convulsions, and severe back pain during the procedure may occur. Meningitis, spinal headache, subdural or epidural abscess, intrathecal hemorrhage, arachnoiditis, nerve root injury, paravertebral muscle pain and contusions, postprocedural pain exacerbation, vasovagal reactions, allergic reactions, and damage to the disk including but not limited to herniation are other possible complications.

Anderson MW. Lumbar discography: an update. *Semin Roentgenol.* 2004;39:52. [PMID: 14976837]

Olmarker K et al. Selective inhibition of tumor necrosis factor-alpha prevents nucleus pulposus-induced thrombus formation, intraneural edema, and reduction of nerve conduction velocity: possible implications for future pharmacologic treatment strategies of sciatica. *Spine.* 2001;26:863. [PMID: 11317106]

Willems PC et al. Lumbar discography: should we use prophylactic antibiotics? A study of 435 consecutive discograms and a systematic review of the literature. *J Spinal Disord Tech.* 2004;17:243. [PMID: 15167324]

SELECTIVE SYMPATHETIC BLOCKS

Selective sympathetic blockade interrupts the efferent sympathetic fibers that are sometimes pathologically involved in a number of medical conditions, including CRPS, neuropathic pain (mononeuropathy, plexopathy), cranial neuralgia, hyperhidrosis, and many other conditions. Surgical or chemical sympathectomy is used to manage a variety of syndromes, yet relief following sympathetic blockade is not consistent, and relapses are common.

1. Cervicothoracic Ganglion Blockade (Stellate Ganglion Block)

 ESSENTIAL CRITERIA

- *CRPS or vascular insufficiency of the upper extremity.*
- *Pain of herpes zoster.*
- *Postherpetic neuralgia.*
- *Congenital prolonged QT syndrome (left cervicothoracic ganglion blockade).*
- *Migraines, tension, and cluster headaches.*
- *Cerebral angiospasm and cerebral thrombosis.*

General Considerations

The cervical sympathetic trunk contains three ganglia: the superior, middle, and inferior cervical ganglia. In 80% of the population, the lowest cervical ganglia is fused with the upper thoracic ganglion to form the cervicothoracic ganglion. The cervicothoracic ganglion lies on or just lateral to the longus colli muscle between the base of the seventh cervical transverse process and the neck of the first rib. The cervicothoracic ganglion receives preganglionic fibers from the lateral gray column of the spinal cord. The preganglionic fibers for the head and neck emerge from the upper five thoracic spinal nerves, ascending in the sympathetic trunk to synapse in the cervical ganglion. The preganglionic fibers supplying the upper extremity originate from the upper thoracic segment between T2–T6, which in turn synapses in the cervicothoracic ganglion. The paradox of accepting Horner syndrome as a gold standard for sympatholysis of the upper extremity is still widely accepted; yet, the presence of Horner syndrome does not indicate complete sympatholysis of the upper extremity. Of the postganglionic sympathetic supply to the upper extremity, 30% passes directly out of the thoracic outlet from the T2–T8 fibers to the brachial plexus and thus escapes the stellate ganglion (fused C7–T1 ganglia).

Patient Selection

The efficacy of stellate ganglion block in conditions such as phantom limb pain, postherpetic neuralgia, and Meniere disease have yielded questionable results.

Duration of Benefit

The duration of relief with diagnostic blocks is variable; however, there is evidence that repeated blocks may overall decrease the level of sympathetically mediated pain. Radiofrequency ablation of the stellate ganglion is generally avoided to prevent a permanent Horner syndrome.

Technique

This block can be performed either blind or by using fluoroscopy. The advantages of fluoroscopy include visualization of the C7 transverse process (which if targeted carries a higher incidence of pneumothorax and intra-arterial injection) and visualization of the local anesthetic spread. Intravenous access is mandatory in this procedure, which may be associated with rare but potentially critical, emergent complications. The patient is placed supine with a small roll or pillow between the shoulder blades to improve extension of the neck. The patient is asked to open his or her mouth in order to relax the neck muscles. After palpation of the cricoid cartilage to determine the level of the C6 transverse process, the carotid pulse is felt and the sheath is then displaced laterally. A 22-gauge, short beveled 5-cm needle is then advanced between the sternocleidomastoid muscle and the trachea until bone is encountered (C6 tubercle); the needle is withdrawn 3 to 5 mm to avoid injecting the substance into the longus coli muscle. A test dose of 0.5 to 1.0 mL is injected to exclude intravascular injection, since as little as 0.5 mL of local anesthetic could result in seizure and loss of consciousness. This is followed by injection of 8 to 12 mL of local anesthetic (local anesthetic concentration can be reduced because autonomic C-fibers are small with no myelin).

Complications

Potential complications include the following:

1. Horner syndrome, which includes ptosis, myosis, and enophthalmos as well as nasal congestion.
2. Seizures and loss of consciousness.
3. Hoarseness, foreign body sensation in the throat resulting from recurrent laryngeal nerve block.
4. Difficulty breathing secondary to phrenic nerve block.
5. Air embolism.
6. Pneumothorax.
7. Epidural, subarachnoid injection.
8. Infection and hematoma formation.

Birklein F. Complex regional pain syndrome. *J Neurol.* 2005;252:131. [PMID: 15729516]

Marples IL, Atkin RE. Stellate ganglion block. *Pain Rev.* 2001;8:3–11.

Pather N et al. The anatomical rationale for an upper limb sympathetic blockade: preliminary report. *Surg Radiol Anat.* 2004;26:178. [PMID: 14730395]

Schurmann M et al. Assessment of peripheral sympathetic nervous system function for diagnosing early post-traumatic complex regional pain syndrome type 1. *Pain.* 1999;80:149. [PMID: 10204727]

2. Lumbar Sympathetic Block

 ESSENTIAL CRITERIA

- *Sympathetically mediated pain of the lower extremity; this type of block could serve as a diagnostic, prognostic as well as therapeutic intervention in such a condition.*
- *Improvement of peripheral circulation in patients with peripheral vascular diseases.*
- *Postherpetic neuralgia, phantom limb pain, and intractable back pain.*

General Considerations

The psoas major muscle and fascia separate the sympathetic chain and ganglia from the somatic nerves at the L2 to the L5 levels; the lumbar sympathetic chain contain both preganglionic and postganglionic fibers to the pelvis and the lower extremities. The sympathetic chain and ganglia are situated close to the anterolateral side of the vertebral bodies at the lumbar level; the best site for the needle tip placement would be the lower one-third of the L2 or the upper third of the L3 body. The rami communicantes course in a fibrous tunnel around the vertebral body; thus, caution is necessary when using a paramedian approach for neurolytic sympathectomy because the neurolytic agent could backtrack and cause ipsisegmental somatic painful neuritis.

Technique

Fluoroscopy is used for optimum needle placement. Accurate diffusion of the local anesthetic is based on the optimal spread of the contrast material. After temperature probes are attached to the feet of the patient to monitor skin temperature, the skin on the patient's back is prepared and draped. The skin is then infiltrated with local anesthetic 7 to 10 cm lateral to the spinous process of L3. A 22-gauge, 6- to 8-inch needle is directed toward the upper or middle third of the L3; the correct positioning of the needle anterior to the psoas fascia is verified using a loss-of-resistance technique. Correct placement of the needle is identified by injecting nonionic contrast showing a linear spread along the anterolateral aspect of the vertebral body. The contrast material is followed by injecting 15 to 20 mL of local anesthetic (may use bupivacaine 0.375%) while monitoring the increase in the lower extremity temperature.

When performing a neurolytic block, a solution of phenol 6% in Conray-420 dye (to add visibility while injecting the neurolytic agent) is used. The injection is performed while the C-arm is in the lateral position to detect any retrograde spread of the dye with resultant somatic neuritis.

Complications

Possible complications associated with lumbar sympathetic block include the following:

1. Bleeding secondary to perforation of the lumbar vessels or the aorta.
2. Orthostatic hypotension.
3. Perforation of abdominal viscera.
4. Subarachnoid or epidural injection.
5. Backache and muscle spasm.
6. Nerve root injury.
7. Hematuria.

3. Celiac Plexus Block

 ESSENTIAL CRITERIA

- *Malignant and nonmalignant pain originating from abdominal organs supplied by the celiac plexus. Although celiac plexus block for nonmalignant abdominal pain has been described, its role as a proven therapy for benign abdominal pain has never been established and may not represent the most effective modality for the treatment of such conditions.*
- *Chronic pancreatitis.*

General Considerations

The celiac plexus is located retroperitoneally in the upper abdomen at the level of T12–L1 vertebrae. This plexus innervates most of the abdominal viscera, including the stomach, liver, biliary system, pancreas, spleen, kidneys, adrenals, and small and large bowel through the splenic flexure. The celiac plexus receives preganglionic sympathetic contribution from the greater (T5–T10 spinal roots), lesser (T10–T11), and least splanchnic (T11–T12) nerves, which relay in the celiac ganglia after running in the posterior mediastinum and traversing the crura of the diaphragm; postganglionic fibers run along the course of blood vessels to innervate the abdominal viscera. The ganglia receive parasympathetic contribution from the vagus nerve. The celiac ganglia are formed by the right and left splanchnic nerves with a network of interconnecting fibers and a great anatomic variability.

Patient Selection

Celiac plexus block has proved both efficient and safe for the treatment of inoperable pancreatic cancer, with patients experiencing sustained pain relief for up to 24 weeks following neurolytic blocks; patients also required fewer medications with resultant decreased side effects related to the medications. This effect extended to other intra-abdominal malignancies of the upper abdomen. Some of the factors that may affect the efficacy of the block include the anatomic site of the tumor, with cancer head of pancreas showing more favorable responses compared with cancer body or tail. As a rule of thumb, celiac plexus block should be implemented early to maximize the benefits to the patient and to avoid technical difficulties related to the late spread of the tumor. The efficacy of celiac plexus block for chronic pancreatitis pain has been less established with studies yielding different results. Patients over 45 years of age and those who had never undergone pancreatic surgery were more likely to experience pain relief.

Technique

Multiple techniques have been described for the celiac plexus block, including the classic retrocrural approach, the transaortic approach, and the anterior approach.

Complications

Following are potential complications of celiac plexus block injections:

1. Orthostatic hypotension.
2. Backache.
3. Diarrhea.
4. Bleeding, aortic dissection, and rupture.

5. Infection.
6. Paraplegia (spasm of the segmental arteries).
7. See Neurolytic nerve blocks later in chapter.

Cunha JE et al. Surgical and interventional treatment of chronic pancreatitis. *Pancreatology.* 2004;4:540. [PMID: 15486450]

Gress F et al. Endoscopic ultrasound-guided celiac plexus block for managing abdominal pain associated with chronic pancreatitis: a prospective single center experience. *Am J Gastroenterol.* 2001;96:409. [PMID: 11232683]

4. Superior Hypogastric Plexus Block

 ESSENTIAL CRITERIA

- *Malignant and nonmalignant pelvic pain.*
- *Cancer pain syndromes that could be amenable to superior hypogastric block include cervical, proximal vaginal, uterine, ovarian, testicular, prostatic, and rectal cancers.*

General Considerations

The superior hypogastric plexus mediates most of the nociceptive afferents from the pelvic organs. It receives preganglionic sympathetic fibers from the aortic plexus and the L2, L3 sympathetic nerves; it also receives preganglionic parasympathetic fibers from S2 and S3. The superior hypogastric plexus is continuous with the intermesenteric plexus and is located retroperitoneally, inferior to the origin of the inferior mesenteric artery. It lies anterior to the lower part of the abdominal aorta, its bifurcation, and the middle sacral vessels; it is located anterior to the L5–S1 vertebrae.

Technique

Despite the paucity of data on the long-term efficacy of the superior hypogastric block, its use as a diagnostic block for chronic nonmalignant pelvic pain syndrome is well established. Conceptually patterned after celiac plexus block, hypogastric plexus block can be used to delineate the source of pain in such conditions as endometriosis, adhesions, interstitial cystitis, and irritable bowel disease. In malignant pelvic pain, sympathetic blocks should be intended as adjuvant techniques to reduce analgesic consumption and not as a panacea, given that multiple pain mechanisms are often involved because progression of disease is able to change the underlying pain mechanisms. Patients who respond favorably to diagnostic blocks have a higher success rate with neurolytic blocks.

Complications

Due to the proximity of the iliac vessels, intravascular injection and vascular injury are possible complications. Other potential complications include epidural, subarachnoid, and intraperitoneal injection as well as discitis with the transdiscal approach.

de Oliveira R et al. The effects of early or late neurolytic sympathetic plexus block on the management of abdominal or pelvic cancer pain. *Pain.* 2004;110:400. [PMID: 15275792]

Erdine S et al. Transdiscal approach for hypogastric plexus block. *Reg Anesth Pain Med.* 2003;28:304. [PMID: 12945023]

Mercadante S et al. Pain mechanisms involved and outcome in advanced cancer patients with possible indications for celiac plexus block and superior hypogastric plexus block. *Tumori.* 2002;88:243. [PMID: 12195764]

5. Ganglion Impar Block

 ESSENTIAL CRITERIA

- *Sympathetically mediated pain as well as visceral pain in the perineum resulting from pelvic malignancy.*
- *Perineal hyperhidrosis.*

General Considerations

Ganglion impar is a single retroperitoneal structure that represents the most caudad ganglia of the sympathetic chain. It is also known as the ganglion of Walther. The location of the ganglion is typically midline, anterior to the sacrococcygeal junction, where it represents the confluence of the two sympathetic chains on each side to form a single structure in the midline. However, the exact location of the ganglion is variable.

Patient Selection

Most of the long-term efficacy data are reported with malignant perineal pain, with reported efficacy of complete relief in 50% of the patients and 60 to 90% pain relief in the remaining 50% of patients in one series. Cryoablation and neurolysis as a means for long-term relief of cancer-related pain should be considered in the armamentarium of pain procedures as a useful adjunct to oral pharmacologic therapy.

Technique

With the patient in a prone position, the area is pre-pared and draped. After making a skin weal, a 20-gauge 1.5-inch needle is inserted through the sacrococcygeal ligament and advanced until the tip is just posterior to the rectum. For diagnostic purposes, 5 to 8 mL of local anesthetic (1% lidocaine or 0.375% bupivacaine) is injected. For neurolysis, 4 to 8 mL of 10% phenol is used.

Complications

This is a relatively safe block; however, potential complications include rectal perforation, infection, and bleeding.

Han KR et al. Effects of neurolysis of the ganglion impar on the hyperhidrosis in the buttock and perineum. *J Korean Pain Res Soc.* 2001;11:114.

Oh CS et al. Clinical implications of topographic anatomy on the ganglion impar. *Anesthesiology.* 2004;101:249. [PMID: 15220800]

■ THERAPEUTIC BLOCKS

EPIDURAL CORTICOSTEROID INJECTION

 ESSENTIAL CRITERIA

- *Symptoms of nerve root irritation, including sciatica.*
- *Patients with herniated disks causing clinically significant nerve root compression or irritation.*
- *Degenerative spinal stenosis.*
- *Tumors infiltrating nerve roots causing radiculopathic pain.*
- *Postural back pain with radiculopathy.*
- *Postherpetic neuralgia.*
- *Discogenic back pain as a temporizing measure until definitive treatment is undertaken.*
- *Acute vertebral compression fractures.*

General Considerations

Epidural corticosteroid injection is intended to deliver the medications in the vicinity of the inflamed nerve root; the therapeutic effects of epidural corticosteroids are attributed to an inhibition of synthesis or release of proinflammatory substances. Corticosteroids block phospholipase A_2, which inhibits the conversion of phospholipids to arachidonic acid. NSAIDs work by a different mechanism, inhibiting the cyclooxygenase pathway. Failure of NSAIDs to produce pain relief, therefore, does not preclude the use of corticosteroids. Local infiltration of betamethasone at a nerve root compression model showed significant decrease in the expression of substance P, which proposes a possible direct effect of corticosteroids on pain mediators as well. Epidural installation of corticosteroids is not hampered by the decrease in local blood flow, which is frequently seen with compressive lesions. This can explain the decreased efficacy of orally administered corticosteroids, since the effectiveness is presumed proportional to the local concentration of the corticosteroids.

Despite the widespread use and acceptance of epidural corticosteroid injection, it remains controversial, especially outside the United States. The question about whether there are long-term benefits for patients remains unanswered.

When epidural corticosteroid injections were given on an outpatient basis to persons with low back pain and sciatica, repeated injections improved the success rate and provided a safe, cost-effective means of treatment without the necessity of hospital admission. Most patients received a series of three epidural corticosteroid injections with progressive improvement after the second and third injection, which is a common pattern of practice in many pain management centers. The reported success rates varied greatly ranging anywhere from 18 to 90%. Selective nerve root injections of corticosteroids were significantly more effective than those of bupivacaine alone. Caudal epidural corticosteroid injections using triamcinolone was superior to placebo, with reported better pain control and mobility at 4 weeks.

Patient Selection

The choice of the patient and the technique used is pivotal when epidural corticosteroid injection is considered. Patients who report superior pain relief include those with a higher educational background, a primary diagnosis of radiculopathy, and pain duration of less than 6 months. Those patients involved in litigations, who were unemployed, had constant back pain, and were symptomatic for 6 to 24 months historically had higher failure rates.

Technique

The choice of the technique should be symptom oriented. Patients with unilateral radicular symptoms are good candidates for transforaminal epidural corticosteroid injections, whereas the interlaminar or caudal approach is more appropriate for patients with axial back pain resulting from degenerative spinal stenosis or for patients with bilateral radicular symptoms.

The transforaminal approach is showing very encouraging results, with long-term success rates of 71 to 84%. The advantages of this approach include decreased risk of dural puncture and delivery of the medications in the anterior epidural space very close to the irritated nerve root. Transforaminal approach is particularly beneficial in large disk herniation, foraminal stenosis, and lateral disk herniations.

Different approaches to the epidural space have been described. Traditionally, two techniques have been used: the interlaminar and the caudal approaches. The transforaminal approach as mentioned above is a novel approach that has proved effective in the hands of experienced clinicians.

Regardless of the technique used, the use of fluoroscopy seems to play a crucial role as far as corticosteroid delivery and minimizing risks. Epidural corticosteroid injections have been demonstrated to be very safe, although inhibition of the hypothalamic-pituitary axis is possible. It is generally considered safe to repeat the injections. In a national survey, the average number of epidural corticosteroid injections a single patient received was 5 to 7 per year; this survey included both academic as well as private practice pain centers.

Complications

Central neuraxial injections generally can result in the following:

1. Infection and abscess formation.
2. Bleeding, including epidural hematoma.
3. Backache, lightheadedness, diaphoresis, and vasovagal reaction.
4. Cardiovascular collapse.
5. Neurologic complications include aseptic meningitis, paraplegia, quadriplegia, and arachnoiditis.
6. Postdural puncture headache can result from dural encroachment; this particular complication is more common with interlaminar approach and less likely with caudal and transforaminal approaches. The incidence of postdural puncture headache < 1%.
7. Transforaminal epidural corticosteroid injection may result in intravascular injection into the artery of Adamkiewicz with subsequent anterior spinal artery syndrome and paraplegia.
8. Systemic complications related to corticosteroid and local anesthetic injection, which is mentioned later in this chapter.

NEUROLYTIC NERVE BLOCKS

 ESSENTIAL CRITERIA

- *Best method for treating pain that is localized and of somatic or visceral origin.*
- *Candidates should have limited life expectancy.*

General Considerations

Visceral cancer pain can be very difficult to treat; neurolytic sympathetic blocks can be effective. In one study, despite optimized systemic analgesic therapy (SAT), patients with unresectable pancreatic cancer treated with SAT only did not have as effective pain control as a comparable group that received neurolytic celiac plexus block.

Patient Selection

Because of possible side effects that can adversely alter the quality of life, candidates for neurolysis should have limited life expectancy.

Technique

Solutions used for neurolytic block include phenol or ethyl alcohol. Phenol, in a concentration of 5 to 6%, has the advantage of being painless on injection, as well as the fact that it can be mixed with contrast material.

Ethyl alcohol is usually used in an undiluted form (95% and above). Alcohol injection may be painful secondary to irritation of the perineurium; therefore, some clinicians inject local anesthetic prior to the neurolytic block.

Complications

The most ominous complication related to alcohol neurolytic blocks includes alcohol-induced neuritis, which can occur during sympathetic blocks secondary to retrograde spread of the neurolytic agent injuring the somatic nerves. Therefore, neurolytic blocks should only be performed by an experienced interventional pain specialist. Pain related to alcoholic neuritis subsides within weeks to months in most cases.

LOCAL ANESTHETIC TOXICITY

Since local anesthetic is used in all the above-mentioned blocks, it is important to be aware of the possible complications related to local anesthetic overdose and toxicity, including neurotoxicity, cardiac toxicity, allergies, and methemoglobinemia.

Neurotoxicity can range from mild toxicity (including ringing in the ears, circumoral numbness, metallic taste, lightheadedness, and confusion) to severe toxicity (progressing from grand-mal seizures to coma and death).

Local anesthetics cause a dose-dependent inhibition of cardiac contractility and conduction, which may result in cardiovascular collapse and cardiac arrest. Guidelines of maximum dosage should be strictly followed, and intravascular injection should be avoided.

Allergy to local anesthetics is very rare; however, allergy to aminoester local anesthetics has been reported. These drugs are derivatives of *p*-aminobenzoic acid, which is known to be allergenic.

A unique systemic side effect associated with a specific local anesthetic is the development of methemoglobinemia after the administration of large doses of prilocaine. In most cases, this condition does not necessitate treatment and usually resolves spontaneously; however, intravenous administration of methylene blue can be used.

Botwin KP et al. Complications of fluoroscopically guided transforaminal lumbar epidural injections. *Arch Phys Med Rehabil.* 2000;81:1045. [PMID: 10943753]

Botwin KP et al. Fluoroscopically guided lumbar transforaminal epidural steroid injections in degenerative lumbar stenosis: an outcome study. *Am J Phys Med Rehabil.* 2002;81:898. [PMID: 12447088]

Cluff R et al. The technical aspects of epidural steroid injections: a national survey. *Anesth Analg.* 2002;95:403. [PMID: 12145061]

Furman MB et al. Is it really possible to do a selective nerve root block? *Pain.* 2000;85:526. [PMID: 10866568]

Mulligan KA et al. Epidural steroids. *Curr Pain Headache Rep.* 2001;5:495. [PMID: 11676883]

Riew KD et al. The effect of nerve-root injections on the need for operative treatment of lumbar radicular pain. A prospective, randomized, controlled, double-blind study. *J Bone Joint Surg Am.* 2000;82-A:1589. [PMID: 11097449]

Stojanovic MP et al. The role of fluoroscopy in cervical epidural steroid injections: an analysis of contrast dispersal patterns. *Spine.* 2002;27:509. [PMID: 11880836]

Vad VB et al. Transforaminal epidural steroid injections in lumbosacral radiculopathy: a prospective randomized study. *Spine.* 2002;27:11. [PMID: 11805628]

Wong GY et al. Effect of neurolytic celiac plexus block on pain relief, quality of life, and survival in patients with unresectable pancreatic cancer: a randomized controlled trial. *JAMA.* 2004;291:1092. [PMID: 14996778]

Wong HK et al. Effects of corticosteroids on nerve root recovery after spinal nerve root compression. *Clin Orthop Relat Res.* 2002;(403):248. [PMID: 12360034]

Psychological Interventions

5

Dennis C. Turk, PhD, Tasha Burwinkle PsyD, PhD, & Kati Thieme, PhD

ESSENTIAL CRITERIA

- *Patients with ongoing, persistent pain.*
- *Patients for whom standard medical care has been unsuccessful or only moderately successful.*
- *Patients with comorbid mood disorders (anxiety, depression).*
- *Patients who have consulted numerous medical professionals in search of pain relief.*
- *Patients whose pain has resulted in social and occupational difficulties (eg, social isolation, job loss).*
- *Patients considering surgery or other invasive procedures to treat chronic pain.*
- *Patients being considered for long-term opioid therapy.*

General Considerations

A number of psychological interventions have been developed for people with chronic pain, with a large body of research supporting their efficacy. Before reviewing the approaches with the greatest empiric support, it is important to consider the plight of the chronic pain sufferer, the role of psychological factors, and the mechanisms involved in the experience of chronic pain because these serve as the basis for the development of treatment modalities.

The Plight of the Person with Chronic Pain

People with chronic and recurrent acute pain (eg, migraine) often become frustrated and irritated and lose faith when the medical system, which may initially create expectations for cure, turns its back on them when treatments prove to be ineffective.

Although those with acute pain can often receive relief from primary health care providers, people with persistent pain become enmeshed in the medical community as they trek from doctor to doctor, laboratory test to laboratory test, and imaging procedure to imaging procedure

in a frustrating search to have their pain diagnosed and successfully treated. In addition, at the same time that returning to work and earning a full income becomes less of a possibility, medical bills for unsuccessful treatments abound. This experience of "medical limbo"—the presence of a painful condition that eludes diagnosis and carries the implication of either psychiatric causation or malingering on the one hand, or an undiagnosed life-threatening disease on the other—is itself a source of stress that can initiate psychological distress or aggravate a premorbid psychiatric condition.

The person who has a chronic pain condition resides in a complex and costly world that is populated not only by the large number of other sufferers but also by their family members, health care providers, employers, and third-party payers. Family members feel increasingly hopeless and distressed as medical costs, disability, and emotional suffering increase while income and available treatment options decrease. Health care providers grow increasingly frustrated as available medical treatment options are exhausted while the pain condition worsens. Employers, who are already resentful of growing workers' compensation costs, pay higher costs while productivity suffers because the employee frequently calls in sick or is unable to perform at his or her usual level. Third-party payers watch as health care costs soar with repeated diagnostic testing for the same chronic pain condition. In time, the legitimacy of the person's reports of pain may be questioned, since a medical etiology often fails to substantiate the complaint.

People with chronic pain may begin to feel that their physicians, employers, and even family members are blaming them when their condition does not respond to treatment. Some may suggest that the individual is complaining in an attempt to receive attention, avoid undesirable activities, or seek disability compensation. Others may suggest that the pain is not real and is simply psychological. Third-party payers may even suggest that the individual is exaggerating the pain in order to receive financial gain. As a result, pain sufferers may withdraw from society, lose their jobs, alienate family and friends, and become more and more isolated.

Given the background provided, it is hardly surprising that the consequences of chronic pain can include demoralization leading to depression, frustration, anger, anxiety, self-preoccupation, and isolation. This emotional distress, however, can be exacerbated by a variety of other factors, including fear, inadequate or maladaptive support systems, inadequate personal and material coping resources, treatment-induced (iatrogenic) complications, overuse of potent drugs, inability to work, financial difficulties, prolonged litigation, disruption of usual activities, and sleep disturbance.

Fear of pain or movement and reinjury is an important contributor to disability associated with several chronic pain disorders, including back pain and fibromyalgia syndrome. People with chronic pain often anticipate that certain activities will increase their pain or induce further injury. These fears may contribute to avoidance of activity and subsequently greater physical deconditioning and greater disability. Their failure to engage in activities prevents them from obtaining any corrective feedback about the associations among activity, pain, and injury. For example, even if their pain does increase with activity, this does not necessarily indicate that *hurt* and *harm* are equivalent.

In addition to fear of movement, people with persistent pain may be anxious about the meaning of their symptoms for the future—will their pain increase, will their physical capacity diminish, will they have progressive disability where they ultimately end up in a wheelchair or bedridden? In addition to these sources of fear, pain sufferers may fear that people will not believe that they are suffering and they may be told that they are beyond help and will "just have to learn to live with it." Such fears can contribute to additional emotional distress and to increased muscle tension and physiologic arousal that may exacerbate and maintain pain. Living with persistent pain conditions requires considerable emotional resilience and tends to deplete people's emotional reserves, taxing not only the individual sufferer but also the capacity of family, friends, coworkers, and employers to provide support.

We want to draw attention to an important point; throughout this chapter we refer to the *person* with chronic pain, not the chronic pain *patient*. Our goal is to sensitize clinicians to the fact that a patient is someone who is being cared for in a clinic, hospital, or practitioner's office; the patient role is only part of the life of the person with chronic pain. As we will note, it is important to consider the prior history and current circumstances of a person with chronic pain and not just the patient with pain ascribed to a problem in some isolated body part.

Despite advances in knowledge of the neurophysiology of pain and the development of new pharmacologic agents with analgesic properties, sophisticated surgical interventions, and the use of advanced technologies (eg, spinal cord stimulation, implantable drug delivery systems), cure of pain has eluded the best efforts of health care providers. Regardless of the treatment, the amount of pain reduction averages only about 33% and less than 50% of patients treated with these interventions obtain even this result.

Chronic pain is by definition incurable; it is a chronic disease much like diabetes. Unlike diabetes, however, those with chronic pain constantly confront noxious sensations and other aversive symptoms. Thus, persons with chronic pain are faced with managing their symptoms on their own. Faced with this task, the common response is "How?"

It is important to consider the prior history and current circumstances of a person with chronic pain. The importance of this whole-person approach is addressed by Bonica who emphasizes the relationship between psychological and environmental factors and the experience of pain. He asserts that the pain cycle is subject to the influence of the "mind."

Based on the overview provided, two conclusions should be obvious:

1. Psychological factors play a significant role in the experience, maintenance, and exacerbation, if not the cause, of pain.
2. Since there are no cures for chronic pain and some level of pain will persist in most pain sufferers regardless of treatment, psychological approaches may be useful complements to more traditional medical and surgical approaches.

Bonica JJ. Preface. In: Bonica JJ, Loeser JD, Chapman CR, Fordyce WE, eds. *The Management of Pain.* 2nd ed. Philadelphia: Lea & Febiger; 1990.

Turk DC. Clinical effectiveness and cost effectiveness of treatments for chronic pain patients. *Clin J Pain.* 2002;18:355. [PMID: 12441829]

Vlaeyen JWS et al. Fear-avoidance and its consequences in chronic musculoskeletal pain: a state of the art. *Pain.* 2000;85:317. [PMID: 10781906]

Psychological Formulations of Chronic Pain

A number of different psychological perspectives on the chronic pain sufferer have evolved. It is important to briefly consider these because psychological treatments are based on different and at times competing psychological principles.

A. PSYCHOGENIC VIEW

Psychodynamic perspectives of chronic pain were first described in the 1960s, when people with pain were viewed as having compulsive and masochistic tendencies, inhibited aggressive needs, and feelings of guilt—"pain-prone personalities." It was commonly believed that people with pain had childhood histories fraught with emotional abuse, family dysfunction (eg, parental quarrels, separation, divorce), illness or death of a parent, early responsibilities, and high orientation toward achievement. Some current research has reported associations between chronic pain and childhood trauma, although the research is not consistent.

Based on the psychogenic perspective, assessment of patients with chronic pain is directed toward identifying the psychopathologic tendencies that instigate and maintain pain. Although the evidence to support this model is scarce, The American Psychiatric Association has created a psychiatric diagnosis, somatoform pain disorder. Diagnosis of a pain disorder requires the following:

1. The patient's report of pain must be inconsistent with the anatomic distribution of the nervous system.
2. If the pain mimics a known disease entity, organic pathology does not account for the pain.

Even in the presence of a medical condition that may cause pain, psychological factors may be implicated, and thus, the patient may receive a psychiatric diagnosis of pain disorder associated with **both** psychological factors and a general medical condition.

B. Behavioral Formulations

According to the classic or respondent conditioning model, if a painful stimulus is repeatedly paired with a neutral stimulus, the neutral stimulus will come to elicit a pain response. For example, a person who experienced pain after performing a treadmill exercise may become conditioned to experience a negative emotional response to the presence of the treadmill and to any stimulus associated with it (eg, physical therapist, gym). The negative emotional reaction may instigate muscle tensing, thereby exacerbating pain and further reinforcing the association between the stimulus and pain. Based on this conditioned correlation, people with chronic pain may avoid activities previously associated with pain onset or exacerbation.

In 1976, psychologist Wilbert Fordyce introduced an extension of operant conditioning to the thinking about chronic pain. This view proposes that acute pain behaviors (such as avoidance of activity to protect a painful area from additional pain) may come under the control of external contingencies of reinforcement (responses increase or decrease as a function of their reinforcing consequences) and thus develop into a chronic pain problem. Overt pain behaviors include the following:

1. Verbal reports.
2. Paralinguistic vocalizations (eg, sighs, moans).
3. Motor activity.
4. Facial expressions.

5. Body postures and gesturing (eg, limping, rubbing a painful body part).
6. Functional limitations (reclining for extensive periods of time, inactivity).
7. Behaviors designed to reduce pain (eg, taking medication, use of the health care system).

These behaviors may be positively reinforced directly; for example, patients may receive attention from a spouse or health care provider or monetary compensation or they may be able to avoid an undesirable activity. Pain behaviors may also be maintained by the escape from noxious stimulation through the use of drugs or rest, or the avoidance of undesirable activities such as work. In addition, "well behaviors" (eg, activity, working) may not be positively reinforcing and the more rewarding pain behaviors may, therefore, be maintained.

The development and maintenance of pain behaviors can also occur by means of observational learning. That is, people can acquire responses that were not previously in their behavioral repertoire by the observation of others performing these activities. Expectancies and actual behavioral responses to nociceptive stimulation are based, at least partially, on prior social learning history. Complicating the issue is that cultural factors may influence how patients interpret, respond to, and cope with illness. This may contribute to the marked variability in response to objectively similar degrees of physical pathology noted by health care providers.

The operant conditioning model does not concern itself with the initial cause of pain. Rather, it considers pain an internal subjective experience that can be directly assessed and may be maintained even after an initial physical basis of pain has resolved. The pain behavior originally elicited by organic factors caused by injury or disease may come to occur, totally or in part, in response to reinforcing environmental events.

It is important, however, not to make the mistake of viewing pain behaviors as being synonymous with malingering. Malingering involves consciously and purposely faking a symptom such as pain for some gain, usually financial. Contrary to the beliefs of many third-party payers, there is little support for the contention that outright faking of pain for financial gain is prevalent.

C. Gate Control Model

Although not a psychological formulation itself, the Gate Control model was the first to popularize the importance of central, psychological factors in pain perception. This model contradicts the notion that pain is either somatic or psychogenic. Instead, it postulates that both factors have potentiating and moderating effects. According to this model, both the central and peripheral nervous systems interact to contribute to the experience of pain. It is not only these physical factors that guide the brain's interpretation of painful stimuli that is at the center of this model but also that psychological factors (eg, thoughts, beliefs, emotions) also play a role in determining the pain experience resulting from painful stimuli.

Prior to the Melzack and Wall formulation of the Gate Control theory, psychological processes were largely dismissed as reactions to pain. Although the physiologic details of the Gate Control model have been challenged, it has had a substantial impact on basic research and in generating treatment modalities.

D. COGNITIVE-BEHAVIORAL PERSPECTIVE

The cognitive-behavioral model, perhaps the most commonly accepted model for the psychological treatment of persons with chronic pain, suggests that behaviors and emotions are influenced by interpretations of events and emphasis is placed on how persons' beliefs and attitudes interact with physical, affective, and behavioral factors. The cognitive-behavioral view suggests that conditioned reactions are largely activated by learned *expectations* rather than being automatically evoked. In other words, it is the person's information processing that results in anticipatory anxiety and avoidance. The critical factor, therefore, is that people learn to anticipate and predict events and to express appropriate reactions.

A number of studies have attempted to identify cognitive factors that contribute to pain and disability. These studies have consistently demonstrated that a person's attitudes, beliefs, and coping strategies as well as his or her expectations about the health care system affect reports of pain, activity, disability, and response to treatment. For example, persons respond to medical conditions in part based on their subjective ideas about illness and their symptoms. When pain is interpreted as signifying ongoing tissue damage or a progressive disease, it is likely to produce considerably more suffering and behavioral dysfunction than if it is viewed as being the result of a stable problem that is expected to improve.

Once beliefs and expectancies are formed, they become stable and rigid and relatively impervious to modification. Pain sufferers tend to avoid experiences that could invalidate their beliefs (disconfirmations) and guide their behavior in accordance with these beliefs, even in situations where these beliefs are no longer valid. Therefore, it is essential for persons with chronic pain to develop adaptive beliefs about the relationships between impairment, pain, suffering, and disability and to deemphasize the role of experienced pain in their regulation of functioning.

Self-efficacy, a personal expectation that one can successfully perform a behavior to produce a desired outcome, is particularly important among persons with chronic pain. Given sufficient motivation to engage in a behavior, it is a person's self-efficacy beliefs that determine the choice of activities that he or she will initiate, the amount of effort that will be expended, and how long he or she will persist in the face of obstacles and aversive experiences. In this way, self-efficacy plays an important role in therapeutic change.

Distorted thinking can also contribute to the maintenance and exacerbation of pain. A particularly potent and pernicious thinking style that has been observed among persons with chronic pain is catastrophizing (holding negative thoughts about one's situation and interpreting even minor problems as major catastrophes). Research has indicated that people who spontaneously use more catastrophizing thoughts report more pain than those who do not catastrophize.

Coping strategies, or a person's specific ways of adjusting to or minimizing pain and distress, act to alter both the perception of pain intensity and the ability to manage or tolerate pain and continue everyday activities. Overt behavioral coping strategies include rest, medication, and use of relaxation, among others. Covert coping strategies include various means of distracting oneself from pain, reassuring oneself that the pain will diminish, seeking information, and problem solving, to list some of the most prominent.

Studies have found that active coping strategies (efforts to function in spite of pain or to distract oneself from pain) are associated with adaptive functioning, while passive coping strategies (depending on others for help with pain control, avoiding activities because of fear of pain and injury, self-medication, alcohol) are associated with greater pain and depression. Regardless of the type of coping strategy, if persons with chronic pain are instructed in the use of adaptive coping strategies, their rating of pain intensity decreases and pain tolerance increases.

E. BIOPSYCHOSOCIAL MODEL

Although the Gate Control model introduced the role of psychological factors in the maintenance of pain symptoms, it focused primarily on the basic anatomy and physiology of pain. The biopsychosocial model, which expands the cognitive-behavioral model of pain, views illness as a dynamic and reciprocal interaction between biologic, psychological, and sociocultural variables that shape the person's response to pain.

This model is unique because it takes into consideration the influence of higher order cognitions, including perception and appraisal. It accepts that persons are active processors of information and that behavior, emotions, and even physiology are influenced by interpretations of events, rather than solely by physiologic factors. Persons with chronic pain may therefore have negative expectations about their own ability and responsibility to exert any control over their pain. Moreover, pain sufferers' behaviors elicit responses from significant others that can reinforce both adaptive and maladaptive modes of thinking, feeling, and behaving.

The biopsychosocial model presumes some form of physical pathology or at least physical changes in the muscles, joints, or nerves that generate nociceptive input to the brain. At the periphery, nociceptive fibers transmit sensations that may or may not be interpreted as pain. Such sensation is not yet considered pain until subjected to higher order psychological and mental processing that involves perception, appraisal, and behavior. Perception involves the interpretation of nociceptive input and identifies the type of pain (ie, sharp, burning, and punishing). Appraisal involves the meaning that is attributed to the pain and influences subsequent behaviors. A person may choose to ignore the pain and continue working, walking, socializing, and engaging in previous levels of activity or may choose to leave work, refrain from all activity, and assume the sick role. In turn, this interpersonal role is shaped by responses from significant others that may promote either the healthy response or the sick-role. The biopsychosocial model has been instrumental in the development of cognitive-behavioral treatment approaches for chronic pain, including assessment and intervention.

American Psychiatric Association. *Diagnostic and Statistical Manual of Mental Disorders.* 4th ed. Text Revision. Washington, DC: APA Press; 2000.

Davis DA, Luecken LJ, Zautra AJ. Are reports of childhood abuse related to the experience of chronic pain in adulthood? A meta-analytic review of the literature. *Clin J Pain.* 2005;21:398.

Dickenson AH. Gate control theory of pain stands the test of time. *Br J Anaesth.* 2002;88:755. [PMID: 12173188]

Engel GL. Psychogenic pain and the pain-prone patient. *Am J Med.* 1959;26:899. [PMID: 13649716]

Fordyce WE. *Behavioral Methods for Chronic Pain and Illness.* St. Louis: Mosby; 1976.

Frischenschlager O et al. Psychological management of pain. *Disabil Rehabil.* 2002;24:416. [PMID: 12033996]

Melzack R, Wall PD. Pain mechanisms: a new theory. *Science.* 1965;50:971. [PMID: 5320816]

Morley S et al. Systematic review and meta-analysis of randomized controlled trials of cognitive behaviour therapy and behaviour therapy for chronic pain in adults, excluding headache. *Pain.* 1999;80:1. [PMID: 10204712]

Sullivan MJL et al. Catastrophizing, depression and expectancies for pain and emotional distress. *Pain.* 2001;91:147. [PMID: 11240087]

Thieme K et al. Predictors of pain behaviors in fibromyalgia patients. *Arthritis Rheum.* 2005;53:343. [PMID: 15934120]

Turk DC. Cognitive-behavioral approach to the treatment of chronic pain patients. *Reg Anesth Pain Med.* 2003;6:573. [PMID: 14634950]

Turk DC. Understanding pain sufferers: The role of cognitive processes. *Spine J.* 2004;4:1. [PMID: 14749188]

Turk DC et al. Psychological factors in chronic pain: evolution and revolution. *J Consult Clin Psychol.* 2002;70:678. [PMID: 12090376]

Assessment & Evaluation

In order to understand and appropriately treat a person whose primary symptom is pain, clinicians must begin with a comprehensive history and physical examination. Physical examination procedures and sophisticated laboratory and imaging techniques are readily available for use in detecting organic pathology. Physical and laboratory abnormalities, however, correlate poorly with pain complaints, and it is often not possible to make any precise pathologic diagnosis or even to identify an adequate anatomic origin for the pain. Thus, an adequate pain assessment also requires clinical interviews, observation, and use of pain assessment tools to assist in the evaluation of the myriad psychosocial and behavioral factors that influence the subjective report (see Chapter 2).

Because there is no tool that can provide an objective quantification of the amount or severity of pain experienced by a person, it can only be assessed indirectly based on a pain sufferer's verbal and behavioral communication. Patients are usually asked to describe the characteristics (for example, stabbing, burning), location, and severity of their pain. However, even a person's communications make pain assessment difficult, since pain is a complex, subjective phenomenon composed of a range of factors and is uniquely experienced by each individual. Wide variability in pain severity, quality, and impact may be noted in reports of people with pain as they attempt to describe what appear to be objectively identical phenomena. People's descriptions of pain are also affected by cultural and sociologic influences.

A. INTERVIEW

Topics that can be covered in an assessment interview are listed in Table 5–1. A functional assessment of the patient's pain can also be used. Patients can be asked about their current level of pain or pain over the past week or month, or they can maintain regular diaries of pain intensity with ratings recorded several times each day for several days or weeks. Asking about the characteristics of pain, while necessary, is not sufficient. The use of diaries can provide more information than just the varying pain intensity. A clinician can use information about pain obtained during the interview and diaries to identify patterns in behavior, including potential antecedents and consequences to pain exacerbation.

Pain sufferers' beliefs about the cause of symptoms, their trajectory, and beneficial treatments will have important influences on coping with pain and adherence to therapeutic interventions. Thus, when conducting a patient interview, attention should focus on the individual's specific thoughts, behaviors, emotions, and physiologic responses that precede, accompany, and follow pain episodes or exacerbations, including environmental and temporal conditions and consequences

Table 5–1. Areas Covered in Clinical Interviews.

- Patient's perception about the cause of pain
- Patient's experience of pain (how often and when it occurs) and related symptoms
- Treatments received and currently receiving
- Impact of pain on daily activities
- Impact of pain on interpersonal relationships
- Level and nature of emotional distress
- Current stressors and areas of conflict
- Methods used to cope with symptoms
- Alcohol and substance abuse history and current use
- Behaviors used to let others know pain is present
- Responses by significant others
- Social history
- Education and vocational history
- Receiving or seeking compensation and involvement in litigation
- Concerns and expectations

associated with the patient's responses (cognitive, emotional, and behavioral, including frequency and specificity/generality across situations). Any patterns of maladaptive thoughts should be noted, since they may contribute to a sense of hopelessness, dysphoria, and unwillingness to engage in activity.

Determining the patient's (and family's) expectations and goals of therapy is important. For example, an expectation that pain will be eliminated completely may be unrealistic and should be addressed to prevent discouragement if this outcome does not occur. In addition, formulating treatment goals (including symptom reduction; reduced emotional distress; improved physical, social, and vocational functioning; reduction of inappropriate use of the health care system) is helpful in returning someone to optimal functioning given their age, sex, education, and presence of physical impairments.

B. Behavioral Observation

A number of different observational procedures have been developed to quantify pain behaviors. Behavioral checklists have been developed to identify the frequency and type of pain behaviors exhibited by a patient. Such checklists can be self-reports or reports by others; for example, behavioral observation scales can be used by significant others, and health care providers can use observational methods to systematically quantify various pain behaviors (eg, observing the patient in the waiting room, while being interviewed, or during a structured series of physical tasks). Noting the type and frequency of pain behaviors can provide detailed information about when someone performs pain behaviors, around whom

the behaviors are elicited, and the responses of others to the pain behaviors. Persons with chronic pain tend to perform more pain behaviors around others who positively reinforce the pain behavior (such as providing soothing statements, physical intimacy, assistance in performing tasks). Obtaining details about what factors increase and decrease (eg, patterns) behavior can be used when developing treatment goals.

C. Self-Report Questionnaires

A number of assessment instruments designed to evaluate a person's attitudes, beliefs, and expectancies about themselves, their symptoms, and the health care system have been developed. There are many advantages to the use of standardized instruments: they are easy to administer, require minimal time, assess a wide range of behaviors, obtain information about behaviors that may be private (sexual relations) or unobservable (thoughts, emotional arousal), and most importantly, they can be submitted to analyses that permit determination of their reliability and validity. These instruments should not be viewed as alternatives to interviews; rather, they may suggest issues to be addressed in more depth during an interview or investigated with other measures. In addition, they allow comparison among groups of patients with pain and provide valuable information about the functional status of individuals in relation to others with the same condition.

Questionnaires have been developed to assess patients' reports of their abilities to engage in a range of functional activities, such as the ability to walk up stairs, to sit for specific periods of time, the ability to lift specific weights, performance of activities of daily living, as well as the severity of the pain experienced upon the performance of these activities.

A number of psychosocial screening tools have been developed (see Table 6–6) to assess patients with chronic pain for psychological distress; the impact of pain on their lives; feeling of control; coping behaviors; and attitudes about disease, pain, and health care providers as well as his or her plight. It should be noted, however, that patient's responses may be distorted as a function of the pain or the medications that they take. For example, common measures of depression ask people about their appetites, sleep patterns, and fatigue. Since disease status and medication can affect responses to such items, individuals' scores may be elevated, distorting the meaning of the responses. As a result, it is always best to corroborate information gathered from the instruments with other sources, such as interviews with the patient, their significant others, and chart review.

D. Referral for Psychological Intervention

The health care provider should be alert for *red flags* that may serve as an impetus for more thorough evaluation by a psychologist who specializes in the treatment of pain.

Table 5–2 lists questions worthy of asking patients who report persistent or recurring pain. The positive responses to any one or a small number of these questions should not be viewed as sufficient to make a referral for more extensive evaluation, but referral should be *considered* when several questions are answered positively. In general, a referral for evaluation may be indicated when the following circumstances are present:

1. Disability greatly exceeds what would be expected based on physical findings alone.
2. Persons with pain make excessive demands on the health care system.
3. Persons persist in seeking medical tests and treatments when they are not indicated.
4. Persons display significant psychological distress (eg, depression or anxiety).
5. Persons show evidence of addictive behaviors such as continual nonadherence to the prescribed regimen.

Turk DC. Clinical effectiveness and cost effectiveness of treatments for chronic pain patients. *Clin J Pain.* 2002;18:355. [PMID: 12441829]

Turk DC, Burwinkle TM. Assessment of pain sufferers: outcomes measures in clinical trials and clinical practice. *Rehab Psychol.* 2005;50:56.

Therapeutic Interventions

There are a number of different clinical approaches to the treatment of chronic pain that have been developed based on the models described, including insight-oriented approaches, behavioral approaches, biofeedback, guided imagery, and hypnosis. Perhaps the most commonly used approach, however, is cognitive-behavioral therapy, which incorporates many techniques from other approaches.

A. INSIGHT-ORIENTED THERAPIES

Therapy based on the psychodynamic view and insight-oriented approaches are primarily focused on early relationship experiences that are reconstructed within the context of the therapeutic relationship. The therapeutic relationship is meant to "correct" the person's prior maladaptive experience via reintegrating emotions into symbolic and available mental processes, resulting in improved emotional regulation. This approach is often supplemented by relaxation therapy and long-term involvement in the therapeutic process. It is thus important for the person with pain and his or her therapist to have a supportive and trusting relationship. Although insight-oriented psychotherapy may be useful with selected individuals, this approach has rarely been shown to be

Table 5–2. Screening Questions.

Clinical Issues
• Has the pain persisted for 3 months or longer despite appropriate interventions and in the absence of progressive disease?
• Does the patient report nonanatomic changes in sensation (eg, glove anesthesia)?
• Does the patient seem to have unrealistic expectations of the health care provider or treatment offered?
• Does the patient complain vociferously about treatments received from previous health care providers?
• Does the patient have a history of previous painful or disabling medical problems?
• Does the patient have a history of substance abuse?
• Does the patient display many pain behaviors (eg, grimacing, moving in a rigid and guarded fashion), and do they increase when a significant other is present?
• Does the patient have a history of repeatedly and excessively using the health care system?
Legal and Occupational Issues
• Is litigation pending?
• Is the patient receiving disability compensation?
• Was the patient injured on the job?
• Does the patient have a job to which he or she can return?
• Does the patient have a history of frequently changing jobs?
Psychological Issues
• Does the patient report any major stressful life events just prior to the onset or exacerbation of pain?
• Does the patient demonstrate inappropriate or excessive depressed or elevated mood?
• Has the patient given up many activities (social, recreational, sexual, occupational, physical) because of pain?
• Is there a high level of marital or family conflict?
• Does the patient's significant other provide positive attention to pain behaviors (eg, taking over chores, providing back rubs)?
• Is there anyone in the patient's family who has chronic pain?
• Does the patient fail to use coping efforts, or are the efforts to cope with pain maladaptive or inappropriate?
• Does the patient have plans for increased or renewed activities if pain is reduced?

effective in reducing symptoms for most patients with chronic pain.

B. RESPONDENT-BEHAVIORAL APPROACH

As stated previously, in the classic or respondent conditioning model, if a nociceptive stimulus is repeatedly paired with a neutral stimulus in close temporal proximity, the neutral stimulus will come to elicit a pain response. In chronic pain, many activities that were neutral or even pleasurable may come to elicit or exacerbate pain and are thus experienced as aversive and actively avoided. Over time, a growing number of stimuli (eg, activities and exercises) may be expected to elicit or exacerbate pain and will be avoided (a process known as **stimulus generalization**). Thus, the anticipatory fear of pain and restriction of activity, and not just the actual nociception, may contribute to disability. Anticipatory fear can also elicit physiologic reactivity that may aggravate pain. Thus, conditioning may directly increase nociceptive stimulation and pain.

As long as activity-avoidance succeeds in preventing pain initiation or exacerbation, the conviction that pain sufferers hold that they remain inactive is difficult to modify. Treatment of pain from the classic conditioning model includes repeatedly engaging in behavior (**exposure**) that produces progressively less pain than was predicted (**corrective feedback**), which is then followed by reductions in anticipatory fear and anxiety associated with the activity. Such transformations add support to the importance of quota-based physical exercise programs, with participants progressively increasing their activity levels despite fear of injury and discomfort associated with use of deconditioned muscles.

C. OPERANT APPROACH

Operant approaches focus on the elimination of pain behaviors by withdrawal of attention and increasing well behaviors by positive reinforcement. The operant learning paradigm does not uncover the etiology of pain but focuses primarily on the maintenance of pain behaviors and deficiency in well behaviors. Target pain behaviors are identified, as are their controlling antecedents and consequent reinforcers or punishments, such as helpful, distracting, or ignoring behaviors by a spouse.

Techniques such as extinction (eg, removing the contingent relationship between overt pain behaviors and its consequences) and positive and negative reinforcement are then used to increase desired behaviors and decrease pain-compatible behaviors (eg, with operant behavioral treatment because patients are expected to be active in setting treatment goals and follow through with recommendations). The efficacy of operant treatment has been demonstrated in several studies of patients with various chronic pain disorders, especially low back pain and fibromyalgia syndrome.

D. BIOFEEDBACK

Biofeedback has been used successfully to treat a number of chronic pain states such as headaches and back pain, among others (see Chapter 6). The purpose of biofeedback is to teach a patient to exert control over his or her physiologic processes. When a patient undergoes biofeedback, he or she is connected by electrodes to equipment that records physiologic responses, including skin conductance, respiration, heart rate, skin temperature, and muscle tension. The biofeedback equipment converts the readings of physiologic responses into visual or auditory signals on a monitor that the patient can observe. In this way, the physiologic information is *fed back* to patients so that they can learn to alter it using their thoughts or breathing.

With practice, most people can learn to voluntarily control important physiologic functions that may be associated directly with pain and stress. Biofeedback generates a state of general relaxation. Typically, patients being treated with biofeedback are instructed to practice relaxing using the methods that have been successful in altering physiologic parameters in the clinic.

The actual mechanisms involved in the success of biofeedback are open to question. The assumption of biofeedback treatment is that the level of pain is maintained or exacerbated by autonomic nervous system parameters believed to be associated with the production of nociceptive stimulation (eg, muscle tension in a person with low back pain). However, in addition to the physiologic changes accompanying biofeedback, patients gain a sense of control over their bodies. Given the high levels of helplessness observed in persons with chronic pain problems, the perception of control may be as important as the actual physiologic changes observed. A general sense of relaxation is also an important feature of biofeedback. Again, it is not clear whether the alterations of specific physiologic parameters putatively associated with pain is the most important ingredient of biofeedback compared with the broader relaxation created.

There are a large number of relaxation techniques that have been used in combination with biofeedback and on their own. The literature is mixed as to whether biofeedback is any more effective than relaxation. The pain condition being treated may differ as far as which of the possible components (relaxation, sense of control, general relaxation) contributes most. Moreover, the components may not be mutually exclusive and may even be synergistic.

E. GUIDED IMAGERY

Guided imagery can be a useful strategy for helping people with pain to relax, achieve a sense of control, and distract themselves from pain (see Chapter 6). Although guided imagery has been advocated as a stand-alone intervention to reduce presurgical anxiety and postsurgical pain, it is most often used in conjunction with other treatment interventions such as cognitive-behavioral therapy or relaxation.

With guided imagery, patients are asked to identify specific situations that they find pleasant and engaging. In this way, a detailed image that is tailored to the person can be created. When the person with chronic pain is feeling pain or is experiencing pain exacerbation, they can use imagery to redirect their attention away from their pain.

The most successful images tend to be those that involve all of the senses (vision, sound, touch, smell, and taste). Persons with chronic pain are thus encouraged to use images that evoke these senses. Some patients, however, may have difficulty generating a particularly vivid visual image and may find it helpful to listen to a taped description or purchase a poster that they can focus their attention upon as a way of assisting their imagination.

F. HYPNOSIS

Hypnosis has been used as a treatment intervention for chronic pain for many years. It has been shown to relieve pain in people with headache, burn injury, arthritis, cancer, and chronic back pain (see Chapter 6). As with imagery, relaxation, and biofeedback, it is rarely used alone; practitioners often use hypnosis concurrently with other treatment interventions. Hypnotic suggestions have been used to instill positive attitudes in patients, facilitate compliance with treatment, foster distraction from negative thoughts or stimuli, alleviate anxiety related to medical procedures, reduce reliance on medication, and promote relaxation and rehearsal of adaptive behaviors.

A meta-analysis suggests an overall benefit of the addition of hypnosis to nonhypnotic pain management strategies, although this may be mediated by a person's level of hypnotic suggestibility. Furthermore, there are discrepancies in the literature with regard to the methods used to induce hypnosis, making it difficult to accurately evaluate the efficacy of this intervention. Finally, it has been suggested that hypnosis has more utility in the treatment of acute pain than chronic pain. Thus, the degree to which hypnosis is effective above and beyond other interventions and for which populations is yet to be determined.

G. MOTIVATIONAL INTERVIEWING

Most persons with chronic pain adhere to a biomedical model; for example, the nature of their symptoms is closely aligned with physical pathology. As pain persists, some patients may become aware of the role of factors, such as emotional stress, in their experience of pain. This latter group may begin to entertain the possibility that they can learn and use self-management techniques to help them adapt to life with a chronic pain condition. Other chronic pain sufferers have difficulty with this expanded perspective. The stage of acceptance of self-management is important, since those who are not ready for the use of psychological techniques tend to avoid and dismiss such methods. Thus, the clinician needs to be aware of an individual's readiness for self-management. The assessment process should help the health care provider determine the person's motivation for the use of nonphysical approaches.

Motivational interviewing as a treatment intervention was initially developed for populations with substance abuse disorders, although it has been increasingly used with patients who have chronic pain. Specific stages of change have been postulated, and the tasks of intervention are tailored to each stage.

In the **precontemplation** stage, persons with chronic pain have not yet begun to consider changing from a purely somatic view of pain with the passive role they adopt as they wait for the health care provider to identify and provide the appropriate treatment. The clinician attempts to assist the patient by fostering acknowledgment of risks and problems due to inactivity, such as increased pain and physical deconditioning.

Once persons with chronic pain take responsibility for their prior inactivity, they enter the next of the proposed stages, **contemplation.** At this stage, the clinical goal is to encourage the patient to conclude that the risks of inactivity outweigh the perceived benefits. When they are ready to become more active (**preparation** stage), the clinician helps the patient outline appropriate structured physical activities in which the person is willing to participate. Finally, in the **action** stage, the clinician helps the patient increase their activity. This is followed by maintenance, geared toward the person's ongoing motivation and commitment.

As patients move through the stages, it is important for clinicians to be tolerant. Clinicians can encourage transition to different stages by providing motivational statements, listening with empathy, asking open-ended questions, providing feedback and affirmation, and handling resistance. Because motivational interviewing has only been applied to chronic pain in recent years, the efficacy of this intervention with different chronic pain populations is not well documented. Motivational interviewing is a general framework for preparing patients for treatment and for adhering within the cognitive-behavioral perspective and can be readily used with cognitive-behavioral therapy.

H. COGNITIVE-BEHAVIORAL THERAPY

It is important to make a distinction between the cognitive-behavioral perspective and cognitive and behavioral techniques. The perspective is based on several key assumptions (Table 5–3). The techniques used can

Table 5–3. Assumptions of the Cognitive-Behavioral Perspective.

- Persons are active processors of information and not passive reactors
- Thoughts (eg, appraisals, expectancies, beliefs) can elicit and influence mood, affect physiologic processes, have social consequences and can also serve as an impetus for behavior; conversely, mood, physiology, environmental factors and behavior can influence the nature and content of thought processes
- Behavior is reciprocally determined by *both* the individual and environmental factors
- Persons can learn more adaptive ways of thinking, feeling, and behaving
- Persons should collaborate actively in changing their thoughts, feelings, behavior, and physiology

be drawn from among those described previously as well as more specific ones noted below.

Cognitive-behavioral therapy is based on the idea that people hold beliefs that they are unable to function because of their pain and that they are helpless to improve their situation. Thus, treatment goals focus on helping the person with pain to realize that he or she can, in fact, manage their problems as well as provide them with skills to respond in more adaptive ways that can be maintained after treatment has ended.

The cognitive-behavioral therapy approach combines cognitive and behavioral techniques, including assertiveness, stress management, relaxation training, goal-setting, and pacing of activities. Psychologists assist patients with their concerns about the future, returning to work, and physical limitations. Furthermore, psychologists help patients build their communication skills; gain a sense of control over their pain; and cope with fear of pain, reinjury, or frustrations due to the responses of others (significant others, physicians, insurance companies, employers) toward the patients' pain reports or behaviors. Patients are educated in developing positive coping strategies and are encouraged to increase their activities in a graded fashion. It is expected that patients will gain mastery over their pain, which will then result in improved mood.

Four components of cognitive-behavioral therapy have been postulated: education, skills acquisition, skills consolidation, and generalization and maintenance. The education component is composed of helping the patient challenge his or her negative perceptions regarding abilities to manage pain through a process called **cognitive restructuring,** which makes the patient aware of the role thoughts and emotions play in potentiating and maintaining stress and physical symptoms.

Steps in cognitive restructuring include the following:

1. Identifying maladaptive thoughts during problematic situations (eg, during pain exacerbations, stressful events).
2. Introducing and practicing coping thoughts.
3. Shifting from self-defeating to coping thoughts.
4. Introducing and practicing positive or reinforcing thoughts.
5. Finally, home practice and follow-up.

Using these steps, the therapist encourages the patients to test the adaptiveness (not the so-called rationality) of individual thoughts, beliefs, expectations, and predictions. The crucial element in successful treatment is bringing about a shift in the person's repertoire from well-established, habitual, and automatic but ineffective responses toward systematic problem-solving and planning, control of affect, behavioral persistence, or disengagement when appropriate.

The goals of skills acquisition and skills consolidation are to help patients learn new pain management behaviors and cognitions, including relaxation skills, problem-solving training, distraction skills training, activity pacing, and communication skills. Using role-playing techniques and homework assignments, patients can practice emerging skill sets and evaluate their usefulness in the management of their pain.

Finally, generalization and maintenance is geared toward solidifying skills and preventing relapse. Problems that arise throughout treatment are viewed as opportunities to assist patients with learning how to handle setbacks and lapses that may occur following treatment. In this phase, it is helpful to assist patients in anticipating future problems and high-risk situations so that they can think about and practice the behavioral responses that may be necessary for successful coping. The goal during this phase, then, is to enable patients to develop a problem-solving perspective where they believe that they have the skills and competencies within their repertoires to respond in an appropriate way to problems as they arise. In this manner, attempts are made to help the person learn to anticipate future difficulties, develop plans for adaptive responding, and adjust his or her behavior accordingly.

The efficacy of cognitive-behavioral therapy has been demonstrated in a large number of studies of patients with various chronic pain disorders. There is a wealth of evidence that both individual and group cognitive-behavioral therapy can help restore function and mood as well as reduce pain and disability-related behaviors. Despite the fact that cognitive-behavioral therapy is undoubtedly the most used intervention for patients with chronic pain, there are limitations. For example, although cognitive-behavioral therapy has been found to be helpful for a number of individuals, there are some for whom cognitive-behavioral therapy is not beneficial. Researchers are just beginning to explore different aspects of cognitive-behavioral treatment to answer the question "What works for whom?"

Cano A et al. Spousal congruence on disability, pain, and spouse responses to pain. *Pain.* 2004;109:258. [PMID: 15157686]

Frischenschlager O et al. Psychological management of pain. *Disabil Rehabil.* 2002;24:416. [PMID: 12033996]

Halpin LS et al. Guided imagery in cardiac surgery. *Outcomes Manage.* 2002;6:132. [PMID: 12134377]

Jensen MP et al. Toward the development of a motivational model of pain self-management. *J Pain.* 2003;4:477. [PMID: 14636816]

McCracken LM et al. Behavioral and cognitive-behavioral treatment for chronic pain: Outcomes, predictors of outcome, and treatment process. *Spine.* 2002;27:2564. [PMID: 12435995]

Montgomery GH et al. A meta-analysis of hypnotically induced analgesia: How effective is hypnosis? *Int J Clin Exp Hypn.* 2000;48:138. [PMID: 10769981]

Morley S et al. Systematic review and meta-analysis of randomized controlled trials of cognitive behaviour therapy and behaviour therapy for chronic pain in adults, excluding headache. *Pain.* 1999;80:1. [PMID: 10204712]

Novy DM. Psychological approaches for managing chronic pain. *J Psychopathol Behav Assess.* 2004;26:279.

Ostelo RW et al. Behavioural treatment for chronic low-back pain. *Cochrane Database Syst Rev.* 2005;(1):CD002014. [PMID: 15674889]

Patterson DR et al. Hypnosis and clinical pain. *Psychol Bull.* 2003;129:495. [PMID: 12848218]

Pinnell CM et al. Empirical findings on the use of hypnosis in medicine: A critical review. *Int J Clin Exp Hypn.* 2000;48:170. [PMID: 10769983]

Thieme K et al. Operant behavioral treatment of fibromyalgia: a controlled study. *Arthritis Rheum.* 2003;49:314. [PMID: 12794785]

Turk DC. Clinical effectiveness and cost effectiveness of treatments for chronic pain patients. *Clin J Pain.* 2002;18:355. [PMID: 12441829]

Turk DC. Cognitive-behavioral approach to the treatment of chronic pain patients. *Reg Anesth Pain Med.* 2003;6:573. [PMID: 14634950]

Turner-Stokes L et al. Outpatient cognitive behavioral pain management programs: a randomized comparison of a group-based multidisciplinary versus an individual therapy model. *Arch Phys Med Rehabil.* 2003;84:781. [PMID: 12808527]

Vlaeyen JWS et al. Cognitive-behavioral treatments for chronic pain: what works for whom? *Clin J Pain.* 2005;21:1. [PMID: 15599126]

Interdisciplinary Pain Rehabilitation Programs

Although cognitive-behavioral approaches on their own have found strong support in the literature, it is worthwhile to discuss the efficacy of interdisciplinary pain rehabilitation programs (IPRPs) since the cognitive-behavioral perspective and cognitive and behavioral techniques are frequently important ingredients in these programs. The premise underlying the development of IPRPs is that patients with complex pain problems are best served by the collaborative efforts of a team of specialists that often includes physicians, nurses, physical therapists, occupational therapists, vocational counselors, and psychologists. IPRPs operate under the assumption that pain is not just the result of body damage but that pain has psychological and environmental origins as well. In other words, IPRPs treat more than pain: they treat the whole person.

The primary goal of IPRPs is to improve physical performance and coping skills, and to transfer the responsibility for pain management from the health care provider to the individual. This treatment plan is rehabilitative rather than curative, and encourages people to take a more active role in the management of their pain.

IPRPs adopt the biopsychosocial model of chronic pain, which assumes that all human behavior, including the report of pain, reflects a combination of the events occurring within the person's body, the recognition of these events, appraisal of these events, the affective responses to these events, and the influence of the environment. Comprehensive and concurrent treatment interventions may include drug detoxification, psychological treatment (eg, relaxation training, problem solving, coping skills training, functional restoration, and rehabilitation), physical conditioning, acquisition of coping and vocational skills, and education about pain and how the body functions.

There have been a large number of published studies and several meta-analyses supporting the clinical effectiveness of IPRPs. In general, compared with pharmacologic, medical, and surgical alternatives, IPRPs appear to be equally effective in reducing pain and significantly more effective in reducing health care consumption, leading to closure of disability claims, increasing functional activities, and returning patients to work. Even at long-term follow-up, patients who are treated in IPRPs appear to maintain their reductions in pain and emotional distress. An additional benefit of IPRPs is that they cost substantially less per person per year than medications and surgeries, rendering treatment more cost-effective.

Guzman J et al. Multidisciplinary rehabilitation for chronic low back pain: systematic review. *BMJ.* 2001;322:1511. [PMID: 11869581]

Loeser JD, Turk DC. Multidisciplinary pain management. *Semin Neurosurg.* 2004;15:13–29.

McCracken LM et al. Behavioral and cognitive-behavioral treatment for chronic pain: Outcomes, predictors of outcome, and treatment process. *Spine.* 2002;27:2564. [PMID: 12435995]

Morley S et al. Systematic review and meta-analysis of randomized controlled trials of cognitive behaviour therapy and behaviour therapy for chronic pain in adults, excluding headache. *Pain.* 1999;80:1. [PMID: 10204712]

Olason M. Outcome of an interdisciplinary pain management program in a rehabilitation clinic. *Work.* 2004;22:9. [PMID: 14757900]

Storro S et al. Effects on sick-leave of a multidisciplinary rehabilitation programme for chronic low back, neck, or shoulder pain: comparison with usual treatment. *J Rehabil Med.* 2004;36:12. [PMID: 15074433]

Turk DC. Clinical effectiveness and cost effectiveness of treatments for chronic pain patients. *Clin J Pain.* 2002;18:355. [PMID: 12441829]

Rehabilitation Issues: Pain Control 6

Steven P. Stanos, DO, & Mark D. Tyburski, MD

ESSENTIAL CRITERIA

- *The ultimate goal of a rehabilitation-based approach to acute and chronic pain is reduction of pain and restoration of function.*
- *Chronic pain states may represent a more integrated biologic, psychological, and social constellation of problems including environmental and social context as well as the patient's emotions, personal meaning, beliefs, and attitudes.*
- *A unidimensional biomedical model approach to pain focuses on pain as a sensory event reflecting underlying disease or tissue damage.*
- *Multidisciplinary pain treatment programs embody a biopsychosocial approach to assessment and treatment and may be a more appropriate setting for management of complex chronic pain conditions.*
- *Realistic treatment goals for patients with acute and chronic pain are essential.*

GENERAL CONSIDERATIONS

The subjective experience of pain results from a complex interaction of physical, emotional, and social factors. For example, two patients with similar diagnostic findings on lumbar magnetic resonance imaging (degenerative disc disease, small annular tear) may have significantly different levels of pain and functional disability. One patient may complain of localized lumbar pain with minimal effect on daily activities. The other patient may be more impaired, reporting elevated pain scores and affective distress, functional decline, and disturbed nonrestorative sleep. Although functional restoration is a goal for both patients, the treatment approaches may differ drastically. In addition to a general understanding of pain as an individual experience, a general working knowledge of common clinically used pain terms is essential for appropriate assessment, documentation, and treatment (Table 6–1).

Rehabilitation professionals are frequently involved in the care of patients suffering from both acute and persistent pain conditions. For patients with acute pain result-

ing from discrete posttraumatic tissue injury or surgery, treatment may include a short course of physical or occupational therapy combined with oral pain medications. For patients complaining of persistent pain, coordinated, multidisciplinary assessment and management may be required.

THE REHABILITATION TEAM

The physiatrist plays a critical role in assessing and treating patients with acute and chronic pain and leads the team of health care professionals. Physical and occupational therapists are the principal members of the rehabilitation team; they help restore structure and function to injured patients suffering from painful conditions (Table 6–2). Physical and occupational therapists use passive and active exercises and passive modalities to guide patients through the process of recovery and rehabilitation. Targeted therapeutic exercises are used to address specific deficits in posture, flexibility, strength, balance, neuromuscular coordination, and endurance. Passive modalities such as cryotherapy, heat, and electrical stimulation are commonly used to address pain, alter tissue distensibility, and control inflammation (see Treatment section).

Occupational therapists focus on educating patients regarding proper posture and ergonomics related to functional activities. Family and caregiver education may be an additional component of the long-term rehabilitation program.

Pain psychologists focus on both cognitive and behavioral factors related to pain. A person's thoughts may impact mood, behavior, and function. Psychological intervention focuses on unlearning maladaptive responses and reactions to pain while fostering wellness, improving coping and perceived control, as well as decreasing catastrophic thoughts.

Therapeutic recreation therapists are important members of the rehabilitation team. They evaluate and plan leisure activities that serve to promote mental and physical health. Recreational therapists help patients establish and incorporate strategies learned from various disciplines of treatment into social and community functions. Application of these techniques (ie, correct biomechanics, pacing, relaxation techniques) leads to the reduction of stress, fear of movement, and depression

Table 6–1. Common Clinical Terms Used to Describe Pain.

Term	Description
Allodynia	Pain due to a stimulus that does not normally provoke pain
Analgesia	Absence of pain in response to stimulation that would normally be painful
Anesthesia dolorosa	Pain in an area or region that is anesthetic
Central pain	Pain initiated or caused by a primary lesion or dysfunction in the central nervous system
Dysesthesia	An unpleasant abnormal sensation, whether spontaneous or evoked
Hyperalgesia	An increased response to a stimulus that is normally painful
Hyperesthesia	Increased sensitivity to stimulation, excluding the special senses
Hyperpathia	A painful syndrome characterized by an abnormally painful reaction to a stimulus, especially a repetitive stimulus, as well as an increased threshold
Hypoalgesia	Diminished pain in response to a normally painful stimulus
Hypoesthesia	Decreased sensitivity to stimulation, excluding the special senses
Neuropathic pain	Pain initiated or caused by a primary lesion or dysfunction in the nervous system
Neuropathy	A disturbance of function or pathologic change in a nerve: in one nerve, mononeuropathy; in several nerves, mononeuropathy multiplex; if diffuse and bilateral, polyneuropathy
Nociceptor	A receptor preferentially sensitive to a noxious stimulus or to a stimulus that would become noxious if prolonged
Noxious stimulus	A noxious stimulus damages normal tissues
Pain threshold	The least experience of pain that a person can recognize (subjective experience of the individual)
Pain tolerance level	The greatest level of pain that a person is prepared to tolerate (subjective experience of the individual)
Paresthesia	An abnormal sensation, whether spontaneous or evoked
Peripheral neuropathic pain	Pain initiated or caused by a primary lesion or dysfunction in the peripheral nervous system

Reprinted, with permission, from Classification of Chronic Pain, 2nd ed. IASP Task Force on Taxonomy. Merskey H, Bogduk N (editors). IASP Press, Seattle. 1994:209–214.

while fostering a feeling of self-efficacy and confidence. In addition, therapeutic recreation therapists facilitate the recovery of motor function and reasoning skills, increase social awareness, and promote integration of patients with disabilities back into the community.

REHABILITATION FRAMEWORK

Acute Pain

In cases of acute pain, in which the type of injury has been accurately determined, the rehabilitation plan progresses through three major stages as the injury heals: acute, recovery, and functional (Table 6–3). The framework for rehabilitation is intimately related to the injury cycle. The injury cycle comprises the following categories: method of presentation, clinical symptom complex, tissue overload complex, functional biomechanical deficit complex, and subclinical adaptation complex. While this rehabili-

tation framework is commonly applied to sports injuries, it is applicable to general acute musculoskeletal injuries (such as shoulder impingement syndrome and discogenic low back pain with radicular leg pain) sustained by nonathletes.

Care must be taken to ensure that the focus is not principally applied to the acute stage of rehabilitation, in which the patient is experiencing acute pain from the tissue injury complex. Failure to remain dedicated to the recovery and functional stages of rehabilitation may lead to maladapted biomechanical alterations and continuation of the injury cycle, resulting in chronic injury and persistent pain conditions.

Chronic Pain

Multidisciplinary functional restoration programs based on cognitive and behavioral principles have been increasingly used in the treatment of patients with

Table 6–2. Rehabilitation Professionals and Their Areas of Expertise.

Therapist	Areas of expertise
Physical	Cervical spine Lumbar spine Lower extremity Upper extremity (large joint) Gait analysis and training Lower extremity bracing Provide adaptive equipment Instruct family and caregivers
Occupational	Upper extremity (large and small joint) Fine motor skills Vision Memory and reasoning skills ADL evaluation and training Work site evaluation Fabrication of upper extremity splints Provide adaptive equipment Instruct family and caregivers
Recreational	Evaluation and application of leisure interests Group or individual based therapy Community reintegration and function Encourage functional independence Pacing during activities Relaxation strategies Use of adaptive equipment

Table 6–3. The Three Stages of Rehabilitation for Musculoskeletal Injury.

ACUTE

Treatment focus
  Clinical symptom complex
  Tissue injury complex

Tools
  Rest or immobilization, or both
  Physical modalities
  Medications
  Manual therapy
  Initial exercise
  Surgery

Criteria for advancement
  Pain control
  Adequate tissue healing
  Near-normal range of motion
  Tolerance for strengthening

RECOVERY

Treatment focus
  Tissue overload complex
  Functional biomechanical deficit complex

Tools
  Manual therapy
  Flexibility
  Proprioception/neuromuscular control training
  Specific, progressive exercise

Criteria for advancement
  No pain
  Complete tissue healing
  Essentially full, pain-free range of motion
  Good flexibility
  75–80% or greater strength compared with uninjured side
  Good strength balance

FUNCTIONAL

Treatment focus
  Functional biomechanical deficit complex
  Subclinical adaptation complex

Tools
  Power and endurance exercises
  Sports or activity-specific functional progression
  Technique/skills instruction

Criteria for return to play/previous recreational activity/activities of daily living
  No pain
  Full, pain-free range of motion/normal flexibility
  Normal strength and strength balance
  Good general fitness
  Normal sports/activity mechanics
  Demonstration of sport- or activity-related skills

chronic pain and related psychosocial dysfunction. Members of these comprehensive teams include physiatrists; physical, occupational, and recreational therapists; pain psychologists; biofeedback specialists; social workers; nursing educators; and vocational counselors (Table 6–4). These comprehensive programs have shown clear benefits over conventional management in regard to decreasing pain behavior, improving mood, and restoring function. Scope and intensity varies, with most outpatient-based centers offering part time (2 days per week) or full-time (5 days per week, 6–8 hours per day) programs lasting 4–6 weeks. Goals of treatment include reduction in pain, maximal restoration of function, return to leisure activities, reduction in medication and health care resources, return to work, and possible vocational retraining.

Frontera WR. Exercise and musculoskeletal rehabilitation: restoring optimal form and function. *Phys Sports Med.* 2003;31(12):39.

Turner-Stokes L et al. Outpatient cognitive behavioral pain management programs: a randomized comparison of a group-based multidisciplinary versus an individual therapy model. *Arch Phys Med Rehabil.* 2003;84:781. [PMID: 12808527]

Kibler WB et al. Functional rehabilitation of sports and musculoskeletal injuries. Aspen Publishers. 1998.

Table 6–4. Members of a Comprehensive Multidisciplinary Pain Treatment Team.

Physiatrist
Physical therapist
Occupational therapist
Pain psychologist
Biofeedback and relaxation training specialist
Therapeutic recreation therapist
Social worker
Vocational counselor
Nurse facilitator/educator

■ ASSESSMENT

The diverse nature of any pain condition requires a comprehensive assessment in order to direct a tailored treatment plan. Identification of the injury type and method of presentation is the first step in the treatment of pain and rehabilitation of injury, since appreciably different approaches may be required for successful intervention. Understanding the injury cycle will help facilitate this process (see above section Rehabilitation Framework).

Injuries are typically classified as acute, subclinical adaptation to repetitive activity, chronic, or acute exacerbation of chronic injury. Table 6–5 compares acute and chronic pain. Most acute musculoskeletal injuries are generally identified and successfully treated before they progress to a subacute or chronic phase. Acute pain generally results from posttraumatic injuries, such as muscle strain, ligament sprain, muscular contusion, or fracture.

Subclinical adaptation to repetitive activity is a type of injury that may not produce significant symptoms in patients but should be identified and addressed in order to avoid future injury. Adaptations include postural abnormalities, joint contractures, and muscle weakness. For example, many athletes who throw a ball overhand display strength imbalances (weak external rotators) and alterations in flexibility (glenohumeral internal rotation deficit) before seeking medical attention for shoulder pain. Functional exercises to address these biomechanical abnormalities may decrease the risk of future rotator cuff injury.

The assessment and treatment of patients with chronic pain complaints is much more complex. In many cases, chronic pain is not a simple biomedical problem, and isolated unimodal medical and surgical treatment interventions may be unsuccessful. Since complete alleviation of pain is usually not possible, treatment strategies must focus on functional restoration and psychosocial distress.

Therefore, the practitioner should use a comprehensive assessment that focuses on functional impairments

Table 6–5. Comparison of Acute and Chronic Pain.

Acute pain	Chronic pain
Result of acute macrotrauma	Result of microtrauma, secondary adaptions with injury to other tissues
Focused diagnosis	Complex diagnosis
Responds to biomedical treatment model	Requires biopsychosocial assessment and management model
Minimal psychosocial interference	Comorbid depression, anxiety, avoidance behavior, maladaptive cognitions
Medications target pain and inflammation	Multimodal pharmacologic treatment addresses pain, affective distress, and disturbed sleep
NSAIDs, nonopioid and opioid analgesics, muscle relaxants	Nonopioid analgesics, judicious use of opioids, antidepressants, anticonvulsants
Low addiction risk	Polyaddiction risk
Complete resolution of pain likely	"Cure" unlikely; adjust expectations to management with reduced pain levels
Focused functional rehabilitation approach	Multidisciplinary approach incorporating functional restoration and cognitive behavioral interventions

NSAIDs, nonsteroidal anti-inflammatory drugs.

Table 6–6. General Psychosocial Screening Tools.

Category	Screening tool
Psychosocial history	Comprehensive pain questionnaire CAGE questionnaire Michigan Alcoholism Screening Test (MAST) Self-Administered Alcohol Screening Test (SAAST) Structured Clinical Interview for DSM-IV (SCID)
Pain intensity	Numerical rating scales (NRS) Visual analogue scales (VAS) Verbal rating scales (VRS) Pain drawings
Mood and personality	Minnesota Multiphasic Personality Inventory (MMPI) Symptom Checklist 90 (SCL-90) Millon Behavioral Health Inventory (MBHI) Beck Depression Inventory (BDI) McGill Pain Questionnaire (MPQ) Jung-Myers-Briggs Typology Test
Functional capacity	Sickness Impact Profile (SIP) Short Form Health Survey (SF-36) Multidimensional Pain Inventory (MPI) Pain Disability Index (PDI)
Pain beliefs and coping	Coping Strategies Questionnaire Pain Management Inventory (PMI) Pain Self-Efficacy Questionnaire (PSEQ) Survey of Pain Attitudes (SOPA) Inventory of Negative Thought in Response to Pain (INTRP)

of the musculoskeletal system as well as appropriate psychosocial screening tools (Table 6–6). In addition to the standard components of the physical examination (Table 6–7), the physiatric assessment includes the directed examination of the suspected tissue injury complex, a comprehensive functional kinetic chain evaluation, and identification of postural imbalances.

Observation of **pain behavior** is an important part of the multidimensional assessment. Pain behaviors include verbal complaints (eg, moaning), motor behaviors (eg, guarding affected body part, limping), and help seeking (eg, requesting medications and rest). Pain behaviors serve to communicate to others the pain and suffering that is being experienced and is based on contingencies of positive and negative reinforcement.

Selection of appropriate psychosocial tools may be patient specific. For the young, athletic patient with an obvious acute musculoskeletal injury due to macrotrauma (ie, ankle sprain), the use of a visual analogue scale and pain drawing may be sufficient when combined with social history, medical and surgical histories, medication history, and general review of systems. Alternatively, a more in-depth psychological assessment may be required for a 35-year-old physical laborer who has had several episodes of back pain over the course of 1 year, who reports depression and increased fear of reinjury, who has poor compliance with his active home exercise program, and who requests early refills for pain medication.

Table 6–7. Comprehensive Physical Assessment.

Pain behavior
Postural abnormalities
Gait assessment
Motor strength
Muscle stretch reflexes
Range of motion
Sensory exam
Soft tissue assessment

Hills CE. Adult physiatric history and examination. eMedicine.com 2003. http://www.emedicine.com/pmr/ topic146.htm.
International Association for the Study of Pain IASP Pain

Terminology http://www.iasp-pain.org/terms-p.html

Keefe FJ et al. Psychological aspects of persistent pain: current state of the science. *J Pain.* 2004;5:195. [PMID: 15162342]

Kibler WB. A framework for sports medicine. *Phys Med Rehabil Clin North Am.* 1994;5:1–8.

Stanos SP, Muellner PM, Harden RN. The physiatric approach to low back pain. *Semin Pain Med.* 2004;2:186–196.

Turk DC et al. Psychological factors in chronic pain: evolution and revolution. *J Consult Clin Psych.* 2002;70:678. [PMID: 12090376]

■ TREATMENT

PASSIVE PHYSICAL MODALITIES

Physical modalities are an integral part of the management and rehabilitation of both acute and persistent pain conditions. A **modality** is a physical agent used to produce a physiologic response in a targeted tissue. Commonly prescribed passive physical modalities for the treatment of acute and chronic pain include cryotherapy, heat, and electrical stimulation. Modalities are initially incorporated into therapy sessions by physical or occupational therapists, with a goal of educating the patient on appropriate application and use at home. Depending on the specific pain complaint, modalities may be used as part of a daily treatment regimen (cryotherapy for osteoarthritic knee after exercise, electrical stimulation for low back pain resulting from prolonged upright postures) or as a rescue treatment for flare-ups.

Cryotherapy

A. PHYSIOLOGY

Most forms of cryotherapy (eg, ice, cold packs, cold whirlpool baths, cryotherapy-compression units, vapocoolant spray) provide transfer of thermal energy by conduction, with the exception of vapocoolant sprays (evaporative cooling) and whirlpool baths (convective cooling). The physiologic effects of cold application include immediate vasoconstriction with reflexive vasodilation, decreased local metabolism and enzymatic activity, and decreased oxygen demand. Cold decreases muscle spindle fiber activity and slows nerve conduction velocity, therefore it is often used to decrease spasticity and muscle guarding.

B. PATIENT SELECTION

1. Indications—Because connective tissue stiffness and muscle viscosity are increased with cold application, cryotherapy should be used during the first 48 hours after a musculoskeletal injury. In addition, cryotherapy plays an important role in the management of many per-

Table 6–8. Indications for Cryotherapy.

Acute trauma
Edema
Hemorrhage
Pain (eg, osteoarthritis)
Muscle spasm
Spasticity
Reduction of metabolic activity

sistent pain problems such as osteoarthritis. Other indications include edema, hemorrhage, muscle spasm, spasticity, and reduction of metabolic activity (Table 6–8).

2. Contraindications—Cryotherapy should be avoided in patients with cryoglobulinemia, paroxysmal cold hemoglobinuria, cold hypersensitivity, ischemia, and Raynaud disease or phenomenon (Table 6–9).

3. Precaution—Cryotherapy may be considered in patients with arterial vascular disease, impaired sensation, cold intolerance, peripheral neuropathy, and cognitive deficits (ie, inability to report pain) but must be used cautiously (Table 6–9).

C. TECHNIQUE

Care must be taken when considering the application of cold therapy to areas overlying superficial nerves and areas of reduced or absent sensation. Cold application should not exceed 30 minutes, and peripheral nerves should be protected in the area of treatment. Cold packs and ice massage applied over 20 minutes have been shown to

Table 6–9. Contraindications and Precautions for Cryotherapy.

Contraindications
Cryoglobulinemia
Paroxysmal cold hemoglobinuria
Cold hypersensitivity
Ischemia
Raynaud disease or phenomenon
Precautions
Arterial vascular disease
Impaired sensation
Cold intolerance
Peripheral neuropathy
Cognitive deficits/inability to report pain

cool muscle by 4 to 5°C at a depth of 2 cm. Cryostretch and cryokinetics are approaches used by therapists to facilitate joint motion. By decreasing pain and muscle guarding, improvements in flexibility and function may be achieved.

D. COMPLICATIONS

Cryotherapy accounts for the majority of complications reported due to the use of passive physical modalities. The most common complications include local skin allergic reactions, burns, and intolerance. Other potential complications include exacerbation of Raynaud phenomenon, frostbite, and diaphoresis.

Heat

A. PHYSIOLOGY

Commonly used mechanisms of heat transfer include conduction, convection, and conversion. **Conduction** is the transfer of heat directly from one surface to another; examples include hydrocollator packs and paraffin baths. **Convection** is the transfer of heat due to movement of air or water across a body surface; examples include hydrotherapy and fluidotherapy. **Conversion** involves the transformation of energy to heat; examples include infrared lamps, electromagnetic microwaves, and most commonly ultrasound.

The heating of a structure results in both local and distant effects. Vasodilation, increased capillary permeability, and increased metabolic demands promote increased blood flow with the delivery of oxygen and leukocytes.

B. PATIENT SELECTION

1. Indications—Heat therapy is used to treat pain, contracture, hematoma, chronic inflammation, muscle spasm, and arthritis. It is also used to increase collagen extensibility before a stretching program (Table 6–10).

2. Contraindications—Avoid heat therapy under the following clinical circumstances: acute trauma and inflammation, hemorrhage, and bleeding diathesis (Table 6–11).

Table 6–10. Indications for Heat Therapy.

Pain
Contracture
Hematoma
Chronic inflammation
Muscle spasm
Increase collagen extensibility prior to stretching program
Arthritis

Table 6–11. Contraindications and Precautions for Heat Therapy.

Contraindications
Acute trauma and inflammation
Hemorrhage
Bleeding diathesis
Precautions
Impaired sensation
Altered thermal regulation (eg, spinal cord injury, traumatic brain injury, multiple sclerosis)
Malignancy
Ischemia
Atrophic or scarred skin
Cognitive deficits (ie, inability to report pain)

3. Precautions—Heat therapy may be considered in patients with impaired sensation, altered thermal regulation, malignancy, ischemia, atrophic or scarred skin, and cognitive deficits (inability to report pain) but should be used with caution.

C. BENEFITS

Heat therapy is beneficial for assisting with pain control, facilitating muscle relaxation, and promoting collagen extensibility.

D. TECHNIQUE

The heat modalities are generally classified as either superficial or deep.

1. Superficial heat—Direct heat penetration is greatest at a depth of 0.5 to 2 cm from the skin surface and depends on the amount of adipose tissue. The most commonly used superficial heat modalities for musculoskeletal rehabilitation include hydrocollator packs, hydrotherapy, paraffin baths, and fluidotherapy.

a. Hydrocollator packs—Available in three standard sizes and are heated in stainless steel containers in water at temperatures between 65 and 90°C. The highest temperatures found during the use of packs are at the surface of the skin. Towels are applied between the skin and pack to minimize skin trauma and maintain heat insulation. Common duration of treatment sessions ranges from 20 to 30 min.

b. Hydrotherapy—Treatment entails submerging small or large body surface areas. The risk of elevating core body temperature increases with the amount of surface area heated. Water temperature should not exceed 40°C for large body surfaces and 43°C when a limb is submerged. Hydrotherapy provides a gravity-eliminated environment that facilitates joint range of motion. Agitation provided by water flow provides sensory input.

c. Paraffin baths—A mixture of paraffin and mineral oil deliver heat to small joints such as those in the hand. Mineral oil creates a lower melting point for the paraffin, providing increased thermal release when compared with water. Temperatures are maintained at 52 to 58°C for upper limb applications and 45 to 52°C for lower limb treatments. Paraffin baths are contraindicated for patients with open wounds and severe peripheral vascular disease.

d. Fluidotherapy—This modality is dry heat therapy. It involves placing an extremity into a fluidotherapy unit in which Cellex medium (a dry powder of glass beads) is circulated using hot air, resulting in warm massage. Mechanical stimulation is thought to augment the heat for increased pain control.

2. Deep heat—The process of conversion is used to heat deep tissue structures. These modalities include ultrasound (most common), phonophoresis, and short wave and microwave diathermy.

a. Ultrasound (US)—Ultrasound therapy may be used in the treatment of contractures, tendinitis, degenerative arthritis, and subacute trauma (Table 6–12).

Ultrasound is defined as acoustic vibration with frequencies above the audible range of 20,000 Hz. The production of heat occurs by applying an electric current to a quartz crystal (or synthetic ceramic), which produces vibration at a specified frequency. The ultrasonic energy

Table 6–12. Indications and Precautions for Ultrasound Therapy.

Indications
Contractures (muscular, tendinous, capsular)
Tendinitis
Degenerative arthritis
Subacute trauma
Precautions
Malignancy
Open epiphysis
Pacemaker
Near spine, laminectomy site
Radiculopathy
Near brain, eyes, or reproductive organs
Pregnant or menstruating women
Arthroplasties, which often use methyl methacrylate or high-density polyethylene
General heat therapy precautions

is absorbed by the tissue and ultimately converted to heat. Selective heating is greatest when acoustic impedance is high, such as at the bone-muscle interface. Conversely, ultrasonic energy is readily conducted through homogeneous structures such as subcutaneous adipose or metal implants with minimal thermal effects due to rapid removal of heat energy.

Ultrasound can be used safely near metal implants. However, in the presence of methyl methacrylate and high-density polyethylene, which are often used in total joint replacements, a higher amount of ultrasound energy is absorbed, contributing to a potential for overheating (Table 6–12). Ultrasound can heat to depths of 5 cm below the skin surface, providing a therapeutic benefit to bone, joint capsule, tendon, ligament, and scar tissue.

In addition to thermal transfer, ultrasound produces other physiologic effects. Gaseous cavitation involves gas bubbles created by high frequency sound or turbulence, which may cause pressure changes within tissues leading to mechanical distortion, changes in cellular function, and cell death. Acoustic streaming causes movement of material due to pressure asymmetries produced by sound as it passes through the medium. Ultrasound physiology effects have the potential to creat plasma membrane damage and acceleration of metabolic processes. Standing waves are produced by superimposition of sound waves and can cause heating at tissue interfaces at different densities.

Ultrasound dosage is measured in W/cm^2. Intensities of 0.8 to 3.0 W/cm^2 are most commonly used. Application is started at approximately 0.5 W/cm^2 and gradually increased while the practitioner monitors patient response. Treatment duration of 5 to 10 min is common and is based on the size of treatment area.

b. Phonophoresis—Medication is delivered into the deeper layers of the skin using US. Phonophoresis is helpful in treating postinjury conditions (eg, dislocations, distortions of joints), pain caused by rheumatic diseases, and low back pain that has a neurologic origin (eg, root pain, discopathies).

c. Short wave and microwave diathermy—**Short wave diathermy** uses an oscillating electromagnetic field of high frequency to heat large areas of the body surface. It heats to a tissue depth of 2 to 3 cm. **Microwave diathermy** uses electromagnetic radiation by microwaves and heats to a greater tissue depth than short wave diathermy. It is particularly useful in heating tissues with high water content, such as muscles, subcutaneous fat, and fluid-filled cavities.

Electrical Stimulation

The most commonly applied electrical modalities in the treatment of pain include transcutaneous electrical nerve stimulation (TENS) and interferential current therapy (ICT). TENS and ICT involve the transmission of electrical energy to the peripheral nervous system via an external stimulator and conductive gel pads on the skin.

A. PHYSIOLOGY

There are multiple presumed mechanisms of action at the peripheral, spinal, and supraspinal levels. Stimulation of large myelinated fibers may block nociceptive transmission at the level of the spinothalamic tract cell bodies via stimulation of inhibitory interneurons (gate control theory). The three routes of neuromodulation include presynaptic inhibition of the spinal cord, direct inhibition of excited abnormally firing nerves, and facilitation of afferent input. Other postulated mechanisms of analgesia include direct peripheral effects of stimulation as well as increased release of endogenous opioids within the central nervous system with suppression of transmission and perception of noxious stimuli from the periphery. The indications for the use of TENS and ICT are similar, and the decision to use one form of electrical stimulation over another is largely based on clinical preference.

B. TECHNIQUE

1. TENS—This treatment is typically applied in two manners: low-intensity, high-frequency "conventional" TENS (1 to 2 mA, 50 to 100 Hz) and high-intensity, low-frequency "dense-disperse" TENS (15 to 20 mA, 1 to 5 Hz).

High-frequency TENS is used to achieve quick analgesia for acute pain states. Treatment duration is 1 to 20 minutes for rapid analgesia and 30 minutes to 2 hours for short analgesia. Treatment should occur as frequently as needed to maintain a pain free state. Adaptation com-

Table 6–13. Indications for Electrical Stimulation Therapy.

Rheumatoid and osteoarthritis pain
Myofascial pain
Dysmenorrhea
Visceral pain
Deafferentiated pain syndromes (phantom limb)
Sympathetically mediated pain
Tension headache
Acute postoperative pain
Raynaud disease
Ischemic pain
Urogenital dysfunction

Table 6–14. Contraindications and Precautions for Electrical Stimulation Therapy.

Contraindications
TENS and ICT
Demand-type cardiac pacemaker
Avoid carotid sinus, laryngeal or pharyngeal muscles, eyes, and mucosal membranes
Incompetent patients
Myocardial disease or arrhythmias without proper monitoring
ICT
Should not be used over rib-cage in children with small body mass
Arterial or venous thrombosis or thrombophlebitis
Abdominal, lumbosacral, or pelvic areas of pregnant women
Precautions
TENS
Safety during pregnancy has not been established
Skin irritation (avoid by rotating treatment area)
ICT
Skin irritation (avoid by rotating treatment area)
Can increase metabolism and may exacerbate fever, infection, tuberculosis, neoplasm
Avoid areas of extreme edema
Avoid open wounds

TENS, transcutaneous electrical nerve stimulation; ICT, interferential current therapy.

monly occurs, so an increase in amplitude or pulse width may be necessary to maintain paresthesia.

Low-frequency TENS is more commonly used for chronic pain conditions. Treatment times range from 30 minutes for slower analgesia effect to 2 to 6 hours for long duration analgesia. Adaptation is minimal and treatment frequency is typically once daily. TENS has shown beneficial effects in numerous conditions and has been shown to decrease the amount of analgesic medication needed after surgical procedures. Indications and precautions are summarized in Tables 6–13 and 6–14.

2. ICT—A variant of TENS, ICT involves the mixing of two unmodulated sine waves with different frequencies (one at 4 kHz, and a second within a variable range) to generate frequencies between 4 and 250 Hz. This allows for the stimulation of deeper tissues with decreased discomfort. The proposed mechanism of action involves the direct stimulation of muscle fibers, as opposed to nerve fibers, to achieve improved muscle blood flow and promotion of the healing process. Variable frequency helps prevent adaptation. Compared with TENS, there is less scientific evidence for the use of ICT. Indications and precautions are similar to those for TENS (Tables 6–13 and 6–14).

Brosseau L et al. Thermotherapy for treatment of osteoarthritis. *Cochrane Database Syst Rev.* 2003;(4):CD004522. [PMID: 14584019]

Cheing GLY et al. Analgesic effects of transcutaneous electrical nerve stimulation and interferential currents on heat pain in healthy subjects. *J Rehabil Med.* 2003;35:15. [PMID: 12610843]

Klein MJ. Deep heat. eMedicine. 2001 http://www.emedicine.com/pmr/topic203.htm

Klein MJ. Superficial heat and cold. eMedicine 2004. http://www.emedicine.com/pmr/topic201.htm

Nadler SF et al. Complications from therapeutic modalities: results of a national survey of athletic trainers. *Arch Phys Med Rehabil.* 2003;84:849. [PMID: 12808537]

ACTIVE ADJUNCTIVE THERAPIES

1. Mind-Body Techniques

Mind-body techniques play an important role in the management of persistent pain conditions and are often incorporated into comprehensive multidisciplinary treatment programs. Biofeedback is often used in acute pain conditions. For example, biofeedback training following surgery to repair the anterior cruciate ligament may help improve motor recruitment of the vastus medialis muscle in an attempt to improve patellofemoral joint stability and function. Patients can be trained in mind-body techniques by health care providers who are certified in the specific field or by licensed therapists (ie, physical, occupational, or recreational therapists and psychologists).

Biofeedback

A. PHYSIOLOGY

Biofeedback is most concisely defined by Olton and Noonberg as "any technique [that] increases the ability of a person to control voluntarily physiological activities by providing information about those activities." Common physiologic target responses include muscle tension, heart rate, blood pressure, skin temperature, and skin conductance. Through the use of specific instrumentation and computers, these physiologic responses are brought closer to conscious awareness and control by their conversion into auditory or visual feedback.

B. BENEFITS

The beneficial actions of biofeedback stem from the ability to decrease overall arousal and muscle tension, improve blood flow to tissue, and promote a generalized state of relaxation. The numerous clinical approaches described for biofeedback training apply equally to relaxation therapy and include diaphragmatic breathing, imagery, and autogenic training. Biofeedback has been shown to be effective in low back pain, upper extremity disorders, headache, temporomandibular disorders, and fibromyalgia. Regardless of the technique used, successful incorporation of relaxation techniques into a patient's treatment plan, offers the patient more active self-management tools. The techniques are applicable to daily self-management of chronic pain, as well as during more problematic periods of flare-ups.

Relaxation Therapy

A. PATIENT SELECTION

Patients with persistent pain and elevated levels of anxiety and related muscle tension may find relief in relaxation therapy.

B. BENEFITS

Relaxation therapies are easy to learn, use minimal health care resources, and have no side effects.

C. TECHNIQUE

The two chief methods of relaxation therapy are categorized as deep and brief. Deep methods include autogenic training and progressive muscle relaxation; brief methods include paced respiration and self-control relaxation.

1. Autogenic training—The patient imagines being in a peaceful place with pleasant body sensations. Breathing is centered and the pulse is regulated. The patient focuses on his or her body and attempts to make differing parts of the body feel heavy, warm, or cool.

2. Progressive muscle relaxation—The patient focuses on contracting and relaxing each of the major muscle groups in an attempt to better understand the feeling of tension, which can then facilitate subsequent relaxation.

3. Self-control meditation—This can be best described as a shortened form of progressive muscle relaxation (see above).

4. Paced respiration—The patient breathes slowly and deliberately for a specific time period.

5. Deep breathing—The patient takes a deep breath, holds it for 3 to 5 seconds, then slowly releases it. The sequences may be repeated several times to achieve a more relaxed state.

Meditation

Common forms of meditation include mindfulness meditation, transcendental meditation, yoga, and walking meditation.

A. Patient Selection

Patients with chronic pain can perform meditation daily to help maintain a basal level of pain control. It can also be useful in the management of flare-ups.

B. Technique

The ultimate goal is mind-body relaxation and the passive removal of harmful thought processes.

1. Mindfulness meditation—Involves the concentration on body sensations and thoughts that occur in the moment. The patient learns to observe these sensations and thoughts without judging them.

2. Yoga and walking meditation—Both are derived from Zen Buddhism and use controlled breathing and slow, deliberate movements and postures to focus the body and mind.

3. Transcendental meditation—Involves focusing on a sound or thought and the repetition of a word, mantra, or sound.

Guided Imagery

A. Patient Selection

Patients with persistent pain typically use guided imagery on a daily basis and may need to increase the number of sessions during acute pain flare-ups.

B. Technique

Guided imagery involves the generation of specific mental images with the goal of evoking a general psychophysiologic state of relaxation. Examples of these visualizations include imagining the immune system attacking cancer cells or the performance of specific daily activities without pain. The visualizations are initially directed by a practitioner, with the goal of eventual self-guidance.

Hypnosis

A. Patient Selection

Studies support the use of hypnosis in the treatment of patients with chronic pain, postoperative pain, anxiety, and tension headache.

B. Technique

Medical hypnosis involves an altered state of consciousness in which the patient assumes a state of heightened awareness and attentive focal concentration, with a relative decrease in peripheral awareness. The three main phases of hypnotherapy include presuggestion, suggestion, and postsuggestion.

The goal of the presuggestion phase is to achieve an altered state in which the patient is relaxed and the mind is susceptible to suggestion. Techniques include distraction, imagery, and relaxation therapy. During the suggestion phase, the practitioner introduces specific goals related to their pain state. The postsuggestion phase occurs when the patient returns to the normal state of consciousness and at this time may practice the new behaviors that were introduced in the suggestion phase.

Techniques used for pain relief include direct and indirect suggestion, interpersonal techniques, hypnoanesthesia, guided imagery, and regression to cause. Typical goals in the treatment of pain states include transformation, alteration or displacement of pain, directly addressing pain and suggesting it to decrease, and the ability of the patient to direct attention away from their pain.

Astin JA et al. Mind-body medicine: state of the science, implications for practice. *J Am Board Fam Pract.* 2003;16:131. [PMID: 12665179]

2. Movement-Based Therapy

Reduction of movement in acute pain is initially thought to serve as a protective function. With the development of chronic pain, reduced movement and guarding the affected extremity or body part serves no adaptive purpose and may contribute to ongoing disability and pain. Two important components are altered biomechanics (secondary to guarding) and fear avoidance behaviors. Guarding the affected limb may lead to compensatory postural imbalances, stressing related muscles and joints most commonly proximal to the original site of injury. These changes may cause an additional source of pain and contribute to a reduction in movement and loss of function.

Important maladaptive psychological aspect of chronic pain syndromes include fear avoidance behaviors and related elevated levels of anxiety. Fear avoidance behavior results in a cyclic cascade of reduced mobility and function. This reduced movement is likely to contribute to an overall decrease in range of motion, muscle strength, and aerobic fitness as well as heightened central nervous system functioning characterized by hypervigilance and increased autonomic arousal. Hypervigilance may predispose patients to attend more closely and self-monitor minor somatic events that would normally be ignored.

Movement-based therapies are instrumental in returning specific subsets of persistent pain patients to more active lifestyles. Through the use of low-level exercise therapies, patients can slowly reintroduce movement back into their lifestyle. These techniques improve balance and teach more efficient ways to use injured joints or muscles to offset loads; improve biomechanical function; and decrease pain, anxiety, and fear of movement or activity.

There are relatively few contraindications for the following movement-based therapies because programs are tailored to the individuals' abilities. Patients with severe osteoporosis or acute joint injuries or fractures should proceed with caution. Pregnant women, those with abdominal or inguinal hernias, and those recovering from recent abdominal surgery should avoid downward straining or holding prolonged postures. Less active patients who do not routinely exercise should avoid overworking when starting a movement-based therapy program. Potential risks include, but are not limited to, muscle soreness, muscle strains, ligament sprains, and back pain.

Yoga

The word yoga is derived from the Sanskrit "yug," which means "to join." The Indian sage Patanjali, who is considered the father of classical yoga philosophy, compiled the Yoga Sutra, a philosophical guidebook for the practice of yoga.

The Yoga Sutra describes the eight major branches of the philosophy:

1. Pranayama (breathing exercises)
2. Asana (physical postures)
3. Yama (moral behavior)
4. Niyama (healthy habit)
5. Dharana (concentration)
6. Pratyahara (sense withdrawal)
7. Dhyana (contemplation)
8. Samadhi (higher consciousness)

There are numerous variations of yoga that are currently practiced, each having different weightings of the eight branches.

A. BENEFITS

Through consistent practice, yoga programs have been reported to reduce blood pressure, heart rate, and anxiety while improving range of motion, muscular endurance, and lung capacity.

B. TECHNIQUE

At its root, yoga consists of the performance of various postures, stretches, and controlled breathing. Yoga can be practiced in groups or on an individual basis.

Tai-Chi

The origins of T'ai Chi Chuan, commonly referred to as Tai-chi, predate the seventeenth century. While T'ai Chi Chuan translates as "supreme ultimate boxing," the method incorporates both a Chinese martial art as well as a health regimen with a common set of principles and movements.

A. PATIENT SELECTION

Recently, Tai-chi has gained more focus in the Western world as a method to improve balance and well-being in various populations, including the elderly and the disabled.

B. BENEFITS

Studies evaluating short-term Tai-chi programs have reported improvements in balance, strength, flexibility, and overall quality of life as well as decreases in pain secondary to osteoarthritis, anxiety, depression, anger, and general pain perception.

Due to the slow, low impact nature of Tai-chi, it can be applied to all categories of pain conditions, especially those in which patients suffer from significant anxiety and fear-avoidance behaviors. Tai-chi aims to establish balance between the mind and the body.

C. TECHNIQUE

Tai-chi is known for its rhythmic, slow, coordinated, dance-like movement sequences performed with sharp mental focus.

Feldenkrais Method

The Feldenkrais method is a system of body retraining that was created by Moshe Feldenkrais, a physicist. The goal is to improve body awareness and psychological well-being through gentle stretching, reaching, and postural change sequences.

A. PATIENT SELECTION

The Feldenkrais method is an appropriate movement-based therapy for the physical rehabilitation of patients with acute or persistent pain.

B. TECHNIQUE

The two complementary components of the Feldenkrais method, awareness through movement and functional integration, may be practiced together or independently of each other. Both components attempt to achieve the same results of improved function, comfort, body awareness, anxiety reduction, and mood improvement.

1. Awareness through movement—Involves group-based sessions led by a Feldenkrais practitioner who guides patients through slow, sequenced movements that include normal activities of daily living as well as abstract

patterns. As patients improve body awareness, they are able to adjust and find patterns and motions of comfort that allow them to perform activities of daily living more efficiently and with reduced discomfort.

2. Functional integration—These sessions are private classes with the Feldenkrais practitioner. Sequenced movements are instructed with hands-on input and feedback from the practitioner, with the goal of finding functional, mechanically efficient ways to perform activities of daily living with less discomfort.

Alexander Technique

This method was developed in the late 1800s by F. M. Alexander, a Shakespearean orator who suffered from recurrent laryngitis. Through careful observation of himself, he realized that poor habitual patterns of posture and movement were the reason for his vocal dysfunction. Through committed reeducation of posture and movement, he was successfully able to solve his vocal problem. He later refined and developed his technique of identification and correction of biomechanical deficits to help others alter poor postural habits and detrimental movement patterns.

Instructors in the Alexander technique use verbal instructions and light touch to guide patients through various movements with the goal of correcting postural and biomechanical imbalances. The position of the head and spine is thought to be important in the determination of overall functioning, and recognition that when a change is made in one body part, the rest of the body is then affected. Through repetition of movements, functional benefits can be achieved through reeducation of mechanics.

Cotter AC. Western movement therapies. *Phys Med Rehabil Clin North Am.* 1999;10:603. [PMID: 10516980]

Garfinkel M et al. Yoga. *Rheum Dis Clin North Am.* 2000;26:125. [PMID: 10680200]

3. Aquatic Therapy

Aquatic therapy is generally provided by physical therapists, occupational therapists, or athletic trainers. Therapy prescriptions should include general safety precautions and one of three categories: "wet to dry" transition, "dry to wet" transition, or "wet only" therapy. Protocols generally are adapted to the functional level of the patient, and home aquatic-based exercise programs can be taught to patients and their caregivers.

A. PATIENT SELECTION

The physical properties of water allow it to be a plausible alternative medium for rehabilitation of selected patients.

While aquatic therapy has classically been promoted for patients with rheumatoid arthritis and osteoarthritis, patients with a wide range of functional impairments are now involved in water-based therapy. Diagnoses include, but are not limited to fibromyalgia, postorthopedic surgery, generalized deconditioning, multiple sclerosis, stroke survivors, and brain injury patients.

B. BENEFITS

The advantages of performing physical and occupational therapy in a pool-based environment are related to the buoyancy and viscosity provided by water. Due to the buoyant force of water, the effective weight of the patient is proportionally decreased as the depth increases. Weight-bearing loads are reduced to 40% of total body weight when standing in chest deep water. And, when floating, the effects of gravity are eliminated. Thus, therapy programs can introduce increased loads to tissue by gradually decreasing the depth at which therapy is performed.

The viscosity of water provides resistance to movement equal to that of the force exerted by the patient. This resistance also varies with the speed of movement performed.

In many cases, patients experience reduced levels of pain while performing passive and active range of motion as well as strengthening exercises in an aquatic environment. Patients can perform closed kinetic chain activities when pain or weight-bearing precautions prohibit land-based therapy. Other benefits include muscle relaxation, improved body awareness, cardiorespiratory fitness, balance, and coordination.

Prins J et al. Aquatic therapy in the rehabilitation of athletic injuries. *Clin Sports Med.* 1999;18:447. [PMID: 10230578]

MEDICATIONS

A complete review of the medications used in treating various pain states can be found in Chapter 3. In this section, the role of medication in the setting of rehabilitation of acute and chronic pain will be discussed briefly. A rational polypharmacologic approach focuses on analgesia, inflammation reduction, relief of muscle spasm, reduction of affective distress, and improved sleep. The scope of medication use may vary depending on chronicity and related medical conditions.

Drugs for Managing Acute Pain

Analgesia and reduction of related muscle spasm and guarding are critical initial steps in the treatment of acute musculoskeletal conditions. Effective use of medications and modalities during the acute phase of rehabilitation may facilitate achieving optimal functional recovery.

A. ANALGESIC DRUGS

Analgesia may be achieved through the judicious use of nonopioid analgesics, such as nonsteroidal anti-inflammatory drugs (NSAIDs), cyclooxygenase (COX-2) inhibitors, acetaminophen, opioid analgesics, muscle relaxants, and tricyclic antidepressants. Practitioners should not hesitate to prescribe a short course of opioid analgesics for acute pain conditions, especially during the acute phase of rehabilitation. Caution should be reserved for those patients with a history of prior substance addiction or abuse. Close monitoring of patients is necessary to avoid or detect adverse sequelae of analgesic medication therapy (ie, bleeding, ulcer, renal or hepatic injury).

B. ANTI-INFLAMMATORY DRUGS

NSAIDs are commonly prescribed medications for acute pain states involving musculoskeletal injury. The rationale stems from the analgesic and anti-inflammatory properties of NSAIDs. However, judicious use is recommended, since inflammation is a necessary component of the healing process during the acute phase of injury. Therefore, excessive reduction of inflammation may be undesirable. In addition, there is insufficient data to support the notion that NSAIDs provide any significant anti-inflammatory action in the setting of acute injury or postoperative swelling. The most significant benefit to patients is likely due to their analgesic properties. Modalities such as ice and compression may be more important in the reduction of edema during the acute phase of injury.

C. MUSCLE RELAXANT DRUGS

Reflex guarding of injured musculoskeletal structures is manifest as the production of local muscular spasm. Short-term use of muscle relaxants (metaxalone and methocarbamol), during the acute rehabilitation phase is appropriate when combined with analgesic medications. Nighttime dosing of more sedating agents (eg, cyclobenzaprine and tizanidine) may also help induce sleep. Prolonged benzodiazepine use is discouraged and may impair sleep architecture as well as lead to the development of tolerance and dependence.

Drugs for Managing Chronic Pain

Drug therapy is a critical component in the treatment of all persistent pain states. The importance of treatment targets may vary considerably from those in acute pain treatment paradigms. While acute pain treatment focuses on analgesia and inflammation control, medication therapy in persistent pain states may need a more comprehensive focus to include related affective distress (depression, anxiety, and anger) and disturbed sleep. A rational polypharmacy approach incorporates the use of various medications including newer generation and traditional antidepressants, anticonvulsants and sleep agents and, in more carefully selected cases, long-term opioid therapy.

Chronic pain-related depression may respond to a number of antidepressants. In general, tricyclic antidepressants help augment serotonin and norepinephrine levels in the brain and may offer both antidepressant and analgesic effects. More selective medications, such as selective serotonin reuptake inhibitors (SSRIs), may have better side-effect profiles but have demonstrated less promising analgesic effects. Tricyclic antidepressants may be taken at night in order to improve sleep and prescribed in conjunction with daily SSRIs for depression. Serotonin-norepinephrine reuptake inhibitors (SNRIs) (eg, venlafaxine and duloxetine) may also provide antidepressant and analgesic effects with less anticholinergic and cardiac side effects as tricyclic antidepressants.

The use of long-term opioid analgesic therapy in chronic pain management should incorporate the use of longer acting medications (sustained release oral medications and transdermal delivery systems) and a more judicious use of short-acting medications for breakthrough pain episodes. Steady serum levels with long-acting agents may help maintain consistent opioid serum levels offering a number of practical advantages including convenient dosing schedules, more sustained analgesia, and uninterrupted sleep, while limiting frequent episodes of breakthrough pain and over-reliance of excessive daily use of short-acting opioids.

Control of inflammation may be less important in the treatment of chronic pain. Numerous studies have shown that chronic musculoskeletal injuries such as those involving the extensor carpi radialis brevis, Achilles tendon, patellar tendon, and rotator cuff tendons have minimal inflammatory properties. Biopsies reveal degeneration and the lack of inflammatory cells. Thus, the long-term use of NSAIDs in these conditions are not recommended, and the benefit in pain reduction is likely through the analgesic properties of NSAIDs. Long-term NSAID and COX-2 inhibitor (celecoxib) therapy may decrease the pain and joint stiffness associated with chronic osteoarthritis pain conditions. Recent reports of cardiac and renal effects associated with long-term use of COX-2 inhibitors may limit their use in this population. Careful patient selection and consideration of comorbid medical conditions may need to be considered.

Curatolo M et al. Pharmacologic pain treatment of musculoskeletal disorders: current perspectives and future prospects. *Clin J Pain.* 2001;17:25. [PMID: 11289086]

Stovitz SD et al. NSAIDs and musculoskeletal treatment. What is the clinical evidence? *Phys Sports Med.* 2003;31:35.

Worsowicz GM et al. Rehabilitative management of pain. *Arch Phys Med Rehab.* 1998;79:S60.

PAIN CONCERNS IN SELECTED REHABILITATION CONDITIONS

Acute and chronic pain are common comorbidities in rehabilitation patients. It has been speculated that patients with disabilities may be at higher risk for developing persistent pain states when compared with the general population. The following section highlights some basic issues to consider when managing pain in these specific groups.

STROKE

Common pain conditions in stroke survivors include hemiplegic shoulder pain (38 to 84%) and central poststroke pain (2 to 8%). Hemiplegic shoulder pain is usually musculoskeletal in nature and may be secondary to subacromial impingement syndrome, glenohumeral subluxation, and adhesive capsulitis. Other causes of shoulder pain include myofascial pain, spasticity, and complex regional pain syndrome (formerly called reflex sympathetic dystrophy).

Careful examination is critical because myofascial pain and central poststroke pain can mimic or present concurrently with pure musculoskeletal etiologies of shoulder pain. Musculoskeletal pain complaints in stroke survivors appear to be less common in patients with longer poststroke duration, and symptoms are typically aggravated by passive and active movements of the affected limb. Treatment of musculoskeletal shoulder pain involves taping or bracing for joint positioning, physical therapy for range of motion, stretching and scapular stabilization, and oral analgesic medications. Effective treatment of related myofascial pain in proximal muscle groups may help differentiate true musculoskeletal shoulder pain and guide appropriate treatment. Spasticity is managed by bracing, oral medications, and local botulinum toxin injections to the affected muscles.

More debilitating central poststroke pain can occur from months to years after stroke. It appears to be a deafferentation syndrome due to damage associated with spinothalamocortical pathways, usually accompanied by pain and temperature sensory deficits. Pain is typically constant and can affect the entire hemiparetic side. Treatment includes oral anticonvulsant medications, deep brain or motor cortex stimulation, and TENS.

SPINAL CORD INJURY

The disability caused by spinal cord injury varies significantly. Functional disability is related to the level as well as the completeness of the injury sustained. Patients with spinal cord injury typically suffer from both neuropathic and musculoskeletal pain. Neuropathic pain is common at the level of the injury (transitional zone pain) as well as below the level of the injury. Musculoskeletal pain commonly occurs above the injury. Estimates of the prevalence of chronic pain have been reported as high as 94%.

The most common pain sites include hip and buttock region, legs and feet, shoulder, arm and hand, and transitional zone. Musculoskeletal pain is common in the upper extremities and tends to increase with age. Overuse injury to the scapular stabilizers and rotator cuff musculature occurs with wheelchair usage, reliance on upper extremities for transfers, as well as other activities of daily living. This is especially true for patients with low cervical lesions, since they may suffer from more significant muscular imbalances in the scapulothoracic and glenohumeral joints.

Treatment for pain in spinal cord injury is relatively empiric. Shoulder pain typically benefits from scapular stabilization exercises, kinesiotaping, massage, heat modalities, and drug therapy. Related myofascial pain may respond to local injections and active strengthening programs. Treatment of central pain is challenging. Primary strategies consist of oral anticonvulsant and antidepressant medications as well as more comprehensive multidisciplinary treatment programs. Long-term opioid therapy, spinal cord stimulation, and surgical procedures such as dorsal root entry zone lesioning may be of benefit in selected cases.

AMPUTATION

Amputee patients suffer from various types of both acute and chronic pain. As with spinal cord injury, the pain can be both neuropathic and musculoskeletal in nature. In addition to postoperative pain in the residual limb, a large number of patients experience residual limb pain long after the amputation has healed. Up to 85% of amputee patients experience phantom limb pain, which manifests as sharp, tingling, shooting, and stabbing pain in the portion of the limb that was amputated. This must be distinguished from phantom limb sensation, which is not painful and typically does not interfere with normal activities of daily living. In addition to pain directly related to the amputation site, many patients (up to 71%) develop back pain due to inactivity and alteration in biomechanics of ambulation. Upper extremity pain can result from excessive wheelchair locomotion or ambulation with an assistive device. These secondary pain etiologies may interfere more with activities of daily living than phantom limb pain or residual limb pain.

Treatment strategies for amputee patients are geared toward the type of pain experienced. Musculoskeletal pain complaints are best addressed with physical therapy, passive physical modalities, and oral analgesics. While there is minimal literature that describes successful treatments for phantom limb pain, antidepressants and anticonvulsants are the most commonly used oral medications. A current focus on more aggressive perioperative pain management, including preemptive analgesia, as a strategy for prevention of phantom limb pain has revealed inconsistent results.

MULTIPLE SCLEROSIS

Acute and chronic pain are both possible sequelae of multiple sclerosis, occurring in 53 to 82% of affected patients. Acute pain is typically neuropathic in nature and can occur during a multiple sclerosis exacerbation as a result of active inflammatory processes. Chronic pain accounts for approximately 90% of cases. It may be neuropathic or musculoskeletal and presents with symptoms dependent on the location of the lesions. Paresthesias and Lhermitte sign are reported to occur with lesions located in the dorsal horn, while trigeminal neuralgia has been associated with lesions in the trigeminal entry zone in the brainstem. Demyelination in the brainstem or spinal cord can lead to muscle spasms that cause painful cramping. Lesions affecting the corticospinal, corticobulbar, or bulbospinal tracts can lead to spasticity with subsequent biomechanic and postural abnormalities resulting in back and extremity pain.

While there are few controlled clinical trials in the treatment of multiple sclerosis–related pain, there are a number of commonly addressed treatment targets. Newer generation anticonvulsant medications such as gabapentin, lamotrigine, oxcarbazepine, tiagabine, topiramate, and zonisamide are routinely prescribed "off-label" for neuropathic pain complaints. Spasticity is managed by both medication and therapy. Oral medications for spasticity management include baclofen, dantrolene, tizanidine, and diazepam. Injection therapies include botulinum toxin into muscle and phenol nerve blocks. They may be used independently or in conjunction with active physical therapy and bracing. Physical and occupational therapy is used to address spasticity and other biomechanical deficits related to abnormal positioning.

Ehde DM et al. Chronic pain secondary to disability: a review. *Clin J Pain.* 2003;19:3. [PMID: 12514452]

Jensen MP et al. Pain site and the effects of amputation pain: further clarification of the meaning of mild, moderate, and severe pain. *Pain.* 2001;91:317. [PMID: 11275389]

Kong KH et al. Prevalence of chronic pain and its impact on health-related quality of life in stroke survivors. *Arch Phys Med Rehabil.* 2004;85:35. [PMID: 14970965]

Lidbeck J. Central hyperexcitability in chronic musculoskeletal pain: A conceptual breakthrough with multiple clinical implications. *Pain Res Manage.* 2002;7:81. [PMID: 12185372]

Siddall PJ et al. Pain report and the relationship of pain to physical factors in the first 6 months following spinal cord injury. *Pain.* 1999;81:187. [PMID: 10353507]

Pain & Addictive Disease

7

Steven D. Passik, PhD, Kenneth L. Kirsh, PhD, & Russell K. Portenoy, MD

Addiction and drug abuse are very common in the United States; 6 to 10% of the population abuses illicit drugs, 15% abuse alcohol, 25% are addicted to nicotine, and 33% of the population samples illicit drugs at least once. Because substance abuse is a risk factor for some sources of chronic pain, these problems will inevitably be seen in a sizable number of patients with chronic pain. There is no reason to believe that abuse rates would be any lower in patients with chronic pain than in the general population.

Given this notion, there is an interesting phenomenon concerning the perception of opioid medications both in the United States and within the health care system. Some members of the medical community (in general, specialists in addiction) consider opioids to be a major cause of abuse, associated with dire consequences to the individual and society at large; whereas, others (usually pain specialists) view opioids as essential medications to relieve pain and suffering. Given the opposing nature of these perspectives, it is not surprising that historically there has been little communication between these two groups.

The Traditional Addiction Specialist Perspective

Specialists in addiction have defined such terms as "tolerance" and "dependence," which are useful in nonpain settings. However, such terminology fails to address the meaning and manifestation of these phenomenon in patients treated with analgesics for painful medical disease. The perspective of addiction specialists is also based on seeing patients who have typically started opioid medications or been exposed to them solely for the purposes of recreational use. In addition, many (if not all) of these patients are vulnerable to the medications, and the addiction specialist is likely to only see the negative consequences of opioids, which can also foster the sense of these medications as being a "gateway" to illicit drug use. Thus, it is typical for these specialists to believe that exposure to the drugs will cause addiction.

The Traditional Pain Specialist Perspective

Pain management professionals have cycled through various stages in their beliefs regarding the abuse potential of opioids. The old mythology stated that addiction was so fearsome and unavoidable that opioids should be withheld until patients were close to death. Luckily, a revolution in pain management, along with the use of opioids that began in oncology and spread to pain of all types, showed that this perception was false. But this myth has been replaced by another, which suggests that patients with chronic pain are somehow immune to problems of aberrant drug-taking, abuse, or diversion. These conclusions were erroneously based on questionable data, such as in the Boston Collaborative Drug Surveillance Project. In that study, the authors evaluated 11,882 inpatients who had no prior history of addiction and were administered an opioid while hospitalized; only four cases of addiction could be identified subsequently. The study focused on treatment of acute pain and was not concerned with chronic pain issues; it must be noted that the Boston Collaborative Drug Surveillance Project was not a developed study but merely a letter to the editor that well-intending professionals used as a rationale to treat more chronic pain with opioids. The potential for opioid addiction is a constant consideration in the management of acute and chronic pain; however, the criteria that define this outcome or the factors that may contribute to it are not well understood.

Thus, there has been a natural divide between these two sets of professionals. However, due to the increased media coverage of the growing abuse of prescription drugs, a new level of discourse has begun. The interaction between pain and addiction specialists has led to the beginning of a shared knowledge that enhances each other's ability to comprehend clinical phenomena and formulate questions for research.

This chapter brings together these two perspectives through an examination of the issues raised by each of two situations commonly encountered in clinical practice: the management of pain in patients with a history of opioid abuse, and the risk of opioid abuse in patients with no such history who are given opioid drugs for medical purposes. Throughout this text, an effort is made to balance the clinical imperative to provide adequate relief of pain with legitimate concerns about the consequences of opioid abuse. Opioids are the focus of this discussion because they have a unique position as both major analgesics and drugs of abuse, and thereby encourage a comprehensive examination of the issues. It should be noted, however, that many of the topics explored herein

78

apply equally to other drug classes, such as the use of benzodiazepines for anxiety and other disorders.

Redefining Abuse & Addiction

Both epidemiologic studies and clinical management depend on an accepted, valid nomenclature for substance abuse and addiction. Unfortunately, this terminology is highly problematic as the pharmacologic phenomena of tolerance and physical dependence are commonly confused with abuse and addiction, as well as sociocultural considerations, which may lead to mixed messages in the clinical setting. The clarification of this terminology is an essential step in improving the diagnosis and management of substance abuse.

A. TOLERANCE

Tolerance, a pharmacologic property defined by the need for increasing doses to maintain effects, has been a particular concern during opioid therapy. Clinicians and patients both commonly express concerns that tolerance to analgesic effects may compromise the benefits of therapy and lead to the requirement of progressively higher, and ultimately unsustainable, doses. In addition, the development of tolerance to the reinforcing effects of opioids, and the consequent need to increase doses to regain these effects, has been speculated to be an important element in the pathogenesis of addiction. Notwithstanding these concerns, an extensive clinical experience with opioid drugs in the medical context has not confirmed that tolerance causes substantial problems. Thus, unlike tolerance to the side effects of the opioids, clinically meaningful analgesic tolerance appears to be a rare phenomenon and is rarely the cause for dose escalation.

Clinical observation also fails to support the conclusion that analgesic tolerance is a substantial contributor to the development of addiction. It is widely accepted that addicts without a medical disorder may or may not have any of the manifestations of analgesic tolerance. Occasionally, a patient treated with opioids may show signs of analgesic tolerance but typically does not show signs of abuse or addiction.

B. PHYSICAL DEPENDENCE

Physical dependence is defined solely by the occurrence of a withdrawal syndrome following abrupt dose reduction or administration of an antagonist. Neither the dose nor duration of administration required to produce clinically significant physical dependence in humans is known. Most practitioners assume that the potential for withdrawal exists after opioids have been administered repeatedly for only a few days.

There is great confusion among clinicians about the differences between physical dependence and addiction. Physical dependence, like tolerance, has been suggested to be a component of addiction, and the avoidance of withdrawal has been postulated to create behavioral contingencies that reinforce drug-seeking behavior. These speculations, however, are not supported by experience acquired during opioid therapy for chronic pain. Physical dependence does not preclude the uncomplicated discontinuation of opioids during multidisciplinary pain management of nonmalignant pain, and opioid therapy is routinely stopped without difficulty in patients with cancer whose pain disappears following effective antineoplastic therapy. Furthermore, indirect evidence for a fundamental distinction between physical dependence and addiction is provided by animal models of opioid self-administration, which have demonstrated that persistent drug-taking behavior can be maintained in the absence of physical dependence.

New Definitions of Abuse & Addiction for the Medically Ill

A. ABUSE

Various definitions of abuse that include the phenomena related to physical dependence or tolerance are not applicable to patients who receive potentially abusable drugs for legitimate medical purposes. A differential diagnosis should be explored if questionable behaviors occur during pain treatment (Table 7–1). A true addiction is only one of several possible explanations but is more likely when behaviors such as multiple unsanctioned dose escalations and obtaining opioids from multiple prescribers occur.

The diagnosis of pseudoaddiction must also be considered if the patient is reporting distress related to unrelieved symptoms. Behaviors such as aggressively complaining about the need for higher doses or occasional unilateral drug escalations may be indications that the patient's pain is undermedicated. Clearly, the diagnosis of addiction is not tenable if pain control eliminates behaviors that would otherwise be considered to reflect loss of control, compulsive use, and continued use despite harm. Aberrant drug-related behaviors may not be infrequent occurrences in the treatment of nonmalignant pain.

Table 7–1. Differential Diagnosis of Aberrant Drug-Taking Attitudes and Behavior.

- Addiction
- Pseudoaddiction (inadequate analgesic)
- Other psychiatric diagnoses
  - Chemical coping
  - Encephalopathy
  - Borderline personality disorder
  - Depression
  - Anxiety
- Criminal intent

Impulsive drug use may also indicate the existence of another psychiatric disorder, the diagnosis of which may have therapeutic implications. For example, patients with borderline personality disorders may be categorized as exhibiting aberrant drug-taking behaviors if they are using prescription medications to express fear and anger or improve chronic boredom. Similarly, patients who use opioids to self-medicate symptoms of anxiety or depression, insomnia, or problems of adjustment may be classified as aberrant drug takers. Occasionally, aberrant drug-related behaviors appear to be causally related to mild encephalopathy, with confusion regarding the appropriate therapeutic regimen. Problematic behaviors rarely imply criminal intent such as when patients report pain but intend to sell or divert medications. These diagnoses are not mutually exclusive and a thorough psychiatric assessment is vitally important in an effort to categorize questionable behaviors properly in both the population without a prior history of substance abuse and the population of known substance abusers who have a higher incidence of psychiatric comorbidity.

B. Addiction

Until recently, all accepted definitions applied to the assessment of addiction had been developed by addiction specialists. These definitions emphasize that addiction is a psychological and behavioral syndrome in which there is drug craving, compulsive use, a strong tendency to relapse after withdrawal, and continued use despite harm to the user or those around him or her. Some of these definitions highlight the development of tolerance or physical dependence in the development of addiction. Although widely accepted, the specifics must be interpreted cautiously if the drug of abuse may be a legitimate therapy for a medical disorder.

According to a recent definition jointly endorsed by professional societies for pain and addiction in the United States, "addiction is a primary, chronic, neurobiologic disease, with genetic, psychosocial, and environmental factors. . . . It is characterized by behaviors that include one or more of the following: impaired control over drug use, compulsive use, continued use despite harm, and craving." This definition does not reference phenomena related to tolerance or physical dependence but rather, focuses on behavior as the relevant assessment for the diagnosis of addiction. Craving may involve rumination about the drug and an intense desire to secure its supply. Compulsive use may be indicated by persistent or escalating consumption of the drug despite physical, psychological, or social harm to the user.

Categories of Substance Abusers

Patients with a history of opioid abuse can be divided into three categories that may predict some of the problems encountered during pain treatment; these categories include the following:

1. Patients with a remote history of opioid substance abuse.
2. Patients with a history of opioid abuse who are currently undergoing methadone maintenance treatment.
3. Patients actively abusing opioid drugs.

Other relevant groups may include those with a remote or present history of addiction to alcohol, nonopioid illicit drugs (eg, cocaine), or nonopioid prescription drugs (eg, benzodiazepines). These distinctions help identify patients at risk for management problems, and this, in turn, may facilitate the assessment process and suggest approaches to therapy.

Unfortunately, there have been no adequate studies to confirm the existence of meaningful differences among these groups or specifically assess the needs and problems posed by each during therapy for pain. Case reports have been helpful in defining the range of concerns and have been particularly useful in highlighting the observation that even a remote history of abuse can stigmatize a patient and complicate pain treatment. Nonetheless, generalizations developed from clinical experience may fail to prepare the clinician for the vagaries of practice, where the experience of pain itself, or other facets of the disease causing the pain, may alter responses in an unpredictable way. They cannot substitute for a comprehensive assessment of each case.

Principles of Pain Assessment

An optimal approach to therapy depends on a comprehensive assessment that clarifies the organic and psychological contributions to the pain and characterizes associated problems that may also require treatment. These associated problems may themselves be medical, psychological (including disorders of personality or affect or profound behavioral disturbances), social, or familial. A history of substance abuse is one such consideration.

Categories of Patients with Pain

Patients with pain can be categorized in several clinically meaningful ways. Some distinctions are particularly relevant to the selection of treatment approaches.

First, patients may be deemed to have acute monophasic pain. These are the most common pains and are acute and self-limited. Most are never evaluated by physicians and demand no therapy beyond simple measures taken by the individual, although some may require clinical intervention. Notwithstanding data documenting the frequent undertreatment of these syndromes, the short-term administration of opioid drugs is widely considered to be medically appropriate treatment for acute severe pain.

The second category, recurrent acute pain, is also extremely prevalent. These disorders also range in severity and need for clinical intervention (eg, headache, dysmenorrhea, sickle cell anemia, inflammatory bowel disease, and some arthritides or musculoskeletal disorders).

The third category is chronic pain associated with cancer. Opioid therapy is considered to be the major therapeutic approach to patients with cancer pain.

Chronic pain associated with progressive nonmalignant medical disease is the fourth category. Like pain due to cancer, other pain syndromes are related to progressive medical illness associated with poor prognosis. A recent study, for example, demonstrated striking similarities between cancer and AIDS in the prevalence, characteristics, and impact of pain.

The fifth category is chronic pain associated with a nonprogressive organic lesion. Many patients have an overtly painful organic lesion that is not life-threatening but is presumed to be adequate to explain the pain. Although psychological processes again can have a profound impact on symptoms and associated functional disturbances, the pain is perceived to be commensurate with the underlying organic condition.

The final category includes patients with chronic nonmalignant syndromes. A large group of patients experience pain or associated disability that is perceived by the clinician to be excessive for the degree of organic disease present. Although these pains have been termed "idiopathic," this term usually does not connote the existence of psychiatric comorbidity and disability in the same way. Overall, the array of labels should not obscure the key point, which is that chronic pain may reflect a complex interaction between biomedical factors and psychological factors, and that each patient requires an astute assessment of all these factors as well as comorbidities.

Management of Pain in the Substance Abuser

Regardless of the population in question, there are important differences between the relatively brief use of opioids to manage acute pain and the long-term use to treat patients with persistent pain. The therapeutic use of opioids in the patient with a history of substance abuse raises additional issues in both clinical settings.

A. Chronic Pain

The role of opioid therapy in patients with a history of substance abuse and chronic pain has traditionally varied with the distinction between cancer-related pain and nonmalignant pain. Opioids are accepted in the management of cancer pain, and management of this condition in patients with a history of substance abuse requires

pharmacologic expertise equal to that applied to similar patients without this history. Opioids have generally been discouraged in other populations with chronic pain; this is particularly true when the patient's pain is complicated by a history of substance abuse.

From a critical perspective, this distinction between cancer pain and nonmalignant pain may be difficult to rationalize. Nonmalignant pain syndromes are extraordinarily diverse, and even a simple classification identifies other large groups of patients with chronic, severe pain due to progressive medical disorders that are similar to cancer in terms of prognosis and functional outcomes but are not neoplastic. It is particularly difficult to justify the view that opioids are the first-line drug for cancer pain but are relatively contraindicated in such pain syndromes as AIDS, sickle cell anemia, hemophilia, inflammatory bowel disease, and others. Similar concerns may arise in attempting to discern the medical rationale for the conventional rejection of opioid drugs in other chronic pain populations, some of which may, like the cancer population, experience pain as a consequence of tissue injury or neuropathic lesions, or experience chronic pain without the development of psychiatric comorbidity or disability.

B. Other Considerations in the Substance Abuser with Chronic Pain

Although the basic approach to the management of chronic pain should apply equally to all patients, including substance abusers, it is nonetheless true that problems may be encountered in the latter population that distinguish it from others. As noted previously, clinical experience suggests that there may be salient differences among those with remote history of addiction, those currently treated in methadone maintenance programs, and those actively abusing opioids or other drugs. A small retrospective study suggested that all three groups were at relatively high risk for inadequate pain management, but only those who were actively abusing could not reliably achieve adequate symptom control once they were treated aggressively by pain service personnel. The major issues encountered during the treatment of each of these groups can be summarized in the following sections.

1. Patients with a remote history of substance abuse—Although clinical experience suggests that patients with a remote history of substance abuse respond appropriately to opioids, the empiric data in support of this conclusion are meager. From a theoretical perspective, it could be speculated that the same genetic, psychological, and situational factors that predisposed persons to the addiction syndrome initially could increase the risk of aberrant drug-taking behavior in patients administered opioids for therapeutic purposes. The failure to observe these outcomes in practice suggests that the factors that ultimately combined to eliminate the abuse behaviors—as well as with the situational changes associated with the diagnosis and treatment of the pain syndrome—may reduce the likelihood of iatrogenic addiction.

It has been observed clinically that some patients with chronic pain who have a remote history of substance abuse are poorly compliant with opioid therapy due to a persistent fear of these drugs. Thus, the optimal management of the patient with chronic pain and remote history of addiction must incorporate careful, ongoing assessment of drug-taking behavior and the recognition that successful treatment may be compromised both by the attitudes of practitioners, whose overconcern about addiction can distort analgesic management, and the attitudes of the patient, whose behavior may implicitly or explicitly endorse the concerns of the staff or result directly in undertreatment. Education of the staff and the patient may limit the adverse consequence of these attitudes and thereby improve pain management.

2. Patients in methadone maintenance programs— Like those persons who have a remote history of substance abuse, patients receiving methadone maintenance are at high risk for undertreatment of chronic pain. In this population, negative attitudes held by the medical staff may combine with some degree of tolerance to opioid analgesics to limit the efficacy of therapy. If persistent pain reports are interpreted as a manipulative attempt to obtain opioids for purposes other than analgesia, the therapeutic relationship will become conflicted; the clinician's goals for analgesia will be superseded by the desire to prevent drug abuse. This concern is, of course, legitimate if aberrant drug-taking behaviors return in a patient. If "drug-seeking" reflects only the need for pain relief, however, undertreatment will result from the failure to respond.

The failure to recognize the need for higher starting doses may lead to initial problems with the management of chronic pain in methadone-treated patients. Patients who have not received an opioid for pain before, but have been receiving methadone for some time, may require starting doses substantially higher than those conventionally used at the initiation of chronic pain therapy. In a rather typical scenario, a patient is given an opioid at a dose perceived by the clinician to be effective, but the patient gains no relief and voices a complaint; the persistence of pain, perhaps now combined with a sense of mistrust or acrimony, is interpreted as evidence of addiction, and the patient is managed by the further withholding of opioids rather than by aggressive upward dose titration. This, of course, further undermines the therapeutic alliance and reduces the likelihood of successful treatment.

It is a common misconception that the use of methadone as an analgesic for pain can mirror its use in the therapy of opioid addiction. In pain management, doses must be titrated according to patient response; there is no predefined appropriate dose range. Equally important, the single daily dose that is sufficient for the management of addiction is almost never adequate to sustain analgesia throughout the day. Extensive clinical experience indicates that analgesia usually requires at least three doses per day. Many patients actually achieve more stable analgesia with four or six doses per day, an observation supported by studies that demonstrate a duration of analgesia that is typically much briefer than would be expected from the half-life of this drug.

3. Active drug abusers—The view of opioid therapy in patients with a remote history of drug abuse and those in methadone maintenance is not applicable to the small number of patients in whom chronic pain develops while actively abusing opioids or other drugs. Anecdotally, pain management in many of these patients is complicated by substantial psychopathology and adverse situational factors. The degree of psychopathology may be severe enough that a useful therapeutic alliance is impossible, and both the veracity of the complaints and compliance with prescribed therapies become major problems.

Careful assessment is again critical to appropriate management. Clear-cut abuse behaviors (including continued use of illicit drugs) must be distinguished from other behaviors (such as frequent emergency department visits) that may be more difficult to interpret. Although both types of behaviors may reflect inadequacy of pain treatment as well as psychological dependence on the drug, the former is clear-cut abuse, which cannot be condoned, whereas the latter potentially may indicate a lesser degree of psychopathology and a desire to remain in the medical setting for the treatment of a pain problem. The specific psychopathology of these patients must be carefully evaluated. Sociopathy is relatively common among the addict population, and to the extent possible, the clinician should attempt to determine whether sociopathic behaviors have been characteristic of the patient prior to the diagnosis of chronic pain. Straightforward questioning about illegal practices may yield surprisingly frank answers, from which an assessment of these behaviors can be made. Although it must be emphasized that the studies needed to clarify these issues have not been performed, it is likely that the risk of management problems during analgesic therapy correlates generally with the degree of psychopathology, and more specifically with the severity of sociopathic proclivities.

In some cases, efforts to implement a simple and effective pharmacologic regimen for pain may have to be sacrificed in lieu of interventions designed to maintain therapeutic control. Virtually all patients require greater frequency of monitoring and strict attention to the assessment of efficacy, side effects, and drug-taking behavior. Some clinicians favor the use of a written agreement that is kept in the medical record and both defines the medication regimen and explicitly states the responsibilities of both the patient and clinician. An example of such an agreement can be found at http://www.painmed.org/productpub/statements/pdfs/opioid_consent_form.pdf. These guidelines should include specific reference to the methods that will be used to renew prescriptions as well as the response that a report of lost or stolen drugs will generate. It may be useful to establish a rule that lost or stolen drugs must be reported to the police and that documentation of this must be provided. When such circumstances arise, prescribing drugs that have relatively low street value, such as methadone, may be more appropriate than prescribing other drugs, such as hydromorphone, for which there is greater demand among street addicts.

For some patients, the cardinal principle of opioid dose titration simply cannot be accommodated due to demands that are perceived to be inappropriate. Limits must be set based on the clinician's assessment of the risks and benefits in this difficult situation. In rare cases, the persistence of severe pain in the setting of intractable management problems suggests the immediate use of some approaches, such as neurolytic techniques, that generally are considered only after an optimal opioid therapy fails.

In all of this decision-making, the dictates of humane and compassionate care should support a bias that patients generally are to be believed. Factitious pain complaints and malingering appear to be rare among patients who are not actively abusing drugs (including those with a remote history of addiction) and probably are uncommon among active abusers who have cancer. Rather, most substance abusers are like other patients with pain, whose symptoms reflect some combination of ongoing nociception and psychological distress. Unless the evidence in support of malingering is compelling, the clinician is better served by avoiding an argument about the "reality" of the pain and focusing instead on the possibility that pain may be profoundly influenced by psychological factors, possibly including psychological dependence on opioids. It is more productive simply to believe the patient's complaint and thoughtfully assess the degree to which it can be explained by physical and psychological determinants. In keeping with this view, it may be postulated that the premorbid psychopathology of the addict predisposes to a greater psychological contribution to pain than is usually observed in the cancer population. This, too, must be evaluated in future research.

American Pain Society. Principles of analgesic use in the treatment of acute pain and cancer pain. 5th edition. Glenview, IL: American Pain Society, 2003.

American Psychiatric Association. Diagnostic and Statistical Manual for Mental Disorders–IV. Washington, DC: American Psychiatric Association, 1994.

Breitbart W et al. Pain in ambulatory AIDS patients. I: Pain characteristics and medical correlates. *Pain.* 1996;68:315. [PMID: 9121820]

Cherny NI. The pharmacological management of cancer pain. *Eur J Cancer.* 2001;37 Suppl 7:S265. [PMID: 11888000]

Cohen MJ et al. Ethical perspectives: opioid treatment of chronic pain in the context of addiction. *Clin J Pain.* 2002;18(4 Suppl):S99. [PMID: 12479260]

Dole VP. Narcotic addiction, physical dependence and relapse. *N Engl J Med.* 1972;286:988. [PMID: 4622638]

Fishman SM et al. The opioid contract. *Clin J Pain.* 2002;18 (4 Suppl):S70. [PMID: 12479256]

Fishman SM et al. The trilateral opioid contract. Bridging the pain clinic and the primary care physician through the opioid contract. *J Pain Symptom Manage.* 2002;24:335. [PMID: 12458115]

Goldstein RZ et al. Drug addiction and its underlying neurobiological basis: neuroimaging evidence for the involvement of the frontal cortex. *Am J Psychiatry.* 2002;159:1642. [PMID: 12359667]

Hanks GW et al; Expert Working Group of the Research Network of the European Association for Palliative Care. Morphine and alternative opioids in cancer pain: the EAPC recommendations. *Br J Cancer.* 2001;84:587. [PMID: 11237376]

Jage J. Opioid tolerance and dependence–do they matter? *Eur J Pain.* 2005;9:157. [PMID: 15737807]

Kan CC et al. Determination of the main risk factors for benzodiazepine dependence using a multivariate and multidimensional approach. *Compr Psychiatry.* 2004;45:88. [PMID: 14999658]

Kirsh KL et al. Abuse and addiction issues in medically ill patients with pain: attempts at clarification of terms and empirical study. *Clin J Pain.* 2002;18(4 Suppl):S52. [PMID: 12479254]

Krantz MJ et al. Treating opioid dependence. Growing implications for primary care. *Arch Intern Med.* 2004;164:277. [PMID: 14769623]

Manfredi PL et al. Prescribing methadone, a unique analgesic. *J Support Oncol.* 2003;1:216. [PMID: 12479260]

McCabe SE et al. Nonmedical use of prescription opioids among U.S. college students: prevalence and correlates from a national survey. *Addict Behav.* 2005;30:789. [PMID: 15833582]

O'Brien CP. Benzodiazepine use, abuse, and dependence. *J Clin Psychiatry.* 2005;66 Suppl 2:28. [PMID: 15762817]

Passik SD et al. Opioid therapy in patients with a history of substance abuse. *CNS Drugs.* 2004;18:13. [PMID: 14731056]

Passik SD et al. Managing pain in patients with aberrant drug-taking behaviors. *J Support Oncol.* 2005;3:83. [PMID: 15724951]

Passik SD et al. The need to identify predictors of aberrant drug-related behavior and addiction in patients being treated with opioids for pain. *Pain Med.* 2003;4:186. [PMID: 12873265]

Perry S et al. Management of pain during debridement: a survey of U.S. burn units. *Pain.* 1982;13:267. [PMID: 6126853]

Porter J et al. Addiction rare in patients treated with narcotics. *N Engl J Med.* 1980;302:123. [PMID: 7350425]

Regier DA et al. The NIMH Epidemiologic Catchment Area program. Historical context, major objectives, and study population characteristics. *Arch Gen Psychiatry.* 1984;41:934. [PMID: 6089692]

Rinaldi RC et al. Clarification and standardization of substance abuse terminology. *JAMA.* 1988;259:555. [PMID: 3275816]

Ripamonti C et al. The use of methadone for cancer pain. *Hematol Oncol Clin North Am.* 2002;16:543. [PMID: 12170567]

Rosenblum A et al. Prevalence and characteristics of chronic pain among chemically dependent patients in methadone maintenance and residential treatment facilities. *JAMA.* 2003;289:2370. [PMID: 12746360]

Santiago-Palma J et al. Intravenous methadone in the management of chronic cancer pain: safe and effective starting doses when substituting methadone for fentanyl. *Cancer.* 2001;92:1919. [PMID: 11745266]

Savage SR et al. Definitions related to the medical use of opioids: evolution towards universal agreement. *J Pain Symptom Manage.* 2003;26:655. [PMID: 12850648]

Strain EC. Assessment and treatment of comorbid psychiatric disorders in opioid-dependent patients. *Clin J Pain.* 2002;18 (4 Suppl):S14. [PMID: 12479251]

Swenson JD et al. Postoperative care of the chronic opioid-consuming patient. *Anesthesiol Clin North America.* 2005;23:37. [PMID: 15763410]

Whitcomb LA et al. Substance abuse issues in cancer pain. *Curr Pain Headache Rep.* 2002;6:183. [PMID: 12003688]

Williams RH et al. Cocaine and its major metabolites in plasma and urine samples from patients in an urban emergency medicine setting. *J Anal Toxicol.* 2000;24:478. [PMID: 11043649]

Cancer Pain

Judith A. Paice, PhD, RN

ESSENTIAL CRITERIA

- *Cancer pain is greatly feared, yet in most cases, can be easily managed.*
- *Cancer pain is often due to the direct effects of the tumor, treatment of the malignancy, or other conditions unrelated to the disease and its treatment.*
- *Certain groups have been shown to be at risk for inadequate assessment and treatment, including minorities, children, older adults, individuals with a history of addictive disease, and those who are cognitively impaired.*
- *Pharmacologic therapies include nonopioids, opioids, adjuvant analgesics, cancer therapies, and in some cases, interventional techniques.*
- *Nonpharmacologic treatment can be supportive to pharmacologic intervention and may include cognitive-behavioral approaches, along with physical measures, such as bracing, exercise, heat, cold, and assistive devices.*

GENERAL CONSIDERATIONS

Pain is relatively common in persons in whom cancer has been diagnosed, ranging from 14 to 100%. At the time of diagnosis, approximately 20 to 75% of adults have pain, while 23 to 100% of those with advanced disease report pain. Children with cancer have similar pain experiences. Because the risk of cancer-related pain is high, universal screening should be conducted in all patients with cancer when they seek medical attention at a clinic or when they are hospitalized. Any report of pain warrants a comprehensive assessment.

The consequences of inadequate cancer pain relief are significant, including increased physiologic stress, diminished immunocompetence, decreased mobility, increased risk of pneumonia and thromboembolism, and increased work of breathing and myocardial oxygen requirements. Furthermore, pain may lead to impaired quality of life. Several groups, including children, older adults, minorities, individuals from lower socioeconomic groups and the uninsured, women, non-English speaking persons, persons with a history of substance abuse, and cancer survivors, are at increased risk for undertreatment of pain. Inadequate assessment and management lead to reduced function, increased risk of depression and anxiety, and ultimately, impaired quality of life.

Pain Assessment

Cancer pain can be categorized in several ways, including the **duration** (acute versus chronic), the **intensity** (mild, moderate, or severe), the **quality** of the pain (neuropathic, nociceptive, or mixed), and its **temporal pattern** (continuous, breakthrough, or both). To determine the pain experience of an individual patient, careful assessment is warranted. The assessment techniques, including a detailed pain history and careful physical assessment, described in Chapter 2 are essential. Additional components of pain assessment in those with cancer include the following:

1. Using tools valid in this population, with attention to the age and language needs of the patient.
2. Obtaining a medication history, which includes drugs currently being taken, drugs taken in the past, as well as efficacy and any adverse effects of those drugs.
3. Considering common cancer pain syndromes while conducting the history and physical.
4. Assessing functional impairment and need for safety measures.
5. Incorporating a psychosocial evaluation into the assessment, including determination of the patient's and family's goals of care.
6. Using a pain diary to track effectiveness of therapies and evaluate changes in pain.
7. Ordering diagnostic evaluation (eg, magnetic resonance imaging, computed tomography, laboratory testing) when warranted, and only if it will contribute to the treatment plan.
8. Evaluating patients for the presence of other symptoms, since pain is highly correlated with such conditions as fatigue, constipation, and mood disturbances.

A. Assessment Tools for Cancer Pain and Related Symptoms

Pain assessment generally begins with screening, using one of the available unidimensional tools, such as the 0 to 10 Numeric Pain Intensity Scale. If patients are unable to use this scale, alternatives include a verbal descriptor scale (no pain, mild, moderate, severe). Any patient who identifies having pain, even mild pain, should undergo a more thorough assessment. The Brief Pain Inventory is a valid, clinically useful pain assessment tool that has been used extensively in people with cancer. It includes a diagram to note the location of pain, questions regarding pain intensity (current, average, worst using a 0 to 10 rating scale), as well as items that gauge impairment due to pain (Figure 8–1). The Brief Pain Inventory has been translated into many languages, including French, Italian, Mandarin, and Spanish.

Because pain does not exist in isolation and symptom clusters are common in those with cancer, a comprehensive assessment should include more than pain. Several instruments have been designed to clinically measure multiple symptoms, including the Edmonton Symptom Assessment Scale, the MD Anderson Symptom Inventory, the Memorial Symptom Assessment Scale, and others. A recently developed tool, termed the "Distress Thermometer" is a vertical visual analogue scale designed to look like a thermometer, with 0 meaning "no distress" and 10 (at the top of the thermometer) indicating "extreme distress." Accompanying the thermometer scale is a checklist that includes a variety of physical, psychological, practical, family support, and spiritual/religious concerns. These are brief, clinically useful tools that quantify the intensity of a variety of symptoms common in cancer. These instruments foster the systematic assessment of pain and other symptoms, while assisting the clinician in forming a treatment plan.

B. Medication and Pain History

A complete medication history is critical and includes what has been prescribed for pain, what the patient is actually taking, and why any disparity between the two might exist. Studies suggest that cancer patients have significant barriers to taking pain medication (including adverse effects, lack of efficacy, cost, fears of addiction or tolerance, or other concerns), and as a result, adherence is often limited. Advise patients to bring all pill bottles with them to the clinic or hospital, including over-the-counter and herbal medications. This obviates confusion about which drugs are used for pain relief and which are used for other conditions. Patients should also be asked about past and current use of recreational drugs and alcohol. Persons with a past history of substance abuse may be extremely reluctant to take opioids for pain relief, believing that the drugs may cause them to again

lose control. Patients with a current history of addictive disease present more complex challenges, although pain treatment is usually possible. Input from addiction specialists and others with expertise in this area can be useful (see Chapter 7 for more information).

During the pain history, patients and their families may reveal their perceptions regarding the meaning of pain. Pain in cancer may signal progressive disease, loss of independence, or perceived punishment for some past indiscretion. Honest and clear discussions of the disease state are warranted, along with revisiting the patient and family's goals. Reframing may be needed (reinterpreting the meaning of the pain), along with referral to therapists, religious figures, social workers, or other support personnel. Consider cultural influences that may affect pain reporting and treatment. For example, in some cultures, admitting to having pain implies weakness.

C. Physical Assessment

The comprehensive physical evaluation of pain in cancer includes particular attention to the neurologic examination, including the sensory, motor, and autonomic systems. Observe sites of pain for evidence of infection, trauma, skin breakdown, changes in bony structures, or cutaneous malignant lesions. Sensory evaluation, particularly in patients receiving chemotherapy, can differentiate large fiber versus small neuronal fiber damage. Reduced sensation to vibration or altered proprioceptive ability suggests the large neuronal fiber damage seen with cisplatin and oxaliplatin therapy. Changes in temperature sensation in the affected region and increased pain response (observed by an exaggerated response to pin prick) are indicators of small fiber dysfunction, relatively common after treatment with paclitaxel, docetaxel, and vincristine. Autonomic nervous system dysfunction can occur, particularly when patients have received vincristine, and can be assessed by comparing blood pressure and pulse rate while lying and sitting or standing. In autonomic nervous system dysfunction, the blood pressure drops when the patient is upright, while the heart rate stays relatively constant (unlike hypotension, which results in reduced blood pressure and elevated heart rate). These findings during active cancer treatment often warrant dose reduction or modification of the chemotherapeutic regimen.

Another component of the neurologic examination is evaluation of cranial nerves, particularly with reports of pain in the head or neck. For example, metastases to the base of the skull (more common in breast, lung, or prostate cancer) can lead to eye pain, headache, hearing loss, and other findings depending on the site of the lesion. Leptomeningeal metastases (more common in breast, lung, and non-Hodgkin lymphoma) present as headache, neck or back pain, consistent with the level of the lesion. Both of these syndromes suggest a poor

STUDY ID# ____________ HOSPITAL # ____________

DO NOT WRITE ABOVE THIS LINE

Brief Pain Inventory (Short Form)

Date: ____/____/____ Time: ____

Name: ________________ ________________ ________________

Last First Middle Initial

1. Throughout our lives, most of us have had pain from time to time (such as minor headaches, sprains, and toothaches). Have you had pain other than these every-day kinds of pain today?

1. Yes 2. No

2. On the diagram, shade in the areas where you feel pain. Put an X on the area that hurts the most.

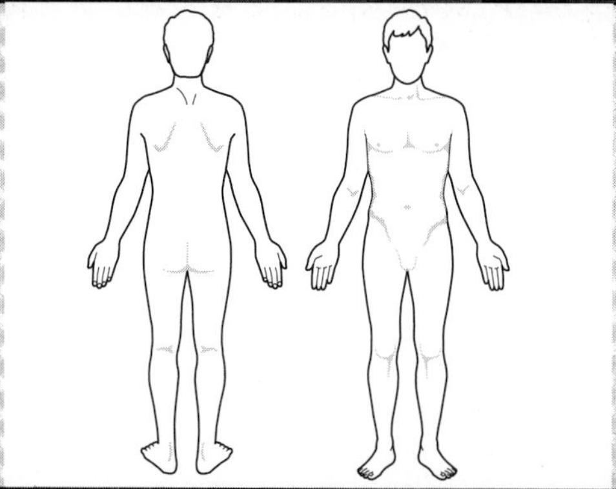

3. Please rate your pain by circling the one number that best describes your pain at its worst in the last 24 hours.

0	1	2	3	4	5	6	7	8	9	10
No Pain										Pain as bad as you can imagine

4. Please rate your pain by circling the one number that best describes your pain at its least in the last 24 hours.

0	1	2	3	4	5	6	7	8	9	10
No Pain										Pain as bad as you can imagine

5. Please rate your pain by circling the one number that best describes your pain on the average.

0	1	2	3	4	5	6	7	8	9	10
No Pain										Pain as bad as you can imagine

6. Please rate your pain by circling the one number that tells how much pain you have right now.

0	1	2	3	4	5	6	7	8	9	10
No Pain										Pain as bad as you can imagine

Figure 8–1. Brief Pain Inventory (short form). (Reproduced, with permission, from Charles S. Cleeland, PhD, Pain Research Group, Copyright 1991.)

7. What treatments or medications are you receiving for your pain?

8. In the last 24 hours, how much relief have pain treatments or medications provided? Please circle the one percentage that most shows how much relief you have received.

0%	10%	20%	30%	40%	50%	60%	70%	80%	90%	100%
No Relief										Complete Relief

9. Circle the one number that describes how, during the past 24 hours, pain has interfered with your:

A.   General Activity

0	1	2	3	4	5	6	7	8	9	10
Does not Interfere										Completely Interferes

B.   Mood

0	1	2	3	4	5	6	7	8	9	10
Does not Interfere										Completely Interferes

C.   Walking Ability

0	1	2	3	4	5	6	7	8	9	10
Does not Interfere										Completely Interferes

D.   Normal Work (includes both work outside the home and housework)

0	1	2	3	4	5	6	7	8	9	10
Does not Interfere										Completely Interferes

E.   Relations with other people

0	1	2	3	4	5	6	7	8	9	10
Does not Interfere										Completely Interferes

F.   Sleep

0	1	2	3	4	5	6	7	8	9	10
Does not Interfere										Completely Interferes

G.   Enjoyment of life

0	1	2	3	4	5	6	7	8	9	10
Does not Interfere										Completely Interferes

Figure 8–1. (*Continued*)

prognosis and pain management is crucial to enhance quality of life.

Allodynia, when normal stimulation is perceived as painful, is a relatively common finding in neuropathy. Examples include tactile allodynia in postherpetic or chemotherapy-induced peripheral neuropathy. The evaluation of tactile allodynia includes lightly stroking the area with a brush or cotton ball. Thermal allodynia is evaluated by holding a cool or warm item lightly against the skin. It is an acute neurotoxicity that is commonly seen during infusion of oxaliplatin; patients describe touching a cold item as burning. Thermal allodynia occurs in 85 to 95% of patients and may also include jaw pain, eye pain, ptosis, and pain in the infusion arm. A small percentage of patients, 1 to 2%, may experience pharyngolaryngeal dysesthesia. To prevent this, patients are advised to avoid drinking cold fluids during and a few days after the infusion.

Reflexes may be reduced or absent in affected areas. Standard motor evaluation should include observation of gait as well as assessment of strength and tone. This also provides baseline safety information to begin planning for assistive devices if the patient is unsteady as well as the need for other safety measures in the home. For example, simple ankle braces can prevent falls in patients with foot drop due to spinal metastases and resultant motor weakness. While conducting the physical examination, observe for possible safety concerns. Is ambulation limited, and is use of a cane or other assistive device warranted? Does the patient have significant paresthesias, placing them at risk for trauma, in much the same way the diabetic patient is at risk for infection after minor injury to the feet or hands? Referral to an occupational therapist can determine functional level and need for assistive devices. Home health nurses can make visits to the home to assess for safety in the living environment; in general, one such visit is reimbursed by most third party payers.

D. Diagnostic Evaluation

Radiographic studies and laboratory analyses can contribute essential information in the care of patients with cancer pain. For example, back pain that is found on magnetic resonance imaging to be a sign of impending spinal cord compression should be aggressively treated to prevent complete compression with paralysis. Bone scans can identify the presence of metastases causing pain, and tumor markers may provide evidence for the spread of a malignancy.

In addition, laboratory data may reveal other conditions that can complicate pain therapy, such as elevated calcium levels as a potential cause of confusion. The extent of the diagnostic evaluation is based on the course of the patient's illness as well as his or her goals for care. Pain may be managed empirically in patients with cancer

Table 8–1. Examples of Acute Pain Syndromes Seen in Cancer.

- Hormonal therapy–induced bone pain flare
- Mucositis
- Postoperative pain
- Procedural pain
  - Bone marrow aspiration or biopsy
  - Chest tube insertion for malignant effusion
  - Lumbar puncture
- Radiation-induced skin reactions
- Radiopharmaceutical-induced pain flare (eg, strontium-89)

who have advanced disease, who are no longer considering curative therapy, and who wish to forgo extensive diagnostic evaluation.

Specific Cancer Pain Syndromes

Cancer pain syndromes can be grouped in a variety of categories: acute versus chronic, nociceptive (also called somatic) versus neuropathic, and disease- versus treatment-related. Breakthrough pain is a particularly challenging cancer pain syndrome, and several types of breakthrough pain have been identified.

A. Acute versus Chronic

Acute pain is generally due to invasive procedures, such as diagnostic or surgical interventions, or to the effects of chemotherapy and other treatment, including mucositis or bone pain flair after hormonal therapy. The management is not unlike the techniques used to manage acute pain in patients with nonmalignant disease. Table 8–1 lists examples of treatment-related acute pain unique to persons with cancer.

Chronic pain syndromes often include involvement of bone, soft tissue, the viscera, and the nervous system. Bone metastases, more common sources of pain in patients with breast, lung, or prostate cancers, are chronic in nature. Lymphedema, occurring in approximately 20% of women who undergo axillary node dissection, is an example of soft tissue pain associated with significant physical and psychological morbidity. Visceral pain, described as cramping, poorly localized, and diffuse, may arise from involvement of tumor within the liver, intestine, kidney, peritoneum, bladder, or other organs (see Chapter 11). Neuropathic pains can evolve from numerous causes, may be difficult for patients to describe, and are often complex to treat. Finally, many people with cancer experience syndromes unrelated to the cancer or its treatment, such as osteoarthritis.

B. Nociceptive versus Neuropathic

Nociceptive pain can be somatic or visceral in nature, is generally described as aching or throbbing, and is frequently due to musculoskeletal complications of cancer. Examples include bone metastases or soft tissue involvement by tumor. Painful flair after hormonal therapy is also nociceptive in nature. Squeezing, gnawing, or cramping pain in the abdomen may be due to pressure on organ capsules or stretching of the mesentery or other visceral structures. Visceral pain may be referred, such as the case of tumor in the liver causing stretching of the capsule surrounding the liver, leading to pain in the right upper quadrant, and often, the right shoulder.

Neuropathic pain, described as tingling, burning, electrical, or shooting, suggests damage to central or peripheral nervous system structures. Examples include peripheral neuropathy due to chemotherapy or radicular pain secondary to spinal metastases with infringement upon nerve roots. Chemotherapeutic agents most closely associated with peripheral neuropathy include the following:

1. Platinum-based agents (eg, cisplatin, oxaliplatin)
2. Taxanes (eg, docetaxel, paclitaxel)
3. Thalidomide
4. Vinca alkaloids (eg, vinblastine, vincristine)

Table 8–2 lists common causes of neuropathic pain seen in persons with cancer. The physician should remember that persons with cancer may have comorbid conditions that lead to neuropathic pain or may place these patients at greater risk for the development of neuropathy. These noncancer causes of neuropathy are listed in Table 8–3. See Chapter 10 for a complete discussion of neuropathic pain.

C. Disease- versus Treatment-Related Pain

Tumor burden often leads to pain (Table 8–4). The treatment of cancer, including surgery, chemotherapy, radi-

Table 8–2. Common Causes of Neuropathic Pain in Cancer.

- Brachial, cervical, or sacral plexopathies
- Cachexia (rapid onset of weight loss)
- Chemotherapy-induced neuropathy
- Cranial neuropathies
- Paraneoplastic sensorimotor neuropathy
- Postherpetic neuropathy
- Postradiation plexopathies
- Surgical neuropathies
  –Phantom pain
  –Postmastectomy syndrome
  –Postthoracotomy syndrome

Table 8–3. Common Noncancer Causes of Neuropathic Pain.[a]

- Alcohol-induced neuropathy
- Atherosclerotic ischemic disease
- Brachial plexus avulsion (trauma)
- Carpal tunnel syndrome
- Complex regional pain syndrome
- Diabetic neuropathy
- Fabry disease
- Failed back syndrome
- Guillain-Barré syndrome
- HIV-associated neuropathy
  –Viral involvement
  –Antiretrovirals
- Poststroke pain
- Trigeminal neuralgia
- Vitamin deficiencies

[a]Preexisting neuropathy may place a patient at significantly greater risk for the development of neuropathy due to cancer treatment.

ation therapy, hormonal, and biological therapies, can also lead to pain (Table 8–4). Careful evaluation is essential, along with consideration of goals of care. Treatment-related pain may lead to interruptions in therapy, changes in the cancer regimen, and in some cases, cessation of therapy.

D. Breakthrough Pain

Intermittent episodes of moderate to severe pain that occur in spite of control of baseline continuous pain are very common in patients with cancer pain. Despite the prevalence of breakthrough pain, studies suggest that short-acting analgesics are frequently not provided, and patients do not take as much as are allowed. Patients with cancer experience breakthrough pains a few times a day, which last a few moments to many minutes, often occurring without warning. Three general types of breakthrough pain have been described: incident pain, spontaneous pain, and end-of-dose failure.

1. Incident pain—Incident pain is associated with specific activities, such as coughing or walking. In one study of patients with cancer who were near the end of life, 93% had breakthrough pain; 72% of the episodes were related to movement or weight bearing. Patients should be encouraged to use a rapid-onset, short-duration analgesic formulation in anticipation of pain-eliciting activities or events. When possible, use the same drug that the patient is taking for baseline pain relief for incident pain (eg, long-acting morphine and immediate-release morphine). Adjust and titrate the breakthrough pain medication dose

Table 8–4. Common Pain Syndromes Seen in Patients with Cancer.

Cancer–related pain syndromes	Example
Bone metastases	Bone marrow expansion Vertebral syndrome Local infiltration Base of skull involvement
Visceral	Hepatic capsule distention Retroperitoneal syndrome Intestinal obstruction Ureteral obstruction
Neuropathies/plexopathies	Mononeuropathies Polyneuropathies Cauda equina syndrome
Paraneoplastic syndrome	Osteoarthropathy Gynecomastia
Treatment-related pain syndromes	
Postradiotherapy	Enteritis Radiation fibrosis Osteoradionecrosis Myelopathy Neuropathy
Postchemotherapy	Avascular necrosis Chronic abdominal pain Mucositis Neuropathy
Posthormonal	Bone pain flare
Postoperative	Phantom limb pain Postamputation pain Postnephrectomy syndrome Postmastectomy syndrome Postthoracotomy syndrome Postradical neck dissection Pelvic floor myalgia

to the severity of anticipated pain or the intensity and duration of the pain-producing event.

2. Spontaneous pain—Spontaneous pain occurs in an unpredictable fashion and is not temporally associated with any activity or event. These pains are more challenging to control. The use of adjuvant analgesics for neuropathic pains may help diminish the frequency and severity of these types of pain. Otherwise, immediate treatment with a potent, rapid-onset opioid analgesic is indicated.

3. End-of-dose failure—End-of-dose failure describes pain that occurs toward the end of the usual dosing interval of a regularly scheduled analgesic. In this case, the patient taking an oral long-acting opioid formulation consistently reports pain several hours prior to the next dose (or in the case of the fentanyl patch describes pain the day before patch change). This results from declining blood levels of the long-acting analgesic prior to administration or uptake of the next scheduled dose. Pain diaries and questioning about the onset of pain will assist with rapid diagnosis of end-of-dose failure. Strategies include increasing the dose of around-the-clock medication or shortening the dose interval to match the onset of this type of breakthrough pain. For instance, a patient who is taking continuous-release morphine every 12 hours and whose pain "breaks through" after about 8 to 10 hours is experiencing end-of-dose failure. The dose should be increased by 25 to 50%, if this is tolerated, or the dosing interval should be increased to every 8 hours.

Bosompra K et al. Swelling, numbness, pain, and their relationship to arm function among breast cancer survivors: a disablement process model perspective. *Breast J.* 2002;8:338. [PMID: 12390356]

Caraceni A et al. Classification of cancer pain syndromes. *Oncology (Williston Park).* 2001;15:1627. [PMID: 11780704]

Caraceni A et al. Gabapentin for neuropathic cancer pain: a randomized controlled trial from the Gabapentin Cancer Pain Study Group. *J Clin Oncol.* 2004;22:2909. [PMID: 15254060]

Chang VT et al. Validation of the Edmonton Symptom Assessment Scale. *Cancer.* 2000;88:2164. [PMID: 10813730]

Cleeland CS et al. Assessing symptom distress in cancer patients: the M.D. Anderson Symptom Inventory. *Cancer.* 2000;89:1634. [PMID: 11013380]

Clohisy DR et al. Bone cancer pain. *Cancer.* 2003;97:866. [PMID: 12548588]

Drake PA. Hemorrhage after bone marrow harvest: a case presentation. *Clin J Oncol Nurs.* 2000;4:29. [PMID: 10865581]

Forcina JM. Re: National Institutes of Health: State-of-the-Science Conference Statement: Symptom Management in Cancer: Pain, Depression and Fatigue, July 15–17, 2002. *J Natl Cancer Inst.* 2002;95:110. [PMID: 15265975]

Hwang SS et al. Dynamic cancer pain management outcomes: the relationship between pain severity, pain relief, functional interference, satisfaction and global quality of life over time. *J Pain Symptom Manage.* 2002;23:190. [PMID: 11888717]

Kanner R. Diagnosis and management of neuropathic pain in patients with cancer. *Cancer Invest.* 2001;19:324. [PMID: 11338889]

Mercadante S et al. Episodic (breakthrough) pain: consensus conference of an expert working group of the European Association for Palliative Care. *Cancer.* 2002;94:832. [PMID: 11857319]

Miaskowski C et al. Guideline for the management of cancer pain in adults and children. Glenview, IL: American Pain Society; 2005.

Paice J. Mechanisms and management of neuropathic pain in cancer. *J Support Oncol.* 2003;1:107. [PMID: 15352654]

Paice J. Pain. In: Yarbro C, Frogge M, Goodman M, editors. *Cancer Symptom Management.* 3rd ed. Boston: Jones & Bartlett Publishers; 2004:77–96.

Portenoy RK, Conn M. Cancer pain syndromes. In: Bruera E, Portenoy RK, editors. Cancer Pain: Assessment and Management. Cambridge: Cambridge University Press; 2003. pp. 89–108.

Potter VT et al. Patient barriers to optimal cancer pain control. *Psychooncology.* 2003;12:153. [PMID: 12619147]

Quasthoff S et al. Chemotherapy-induced peripheral neuropathy. *J Neurol.* 2002;249:9. [PMID: 11954874]

Soares LG. Poor social conditions, criminality and urban violence: Unmentioned barriers for effective cancer pain control at the end of life. *J Pain Symptom Manage.* 2003;26:693. [PMID: 12906953]

Thomas RR et al. Hypersensitivity and idiosyncratic reactions to oxaliplatin. *Cancer.* 2003;97:2301. [PMID: 12712487]

Wilson RH et al. Acute oxaliplatin-induced peripheral nerve hyperexcitability. *J Clin Oncol.* 2002;20:1767. [PMID: 11919233]

TREATMENT

The management of cancer pain includes pharmacologic interventions, cancer therapies, and nonpharmacologic techniques.

Pharmacologic Therapies

Pharmacologic therapies include nonopioids (acetaminophen and nonsteroidal anti-inflammatory drugs [NSAIDs]), opioids, and adjuvant analgesics. These are discussed in depth in Chapter 3. Specific cancer-related applications of each of these agents are addressed below. Because of the complexity of many cancer pain syndromes, multimodal therapies are indicated. This may include the use of nonopioids, opioids, and adjuvants, along with nonpharmacologic techniques. These combinations, such as morphine and gabapentin, have been shown to provide better relief than when given individually.

A. NONOPIOIDS

1. Acetaminophen—The mechanism of action of acetaminophen is unknown. Acetaminophen is analgesic and antipyretic but has limited anti-inflammatory effect. Available in oral administration, the maximum recommended dose is 4000 mg/d. Inadvertent overdose is common since acetaminophen is found in many combination over-the-counter products, including cold medications and sleep agents. Dose adjustment should be made for persons with hepatic dysfunction, including those patients with liver metastases.

2. Nonsteroidal anti-inflammatory drugs—NSAIDs are analgesic, antipyretic, and anti-inflammatory. This class of compounds includes older nonselective agents and selective cyclooxygenase (COX)-2 inhibitors.

The nonselective NSAIDs, such as ibuprofen and naproxen, inhibit COX enzymes, theoretically leading to analgesia as well as adverse effects. These adverse effects are not trivial and include gastrointestinal bleeding, renal dysfunction, and clotting abnormalities. Given these risks and benefits, NSAIDs are an effective component of the multimodal therapy necessary to treat cancer pain in carefully selected patients.

Currently, NSAIDs are available by the oral route in the United States, except for ketorolac, which can be administered parenterally. Because of its potent effects on renal prostaglandins and the gastrointestinal mucosa, potentially leading to renal failure or gastrointestinal bleeding, ketorolac has a very limited role in cancer pain control outside of short-term use after a surgical or other invasive procedure.

Selective COX-2 inhibitors, introduced in 1999, were believed to provide protection from the gastrointestinal effects commonly associated with NSAIDs, of particular concern in people with cancer. Furthermore, celecoxib was being tested as a chemopreventive agent in colorectal and other cancers. However, concern arose regarding the cardiovascular effects of the COX-2 inhibitors, leading to the withdrawal of rofecoxib and valdecoxib from the US market. This concern was based on data suggesting an increased risk of cardiovascular events, including acute myocardial infarction, associated with the use of higher doses (>25 mg) of this drug. And although celecoxib remains available, the National Institutes of Health announced that it suspended the use of celecoxib in a large colorectal cancer prevention clinical trial conducted by the National Cancer Institute. The Adenoma Prevention with Celecoxib (APC) trial incorporated celecoxib at doses of 400 to 800 mg/d versus placebo. The trial was stopped because interim analysis demonstrated a 2.5-fold increased risk of major cardiovascular events for participants taking the drug compared with those receiving placebo (see http://www.nih.gov/news/pr/dec2004/od-17.htm). The underlying mechanism of these cardiovascular events is unclear, although one hypothesis includes the role of prostacyclins and thromboxane. Nonselective COX-2 inhibitors, or traditional NSAIDs, suppress both prostacyclins (which prevents platelet formation and clumping, as well as fosters vasodilation) and thromboxane (which enhances platelet clumping and causes vasoconstriction). Selective COX-2 inhibitors block only prostacyclins, hypothetically leading to increased risk of clots. However, alternate mechanisms have also been postulated. When considering therapy with celecoxib, carefully weigh the risks and benefits, the anticipated duration of therapy, and the goals of care.

B. OPIOIDS

The pharmacology of opioids has been thoroughly reviewed in Chapter 3. Pure opioid agonists are the mainstay of cancer pain management. There is no role for partial or mixed agonist-antagonist agents in cancer pain control.

Multiple routes of administration are warranted in cancer care. For example, mucositis or dysphagia due to irradiation of a tumor in the aerodigestive system can lead to inability to tolerate oral administration of opioids. Alternatives to oral opioid administration include the following:

1. Enteral (*via* feeding tube, rectal, or -ostomy).
2. Parenteral (including intravenous and subcutaneous) may incorporate intermittent injections, continuous infusions, and patient-controlled analgesia; the intramuscular route is not recommended due to the lack of muscle mass in most cachectic patients, the variability in uptake of the drug, and the pain caused by this route of administration.
3. Spinal delivery (including epidural and intrathecal, often in combination with local anesthetics or other agents) entails significantly lower doses of drug, although this route requires the expertise of clinicians skilled in placing these catheters and often expensive external or internal devices to deliver the drug.
4. Transdermal fentanyl is commercially available in 12.5, 25, 50, 75, and 100 mcg/h formulations. Because morphine is hydrophilic, it is unlikely to cross the skin readily. There is no evidence to support the use of topical morphine or other opioids applied to intact skin for pain control.
5. Transmucosal fentanyl. (Although liquid morphine is often given sublingually to patients who cannot swallow, evidence suggests the medication is not being absorbed by this route, in part due to its hydrophilic nature. Rather, the liquid is gradually trickling down the back of the throat and absorbed enterally.)
6. Nasal administration is currently not available for people with cancer (the only commercially produced product, butorphanol, is contraindicated). Studies are under way examining the use of intranasal fentanyl.

Long-acting (or sustained-release) formulations are the mainstay of cancer care. First, the dosage is titrated using an immediate-release compound until an effective dose is determined. That dose is then converted to one of the available long-acting formulations. Selection is based on the patient's ability to obtain relief with a particular opioid; the need for an oral, enteral, or transdermal delivery method; support in the home to adhere to a particular regimen; and preference.

Long-acting morphine (MS Contin and generic equivalents) is administered every 12 hours, although some patients require 8-hour dosing. Avinza and Kadian can be administered daily, can be opened and sprinkled in applesauce for patients who can swallow soft items but not pills, and they can also be placed in some enteral feeding tubes.

Long-acting oxycodone (OxyContin and generic equivalents) can be administered every 12 hours; 8-hour delivery is rarely necessary.

Transdermal fentanyl (Duragesic and generic equivalents) can be administered every 72 hours, although some patients require more frequent patch changes.

Methadone has a long half-life (approximately 15 to 60 hours), thus allowing administration every 8 hours to provide analgesia. In addition to binding to μ opioid receptors, it is an antagonist at the *N*-methyl-D-aspartate (NMDA) receptor, which may allow improved neuropathic pain control. These attributes, coupled with its low cost, have led to an increase in the use of methadone for pain control.

The equianalgesic dosing of methadone is complicated. In opiate naïve patients, the conversion with morphine may be 1:1. However, when patients are receiving higher doses of morphine (or other opioids), the ratio increases. Few studies have been conducted, thus conversions are approximations:

<100 mg oral morphine equivalents	3:1
101–300 mg oral morphine equivalents	5:1
301–600 mg oral morphine equivalents	10:1
601–800 mg oral morphine equivalents	12:1
800–1000 mg oral morphine equivalents	15:1
>1000 mg oral morphine equivalents	20:1

(www.eperc.mcw.edu, Fast Fact #75)

Titration should be undertaken slowly in most cases, with increases occurring no more frequently than every 1 to 5 days. Several different conversion schema can be found at www.cancer.gov/cancerinfo/pdq/supportivecare/pain.

Intravenous and subcutaneous administration of methadone are alternative routes, although there are reports of irritation with subcutaneous delivery. There have been reports of prolonged Q–T wave interval noted with high-dose intravenous delivery of methadone, with the concern that this may be due to additives in the parenteral formulation. However, more recent information suggests this effect may also occur with high-dose oral administration, although others suggest the effect may be due to prolonged administration rather than a high dose.

Methadone is metabolized primarily by CYP3A4 but also by CYP2D6 and CYP1A2. Therefore, drugs that induce CYP enzymes accelerate the metabolism of methadone, resulting in reduced serum levels of the drug (Table 8–5). The patient may experience shortened duration of analgesia or reduced overall pain relief. Examples of these drugs often used in palliative care include several antiretroviral agents, dexamethasone, carbamazepine, phenytoin, and barbiturates. Drugs that inhibit CYP enzymes slow methadone metabolism,

Table 8–5. Agents That Interact with Serum Methadone Levels.

Drugs that may lower serum methadone levels (CYP3A4 inducers)	Drugs that may increase serum methadone levels (CYP3A4 inhibitors)
Abacavir	Cimetidine
Amprenavir	Ciprofloxacin
Barbiturates	Clarithromycin
Carbamazepine	Delavirdine
Cocaine	Diazepam
Dexamethasone	Dihydroergotamine
Efavirenz	Diltiazem
Ethanol (long-term use)	Disulfiram
Fusidic acid	Erythromycin
Heroin	Fluconazole
Lopinavir + ritonavir	Grapefruit (juice or whole)
Nelfinavir	Haloperidol
Nevirapine	Ketoconazole
Oxcarbazepine	Moclobemide
Phenytoin	Norfloxacin
Rifampin	Omeprazole
Risperidone	SSRIs
St. John's wort	Troleandomycin
Spironolactone	Thioridazine
Topiramate	Sodium bicarbonate (alkalinizes urine)
Vitamin C in high doses	Venlafaxine
	Verapamil

SSRIs, selective serotonin reuptake inhibitors.

potentially leading to sedation and respiratory depression. These include ketoconazole; cimetidine; omeprazole; and selective serotonin reuptake inhibitors, such as fluoxetine, paroxetine, and sertraline.

Cross-tolerance to opioids develops in patients who are enrolled in a methadone maintenance program for addictive disease. These patients require higher doses than opioid naïve patients. Prescribing methadone for addictive disease requires a special license in the United States. Therefore, prescriptions provided for methadone to manage pain in cancer care should include the statement "for pain."

Along with a long-acting opioid, short-acting opioids are indicated to manage breakthrough pain. Break-through dosing of oral opioids is generally 10 to 20% of the 24-hour oral dose. This can be administered as frequently as every hour.

Side effects of opioids are generally preventable or easily managed. See Chapter 3 for additional information. Constipation occurs in most persons requiring opioids for pain control. Prevention is usually effective using a combination stimulant laxative/softener, such as senna and docusate. As the dose of opioid is titrated upward, the dose of laxative/softener generally needs to be increased. Dietary changes, bulking agents such as methylcellulose, and increased fluid intake are rarely sufficient to counteract the constipating effects of opioid therapy in people with cancer.

Nausea is more common in opioid-naïve persons. Prescribing an around-the-clock antiemetic for the first 24 to 48 hours in patients who have experienced this adverse effect of opioids in the past can obviate this effect. Some patients may require longer-term antiemetic therapy of 1 week or longer. Since many people with cancer have already been treated with an antiemetic during chemotherapy administration, select an antiemetic that has been well-tolerated by the patient in the past, such as phenothiazines (including prochlorperazine) or prokinetic agents (such as metoclopramide). Serotonin 5-HT$_3$ receptor antagonists, such as ondansetron and others in this class, likely have limited usefulness in the management of prolonged opioid-induced nausea and vomiting.

Sedation related to opioid administration is generally managed by switching to an alternate opioid (opioid "rotation" or "switching") or adding a psychostimulant, such as methylphenidate. In one study that allowed doses up to 20 mg/d taken at any time (morning, afternoon, or evening), patients were found to have relief of sedation, reduced fatigue, improved appetite, as well as deeper sleep. Others have been described safely and effectively using doses of 60 mg and higher.

Myoclonus is a neurotoxicity of opioid administration, usually seen with higher doses of opioid, with concomitant renal dysfunction, often in cases of advanced malignancy. Adding a benzodiazepine, such as clonazepam 0.5 mg orally twice daily, or switching to an alternate opioid may relieve the myoclonic jerking that can occur. Chapter 9 details the management of opioid-induced myoclonus.

C. ADJUVANT ANALGESICS

Adjuvant analgesics include antidepressants, anticonvulsants, corticosteroids, and local anesthetics. These are key components of the multimodal therapy necessary to treat cancer pain, generally in combination with opioids.

1. Antidepressants—Tricyclic antidepressants appear to provide analgesia through inhibition of norepinephrine and serotonin reuptake. A recent consensus panel listed this category as one of five first-line therapies for the management of general neuropathic pains. Side effects often limit the use of these agents in cancer care. Cardiac arrhythmias, conduction abnormalities, narrow-angle glaucoma, and clinically significant prostatic hyperplasia are relative contraindications to the tricyclic antidepressants. The delay in onset of pain relief of days to weeks may preclude the use of these agents for pain relief in patients with limited life expectancy. On the other hand, their sleep-enhancing and mood-elevating effects may be of benefit.

Venlafaxine, a newer, atypical antidepressant, has been shown to reduce neuropathy associated with cisplatin-induced neuropathy and has the added advantage of treating hot flashes. Case studies suggest venlafaxine is also useful in reducing oxaliplatin-associated neuropathy.

2. Anticonvulsants—The older anticonvulsants, such as carbamazepine and clonazepam, relieve pain by blocking sodium channels, and as a result, often are referred to as membrane stabilizers. Anticonvulsants are very useful in the treatment of neuropathic pain and may be effective in reducing neuropathic pain associated with chemotherapy. Gabapentin is believed to have several different mechanisms of action, including acting as an NMDA antagonist among other analgesic activities. The analgesic doses of gabapentin reported to relieve pain in noncancer and cancer pain conditions ranged from 900 mg/d to 3600 mg/d in divided doses. A common reason for inadequate relief is failure to titrate upward after prescribing the usual starting dose of 100 mg orally three times daily. Gradual downward titration from gabapentin is critical to prevent possible seizures. Other anticonvulsants have been used with success in treating neuropathies, including lamotrigine, levetiracetam, tiagabine, topiramate, and zonisamide, yet no randomized controlled clinical trials in cancer are currently available. Table 8–6 lists dosing information and adverse effects.

3. Corticosteroids—Corticosteroids inhibit prostaglandin synthesis and reduce edema surrounding neural tissues. This category of drug is particularly useful for neuropathic pain syndromes, including plexopathies and pain associated with stretching of the liver capsule due to metastases. Corticosteroids are also highly effective at treating bone pain due to their anti-inflammatory effects, as well as relieving pain due to malignant intestinal obstruction. Dexamethasone produces the least amount of mineralocorticoid effect, and is available in oral, intravenous, subcutaneous, and epidural formulations. The standard dose is 12 to 24 mg/d and can be administered once daily due to the long half-life of this drug. Intravenous bolus doses should be pushed slowly, to prevent uncomfortable perineal burning and itching.

4. Local anesthetics—Local anesthetics work in a manner similar to the older anticonvulsants, by inhibiting the movement of ions across the neural membrane and are useful for relieving neuropathic pain. Local anesthetics can be given orally, topically, intravenously, subcutaneously, or spinally. Local anesthetic gels and patches have been used to prevent the pain associated with needle stick and other minor procedures. Both gel and patch versions of lidocaine have been shown to reduce the pain of postherpetic neuropathy, a syndrome common in malignancy. Intravenous lidocaine at 1 to 2 mg/kg (maximum 500 mg) administered over 1 hour, followed by a continuous infusion of 1 to 2 mg/kg/h has been reported to reduce intractable neuropathic pain in patients who are in inpatient palliative care and home hospice settings. Epidural or intrathecal lidocaine or bupivacaine delivered with an opioid can reduce neuropathic pain.

5. *N*-methyl-D-aspartate antagonists—NMDA antagonists are believed to block the binding of excitatory amino acids, such as glutamate, in the spinal cord and brain. Ketamine, a dissociative anesthetic, is thought to relieve severe neuropathic pain by blocking these NMDA receptors. Routine use often is limited by cognitive changes and other adverse effects and a recent Cochrane review found insufficient trials conducted to determine safety and efficacy in cancer pain. Oral compounds containing dextromethorphan have been tested but have been found to be ineffective in relieving cancer pain.

D. Anticancer Therapies

1. Bisphosphonates—Bisphosphonates may reduce pain related to metastatic bone disease by inhibiting osteoclast-mediated bone resorption (Table 8–7). These drugs are also used to prevent skeletal complications and to treat hypercalcemia. They should not be used in patients without evidence of bony metastases. Pamidronate disodium reduces pain, hypercalcemia, and skeletal morbidity associated with breast cancer and multiple myeloma, although a recent study of prostate cancer failed to demonstrate any benefit. The drug is administered as an intravenous infusion and dosing is generally repeated every 4 weeks. The analgesic effects occur in 2 to 4 weeks. Zoledronic acid, a newer bisphosphonate, has been shown to relieve pain due to metastatic bone disease and is somewhat more convenient in that it can be infused over a shorter duration of time. Clodronate and sodium etidronate appear to provide little or no analgesia. A recent report suggests osteonecrosis of the jaw may occur in patients who have been given bisphosphonates, then undergo dental extraction or other oral surgery procedures, even at a time distant from the bisphosphonate administration. Patients with poor dentition should undergo dental work prior to bisphosphonate therapy.

Table 8–6. Selected Antidepressants and Anticonvulsants Used in the Management of Malignant Neuropathic Pain.

Drug	Dose	Comments
Tricyclic Antidepressants		
Nortriptyline	10–25 mg orally at bedtime; increase gradually to 150 mg	*Adverse effects:* Sedation Anticholinergic effects (dry mouth, urinary retention, constipation) Orthostatic hypotension
Desipramine	10–25 mg orally at bedtime; increase gradually to 150 mg	*Adverse effects:* Sedation Anticholinergic effects (dry mouth, urinary retention, constipation) Orthostatic hypotension
Atypical Antidepressants		
Venlafaxine	37.5 mg orally twice daily; increase gradually to maximum 375 mg/d	Also effective in relief of hot flashes Adjust dose in renal impairment *Adverse effects:* Nausea Dry mouth Sedation Constipation Sexual dysfunction
Duloxetine	60 mg orally daily; maximum 60 mg/d	Adjust dose in renal impairment *Adverse effects:* Nausea Dry mouth Constipation Insomnia
Anticonvulsants		
Gabapentin	100–300 mg 2–3 times daily; 100–300 mg daily if frail; advance by 50--100% every 3–5 days or as tolerated; usual maximum dose 3600 mg/d	Adjust dose in renal impairment Taper when discontinuing drug *Adverse effects:* Somnolence Dizziness Ataxia Fatigue
Lamotrigine	25–50 mg orally daily; titrate gradually to 200 mg/d	Taper when discontinuing drug *Adverse effects:* Fatigue Dizziness Headache Rash
Levetiracetam	250–500 mg orally twice; titrate gradually to 3000 mg/d	Adjust dose in renal impairment *Adverse effects:* Somnolence Dizziness Ataxia Incoordination Anxiety

Continued

Table 8–6. Selected Antidepressants and Anticonvulsants Used in the Management of Malignant Neuropathic Pain. (*Continued*)

Drug	Dose	Comments
Anticonvulsants		
Topiramate	25 mg orally twice daily; titrate to maximum 200 mg/d	Also used in migraine prophylaxis Adjust dose in renal impairment *Adverse effects*: Metabolic acidosis Dizziness Somnolence Fatigue Anorexia

2. Radiation therapy and radiopharmaceuticals— Radiotherapy can be enormously beneficial in relieving pain due to bone metastases or other lesions. In many cases, single fraction external beam therapy can be used to facilitate treatment. Radiolabeled agents such as strontium-89 and samarium-153 have been shown to be effective at reducing metastatic bone pain. Thrombocytopenia and leukopenia are relative contraindications since strontium-89 causes thrombocytopenia in as many as 33% of those treated and leukopenia in up to 10%. Therapy should be considered only in those patients with a projected lifespan of greater than 3 months since there is

Table 8–7. Bisphosphonates and Calcitonin for Malignant Bone Pain.

Drug	Dose	Comments
Alendronate	35–70 mg orally every week	Inhibits osteoclast bone resorption. Take with water at least 30 minutes before eating food or other medications. Do not lie down for at least 30 minutes.
Calcitonin	100 international units SC/IM daily or 3 times/week	Not a true bisphosphonate but used to treat bone pain. Use with oral calcium and vitamin D.
Clodronate	1600 mg orally daily	Not available in the United States. Shorter duration of analgesia compared with pamidronate. Can be given in small volume subcutaneous dose.
Ibandronate	150 mg orally every month or 2 to 4 mg IV	Inhibits osteoclast bone resorption. Take with water at least 60 minutes before eating food or other medications. Do not lie down for at least 30 minutes.
Pamidronate	60–90 mg via infusion over 2–4 hours every 2–4 weeks	Inhibits osteoclast bone resorption. 2–3 doses necessary to determine efficacy. Use with caution in renal impairment. Only bisphosphonate approved in the United States for use in bone metastases.
Risedronate	5 mg orally daily or 35 mg orally every week	Inhibits osteoclast bone resorption. Take with water at least 30 minutes before eating food or other medications. Do not lie down for at least 30 minutes.
Zoledronic Acid (Zometa)	4 mg via infusion over 30–90 minutes every 3–4 weeks	Inhibits osteoclast bone resorption. Use with oral calcium and vitamin D. Use with caution in renal impairment.

a delay in onset of effect. A transitory pain flare is reported by as many as 10% of persons receiving strontium-89, and additional analgesics should be provided in anticipation, as well as patient education.

3. Chemotherapy—Palliative chemotherapy is the use of antitumor therapy to relieve symptoms associated with malignancy. Patient goals, performance status, sensitivity of the tumor, and potential toxicities must be carefully weighed. Examples of symptoms that may improve with chemotherapy include hormonal therapy in breast cancer to relieve chest wall pain due to tumor ulceration, or chemotherapy in lung cancer to relieve dyspnea.

E. Interventional Therapies

In addition to previously mentioned spinal administration of analgesics, interventional therapies to relieve pain at end-of-life can be beneficial; these therapies include nerve blocks, vertebroplasty, radiofrequency ablation of painful metastases, procedures to drain painful effusions, and other techniques. However, few of these procedures have undergone controlled clinical studies, particularly in cancer pain. One technique, the celiac plexus block, has been shown to be superior to morphine in patients with pain due to unresectable pancreatic cancer. A complete review of many of these procedures can be found in Chapter 4. Choosing one of these techniques depends on the availability of experts in this area who understand the special needs of cancer patients, the patient's ability to undergo the procedure, and the patient's and family's goals of care.

Table 8–8. Cognitive-Behavioral Therapies for Cancer-Related Pain.

Cognitive	Behavioral
Distraction	Exercise/active or passive range of motion
Education	Heat or cold
Hypnosis	Immobilization
Imagery	Massage
Pastoral counseling or prayer	Repositioning
Psychotherapy	Vibration
Reframing	
Relaxation	
Support groups	

Nonpharmacologic Therapies

Nondrug therapies, including cognitive-behavioral techniques and physical measures, can serve as adjuncts to analgesics (Table 8–8). These strategies are particularly useful to address periods of increased pain intensity, while waiting for the onset of the immediate-release analgesic. The patient's and caregivers' abilities to participate must be considered when selecting one of these therapies, including fatigue level, belief in the use of these types of techniques, cognitive ability, and other factors.

Cognitive-behavioral therapy includes strategies that improve coping and enhance relaxation. Examples include guided imagery, music, prayer, and reframing. In a randomized clinical trial of patients undergoing bone marrow transplantation, pain was reduced in those patients who received relaxation and imagery training and in those who received cognitive-behavioral skill development with relaxation and imagery, but not in those patients who received treatment as usual or who were randomized to receive support from a therapist. A recent study of art therapy in an inpatient cancer unit revealed a significant reduction in pain, anxiety, fatigue, and other symptoms.

Physical measures, such as massage, reflexology, heat, chiropractic and other techniques, relieve pain, although the mechanism is unknown. In a study of massage in hospice patients, relaxation resulted as measured by blood pressure, heart rate, and skin temperature. In another study, a 10-minute back massage was found to relieve pain in male cancer patients. These are simple inexpensive procedures that can incorporate family members, who are often seeking strategies to demonstrate support of their loved one.

Complex Cancer Pain Syndromes & Their Management

Several syndromes present unique challenges to the management of cancer-related pain. These include bone pain, malignant bowel obstruction, and pain crisis (Table 8–9).

A. Bone Pain

Pain due to bone metastates or pathologic fractures can be difficult to manage. Bone pain is generally associated with painful breakthrough pain when the patient tries to move in bed, sit, or stand. Although short-acting opioids may be effective, when the patient stops moving, the opioid is no longer necessary as the pain source diminishes, leaving the patient somnolent when at rest. Patient-controlled analgesia may be of benefit while the patient is awaiting surgical repair or fixation of the fracture. If the patient is opioid naïve, a bolus dose should be initiated, with rapid titration to determine the most effective dose to

Table 8–9. Management of Complex Cancer Pain Syndromes.

Malignant Bone Pain
- Dexamethasone 8–20 mg PO, IV, SC every morning (not to be used in conjunction with NSAIDs)
- Opioids
- Bisphosphonates, such as pamidronate or zoledronic acid
- Radiation therapy (may be given as single fraction in some cases)
- Radiopharmaceuticals, such as strontium-89
- Orthotics for braces or slings
- Physical or occupational therapy for assistive devices

Intractable Neuropathic Pain
- Dexamethasone 8–20 mg PO, IV, SC every morning (not to be used in conjunction with NSAIDs)
- Opioids can be effective, but higher doses are often indicated
- Methadone may provide additional benefit over other opioids
- Anticonvulsants
- Antidepressants, including tricyclics and novel or atypical agents (such as venlafaxine)
- Local anesthetics (eg, transdermal lidocaine, intraspinal infusions in combinations with opioids or parenteral infusions)
  - Intravenous lidocaine 1–2 mg/kg over 30–60 minute infusion as diagnostic intervention. If perioral numbness or lightheadedness occurs, slow or stop the infusion. Resume at a lower rate once symptoms subside.
  - If effective, continue infusion 1–2 mg/kg/h IV or SC

Malignant Intestinal Obstruction
- Dexamethasone 8–20 mg PO, IV, SC every morning to reduce inflammation and nausea (not to be used in conjunction with NSAIDs)
- Opioids
- Octreotide 20 mcg/h IV or SC to decrease intestinal secretions; increase dose as needed
- Scopolamine transdermal patches (1.5 mg, up to 2 patches) may reduce upper aerodigestive secretions
- Nasogastric tube or venting gastrostomy if consistent with patient goals

NSAIDs, nonsteroidal anti-inflammatory drugs.

relieve pain. If the pain is persistent, a basal rate may be calculated based on the necessary total bolus dose during an established time period. The bolus is continued along with the basal rate. For patients already taking opioids, the oral dose can be converted to the basal infusion, or the long-acting opioid is continued and the bolus dose is used for rapid-onset breakthrough pain.

Long-acting opioids combined with short-acting agents are the foundation of long-term treatment of persistent pain. However, additional nonopioid therapies are usually warranted, including corticosteroids, bisphosphonates if indicated, radiotherapy or radionuclides. Vertebroplasty may stabilize the vertebrae if tumor invasion leads to instability.

B. Malignant Bowel Obstruction

Bowel obstruction is common in progressive gynecologic (particularly ovarian cancer) and colorectal malignancies. This is a sign of more advanced disease, as the majority of patients with bowel obstruction will die within 6 months. Prevention is sometimes possible by adding corticosteroids to reduce inflammation, along with the aggressive use of stool softeners, laxatives, and agents that stimulate motility, such as metoclopramide. When obstruction cannot be prevented or delayed, several approaches can reduce pain as well as nausea and vomiting. Palliation can include surgery in selected cases, or more commonly, intravenous or subcutaneous octreotide, nasogastric tube suction, and venting gastrostomy, in addition to analgesics and antiemetics. As with all aspects of cancer pain management, the patient's and family's goals must be considered when devising a plan of care. The family's inability to manage external tubes, pumps, or infusion devices may affect the plan of care or result in placement where more assistance can be provided. Hospice usually can provide the support necessary to allow the patient to remain at home.

C. Pain Crisis

Most nociceptive (ie, somatic and visceral) pain is controllable with appropriately titrated analgesic therapy. However, some pain syndromes, such as complicated neuropathic pain or rapidly escalating pain, may be less responsive to conventional analgesic therapies. The following should be considered in the face of a pain crisis:

1. Differentiate terminal agitation, anxiety, or existential distress from "physically" based pain, if possible. If rapid upward titration of the opioids and other analgesics is insufficient, benzodiazepines (eg, diazepam, lorazepam, midazolam) or other sedating agents (eg, propofol) may be warranted. Incorporate other disciplines, including chaplains, psychologists and psychiatrists, social workers, and others, to address existential distress and spiritual issues. (See Chapter 9 for more information.)

2. Consider whether absorption of the medication is adequate. This is particularly true when using the oral route in a patient with bowel obstruction or other gastrointestinal complications but can also include transdermal or other routes of administration. The intravenous route is the only route that can provide consistent drug delivery when oral, enteral, or transdermal delivery is compromised. In most cases, invasive routes of drug delivery are to be avoided unless necessary. Parenteral access should be initiated if there is any question about absorption of analgesics or other necessary palliative drugs.

3. In some cases, radiotherapeutic, anesthetic, or neuroablative interventions may be warranted.

Barrueto F Jr et al. Gabapentin withdrawal presenting as status epilepticus. *J Toxicol Clin Toxicol.* 2002;40:925. [PMID: 12507063]

Bell R et al. Ketamine as an adjuvant to opioids for cancer pain. *Cochrane Database System Rev.* 2003;(1):CD003351. [PMID: 12535471]

Bruera E et al. Methadone use in cancer patients with pain: a review. *J Palliat Med.* 2002;5:127. [PMID: 11839235]

Bruera E et al. Methadone versus morphine as a first-line strong opioid for cancer pain: a randomized, double-blind study. *J Clin Oncol.* 2004;22:185. [PMID: 14701781]

Caraceni A et al. Gabapentin for neuropathic cancer pain: a randomized controlled trial from the Gabapentin Cancer Pain Study Group. *J Clin Oncol.* 2004;22:2909. [PMID: 15254060]

Cherny N et al. Strategies to manage the adverse effects of oral morphine: an evidence-based report. *J Clin Oncol.* 2001;19:2542. [PMID: 11331334]

Doverty M et al. Methadone maintenance patients are cross-tolerant to the antinociceptive effects of morphine. *Pain.* 2001;93:155. [PMID: 11427327]

Durand JP et al. Clinical activity of venlafaxine and topiramate against oxaliplatin-induced disabling permanent neuropathy. *Anticancer Drugs.* 2005;16:587. [PMID: 15846125]

Dworkin RH et al. Advances in neuropathic pain: diagnosis, mechanisms, and treatment recommendations. *Arch Neurol.* 2003;60:1524. [PMID: 14623723]

Ferrari A et al. Methadone–metabolism, pharmacokinetics and interactions. *Pharmacol Res.* 2004;50:551. [PMID:15501692]

Ferrini R et al. How to initiate and monitor infusional lidocaine for severe and/or neuropathic pain. *J Support Oncol.* 2004;2:90. [PMID:15330376]

Gilron I et al. Morphine, gabapentin, or their combination for neuropathic pain. *N Engl J Med.* 2005;352:1324. [PMID: 15800228]

Grothey A. Clinical management of oxaliplatin-associated neurotoxicity. *Clin Colorectal Cancer.* 2005;5 Suppl 1:S38. [PMID:15871765]

Hammack JE et al. Phase III evaluation of nortriptyline for alleviation of symptoms of cis-platinum-induced peripheral neuropathy. *Pain.* 2002;98:195. [PMID:12098632]

Hanks GW et al. Morphine and alternative opioids in cancer pain: the EAPC recommendations. *Br J Cancer.* 2001;84:587. [PMID:11237376]

Indelicato RA et al. Opioid rotation in the management of refractory cancer pain. *J Clin Oncol.* 2002;20:348. [PMID: 11773191]

Juni P et al. Are selective COX 2 inhibitors superior to traditional non steroidal anti-inflammatory drugs? *BMJ.* 2002;324:1287. [PMID:12039807]

Kornick CA et al. QTc interval prolongation associated with intravenous methadone. *Pain.* 2003;105:499. [PMID: 14527710]

Kraeber-Bodere F et al. Treatment of bone metastases of prostate cancer with strontium-89 chloride: efficacy in relation to the degree of bone involvement. *Eur J Nucl Med.* 2000;27:1487. [PMID: 11083537]

Krantz MJ et al. Dose-related effects of methadone on QT prolongation in a series of patients with torsade de pointes. *Pharmacotherapy.* 2003;23:802. [PMID: 12820821]

Lauretti GR et al. Comparison of sustained-release morphine with sustained-release oxycodone in advanced cancer patients. *Br J Cancer.* 2003;89:2027. [PMID: 14647133]

Lucas LK et al. Recent advances in pharmacotherapy for cancer pain management. *Cancer Pract.* 2002;10:S14. [PMID: 12027964]

Maremmani I et al. QTc interval prolongation in patients on long-term methadone maintenance therapy. *Eur Addict Res.* 2005;11:44. [PMID: 15608471]

McNamara P. Opioid switching from morphine to transdermal fentanyl for toxicity reduction in palliative care. *Palliat Med.* 2002;16:425. [PMID: 12380661]

Mercadante S. The use of anti-inflammatory drugs in cancer pain. *Cancer Treat Rev.* 2001;27:51. [PMID: 1123777]

Mercadante S et al. Pain mechanisms involved and outcome in advanced cancer patients with possible indications for celiac plexus block and superior hypogastric plexus block. *Tumori.* 2002;88:243. [PMID: 12195764]

Moryl N et al. Pitfalls of opioid rotation: substituting another opioid for methadone in patients with cancer pain. *Pain.* 2002;96:325. [PMID: 11973005]

Payne R et al. Long-term safety of oral transmucosal fentanyl citrate for breakthrough cancer pain. *J Pain Symptom Manage.* 2001;22:575. [PMID: 11516599]

Prommer E. Guidelines for the use of palliative chemotherapy. *AAHPM Bulletin.* 2004;5:1–4.

Ruggiero SL et al. Osteonecrosis of the jaws associated with the use of bisphosphonates: a review of 63 cases. *J Oral Maxillofac Surg.* 2004;62:527. [PMID: 15122554]

Sarhill N et al. Methadone-induced myoclonus in advanced cancer. *Am J Hosp Palliat Care.* 2001;18:51. [PMID: 11406880]

Sciuto R et al. Metastatic bone pain palliation with 89-Sr and 186-Re-HEDP in breast cancer patients. *Breast Cancer Res Treat.* 2001;66:101. [PMID:11437096]

Small EJ et al. Combined analysis of two multicenter, randomized, placebo-controlled studies of pamidronate disodium for the palliation of bone pain in men with metastatic prostate cancer. *J Clin Oncol.* 2003;21:4277. [PMID: 14581438]

Smith MT. Neuroexcitatory effects of morphine and hydromorphone: evidence implicating the 3-glucuronide metabolites. *Clin Exp Pharmacol Physiol.* 2000;27:524. [PMID: 10874511]

Solomon DH et al. Relationship between selective cyclooxygenase-2 inhibitors and acute myocardial infarction in older adults. *Circulation.* 2004;109:2068. [PMID: 15096449]

Tanaka E et al. Update: the clinical importance of acetaminophen hepatotoxicity in non-alcoholic and alcoholic subjects. *J Clin Pharm Ther.* 2000;25:325. [PMID: 11123483]

Tasmuth T et al. Venlafaxine in neuropathic pain following treatment of breast cancer. *Eur J Pain.* 2002;6:17. [PMID: 11888224]

Watanabe S et al. Opioid rotation to methadone: proceed with caution. *J Clin Oncol.* 2002;20:2409. [PMID: 11981018]

Wong GY et al. Effect of neurolytic celiac plexus block on pain relief, quality of life, and survival in patients with unresectable pancreatic cancer: a randomized controlled trial. *JAMA.* 2004;291:1092. [PMID: 14996778]

Wong R et al. Bisphosphonates for the relief of pain secondary to bone metastases. *Cochrane Database System Rev.* 2002;(2):CD002068. [PMID: 12076438]

Wooldridge JE et al. Corticosteroids in advanced cancer. *Oncology (Williston Park).* 2001;15:225. [PMID: 11252935]

Wright AW et al. Hydromorphone-3-glucuronide: a more potent neuro-excitant than its structural analogue, morphine-3-glucuronide. *Life Sci.* 2001;69:409. [PMID: 11459432]

American Cancer Society http://www.cancer.org/docroot/home/index.asp

American Pain Foundation http://www.painfoundation.org

American Pain Society http://www.ampainsoc.org

Cochrane Pain, Palliative Care and Supportive Care Group http://www.cochrane.org/cochrane/revabstr/ SYMPTAbstractIndex.htm

End of Life, Palliative Education Resource Center - EPERC (Fast Facts) http://www.eperc.mcw.edu/

Federation of State Medical Boards of the United States (for information regarding prescribing controlled substances) http://www.fsmb.org

International Association for the Study of Pain http://www.iasp-pain.org/index.html

National Cancer Institute, PDQ http://cancernet.nci.nih.gov/cancertopics/pdq/supportivecare/pain/

National Comprehensive Cancer Network http://www.nccn.org/

Pain Management in Palliative Care 9

Jamie H. Von Roenn, MD, Judith A. Paice, PhD, RN, & Michael E. Preodor, MD

ESSENTIAL CRITERIA

- *Palliative care is whole-person care for patients with disease that is not responsive to treatment, including cancer, cardiac disease, neuromuscular disorders, and many other illnesses, to achieve the best possible quality of life.*
- *Pain, one of the most feared symptoms at the end of life, can be relieved in most patients.*
- *Anticipate expected opioid side effects and prescribe preventive therapies.*

General Considerations

Internists care for a variety of patients with life-threatening illnesses, including those with cancer, cardiac disease, neuromuscular disorders, and many other illnesses. The number of these patients will grow as the population ages, increasing the need for physicians who can provide care to persons with advanced disease. Although usually provided in the context of an interdisciplinary team of physicians, nurses, social workers, chaplains, and other professionals, these formal services are not yet available in all health care settings. As a result, all physicians must be able to address some of the basic components of palliative care, including aggressive symptom management.

Of the many symptoms that occur during the end of life, pain is one of the most feared. Yet, the majority of patients can obtain relief, even during the final hours of life. In fact, despite concerns that high-dose infusions of parenteral opioids will be necessary, many patients remain on relatively low oral doses of these agents even until the time of death. An awareness of the common pain syndromes seen during this time will assist the physician to determine the underlying cause and devise an appropriate treatment plan.

A. PREVALENCE

Not unexpectedly, the prevalence of pain at the end of life varies with the underlying diagnosis as well as the setting of care. In a retrospective review of 400 patients referred for palliative care services in London, pain was the most common symptom, experienced by 64% of patients; most (90%) had cancer. Other common symptoms in this study included anorexia (34%), constipation (32%), weakness (32%), and dyspnea (31%). This prevalence is consistent with other studies of patients with advanced cancer.

Pain in HIV-infected persons is well documented as is the undertreatment of pain in this population. Unfortunately, the prevalence of pain associated with other life-threatening illnesses has not been studied in sufficient detail.

Patients referred to palliative care or hospice generally have a greater symptom burden, particularly increased prevalence of pain. For example, one study of lung cancer outpatients revealed that 27% had pain, compared with 76% of those referred to palliative care. However, after 2 weeks in hospice, pain usually diminishes significantly.

B. COMMON PAIN SYNDROMES

With the exception of cancer, few studies have explored specific pain syndromes associated with life-threatening illnesses. Table 9–1 lists pain syndromes that are common at the end of life.

Most patients experience continuous pain, with episodes of escalation. Breakthrough or transient pain is common at the end of life in persons with cancer and nonmalignant disease, though rapid escalation of pain in the last days and hours of life is not. Breakthrough pain is often spontaneous (40%) or related to movement (36%), to the analgesic regimen (35%), to coughing (11%), or to other factors (18%). In a recent study of patients seen by a palliative care service, breakthrough pain occurred in 75% of persons who had continuous pain. Of these, 30% were exclusively incidental, 26% were not related to a particular movement or other factors, and 16% were due to end-of-dose failure.

Clinical Findings

A. ASSESSMENT

The assessment of pain in palliative care includes the principles discussed in Chapter 2. A thorough history and physical examination is critical when evaluating a

Table 9–1. Pain Syndromes in Palliative Care.

Pain related to underlying disease

- Tumor-related pain due to pressure or compression
- Chest pain due to end-stage cardiac disease
- Ischemia caused by atherosclerotic disease
- Abdominal pain with referral to thorax and shoulder due to liver failure, cirrhosis
- Abdominal pain due to ascites
- Extremity skin pain due to edema
- Back pain and skin discomfort or pruritus due to end-stage renal disease
- Chest pain due to pulmonary fibrosis, emphysema, other advanced lung disorders
- Central nervous system infection (meningitis, cryptosporidiosis) leading to headache
- Central pain after stroke, particularly affecting thalamus
- Trigeminal neuralgia in multiple sclerosis
- Vasoocclusion leading to bone, muscle, and visceral pain in sickle cell disease
- Rapid onset of cachexia leading to peripheral neuropathy
- Spasticity due to neuromuscular disorders

Pain related to treatment

- Peripheral neuropathy due to chemotherapy, highly active antiretroviral therapy (HAART)
- Surgically induced phantom pain, chronic neuropathy
- Immunocompromise leading to postherpetic neuropathy
- Aseptic necrosis due to prolonged corticosteroid use

Pain unrelated to disease or its treatment

- Pressure ulcers
- Reduced muscle and fat padding at bony prominences
- Muscle atrophy leading to myalgia
- Immobility leading to joint pain
- Contractures

Key aspects of pain assessment in palliative care include the following:

1. Select tools appropriate to the patient's developmental and cognitive state.
2. Differentiate between physical pain and distress.
3. Develop an evaluation and treatment plan consistent with the patient's and family's stated goals of care.

B. ASSESSMENT TOOLS

A variety of circumstances may confound pain assessment in patients with life-threatening illness. Diseases, such as dementia, stroke, Parkinson disease, and others, may limit self-report. As patients approach the end of life, the risk of—or potential for—cognitive impairment (including delirium) increases, making the use of standard, self-report tools difficult. Internists may also see patients in the intensive care unit who are ventilated and unable to respond. There is little research regarding pain assessment in palliative care patients with greater cognitive impairment or in those who have no ability to self-report. In the absence of standardized measures, these challenges can be addressed in several ways:

1. Ask the patient. Many patients with mild cognitive impairment can effectively use standard unidimensional pain intensity tools, such as the 0 to 10 scale.
2. Use nonfamily translators to assist in obtaining pain information when language or cultural issues preclude adequate assessment.
3. Ask the family or other caregivers who know the patient. Of concern, however, is that family members who are distraught at witnessing their loved one during this time may integrate some of their own distress in this report.
4. Review the patient's history for the existence of pre-existing painful conditions.
5. Examine behavioral cues (such as the furrowed brow; posture; and vocalization, such as crying out when moved) that may provide evidence of pain. Empiric management is warranted, as is assessment to rule out other potential contributors, such as impaction or a distended bladder.
6. Conduct a thorough physical assessment to determine possible causes of pain.

C. PAIN VERSUS DISTRESS

For many patients and their families, having a diagnosis of a life-threatening illness leads to significant existential distress. Although some patients and family members find this time a period of great personal growth, for others, futility, hopelessness, and anxiety are common. Spiritual issues and a sense of loss of meaning may arise. These are intertwined with the grief and distress experienced by loved ones and other caregivers.

new pain complaint, with ongoing reassessment as warranted. Laboratory and imaging studies are conducted based on the patient's goals of care. If these tests yield information that will guide and inform treatment, they may be considered. However, if they are not likely to provide meaningful information, empiric management of the pain is warranted. Additionally, these tests can be painful, expensive, and can provide a false sense of hope to patients and families who believe the results may lead to some new cure.

Assessment includes the following:

1. Identifying physical symptoms, such as pain, dyspnea, nausea, fatigue, and others. Distress is highly correlated with the presence of pain and other symptoms.

2. Distinguishing between physical and existential pain. Pain that is not easily explainable or does not respond to aggressive management raises the concern that existential pain is being reported as physical pain. Some persons do not have the language to discuss this distress, or there may be cultural barriers to initiating discussions regarding spiritual pain. Patients may be asked about the meaning of the pain and their illness to begin this discussion.

3. Identifying psychological symptoms, such as anxiety, depression, or delirium.

4. Determining adequacy of care and family support. This includes the patient's level of physical functioning, the home environment, and the availability of family to provide care and emotional support.

5. Ensuring the patient's and family's understanding of the extent of the illness and their awareness of probable treatment outcomes.

6. Establishing goals of care, particularly related to prolonging survival and providing comfort. Conducting a family meeting can be an effective strategy to elicit these goals and develop a plan of care that is based on consensus of the patient and his or her loved ones.

Because physical symptoms, particularly pain, can increase suffering, it is critical to aggressively manage pain. This not only builds trust with patients and their families, but allows them to direct their energies toward addressing the other factors contributing to distress and suffering.

D. SPECIAL CONSIDERATION

Prolonged pain (weeks to months) due to any etiology may change in character with time. For example, chronic abdominal pain due to advanced colon cancer with intraperitoneal spread begins as an achy pain, typical of nociceptive pain. It may assume a squeezing, pulling, neuropathic character that may become less responsive to opioid therapy. This underscores the need for frequent reassessment of pain and its prescribed management. Treatment of pain that has undergone neuropathic transformation follows the same principles of treatment as classic neuropathic pain (see Chapter 10).

Gutgsell T et al. A prospective study of the pathophysiology and clinical characteristics of pain in a palliative medicine population. *Am J Hosp Palliat Care.* 2003;20:140. [PMID: 12693647]

Mercadante S et al. Episodic (breakthrough) pain: consensus conference of an expert working group of the European Association for Palliative Care. *Cancer.* 2002;94:832. [PMID: 11857319]

Potter J et al. Symptoms in 400 patients referred to palliative care services: prevalence and patterns. *Palliat Med.* 2003;17:310. [PMID: 12822846]

World Health Organization. Cancer pain relief and palliative care. Geneva: World Health Organization, 1990.

The EPEC™ Project. Education in Palliative and End-of-life Care. Available at http://www.epec.net (accessed August 27, 2005).

■ TREATMENT

Pain is by far a more complex phenomenon than once believed. A number of factors (ie, personal, social, and cultural) interact to impact the perception of pain. Relieving pain in palliative care requires knowledge and utilization of multiple therapeutic modalities. Pharmacologic interventions, extensively discussed here, are more efficacious if used in combination with other modalities (Table 9–2).

Table 9–2. Multiple Treatment Modalities for Pain.

Modalities	Examples
Disease modifying	Medical therapy Chemotherapy Radiation therapy Surgery
Pharmacologic	Opioids Nonopioids Adjuvants Other
Physical therapy	Exercise Stretching
Psychological	Psychodynamic Cognitive-behavioral
Spiritual	Prayer Meditation
Alternative therapies	Healing touch Aromatherapy
Relaxation	Guided imagery Music and art therapies
Other complementary	Acupuncture Transcutaneous electrical nerve stimulation Heat and cold therapies Massage

Table 9–3. Palliative Medical Therapies.

Condition	Therapy
Thrombophlebitis	Anticoagulation
Pulmonary emboli	Venous filter
Arthritis (eg, gout, rheumatoid arthritis, osteoarthritis)	Anti-inflammatory medication Methotrexate Corticosteroids
Angina	β-Blockers, nitrates, calcium channel blockers
Peptic ulcer disease	H$_2$-blockers, pump blockers *Helicobacter pylori* eradication

Table 9–4. Palliative Surgical Therapies.

Goal	Procedure
Relief of gastrointestinal or biliary obstruction	Diversion or venting Stent placement
Relief of effusions	Pleural or peritoneal catheter placement Paracentesis/ thoracentesis Pleurodesis Pericardiocentesis, "window" placement
Urologic obstruction	Urinary catheter placement Suprapubic catheter Ureteral stent Percutaneous stent
Bone pain	Stabilize impending or pathologic fracture Spinal cord or cauda equina lesions
Abscess	Percutaneous drainage
Treatment of symptomatic metastases	Tumor ablation (eg, radiofrequency, cryotherapy)

While some modalities, such as rigorous physical therapy, may be difficult or seemingly impossible due to advanced illness and poor functional status, similar interventions, such as massage and gentle stretching, can complement pharmacologic interventions.

Effective pain management is complemented by concurrent disease-modifying treatment. For example, ongoing medical management of painful, preexisting, chronic conditions, such as gout or osteoarthritis, is an essential component of optimal pain management in palliative situations (Table 9–3). Complications of advanced illness, such as bowel, biliary, or urinary tract obstruction, may require surgical intervention to effectively relieve pain (Table 9–4).

Prophylactic therapies also may provide a measure of palliation. For example, ablation of the celiac plexus at the time of exploration for pancreatic cancer reduces the likelihood and severity of subsequent abdominal pain. Antimicrobial prophylaxis for opportunistic infections such as *Mycobacterium avium-intracellulare* (MAC) in patients with advanced HIV disease may prevent MAC-associated abdominal pain.

NONOPIOID ANALGESICS

Nonopioid analgesics (Table 9–5) are the initial treatment of choice for mild pain. These agents are free of significant central nervous system (CNS) adverse effects. When caring for patients with advanced illness, there is often a rush to initiate opioids before a trial of nonopioids. Aspirin, acetaminophen, and NSAIDs have proved effective for mildly painful conditions.

Acetaminophen

Acetaminophen is an effective analgesic at standard doses, though not an anti-inflammatory agent. Because of its relative safety, acetaminophen is a useful tool to manage mild pain in the palliative and end-of-life care setting. It is effective for the musculoskeletal aches and pains that often accompany advanced age and, in particular, is useful for the generalized stiffness associated with reduced mobility in the frail elderly or bedridden patient.

Acetaminophen is available as tablets, a liquid, or as rectal suppositories. No parenteral preparation is available. Use the minimally effective dose of acetaminophen. Efficacy increases little above the ceiling dose of 2.6 g/d. The maximally tolerated dose is 4 g/d in healthy persons. The likelihood of liver or renal toxicity increases with higher doses. This may or may not be an important consideration, depending on the patient's overall medical condition. The dose is reduced by 50 to 75% if the patient has a history of chronic alcohol intake (more than three drinks per day) or significant hepatic impairment.

Nonsteroidal Anti-Inflammatory Drugs

The NSAIDs are analgesic via their inhibition of prostaglandins (Table 9–5). Like acetaminophen, NSAIDs are widely used in combination with opioids for patients with moderate to severe pain at the end of life. Their usefulness, especially for bone pain and inflammatory syndromes, is well established. NSAIDs are also appropriate for treating the generalized body aches, joint stiffness, and pain due to periods of immobility that are common in advanced illness.

***Table* 9–5.** Nonopioids: Nonsteroidal Anti-Inflammatory Drugs and Acetaminophen.[a]

Drug	Trade name	Dosage[b]	Maximum dose
Acetaminophen	Tylenol	650–1000 mg PO q4h	4 g/d
Celecoxib	Celebrex	100–200 mg PO bid	400 mg/d
Diclofenac	Voltaren	50–75 mg PO tid	200 mg/d
Ibuprofen	Motrin Advil	600–800 mg PO qid	3.2 g/d
Ketorolac	Toradol	15–30 mg IV q6h[c]	120 mg/d
Nabumetone	Relafen	500–1000 mg PO bid	2000 mg/d
Naproxen	Naprosyn	375–500 mg PO tid	1.5 g/d
Salsalate	Disalcid	1000–1500 mg PO tid	4.5 g/d

[a]These agents are useful for muscle and bone pain and should be taken with food.
[b]All above doses are based on healthy patients and may need to be adjusted for age, weight, and renal or liver functions.
[c]Ketorolac use should be limited to 5 days; may precipitate renal failure in dehydrated patients.

The analgesic effects are dose-dependent but with a ceiling effect. There are individual variations in the effectiveness of the various products. When faced with diminished or absent effectiveness with one agent, try an alternate preparation.

The use of NSAIDs for palliation may be limited by toxicity. Their toxicity (gastrointestinal and renal) is particularly relevant when used in patients who, due to advanced illness, may be more susceptible to gastric irritation, especially if multiple oral medications accompany NSAID therapy. Careful attention to prior episodes of gastrointestinal upset or bleeding with NSAIDs may prevent inappropriate use of these drugs in sensitive persons. However, a high percentage (75–80%) of patients with gastrointestinal bleeding due to NSAIDs have no prior gastrointestinal symptoms. The renal effects may be problematic due to compromised renal function or decreased renal perfusion as a consequence of longstanding illness, dehydration, or the normal decline in renal function with advancing age.

NSAIDs diminish platelet function and increase the risk of bleeding and bruising. There is also a modest interaction between warfarin and NSAIDs, requiring appropriate monitoring of the international normalized ratio (INR) and adjustment of warfarin dose as necessary, depending on the clinical setting.

The cardiovascular risks of NSAIDs, particularly the cyclooxygenase-2 (COX-2) inhibitors, are well documented. Whether this should preclude their use in end-of-life care depends on the relative benefits and risks in a particular clinical setting and the patient's and family's goals. All NSAIDs are available as oral preparations. Ketorolac is the only parenteral NSAID available in the United States. In the face of opioid toxicity, ketorolac is a good adjunct to opioid therapy. Ketorolac 30 mg IV has the approximate analgesic effect of morphine 12 mg IV. Its renal toxicity limits the recommended duration of use to fewer than 5 days. The dose is reduced to 15 mg in patients over 65 years of age. Oral ketorolac appears to be no more effective than other NSAIDs.

Acetaminophen Plus Opioid Combinations

Acetaminophen is available in fixed combination with multiple opioids (Table 9–6). These agents are effective for treating moderate pain (eg, local pain due to tissue damage without neuropathic qualities). They are widely prescribed in seriously ill patients because of their somewhat lower incidence of sedation and confusion, compared with the stronger opioids. Care should be taken to avoid escalating combination preparations to acetaminophen doses that are toxic. Changing to an opioid without acetaminophen is safer and more effective in this circumstance. As a practical matter, the regulatory environment in many countries (ie, the United States) allows combination products to be ordered by telephone, thus facilitating their use. All combination preparations are oral. Tablet and liquid formulations are available for many. The usual opioid side effects of constipation and, less frequently, nausea may be observed and should be anticipated.

The two adult strengths of acetaminophen, 325 mg and 500 mg (regular and extra strength, respectively), are present in most combination pain products, eg, acetaminophen with codeine (Tylenol #3 and #4) and acetaminophen with hydrocodone (Vicodin). The

Table 9–6. Opioid Equianalgesic Dosing Guidelines.[a]

Generic name	Trade name and formulation	IV/SC (mg)	Oral (mg)	Duration
Codeine/Acetaminophen[b]	Tylenol #3: 30 mg/300 mg (12) (Empirin #3) Tylenol #4: 60 mg/300 mg (12) (Empirin #4)	130 130	200 200	3–4 h 3–4 h
Fentanyl	IV Duragesic patch (12.5, 25, 50, 75, 100 mcg)	0.1		30–60 min 72 hours
Hydrocodone/ Acetaminophen[b]	Lortab or Vicodin: 5 mg/500 mg (8) Vicodin ES: 7.5/500 Vicodin HP: 10/660 Lortab: Elixir 7.5 mg/500 mg/15 mL Norco: 10 mg/325 mg (12)	N/A	30	3–4 h
Hydromorphone	Immediate release: Dilaudid: 2, 4, 8 mg tablets; 5 mg/5 mL oral liquid	2	8	3–4 h
Levorphanol[c]	Levo-Dromoran: 2 mg tablets	2	4	3–4 h
Methadone[d]	Dolophine: 10 mg tablets	–	–	4–6 h
Morphine	Immediate release: MSIR 30 mg Liquid: Roxanol 20 mg/mL Long-acting MS Contin: 15, 30, 60, 100, 200 mg	10 10 10	30 30 30	3–4 h 3–4 h 3–4 h
Oxycodone	Immediate release: Percocet: 5 mg/325 mg (12)[b] Immediate release: Roxicodone: 5 mg tablets or 5 mg/5 mL oral liquid or 20 mg/mL oral liquid Tylox: 5 mg/500 mg (8)[b] Long-acting: OxyContin: 10, 20, 40, 80 mg	N/A N/A N/A N/A	20–30 20–30 20–30 20–30	3–4 h 3–4 h 12 h

[a]Equianalgesic doses are approximate; individualize the dose to meet the patient's needs. Cross tolerance is incomplete; reduce the dose by 25% when converting to another opioid in a patient with well-controlled pain.
[b]Acetaminophen-opioid mixture: give no more than 4000 mg/d to patients with normal liver function. Discharge prescriptions should read: Take 1–2 tablets PO every 4–6 hours PRN pain–not to exceed "#" tablets per day.
[c]Levorphanol has a long elimination half-life; may require dose adjustment to prevent accumulation.
[d]Methadone conversion:
Long, unpredictable half-life, from 13 to 100 + hours
Acute pain: methadone + morphine (1:1)
Chronic pain: ratio depends on previous opioid dose (methadone:morphine)
If the patient is taking less than 90 mg oral morphine equivalents: 1 mg methadone = 5 mg morphine
If the patient is taking 91 to 299 mg oral morphine equivalents/day: 1 mg methadone = 10 mg morphine
If the patient is taking 300 mg or more of oral morphine equivalents: 1 mg methadone = 20 mg morphine
Methadone is not a first-line agent. When discharging a patient with a prescription for methadone, include "for pain" after the dose and frequency. Many pharmacies do not carry methadone.
    If the parenteral route is required, avoid IM injections. Absorption is variable and injection is painful.

acetaminophen component limits the safe dose of these products to 8 tablets per day for products containing 500 mg of acetaminophen and 12 tablets daily for those containing 325 mg of acetaminophen.

OPIOIDS

Since the birth of the modern hospice and palliative care movement, opioids have been an essential element of pain management in patients with life-threatening illness. Oral opioids are effective for controlling pain when administered in adequate doses on a regular schedule rather than on an as-needed basis (see Chapter 3).

Patients and families often worry that use of strong opioids will result in addiction or "feeling high." There also may be reluctance to use adequate doses due to fears that the opioid will become ineffective, thus making it necessary to "save" the drugs for more severe circumstances. Educating and reassuring patients and families about the safety and efficacy of opioids and pointing out the low likelihood of addiction in palliative care settings provide reassurance and may enhance adherence to the opioid regimen.

Use of opioids in advanced illness is safe and effective if prescribed appropriately. The adage, "start low and go slow," is germane. An "opioid naïve" patient (a patient not recently treated with opioids) should be given the lowest possible dose that is then titrated upward. For the patient who has been taking one or more opioids, equianalgesic principles are applied to identify the starting dose. To relieve severe pain, opioids are delivered on an around-the-clock schedule.

Most of the commonly prescribed oral opioids (see Table 9–6) have a 4-hour half-life under usual physiologic circumstances. Therefore, routine oral dosing is every 4 hours; after 4 to 5 half-lives, or slightly less than a day, steady state is achieved. Therefore, if pain control is inadequate after 24 hours, dose adjustment is required. Once the daily dose requirement for pain control is established, patient convenience is enhanced by the introduction of long-acting preparations. There are both 12 hourly and daily long-acting opioid preparations available. If pain is not well controlled, the dose of opioid may be increased by 25 to 50% for mild to moderate pain and by 100% if the pain remains severe. During this titration phase, reassess pain at least every 4 hours and adjust the opioid dose. There is no total dose that is too high. The dose that is effective to control pain is the "right" dose for a given patient. Morphine does not have a ceiling effect. Knowledge of the pharmacology of opioids in this very ill group of patients will provide pain relief without unacceptable toxicity.

Once on a stable opioid dose, breakthrough dosing is generally necessary to allow "rescue" doses of opioid to be given during times of increased activity or pain escalation during the day or night. The recommended dose of opioid for breakthrough pain, based on opioid pharmacodynamics, is equal to 10 to 20% of the 24-hour total dose. The peak analgesic effect occurs when C_{max}, the peak serum concentration, is achieved. For most opioids, the C_{max} occurs 1 hour after oral dosing. Opioids administered by intravenous bolus peak in 10 to 15 minutes, and when delivered subcutaneously, in 15 to 20 minutes. Therefore, a breakthrough dose may be repeated after 1 hour by mouth, 10 to 15 minutes by IV, and after 15 to 20 minutes subcutaneously.

If breakthrough doses are required three or more times in 24 hours, the total dose used in the 24-hour period is added up and the daily dose is adjusted upward. A breakthrough dose of 10 to 20% is recalculated as the new total daily dose for continued effectiveness.

Opioids are the mainstay of therapy for severe pain. Morphine is one of the most versatile drugs available and can be delivered via multiple routes: oral, intravenous, subcutaneous, rectal, intramuscular (although not recommended due to variable uptake and pain upon injection), sublingual, epidural, and intranasal. Intravenous and subcutaneous opioid administration follows first order kinetics; therefore, the opioid blood concentration is in linear proportion to the dose administered. Opioids are metabolized by the liver, and 90 to 95% is excreted by the kidneys. When using the oral route, first-pass metabolism by the liver reduces opioid potency by about two-thirds. As advanced illness, age, or intrinsic disease reduce renal or liver function, the serum level of the opioid rises proportionally. As patients approach death and renal function declines, the opioid dose may require reduction. Opioid metabolites, such as morphine-6 glucuronide and morphine-3 glucuronide, accumulate in patients with renal impairment. Many of these metabolites are centrally acting and have the potential to increase side effects, particularly sedation.

Successful analgesia, defined as adequate pain control without unacceptable adverse effects, is achieved in 70 to 90% of patients. There are several frequently encountered situations in palliative medicine where adverse effects of opioids are more common and may forestall adequate opioid dosing:

1. Significant comorbidities: Patients with CNS disease may be predisposed to drowsiness, nausea or vomiting and may have cognitive impairment prior to opioid therapy. Similarly, metabolic abnormalities or organ failure may mimic or exacerbate opioid-induced adverse effects, including mental status changes and nausea.

2. Drug interactions: Anticholinergic medications, especially tricyclic antidepressants, as well as psychotropics, including benzodiazepines and major tranquilizers, produce sedation and fatigue that is exacerbated by opioids.

3. Treatments: Chemotherapy, radiotherapy, or dialysis may cause nausea and vomiting, drowsiness, or constipation, all of which may be exacerbated by opioids.

Opioids Not Recommended for Use in Palliative Medicine

Table 9–7 lists the opioids that should be avoided. Propoxyphene, a synthetic derivative of methadone, is a weak opioid of limited use in palliative care. It has low analgesic potency and a prolonged half-life. Propoxyphene is biotransformed by the liver to norpropoxyphene, a metabolite with the potential to cause CNS excitation (ie, tremors, myoclonus, twitches, seizures). Because norpropoxyphene is renally excreted, its use is not recommended in persons with renal impairment.

Table 9–7. Opioids Not Recommended.

Drug	Reason
Propoxyphene	• Weak analgesic • Low efficacy at available commercial doses • Longer half-life
Tramadol	• Weak opioid agonist • Psychomimetic effects • Ceiling effect • Expensive
Meperidine	• Poor oral absorption • Normeperidine is a toxic metabolite and has a longer half-life (6 hours) • Psychomimetic adverse effects, myoclonus, seizures • For analgesia, dosing every 3 hours necessary, normeperidine builds up • Toxicity increases with renal insufficiency and old age
Mixed agonist-antagonists	• Pentazocine, butorphanol, nalbuphine, dezocine • Compete with agonists, results in withdrawal syndrome • Analgesic ceiling effect • High risk of psychomimetic adverse effects

Tramadol is a weak opioid agonist and blocks reuptake of serotonin and noradrenalin. The significance of the latter is unclear. Its use in palliative care is limited due to its psychomimetic effect, a ceiling effect (doses greater than 300 to 400 mg/d are not recommended), and significant cost. However, compared with codeine and related compounds, constipation appears to be less prominent with this agent.

Meperidine is an opioid with erratic oral absorption, a relatively short half-life, and toxic metabolites. Meperidine is metabolized in the liver to normeperidine. This metabolite has half the analgesic effect of the parent compound but twice the potential for CNS toxicity. The neurotoxicity of normeperidine may occur rapidly, particularly in the face of renal toxicity. Other factors that may contribute to meperidine-induced CNS excitation include long-term treatment, high-dose therapy, a prior history of seizures, or coadministration with other potentially neurotoxic agents (eg, methylphenidate, phenothiazines).

Mixed agonist-antagonist agents (eg, pentazocine, butorphanol) cannot be recommended. Dose escalation leads to psychomimetic effects for a significant number of patients and, in addition, there is a ceiling to their analgesic effect. Furthermore, all of these agents have the potential to precipitate withdrawal in opioid-dependent patients.

Routes of Administration

The versatility of opioids allows for the provision of adequate analgesia when the oral route of administration is not feasible. For situations in which the oral route is not available, alternatives are indicated and summarized in Table 9–8. Opioids for palliation are currently available in multiple formulations to facilitate administration. The optimal route of opioid administration is oral. In general, the route that is simplest, most cost effective, and most convenient should be used.

A. ORAL OPIOIDS

Most opioids, with the exception of fentanyl and related compounds (eg, sufentanil), are available by mouth. Morphine, hydromorphone, oxycodone, and methadone are available in liquid preparations. Morphine, hydromorphone, and oxycodone are available as long-acting preparations. The long-acting preparations have the added convenience of being taken fewer times a day (one to three times), compared with short-acting preparations that are usually taken six times a day.

B. SUBLINGUAL, BUCCAL, AND TRANSMUCOSAL OPIOIDS

Sublingual and buccal application of opioids may be used with some success. However, the effectiveness of this administration route is primarily from swallowing the opioid rather than through direct oral absorption. This is particularly true for morphine. Due to its low lipid solubility, the bioavailability of sublingual morphine is about 18%. Highly lipid-soluble opioids, such as fentanyl and methadone, have significantly greater transmucosal absorption. For example, oral transmucosal fentanyl citrate, a fentanyl-containing matrix that dissolves when rubbed against the buccal mucosa, provides rapid relief of pain (within 5 to 10 minutes). About 25% of the total fentanyl dose is absorbed through the buccal mucosa, avoiding first-pass metabolism, while the remainder is swallowed.

C. SUBCUTANEOUS OPIOIDS

Continuous subcutaneous administration of opioids is approximately equianalgesic to continuous parenteral

Table 9–8. Alternatives to Oral Administration of Opioids.

Setting	Alternative routes of administration				
	IV	SC	Rectal	Transdermal	Sublingual/transmucosal
Bowel obstruction	+	+	+	+	±
Nausea/vomiting	+	+	+	+	±
Diarrhea	+	+	−	+	+
Constipation	+	+	−	+	+
Inadequately controlled pain	+	+	+	−	+
Anal problems	+	+	−	+	+
Dysphagia	+	+	+	+	±

Key: +, useful route in this setting; −, not useful route in this setting; ±, may or may not be useful route in this setting.

opioid infusions. A cannula can be readily inserted in the subcutaneous tissue of the abdomen or chest without the need for multiple injections or placement of a venous catheter. The ability of the subcutaneous tissue to absorb fluid is the dose-limiting factor. For patients requiring higher opioid doses to maintain effective analgesia, hydromorphone, rather than morphine, is preferred. Hydromorphone is more soluble than morphine, allowing administration of a higher dose, in a smaller volume. For patients with terminal illness who require large doses of opioids for adequate pain relief and who cannot tolerate oral administration, subcutaneous infusion is often the administration route of choice.

D. TRANSDERMAL OPIOIDS

Fentanyl is available as a transdermal patch, releasing an amount of fentanyl per hour proportional to the surface area of the patch. Steady-state blood levels are not reached until 17 to 24 hours after application of the patch. Once achieved, 17 to 24 hours is required after patch removal before the dermal fentanyl deposits are eliminated. Transdermal fentanyl is useful after the opioid requirement for pain control is established but not during the dose titration period. Equipotent conversion to the transdermal system is made after titration (Table 9–9). While the recommended dosing interval is 72 hours, about 25 to 30% of patients experience end-of-dose failure and require a dosing interval of 48 hours to maintain analgesia.

E. RECTAL OPIOIDS

Rectal opioid administration is approximately equivalent to absorption via the oral route. Long-acting morphine matrix preparations may be administered per rectum with the desired sustained-release effect, but higher oral doses may be required. The absorption of rectal opioids is de-

creased by the presence of feces in the rectum and altered by characteristics of the opioid preparation.

F. EPIDURAL, INTRATHECAL, AND INTRAVENTRICULAR OPIOIDS

These routes of administration are options for drug delivery when systemic opioids, in doses necessary to control pain, result in unacceptable side effects. Spinal opioid delivery systems may be especially useful, particularly when combined with a local anesthetic, when pain is present in the lower body. These routes require catheter placement. If prolonged therapy is contemplated (longer than 3 months) and the patient's life expectancy and condition warrant, surgical implantation of an epidural catheter is necessary. This increases the initial cost but has been shown to be cost effective overall when used for more than 3 months.

Important considerations include the following:

1. Dosing and administration: Side effects, including respiratory depression, nausea, and urinary retention, possibly due to supraspinal redistribution.

2. The major complications of spinal opioid administration are infection and catheter migration.

Methadone

Methadone is an atypical opioid. It is particularly useful in patients with opioid toxicity and in situations in which its blocking of *N*-methyl-D-aspartate (NMDA) may provide an advantage (eg, neuropathic pain syndromes). However, it is not generally the first drug of choice; it is frequently given late in the course of illness. Problems arise because of methadone's long half-life (20 to 100 hours). In addition, because it is metabolized by cytochrome P450, plasma levels of methadone can be increased or decreased by other drugs metabolized

Table 9–9. Use of the Fentanyl Patch.

Fentanyl Patch Conversion
- 25 mcg/h topically every 72 h is approximately equal to the following:
  - –Morphine 15 mg IV or 50 mg PO per 24 h
  - –Hydromorphone 3 mg IV or 12 mg PO per 24 h
  - –Oxycodone 50 mg per 24 h
  - –Vicodin or Tylenol #3 ≅ 9 tablets or Norco 10/325 ≅ 4–5 tablets per 24 h

To convert TO a fentanyl patch:
Determine consistent daily opioid use and fentanyl patch equianalgesic dose (see above). Apply patch.
- PCA: reduce basal rate by 50% for first 12 h, then discontinue after 12 h and keep PCA bolus dose for at least first 24 h of patch therapy.
- Parenteral opioid infusion: reduce infusion by 50% for first 12 h, then discontinue after 12 h
  - –Continue breakthrough parenteral opioid dose at 50–100% of hourly rate every 15 min prn
- Oral long-acting (every 12 h) opioid: apply patch with long-acting dose, then discontinue long-acting agent
  - –Continue breakthrough oral opioid dose at 10–20% of daily oral opioid dose every h prn
- If unable to swallow oral tablets/liquids, consider rectal or parenteral administration

To convert FROM a fentanyl patch:
Determine fentanyl patch dose and selected opioid equivalent dose (see above). Remove patch.
- Begin parenteral opioid basal rate or infusion at half dose for first 12 h and increase to full dose after 12 h
  - –Begin breakthrough parenteral opioid dose of 50–100% of final hourly rate every 15 min prn

OR
- Begin oral long-acting opioid at same time as patch removal, start with 50% of the first 12-h dose for first dose and increase to full 12-h dose at next administration
  - –Continue breakthrough oral opioid dose of 10–20% of daily oral opioid dose every h prn

PCA, patient-controlled analgesia.

by this enzyme system. Conversion from standard opioids to methadone does not conform to a fixed dose ratio. When converting an oral morphine equivalent of 20 mg/d to methadone, the conversion is 10 mg/d methadone (1:2). However, when converting oral morphine equivalent of 300 mg/d to methadone, the conversion is 30 to 60 mg/d of methadone (1:5 to 1:10). Monitoring the effects of methadone closely for the first few weeks of treatment is important. Dose adjustments of methadone should not be made more often than every 3 to 5 days.

Management of Opioid Adverse Effects

To manage adverse effects of opioids consider the following:

1. Dose reduction. Consider adding a coanalgesic or adjuvant that allows opioid dose reduction with maintenance of analgesia. If side effects such as sedation are troublesome, consider a trial of opioid dose reduction by 25% if the patient has periods of no pain (both the around-the-clock and rescue dose should be reduced).

2. Consider regional anesthetic interventions or intraspinal opioid administration when appropriate, which may reduce systemic opioid toxicity.

3. Treatment of the underlying cause of the pain, if possible. Antitumor therapy, such as radiation therapy or chemotherapy, or intestinal decompression for the visceral pain of bowel distention, may be useful.

4. Opioid rotation. Persons vary in their responsiveness to side effects from different opioids. Because of incomplete cross-tolerance (see Table 3–3), a dose reduction of 25 to 50% is prescribed when replacing one opioid agonist with another.

5. Symptomatic management of opioid toxicity (Table 9–10).

Respiratory depression, although feared, is extremely uncommon. Tolerance to this adverse effect

Table 9–10. Management of Opioid Toxicity.

Toxicity	Incidence	Treatment
Respiration depression	Rare	Hold opioid Dilute naloxone 0.04 mg IV/SC *only* if patient is unarousable
Sedation	Increased frequency at high doses and at end of life	Methylphenidate 2.5–5.0 mg PO every morning, noon Titrate dose upward
Nausea and vomiting	Generally occurs early or with dose titration and resolves in up to 14 days	
Myoclonic jerks	Usually at high doses	Clonazepam Other benzodiazepines Rotate opioid
Constipation	Universal	Treat with prophylactic laxatives or stool softeners

develops rapidly. Naloxone is effective in reversing respiratory depression but should be used with extreme caution in the opioid-dependent patient with chronic pain to avoid precipitating an acute abstinence syndrome. Naloxone is rarely indicated in the palliative care setting. A patient may be comfortable with a respiratory rate of 10 breaths per minute. If the patient is arousable, naloxone is *not* indicated. However, if naloxone is necessary, start with a very low dose and monitor respiratory status and reoccurrence of pain. Dilute one ampule of naloxone 0.4 mg in 10 mL of normal saline. Give 1 mL (0.04 mg) as a frequent injection, as often as every 5 minutes, or by continuous infusion if necessary until the patient is arousable. Overzealous administration of naloxone will result in an opioid withdrawal syndrome that is highly unpleasant for the patient and associated with reemergence of severe pain.

Sedation is another manifestation of opioid toxicity. Psychostimulation with methylphenidate may be useful. Start with a low dose, 2.5 to 5 mg orally each morning and at noon. Titrate the dose to desired effect or toxicity. Titrate dose by 5 mg/dose to effect.

Nausea and vomiting is covered in detail later in this chapter, since they are frequent symptoms in patients with terminal illness. Opioids are just one potential cause of nausea in the palliative care setting. When opioids do play a role, opioid rotation is sometimes helpful.

Due to the prevalence of **constipation,** anticipating this adverse effect and prescribing softeners and cathartics with initiation of opioid therapy is recommended. This is covered in greater detail later in this chapter.

Myoclonus may occur with any opioid secondary to the accumulation of neuroexcitatory opioid metabolites in the CNS. If an option, a 25% reduction of the opioid dose or opioid rotation may alleviate the symptom. However, if myoclonus is disturbing for the patient, benzodiazepines, such as clonazepam, are useful.

COANALGESICS

Coanalgesics are useful when added to opioids for controlling pain. Coanalgesic medications enhance pain control when opioid therapy is not adequate to control pain. This combination therapy is particularly useful for neuropathic pain and for pain due to pleural disease (Table 9–11). The principles governing their use in the palliative care setting are not significantly different from other situations, except as noted below. The use of coanalgesics is described in detail in Chapter 3.

Corticosteroids

Corticosteroids are potent anti-inflammatory medications. They are effective in treating pain secondary to edema (CNS disease and increased intracranial pressure) and in managing prostaglandin-mediated pain (eg, arthritis, bone metastases). The usual starting dose is dexamethasone 10 mg orally each morning. Other conditions in which 10 mg/d of dexamethasone may be used include capsular distention of the liver from tumor, subcapsular hemorrhage, or liver infiltration.

In addition, corticosteroids enhance appetite (short-term), ameliorate nausea, malaise, and improve sense of well-being. The potential for multiple beneficial effects from a single agent suggests its usefulness in the palliative care setting.

Local Anesthetics

Lidocaine infusion for treatment of neuropathic pain may be used in the palliative care setting. A lidocaine trial using a bolus dose of 100 mg IV (1 to 3 mg/kg), administered over 30 minutes in a concentration of 8 mg/mL, should provide pain relief. Vital signs should

Table 9–11. Adjuvant Analgesics.[a]

Drug	Trade name	Dosage	Maximum dose
Anticonvulsants			
Gabapentin	Neurontin	100 mg PO tid; increase every few days	3600 mg/d
Carbamazepine	Tegretol	200 mg PO bid	1200 mg/d
Antispasm Agents			
Baclofen	Lioresal	2.5–5 mg PO tid	80 mg/d
Tizanidine	Zanaflex	2 mg PO tid	36 mg/d
Clonazepam	Klonopin	0.5 mg PO tid	20 mg/d
Corticosteroids[b]			
Dexamethasone	Decadron	4–12 mg PO every morning	
Local Anesthetics			
25% lidocaine/2.5% prilocaine	EMLA	Apply and cover with occlusive dressing 1 hour before invasive procedure	
5% lidocaine patch	Lidoderm	Apply up to 3 patches to intact skin	
Tricyclic Antidepressants			
Desipramine	Norpramin	25–50 mg PO every morning or at bedtime; increase every few days	Based on therapeutic blood levels
Nortriptyline	Pamelor	10–25 mg PO at bedtime; increase every few days	Based on therapeutic blood levels

[a]These agents, usually approved for other purposes, are often effective for neuropathic and other pain syndromes.
[b]More common in cancer and other chronic pain states.

be monitored at least every 15 minutes during the loading period. An infusion, 0.5 mg/kg, is titrated to comfort. Perioral paresthesias or lightheadedness suggest the need for dose reduction (use therapeutic cardiac levels), but clinical evaluation is generally adequate. Minor sedative adverse effects are noted in 30% of patients with no significant severe adverse reactions. Dose adjustment should take place in obese patients with liver disease.

Abrahm JL. Update in palliative medicine and end-of-life care. *Annu Rev Med.* 2003;54:53. [PMID: 12525669]

Cherny N et al. Strategies to manage the adverse effects of oral morphine: an evidence-based report. *J Clin Oncol.* 2001;19:2542. [PMID: 11331334]

Dean M. Opioids in renal failure and dialysis patients. *J Pain Symptom Manage.* 2004;28:497. [PMID: 15504625]

Ferrini R et al. How to initiate and monitor infusional lidocaine for severe and/or neuropathic pain. *J Support Oncol.* 2004;2:90. [PMID: 15330376]

Gloth FM 3rd. Pain management in older adults: prevention and treatment. *J Am Geriatr Soc.* 2001;49:188. [PMID: 11207874]

■ COMMON NONPAIN SYMPTOMS

In the palliative care setting, particularly at the end of life, patients often carry a significant symptom burden. Pain, and its treatment, may be associated with a multitude of symptoms, including nausea and vomiting, constipation, delirium, and myoclonus. The evaluation and treatment of these symptoms are an essential component of palliative care.

DELIRIUM

General Considerations

Delirium is a frequent neuropsychiatric complication at the end of life, occurring in 28 to 83 of patients depending on the population studied and the criteria used. Delirium has been defined as a transient, global disorder of cognition and attention. It is characterized by an acute onset and a fluctuating course, unlike the insidious, progressive nature of dementia. Impairment of attention is the central feature of delirium, while in dementia, attention is relatively preserved until late in the course. Speech is often incoherent, and the level of consciousness is disturbed with delirium, with decreased ability to focus, sustain, or shift attention.

Delirium may present as one of three major types: hyperactive, hypoactive, or mixed. Hyperactive, or agitated, delirium is characterized by agitation and often hallucinations. In contrast, hypoactive delirium presents as a decreased level of consciousness with somnolence and may be mistaken for sedation secondary to opioids or other medications. The third type, mixed delirium, alternates between agitation and quiet and may be difficult to recognize.

Clinical Findings

The standard approach to the management of delirium involves a search for reversible, underlying causes in concert with management of the symptoms and signs of the disorder (Table 9–12). Reversibility of delirium depends on identification of reversible etiologies. Medications are a common cause of delirium, and opioids, in particular, are a concern in the patient with pain. Adjuvant analgesics, such as tricyclic antidepressants, other anticholinergic agents, neuroleptics, and corticosteroids also may cause delirium. Other psychoactive medications, such as selective serotonin reuptake inhibitors, antihistamines, H_2-blockers, and ciprofloxacin, also are potential culprits.

The laboratory evaluation of a patient with delirium may identify reversible causes of delirium. Laboratory tests include blood counts, as severe anemia may cause delirium; renal function; or alterations in calcium, magnesium, phosphorus, and glucose. Oxygen saturation also should be evaluated because hypoxia is another potential, treatable cause of delirium.

The intensity of the evaluation and treatment of the delirium should depend on the goals of therapy and the patient's status overall. The distress of the delirium needs to be evaluated in the context of the patient's overall symptom complex, and the advantages and disadvantages of evaluation and intervention need to be discussed with the patient's family.

In patients with advanced disease, delirium is often multifactorial, and the likelihood of identifying a reversible, underlying etiology varies but has been reported to be as high as 50 to 60%, even in patients with advanced cancer. In patients with pain, opioids as a cause of alterations in mental status or delirium should always be considered. Particularly in the face of decreased renal function or underlying renal failure, the risk of delirium is high, as active opioid metabolites may lead to delirium.

Table 9–12. Etiology and Work-up of Delirium.

Cause	Work-up
Medications[a]	
Opioids	Recent dose titration? Decreased renal clearance
Corticosteroids	Lowest dose to treat the symptom?
Anticholinergics	New medication? Alternate drug available?
Antiemetics	New agent? Dose increased?
Metabolic	
Elevated calcium levels	Check serum calcium
Decreased or elevated glucose levels	Check serum glucose History of diabetes? Corticosteroids recently initiated? Unable to take oral hypoglycemics?
Decreased magnesium levels	Check serum magnesium
Infection	Check urinalysis, culture and sensitivity, chest radiograph, blood cultures as dictated by history and physical
Organ Failure	
Renal	Not clearing opioid metabolites? Other medications not cleared? Uremic?
Liver	Jaundice? Ascites?
Dehydration	Reduced skin turgor Elevated heart rate Decreased blood pressure Elevated BUN/creatinine
Hypoxia	Check P_{O_2}
Anemia	Check CBC

[a]All medications: decrease or stop if possible; looking for overlapping toxicity.
BUN, blood urea nitrogen; CBC, complete blood count.

Differential Diagnosis

Delirium is often unrecognized and most commonly misdiagnosed as either depression or dementia. Table 9–13 identifies differences in these diagnostic categories.

Table 9–13. Distinguishing Delirium, Dementia, and Depression.

	Onset	Attention	Speech	Course over 24 hours
Delirium	Acute	Impaired	Incoherent	Fluctuating
Depression[a]	Usually slow	Normal	Normal	Stable
Dementia	Slow, insidious	Preserved until late	Slowly deteriorates, difficulty finding words	Stable

[a]Most commonly confused with hypoactive delirium.

According to the criteria of the *Diagnostic and Statistical Manual for Mental Disorders,* 4th edition, published by the American Psychiatric Association, the diagnosis of delirium is characterized by the following:

1. Disturbance of consciousness, with a reduced ability to focus, sustain, or shift attention appropriately.
2. An acute onset with a fluctuating course.
3. The absence of an underlying medical, substance use, or other cause for this acute change in mental status.

Frequently, there are disorders of the sleep/wake cycle, altered psychomotor activity, and emotional lability, but these are not required for the diagnosis.

Recognized risk factors for delirium include advanced age, underlying cognitive impairment, advanced illness, and select clinical findings. A multifactorial model for delirium in the hospitalized elderly distinguishes between "baseline vulnerability" and "precipitating factors or insults." Predisposing factors present at the time of admission to the hospital define the "vulnerability factors" in this model and include visual impairment, severe illness, cognitive impairment, and dehydration. The precipitating factors or insults identified in this model include the use of physical restraints, malnutrition, the addition of more than three new medications, bladder catheter, and iatrogenic events. Additional factors suggested by other studies include age, dementia, depression, alcohol use, and poor functional status.

Underlying neurocognitive dysfunction increases the risk of delirium. Both primary and metastatic tumors of the brain as well as leptomeningeal disease may trigger delirium. A postictal state is occasionally associated with delirium as well. Organ failure of any major organ system, infection, and dehydration are all potential causes of delirium. Delirium may be the presenting sign of life-threatening sepsis.

Other metabolic disorders that may cause or contribute to the development of delirium include hypercalcemia, hyponatremia, hypomagnesemia, and hypoglycemia.

Treatment

Treatment interventions, both pharmacologic and non-pharmacologic, have been used to treat delirium. Non-pharmacologic interventions include supportive measures, such as a well-lighted room, familiar sounds and music, and presence of family members and friends. While these interventions may be helpful, the mainstay of therapy remains as pharmacologic intervention.

Treatment of opioid-related delirium involves decreasing the dose of the opioid if the patient's symptoms will allow. Alternatively, consider opioid rotation, although this is based more on practice and consensus than clinical trial data. Medications that may contribute to the delirium should be changed when possible. For example, discontinue cimetidine and replace it with an alternate H_2-blocker, or taper the corticosteroid dose if feasible.

There is insufficient data to guide the selection of treatment for delirium. Haloperidol is the most widely used agent, though only one randomized, controlled trial suggests its superiority to benzodiazepines for hyperactive and hypoactive delirium in patients with AIDS. Haloperidol has the advantages of having a fairly wide therapeutic window and the availability as an oral, intravenous, intramuscular, subcutaneous, or rectal preparation. Start with 0.5 to 1.0 mg every hour as needed. The drug is associated with minimal risks for respiratory depression and is less sedating than benzodiazepines. Although generally safe, haloperidol is associated with the risk of dystonia and the potential for initial worsening of delirium symptoms, particularly the agitation.

The short-acting benzodiazepines are another choice for the treatment of delirium, either lorazepam or midazolam. However, it is noteworthy that benzodiazepines may actually exacerbate the delirium state and need to be used and titrated with caution.

Casarett DJ et al. Diagnosis and management of delirium near the end of life. *Ann Intern Med.* 2001;135:32. [PMID: 11434730]

Jackson KC et al. Drug therapy for delirium in terminally ill patients. *Cochrane Database Syst Rev.* 2004;(2):CD004770. [PMID: 15106261]

Lawlor PG et al. Delirium in patients with advanced cancer. *Hematol Oncol Clin North Am.* 2002;16:701. [PMID: 12170576]

McNicol E et al. Management of opioid side effects in cancer-related and chronic noncancer pain: a systematic review. *J Pain.* 2003;4:231. [PMID: 14622694]

Ross DD et al. Management of common symptoms in terminally ill patients: Part II. Constipation, delirium and dyspnea. *Am Fam Physician.* 2001;64:1019. [PMID: 11578023]

NAUSEA & VOMITING

General Considerations

Nausea and vomiting are among the most common and distressing symptoms of patients in the palliative care setting and can be particularly disturbing at the end of life. Earlier in the trajectory of disease, the incidence of nausea and vomiting varies somewhat with diagnosis and treatment. In the setting of cancer, chemotherapy- and radiation-related nausea and vomiting are frequent but generally self-limited. In patients with terminal cancer, nausea and vomiting occur in nearly two-thirds of patients, although its prevalence during the last 6 weeks of life is lower than 50% and rarely develops as a new symptom during the last days of life.

Clinical Findings

Nausea is an unpleasant, subjective feeling that can only be determined by self-report. It is generally felt in the back of the throat and the epigastrium and is accompanied by decreased gastric tone, duodenal contractions, and reflux of intestinal contents into the stomach. Many patients describe it as feeling "sick to their stomach." It is frequently associated with loss of appetite and may be described as a vague, unpleasant feeling in the epigastric region. Chronic nausea is defined as nausea lasting for more than 2 weeks without the presence of mechanical bowel obstruction or a well-identified, self-limiting cause of the symptom.

Vomiting is the forceful expulsion of gastric contents from the mouth, resulting from contraction of the abdominal muscles, descent of the diaphragm, and opening of the gastric cardia. Vomiting is an objective phenomenon that can be quantified. Both nausea and vomiting may be associated with other symptoms. A recent study concluded that patients with nausea and dyspnea actually experienced more pain than patients without these symptoms. This may be, in part, due to the frequent use of opioids in patients at the end of life. Clinical evaluation should include identification of potentially readily reversible causes of nausea and vomiting.

The etiology of nausea and vomiting in the palliative care setting varies and is often multifactorial. Blood tests to rule out hyponatremia, renal failure, or hypercalcemia, and liver function tests to rule out liver disease as causes of nausea may be helpful. Imaging studies are ordered as indicated by physical examination.

Bowel obstruction is a clinically important cause of nausea and vomiting in the setting of advanced disease, particularly in patients with advanced ovarian or colon cancer or a history of multiple abdominal surgeries. Characteristic clinical findings include nausea and vomiting without normal bowel movements; frequently, the patient has a distended, tender abdomen with high-pitched bowel sounds on physical examination, and a flat plate of the abdomen demonstrates dilated loops of bowel, with or without air-fluid levels.

Increased intracranial pressure may present with nausea and vomiting, often associated with severe headache occurring upon awakening. Papilledema, or focal neurologic findings, new cranial nerve abnormalities, or evidence of meningeal carcinomatosis may all be associated with nausea and vomiting.

Other findings that may lead to a specific explanation for nausea and vomiting include signs and symptoms of myocardial ischemia. An electrocardiogram would be the evaluation of choice as well as serum troponin levels. Constipation or obstipation, identified by history as well as physical examination, is another cause of nausea and vomiting, particularly in patients with advanced illness.

Review of the patient's current medications often suggests contributing factors. Both anticonvulsants and digoxin are prescribed frequently and may be reversible causes of nausea and vomiting. Patients taking NSAIDs may have gastric irritation, resulting in nausea and vomiting, readily treated with antacids or cytoprotective agents. Similarly, gastrointestinal tract infections may cause nausea and vomiting as well. Specific treatment for the underlying infection is the ultimate treatment for the nausea and vomiting.

Opioid-induced nausea and vomiting is estimated to occur in 10 to 40% of opioid-treated patients. It occurs most frequently shortly after and at the time of initiation of opioids. The mechanism of opioid-induced nausea includes stimulation of the chemoreceptor trigger zone on the floor of the fourth ventricle, gastric stasis, and enhanced vestibular sensitivity. Long-term dosing generally results in decreased nausea and vomiting, usually over 2 weeks of therapy. Slow titration upward of the opioid dose may also prevent nausea. If the nausea is severe and the analgesic cannot be altered or reduced, parenteral administration of an antiemetic is preferred until the symptom is improved. Once improved, the oral route remains the preferred route of opioid administration.

Treatment

Pharmacologic treatment of nausea and vomiting in the palliative care setting, whenever possible, should be selected based on an understanding of the underlying pathophysiology. For nausea and vomiting arising from stimulation of the chemoreceptor trigger zone, such as

Table 9–14. Treatment of Nausea and Vomiting.

Drug	Mechanism of action	Dose	Routes of administration
Prochlorperazine	Antidopaminergic Weak antihistamine	5–20 mg q4–6h	PO, IV, PR
Haloperidol	Antidopaminergic	0.5–5 mg q4–8h	PO, SC, IV, PR
Scopolamine	Anticholinergic	1–2 patches q72h; 0.3–0.6 mg q4–8h	PO, SC Transcutaneous
Cyclizine	Antihistamine	25–50 mg q8h	PO, SC
Diphenhydramine	Antihistamine Weak anticholinergic	25–100 mg q4–6h	PO, IV, PR
Metoclopramide	Prokinetic Antidopaminergic	5–20 mg q6–8h	PO, IV, SC
Lorazepam	Anxiolytic	0.5–2 mg q4–8h	SL, PO, IV, SC
Ondansetron	Antiserotonergic	8–32 mg daily	IV, PO
Dexamethasone	Unclear	4–20 mg daily	IV, PO

with opioid-induced nausea, a dopamine antagonist, such as prochlorperazine or haloperidol, should be considered first. These are cost-effective agents that are generally well-tolerated and available for use by multiple administration routes (Table 9–14). If ineffective, the more expensive serotonin antagonists are also generally useful for chemoreceptor trigger zone–stimulated nausea and vomiting. If gastric stasis appears to be a major component (eg, in the patient with diabetes, ascites, or significant opioid use), then a prokinetic agent is the treatment of choice. Metoclopramide in doses of 10 to 20 mg every 6 hours is generally prescribed, although in patients with decreased creatinine clearance, the dose must be reduced.

For nausea exacerbated by motion or vestibular toxicity, an acetylcholine antagonist, such as transdermal scopolamine, is helpful. Other potentially useful agents are the histamine blockers (diphenhydramine, meclizine, hydroxyzine, hydrochloride, and promethazine).

Small studies have suggested that in ambulatory cancer patients who initiate opioid therapy, labyrinthine hypersensitivity to motion may play a greater role in the initiation of nausea than in those who are bedridden. In a pilot study, the majority of ambulatory cancer patients with opioid-induced nausea responded to scopolamine patches. Similarly, in a study of ambulatory cancer patients with chronic nausea and vomiting, patients identified the histamine antagonist, cyclizine 50 mg, to significantly reduce the incidence of vomiting, though it was less effective for the treatment of nausea.

In general, anticholinergic medications are the choice first-line for patients with nausea and vomiting related to colic or mechanical bowel obstruction. These agents may provide some symptomatic relief for patients with increased intracranial pressure but are secondary agents after corticosteroids. In the older population, anticholinergics may cause cardiovascular toxicity. In ambulatory patients, the xerostomia associated with anticholinergics may be dose limiting.

Corticosteroids are the treatment of choice for increased intracranial pressure but also produce an addictive effect when combined with a variety of other antiemetics. For chemotherapy-induced nausea and vomiting, they are part of the standard antiemetic regimen, in concert with serotonin antagonists. While there is no evidence-based data for identification of a dose of corticosteroid for nausea and vomiting, most people choose doses of dexamethasone in the range of 6 to 20 mg orally once daily. Dexamethasone is generally the corticosteroid of choice due to its limited mineralocorticoid activity, the availability of multiple dosage forms, and its long half-life. In patients with multiple symptoms, particularly pain, dexamethasone may provide an important anti-inflammatory, and therefore analgesic, effect.

For the patient with nausea and vomiting related to bowel obstruction, in addition to anticholinergics, octreotide, a somatostatin analogue, is useful for control of nausea and vomiting as well as abdominal discomfort. Octreotide decreases gastrointestinal secretions, stimulates absorption of water and electrolytes, and inhibits intestinal peristalsis. Octreotide is generally initiated at a dose of 50 to 150 mcg intravenously or subcutaneously every 8 to 12 hours with titration over 24 to 48 hours to maintain maximum benefit.

Nonpharmacologic therapies are an essential component of the treatment and prevention of nausea.

For patients with nausea, the odor of foods may be unpleasant. Room temperature or cold foods tend to have less aroma. In addition, for patients with nausea related to early satiety, small, frequent meals may be better tolerated and result in improved control of symptoms. The major nonpharmacologic antiemetic therapies include acupuncture, acupressure, and transcutaneous electrical acupoint stimulation.

Bruera E et al. Dexamethasone in addition to metoclopramide for chronic nausea in patients with advanced cancer: a randomized controlled trial. *J Pain Symptom Manage.* 2004;28:381. [PMID: 15471656]

McNicol E et al. Management of opioid side effects in cancer-related and chronic noncancer pain: a systematic review. *J Pain.* 2003;4:231. [PMID: 14622694]

Rhodes VA et al. Nausea, vomiting, and retching: complex problems in palliative care. *CA Cancer J Clin.* 2001;51:232. [PMID: 11577489]

Ross DD et al. Management of common symptoms in terminally ill patients: Part I. Fatigue, anorexia, cachexia, nausea and vomiting. *Am Fam Physician.* 2001;64:807. [PMID: 11563572]

CONSTIPATION

General Considerations

Constipation is frequently seen in hospitalized patients and is the most common adverse effect of opioids in patients receiving long-term opioid therapy. While opioids account for only 25% of the constipation identified in terminally ill cancer patients in hospice, the need for laxatives and softeners in those patients who require opioids is greater than 75%. In patients with pain, the most likely etiology of constipation is opioid related, though the cause for a given patient is generally multifactorial.

By definition, constipation is evacuation of hard stools less frequently than is normal for a particular person or a subjective sensation of difficulty or discomfort with bowel movements that occur at decreased frequency compared with baseline.

Treatment focuses on both dietary and fluid changes as well as pharmacologic interventions. Prevention remains an essential component of treatment for patients receiving opioid therapy.

Clinical Findings

First, establish what the patient means by constipation. Are the stools too hard, too infrequent, or too difficult to expel? Is there pain with bowel movements? Is there an incomplete sense of emptying after defecation? Is there intermittent watery stool and hard stool, suggesting impaction with overflow?

Symptoms that may be associated with constipation, and may be the presenting symptoms, include bloating, nausea, loss of appetite, abdominal pain, and even early satiety. Physical examination should focus on the presence of abdominal masses, distention, the quality of bowel sounds and, of course, the rectal examination. In addition, evidence of neurologic symptoms and signs should be sought. Parkinson disease, spinal cord lesions, and autonomic neuropathies are all associated with an increased likelihood of constipation.

Physical examination should consider all causes of constipation in patients with advanced disease. Digital examination of the rectum may reveal an impaction or a mass, rectal ulcerations or anal stenosis, loss of anal sphincter tone, or loss of anal sensation. Palpation of the abdomen may reveal fecal masses in the left iliac fossa. These are usually nontender and relatively mobile and can be altered in shape with gentle pressure, unlike other causes of mass lesions.

If the diagnosis of constipation is not clearly explained by physical examination, an abdominal radiograph is useful to distinguish constipation from obstruction. Assessment also includes a review of the patient's current medications (eg, antidepressants, antiemetics). Many of the medications used for the treatment of symptoms associated with advanced illness cause constipation. Anticholinergics, the serotonin antagonist class of antiemetics, and diuretics all induce constipation. Selective 5-HT$_3$ receptor antagonists cause constipation by antagonizing the ability of 5-HT to stimulate cholinergically mediated contractions of the intestinal longitudinal muscle. The anticholinergic activity of antidepressants and some antihypertensive agents are also important to consider. Patients treated with carbamazepine for neuropathic pain or seizures may develop severe constipation that does not appear to be dose-related. It may be refractory to oral laxatives and necessitate discontinuation of the agent.

In patients with pain, however, opioid-related constipation is the primary concern. Opioids cause constipation by binding to opioid receptors on gut smooth muscle as well as in the CNS. Opioids delay gastric emptying, decrease peristalsis, increase oral cecal transit time, and desiccate the intraluminal contents. It is generally believed that patients do not build tolerance to opioid-induced constipation.

There is no apparent correlation between the dose of opioids and the dose of laxatives, though as opioid doses are titrated up, generally the same is required of the laxatives. There is significant variability among patients with regard to the laxative dose needed with a particular opioid dose. While few data are available, there is at least one prospective, open-label study that compared laxative use and frequency of bowel movements in patients receiving morphine versus transdermal fentanyl. Although the same number of patients had bowel movements in each arm of the trial, lesser amounts of laxative were used by patients in the transdermal fentanyl arm versus the oral morphine-treated group.

Table 9–15. Treatment of Constipation.

Type of oral agent	Mechanism of action	Time to effect	Examples	Side effects
Bulk forming	Increased dietary fiber Increased stool bulk Reduced colon transit time	2–4 d	Methylcellulose psyllium	Flatulence Belching Hyperglycemia in diabetics Ineffective with opioid-induced constipation
Lubricant[a]	Softens fecal mass	Overnight	Mineral oil	Increased prothrombin time Long-term use impairs absorption of vitamins A, D, K absorption
Emollient	Increases water retention in bowel lumen Acts as detergent Increases peristalsis	3–12 h	Ducosate Senna, cascara Castor oil Bisacodyl	Cramps Diarrhea
Hyperosmotic	Increases water retention in bowel lumen Acts as detergent Increases peristalsis		Lactulose Sorbitol Magnesium citrate	Increased salt absorption Na^{2+}, Mg^{2+} may worsen Congestive heart failure or renal insufficiency

[a]Not recommended.

It is important to remember that in the palliative care setting, even in the absence of opioid use, constipation is common, occurring in as many as 64% of patients enrolled in a hospice and not receiving opioid analgesia. This highlights the importance of other contributing factors, such as immobility, dehydration, concomitant medications, and neurologic diseases.

Treatment

Constipation is managed with both pharmacologic and nonpharmacologic measures. In the setting of advanced disease, the nonpharmacologic interventions are generally not helpful. These include increased activity, dietary manipulation (eg, fruit juices, increased fluid intake, bran), and increased dietary fiber. Bulking agents, such as methylcellulose or cilium, are relatively ineffective and may worsen constipation for patients who are bedridden. These agents require physical activity as well as adequate fluid intake to increase stool water content.

Prophylactic laxatives are essential for patients at increased risk for constipation. Commonly identified factors in the setting of palliative care include the use of long-term opioids, being elderly or bedridden, and a variety of medications, as noted above. A low rectal impaction should be evacuated manually. Manual disimpaction is uncomfortable, and the patient should be premedicated either with lorazepam 1 mg intravenously or midazolam

5 mg subcutaneously as well as with analgesics as necessary. After disimpaction, the patient is likely to require enemas to reach stool that is higher up in the colon.

Therapeutic and prophylactic measures for the treatment of constipation can be administered orally or rectally (Table 9–15). The clinical situation, patient preference, and potential side effects dictate which type of medication should be chosen. The osmotic or emollient laxatives are surfactant substances that act as a detergent and facilitate the interface between aqueous and fatty acid components of stool. They increase the luminal water and salt. These agents, which are not absorbed in the gut, are the most commonly prescribed medications to treat constipation. As noted in Table 9–15, representative agents include senna, cascara, bisacodyl, and phenolphthalein. These agents directly stimulate the myenteric plexus, increasing peristalsis and decreasing water absorption in the small and large intestine. Recommended starting doses of commonly prescribed laxatives are shown in Table 9–16.

Lubricant laxatives are used to soften the fecal mass. They are primarily used for fecal impaction but are otherwise of little use for chronic constipation. Mineral oil is a representative of this group. Its use may interfere with the absorption of fat-soluble vitamins, and it may, as a result, increase the prothrombin time if used long term.

Hyperosmotic agents, as with the emollients, are not broken down or absorbed in the small bowel. Laxatives representative of this group include lactulose, sorbitol,

Table 9–16. Recommended Starting Doses of Commonly Prescribed Laxatives.

Agent	Starting dose	Onset of action
Senna	15 mg daily (maximum 8 tablets/d)	6–12 h
Bisacodyl	50–20 mg/d, oral 10–20 mg, rectal	6–12 h 1 h
Docusate	100–800 mg/d	24–72 h
Lactulose	15–60 mL/d	1–2 d
Magnesium citrate	200 mL	0.5–3 h

and magnesium citrate. These agents have the potential to cause significant cramping as well as diarrhea. Lactulose, in particular, may result in bloating, colic, and flatulence. These agents directly stimulate peristalsis and increase water secretion, adding to their effectiveness. They should be used with caution in the face of congestive heart failure or renal insufficiency due to increased absorption of salt and magnesium. If given rectally, these agents work extremely rapidly (within 15 minutes) due to their stimulation of rectal peristalsis.

An overall strategy for use of laxatives is similar philosophically to the treatment of other symptoms. Doses of laxatives should be titrated to effect. The best example of this is opioid-induced constipation. When the dose of opioid is increased, the prescription for laxatives generally needs to be increased as well. Frequently, combination treatment with a softener and stimulant, for example, is most effective for opioid-induced constipation.

Different clinical scenarios suggest alternate approaches. For example, a patient with severe constipation, abdominal distention, nausea, vomiting, and stool palpability, both on abdominal and rectal examination, requires treatment rectally first with a glycerin suppository to soften the fecal mass and oral laxatives as tolerated. Oral laxatives are the treatment of choice if the patient is able to tolerate them. Agents with different modes of action should be used if constipation is not responding to prescribed management. For example, constipation with colicky pain may require either an increase in the softener or use of an osmotic agent, like sorbitol or lactulose. If a stimulant is not working, addition of an osmotic agent is worth considering. As with all symptoms, reassessment is an essential component of management.

Ross DD et al. Management of common symptoms in terminally ill patients: Part II. Constipation, delirium and dyspnea. *Am Fam Physician.* 2001;64:1019. [PMID: 11578023]

Sykes NP. The relationship between opioid use and laxative use in terminally ill cancer patients. *Palliat Med.* 1998;12:375. [PMID: 9924600]

MYOCLONUS

General Considerations

Myoclonus presents as sudden, uncontrollable, non-rhythmic jerking or twitching of the extremities, which initially may be confused with seizure activity or restlessness. While there are multiple causes of myoclonus, a common etiology near the end of life is opioid-induced myoclonus; the prevalence of which ranges anywhere from 2.7 to 87%. It can exacerbate pain significantly in the setting of widespread bone metastases and may progress to more significant neurologic dysfunction, such as grand mal seizures and, therefore, requires rapid identification and treatment.

Pathogenesis

Opioid-induced myoclonus is thought to occur secondary to the formation of neural excitatory metabolites that are poorly excreted in the face of progressive renal dysfunction. The byproducts of opioid glucuronidation, both morphine-3 glucuronide and hydromorphone-3 glucuronide, are believed to be responsible for the excitatory behaviors, myoclonus, and seizures. Limited data suggest that the plasma levels of these glucuronidation byproducts are significantly increased in the presence of renal insufficiency, with the ratio of metabolite to parent compound four times greater than the ratio seen in patients with normal renal function.

Myoclonus and seizures have been seen with other opioid compounds, including methadone and acute administration of fentanyl in the operating room. Other reported nonopioid causes of myoclonus include the following:

1. Brain surgery
2. Placement of an intrathecal catheter
3. AIDS dementia
4. Hypoxia
5. Medications (eg, chlorambucil and metoclopramide)
6. Paraneoplastic syndrome

Treatment

The primary treatment of opioid-related myoclonus is opioid rotation, particularly if the patient has renal insufficiency. Increased use of adjuvant analgesics may reduce the opioid dose necessary for adequate pain control and reduce or eliminate myoclonus. While there are few data, an alternative approach is the use of benzodiazepines, including clonazepam, diazepam, and midazolam. Start with clonazepam 0.5–1.0 mg at night or 0.5 mg two or three times a day for mild myoclonus. For patients with severe myoclonus near the end of life, where opioid rotation or opioid dose reduction is not feasible or appropriate, a continuous infusion of either midazolam or lorazepam may be appropriate. Begin with 0.5 to 1.0 mg per hour and titrate to symptom control.

Cherny N et al. Strategies to manage the adverse effects of oral morphine: an evidence-based report. *J Clin Oncol.* 2001;19:2542. [PMID: 11331334]

Smith MT. Neuroexcitatory effects of morphine and hydromorphone: evidence implicating the 3-glucuronide metabolites. *Clin Exp Pharmacol Physiol.* 2000;27:524. [PMID: 10874511]

Neuropathic Pain

10

R. Norman Harden, MD

ESSENTIALS OF DIAGNOSIS

- *Neuropathic pain can be divided into two types: stimulus-evoked and stimulus-independent.*
- *Stimulus-evoked pain is characterized by signs of hyperalgesia and allodynia that result from mechanical, thermal, or chemical stimulation.*
- *Stimulus-independent pain (ie, spontaneous pain) may be persistent or paroxysmal and is often described as shooting, stabbing, or burning.*
- *Paresthesias (defined as abnormal sensations) and dysesthesias (defined as unpleasant abnormal sensations) may be spontaneous or evoked.*

General Considerations

A. EPIDEMIOLOGY

Chronic neuropathic pain is not uncommon, although estimates of its prevalence vary widely from 2 to 40% of all adults. The estimated 3.75 million cases of chronic neuropathic pain in the United States include conditions as diverse as cancer-associated pain, spinal cord injury, low back pain, and phantom pain. Recurrent and persistent pain ranging from back pain to facial pain was reported by 45% of enrollees in one health maintenance organization in the United States, and in the United Kingdom up to 25% of patients who attended pain clinics experienced neuropathic pain syndromes.

B. ETIOLOGY

Neuropathic pain that is associated with such disorders as diabetes mellitus and herpes zoster is the most frequently described and studied. However, these disorders are certainly not the exclusive causes of neuropathic pain. Radiculopathy, which may be an underlying cause in many cases involving lower back pain, is probably the most frequent peripheral nerve pain generator. A partial list of causes of neuropathic pain is presented in Table 10–1.

C. DIAGNOSTIC ISSUES

Chronic pain should be broadly categorized into two categories: **nociceptive** (ie, stimulus of pain peripheral receptors in skin, joint, and muscle) and **neuropathic** (also called neurogenic, implying that damage to the nervous system is generating the pain). Pain is often multifactorial; there may be multiple primary and secondary pain generators.

Neuropathic pain refers to pain caused by a clinically heterogeneous group of disorders that vary widely in etiology and presentation. It includes signs and symptoms that arise from a primary lesion in the peripheral nervous system or from dysfunction in the central nervous system which occur in the absence of nociceptor stimulation, such as postherpetic neuralgia.

In contrast, nociceptive pain is a response triggered by an unpleasant, damaging, or potentially damaging stimulus in the periphery. It can be acute, such as acute postoperative pain, or it may be chronic, such as the inflammation of arthritis.

This binary categorization has clinical significance; for instance, neuropathic pain may not respond as well to opioids or nonsteroidal anti-inflammatory drugs (NSAIDs) as nociceptive pain, which is usually easily managed with these classes of drugs at least in the short-term. Neuropathic pain may be treated more effectively by drugs that stabilize or modulate central nervous system function (eg, drugs indicated for seizures or depression) or by antiarrhythmic agents (such as sodium channel blockers). While the reasons for correctly diagnosing neuropathic pain are clear, the methods for effectively doing so are not.

At present, the diagnostic approach to neuropathic pain relies on antiquated classification systems based on the etiology of pain and its anatomic distribution. This is less than ideal for several reasons. First, most neuropathic disease states are associated with more than one mechanism of pain and that mechanism may change over time. Second, different syndromes may produce mechanistically identical types of neuropathic pain. Finally, presenting symptoms and signs and diagnostic testing are often diverse within a single neuropathic pain syndrome. All of these problems hinder accurate and efficient diagnosis of neuropathic pain and contrast the

Table 10–1. Causes of Neuropathic Pain.

Cause	Example
Cancer-related	Compressive Iatrogenic Infiltrative Paraneoplastic
Compression/ entrapment syndromes	Carpal tunnel syndrome Chronic radiculopathy Plexus disorders Spinal stenosis Tarsal tunnel
Congenital	Fabry disease Hereditary sensory neuropathies
Immune- mediated	Guillain-Barré syndrome Multiple sclerosis
Infection	Herpes zoster HIV or AIDS Infectious mononucleosis Leprosy Syphilis
Metabolic disturbance	Amyloidosis Diabetes mellitus Hypothyroidism Porphyria Uremia
Nutritional deficiency	Folic acid deficiency Niacin deficiency Pyridoxine deficiency Thiamine deficiency

Toxins	Alcohol
	Arsenic
	Chemotherapy agents, especially
	  vincristine, cisplatin,
	  oxaliplatin, and taxanes
	Glue sniffing
	Gold
	Lead
	Mercury
	Other drugs including hydralazine,
	  isoniazid, nitrofurantoin,
	  phenytoin, thalidomide

Trauma	Amputation (phantom limb pain/stump pain) CRPS type II Crush injuries Spinal cord injury Surgery
Vasculitis/ connective tissue disorders	Cryoglobulinemia Lupus erythematosus Polyarteritis nodosa Rheumatoid arthritis Sjögren syndrome

descriptive diagnoses with the "mechanistic diagnoses" currently recommended in pain circles. However, exist problems with this "mechanistic" diagnostic approach as well.

Postherpetic neuralgia can be used to illustrate the pitfalls in diagnosing neuropathic pain according to mechanism. In postherpetic neuralgia, at least three different mechanisms for pain have been identified, all of which are associated with direct neuronal damage to both the peripheral and central nervous systems (ie, infectious, inflammatory, and ischemic). Each of these mechanisms may be associated with different symptoms. For instance, some patients present with a profound sensory loss in an area of pain. Other patients will have pronounced allodynia and hyperalgesia with minimal or no sensory loss. Still others will have sensory loss *and* allodynia. This multiplicity of potential mechanisms, signs, and symptoms increases the potential for misdiagnosis and may result in complicated or conflicting "mechanistic diagnoses." Consequently, the response to treatment will be unpredictable, and two different patients with postherpetic neuralgia may respond differently to the same treatment. However, it is clear that mechanistically based diagnoses are superior to descriptive diagnoses. With new insights being gained into the biologic mechanisms underlying neuropathic pain, a more valuable way to approach neuropathic pain is not only through a clinical framework that categorizes pain according to the presumed etiology or affected body part, but also according to presenting signs, symptoms, and electrodiagnostic and quantitative sensory testing. The combined power of these complementary tactics may yield a more precise and clinically useful diagnostic target, and this approach has been gaining some acceptance in the pain community.

D. Treatment Issues

Adding to the clinical challenge of treating neuropathic pain is the fact that many currently prescribed therapies lack evidence-based support in the form of prospective, randomized, controlled clinical trials or, in the case of drugs, approval by the US Food and Drug Administration (FDA) for the indication of neuropathic pain. (Exceptions to the latter include carbamazepine, which is approved for trigeminal neuralgia; the lidocaine patch and gabapentin, which are approved for postherpetic neuralgia; and duloxetine, which is approved for painful diabetic neuropathy.) Therefore, medications indicated for the treatment of other syndromes (including depression, seizures, and cardiac arrhythmias) are used off-label for the treatment of neuropathic pain. Without rigorous clinical data to support safety and efficacy in patients with neuropathic pain, formal guidelines for dosage and administration of many of these off-label drugs are not adequately established. These limitations render the current haphazard treatment approaches even more cumbersome and speculative; however, they do provide a modest rationale for interdisciplinary care (ie, with drug treatments of variable effectiveness, nonpharmacologic treatments are more likely to be used). However, it must be noted there is even less evidence for nondrug interventions; at least for interdisciplinary care, the risk part of the risk/benefit ratio is minimal.

Close analysis of the published data reveals some useful information regarding the clinical usefulness of commonly used drugs for specific neuropathic pain symptoms. Though the majority of these studies target descriptive diagnoses (that is, specific drugs were evaluated in patients in a traditional diagnostic model), understanding treatment mechanisms and deriving treatment (nonpharmacologic as well as pharmacologic) from symptoms, signs, and test results as well as the underlying mechanisms they reveal will result in more effective therapy and improved quality of life for the patient. However, the literature providing this type of information is sparse.

Dworkin RH et al. Advances in neuropathic pain: diagnosis, mechanisms, and treatment recommendations. *Arch Neurol.* 2003;60:1524. [PMID: 14623723]

Mannion RJ et al. Pain mechanisms and management: a central perspective. *Clin J Pain.* 2000;16:S144. [PMID: 11014459]

Merskey H, Bogduk N, eds. *Classification of chronic pain: descriptions of chronic pain syndromes and definitions of pain terms.* 2nd ed. Seattle: IASP Press; 1994.

Woolf CJ. Dissecting out mechanisms responsible for peripheral neuropathic pain: implications for diagnosis and therapy. *Life Sci.* 2004;74:2605. [PMID: 15041442]

TYPES OF NEUROPATHIC PAIN

Physiologically, neuropathic pain results from central or peripheral nervous system damage, threat of damage, or dysfunction. Although nervous system damage would logically be expected to cause a sensory loss (negative symptoms)—with the degree of loss approximating the amount of damage—a proportion of cases present with various kinds of pain and dysesthesias (or positive symptoms).

The two relevant types of neuropathic pain are stimulus-evoked pain and stimulus-independent pain (ie, spontaneous pain). Stimulus-evoked pain is characterized by signs of hyperalgesia and allodynia that result from mechanical, thermal, or chemical stimulation. Stimulus-independent pain may be persistent or paroxysmal and is often described as shooting, stabbing, or burning. Paresthesias (defined as abnormal sensations) and dysesthesias (defined as unpleasant abnormal sensations) may be spontaneous or evoked.

Stimulus-Evoked Pain

Within the category of stimulus-evoked pain, hyperalgesia and allodynia are the two main symptoms that may manifest via mechanical, chemical, or thermal stimulation. Hyperalgesia is an exaggerated pain response produced by a normally painful stimulus (eg, pin prick), while allodynia is pain produced by a stimulus that is not usually painful (eg, light touch).

A. HYPERALGESIA

Hyperalgesia can arise from peripheral or central mechanisms, or both. Peripherally, sensitization of primary afferent nociceptors (Aδ and C fibers) may occur due to release of inflammatory mediators, such as bradykinin, histamine, prostaglandins, and substance P. Another peripheral mechanism for stimulus-evoked pain involves formation of a neuroma, a tangled mass of regenerating nervous tissue embedded in scar and connective tissue at the site of nerve injury which may act as a mechanically sensitive site. Neuromas accumulate or "uncover" pathologic and nonpathologic ion channels (eg, sodium channels) and receptors (eg, norepinephrine) that result in foci of hyperexcitability and ectopic activity. The neuroma sign, or Tinel sign, may be elicited by mechanically stimulating the affected area, triggering exquisite, "electrical" pain caused by changes in afferent nerve membrane properties and mechanical threshold.

B. ALLODYNIA

Allodynia may also be evoked by what is usually perceived as innocuous stimuli (usually mechanical or temperature). This may be due to peripheral or central sensitization. Peripheral sensitization occurs due to persistent release and presence of inflammatory or algesic substances in the local environment. In response to ongoing nociception or overstimulation, changes in spinal cord dorsal horn cells can occur, resulting in the central sensitization and central reorganization that finally lead to allodynia. Central sensitization may cause an increase in the size of the sensory receptive field, a reduced threshold for sensory (pain) perception, and hypersensitivity to various innocuous stimuli.

At the molecular level, central sensitization occurs when the excitatory amino acids glutamate and aspartate and substance P bind to receptors located on spinal dorsal horn transmission cells (second-order neurons). Specific glutamate receptors include *N*-methyl-D-aspartate (NMDA) receptors and non-NMDA receptors (α-amino-3-hydroxy-5-methyl-4-isoazolepropionic acid [AMPA], kainate), which may enhance and prolong depolarization. This may increase the responsiveness of the nociceptive system and lead to long-lasting changes in the dorsal horn transmission cells. In addition, NMDA receptors may be involved in potentiating synaptic transmission into the cerebrum, a process that may be responsible for "pain memory," (eg, phantom limb pain). In fact, it is likely that there are pain-associated excitatory amino acid receptors throughout the neuroaxis. Activation of non-NMDA receptors, specifically the AMPA and kainate receptors and neurokinin-1 (substance P) receptors may act to further sensitize the NMDA receptor.

Central changes also occur through reorganization. As the damaged nerve regenerates or begins firing ectopically or ephaptically, Aβ-fiber sprouting into the pain layers (laminae I and II) may occur. When nerves that do not normally transmit pain sprout into these more superficial regions of the dorsal horn—regions where the first synaptic relay in pain transmission usually occurs—pain may result from non-noxious stimuli. Regeneration also causes sensory disorganization, so that the normal somatotropic organization of inputs becomes disordered ("spreading").

Another central change that contributes to the development of allodynia is the loss of inhibitory controls projecting to the superficial spinal cord dorsal horn. This occurs when segmental inhibitory interneurons (mediated by neurotransmitters like γ-aminobutyric acid [GABA], glycine, and endogenous opioids [enkephalins]) or descending inhibitory pathways (mediated by neurotransmitters such as serotonin and norepinephrine) decrease their function. Because this inhibition normally acts as a spinal "gate" for sensory information, reduced inhibition increases the likelihood that the dorsal horn neuron will fire spontaneously or more energetically to primary afferent input. Thus, allodynia may result from any of these three central mechanisms for stimulus-evoked pain: central sensitization, reorganization, or loss of inhibitory controls.

Stimulus-Independent Pain

Stimulus-independent pain, or spontaneous pain occurs without provocation, so symptoms can occur constantly or at any time. Paresthesias and dysesthesias can originate peripherally via ectopic impulses along the Aβ, Aδ, and C fibers, arising as spontaneous activity due to processes such as damaged ("leaky") sodium channels that accumulate along affected nerves, causing a drift toward threshold potential. Paroxysmal shooting or electrical pain (once thought to distinguish ectopic activity in myelinated fibers) as well as continuous burning pain (still thought to be caused by activity in unmyelinated nerves), most likely occur from ectopic or ephaptic discharges arising in any type of fiber. Stimulus-independent pain may also occur as a result of reduced inhibitory input from the brain or spinal cord.

In most neuropathic pain syndromes, stimulus-independent pain occurs along with stimulus-evoked pain; for example, spontaneous burning pain and me-

chanical allodynia present concurrently in complex regional pain syndrome (CRPS). In some syndromes, the activity at the site of injury seems to maintain the peripheral or central sensitivity in some fashion, and blocking the peripheral input may at least temporarily normalize the altered central processing. Thus patients' symptoms cease until peripheral input returns.

ASSESSING PAIN

A careful history, physical examination, and a thoughtful use of testing are necessary to properly and fully define the putative mechanisms involved in a given neuropathic pain syndrome. Detailed medical and surgical histories are essential first steps in understanding pain etiology. A comprehensive physical examination allows the physician to integrate the patient's presenting symptoms and to begin to localize which elements of the neuroaxis are involved. It is particularly important to identify the location, quality, intensity, and pattern of pain. The neurologic examination uses simple bedside tests to assess the patient for the presence or absence of specific stimulus-evoked signs (Tables 10–2 and 10–3). Special attention should be paid to the sensory examination, especially searching for hypoesthesia (numbness) or hyperesthesia (hyperpathia or allodynia or both). A distinction between mechanical and thermal allodynia may have clinical relevance.

Testing of reflexes, a comprehensive motor examination, and autonomic examination are all essential to understanding neuropathies. Testing can complement and corroborate careful history and physical examinations and has the advantage of being quantitative, although all tests have their known limitations. A comprehensive list of diagnostic tests evaluating the motor, sensory, and autonomic systems is presented in Table 10–4. Some highly technical and invasive tests may be necessary, such as immunohistochemical staining of skin-punch biopsy specimens using antibodies specific for small diameter myelinated and unmyelinated peripheral nerves which can be used to quantify nerve fiber density in patients with peripheral neuropathy.

The physician should also be aware of any comorbid conditions affecting the patient's pain experience and quality of life, such as sleep disturbance, anxiety, or depression, which may help guide treatment decisions.

TREATMENT

Once the patient has been thoroughly assessed and a putative mechanism (ie, a working diagnosis) has been developed, a treatment strategy should be formulated targeting each mechanism, with a primary goal of normalizing the underlying dysfunction. Sometimes, the underlying dysfunction can be corrected (eg, the compression

Table 10–2. Bedside Tests for the Assessment of Allodynia.

Stimulus-evoked sign: Allodynia
Definition: Normally nonpainful stimulus evokes a painful sensation.
Control: Identical stimulus in unaffected skin does not evoke pain.

Subtype	Assessment	Pathologic response
Mechanical dynamic	Stroking skin with a brush, gauze, or cotton applicator	Sharp, burning, superficial pain
Mechanical deep somatic	Manual light pressure at the joints	Deep pain at the joints
Mechanical punctate	Light manual pinprick with a sharpened wooden stick or stiff von Frey hair	Sharp superficial pain
Mechanical static	Manual light pressure of the skin	Dull pain Burning pain
Thermal cold	Contact skin with objects at 20°C[a]	Painful, often burning, temperature sensation
Thermal warm	Contact skin with objects at 40°C[a]	Painful burning temperature sensation

[a] As a control, also contact skin with object at skin temperature.

in compressive neuropathy can be relieved by postural correction or a toxic or metabolic insult, such as hyperglycemia). If a direct fix is not possible, then the source or nociceptive generator can be targeted using nonpharmacologic treatments (eg, ice to reduce inflammation) or medications (eg, normalizing pathologic sodium flux with sodium channel blockers).

1. Nonpharmacologic Treatment

Patients with neuropathic pain often require a significant reduction in their pain, but traditional medical treatments, including nerve ablation, nerve blocks, and medication management, achieve only partial success in these goals. Clinicians understand that the efficacy of these interventions is sometimes limited; they also understand the tremendous direct and indirect costs in terms of pain and suffering, health care expenditures, and quality of life, not to mention the costs to society in lost productivity and vocational disability.

In attempts to address the associated emotional, social, and vocational sequelae of chronic pain, interdisciplinary and multidisciplinary pain management programs have been developed (see Chapter 6). Interdisciplinary programs are designed to help patients learn to cope more effectively with pain and help them maintain the highest possible functional level in order to alleviate pain and suffering. These interdisciplinary pain management programs have developed and introduced nonpharmacologic treatments that have actually had a dramatic impact on the biomedical issues.

More than just a physical sensation, a patient's pain is also the emotional, cognitive, and behavioral reactions to that sensation. Patients who have chronic neuropathic pain may become more disabled than their physical impairments can explain. Numerous studies have shown that a one-to-one correspondence does not necessarily exist between the amount of tissue damage and the person's experience of pain. Pain can be aggravated

Table 10–3. Simple Bedside Tests for the Assessment of Hyperalgesia.

Stimulus-evoked sign: Hyperalgesia
Definition: Normally painful stimulus evokes a more intense painful sensation.
Control: Identical stimulus in unaffected skin evokes a less painful sensation.

Subtype	Assessment	Pathologic response
Mechanical pinprick	Manual pinprick of the skin with a safety pin	Sharp superficial pain
Thermal cold	Contact skin with coolants, such as alcohol (evaporation) or cold metal	Painful, often burning, temperature sensation
Thermal heat	Contact skin with objects at 46°C[a]	Painful burning temperature sensation

[a] As a control, also contact skin with object at skin temperature.

Table 10–4. Neurologic Tests Used in the Diagnostic Assessment of Neuropathic Pain.

Type of neurologic test	Functions evaluated	Fibers examined	Anticipated findings
Motor System			
Electromyography (EMG) and motor nerve conduction studies (NCS)	Motor nerve conduction velocity; compound muscle action potential amplitude	Efferent large myelinated motor axons	Velocity and amplitude decreased with reduction in number of large myelinated motor axons or with interruption in myelination
Sensory NCS	Sensory nerve conduction velocity and action potential amplitude	Afferent large myelinated sensory axons (Aβ fibers)	Velocity and amplitude decreased with reduction in number of large myelinated sensory axons
Sensory System			
Algometer	Mechanical pressure and threshold tolerance	Aδ and C fiber activity arising from nociceptors and Aβ fiber activity arising from mechanoreceptors	Lower threshold tolerance or suprathreshold response to stimuli
Microneurography	Presence of ectopic impulses velocity and action potential amplitude	Single fiber activity arising from nociceptors (Aδ and C fibers) and mechanoreceptors (Aβ fibers)	Ectopic impulse generation along sensory axons
Quantitative sensory testing (Peltier device)	Sensory and pain threshold after stimulus with cool and warm temperature	Aδ and C fiber activity arising from nociceptors and mechanoreceptors	Lower threshold and suprathreshold response to stimuli
Vibrometer (QST)	Vibration perception thresholds	Aβ fiber activity arising from mechanoreceptors	Increase thresholds
Von Frey hairs	Mechanical pressure and threshold tolerance	Aδ and C fiber activity arising from nociceptors and Aβ fiber activity from mechanoreceptors	Lower threshold and tolerance or suprathreshold response to stimuli
Autonomic System			
Heart rate	Heart rate variation in response to deep breathing	Autonomic efferent parasympathetic axons (eg, vagus nerve)	Less variation seen with polyneuropathy affecting vagal function
Quantitative sudomotor axon reflex test (QSART)	Sweat gland response to stimulation	Sympathetic postganglionic sudomotor axons	Excess or persistent sweat with reduced latency or reduced sweat volume consistent with peripheral neuropathy
Skin temperature and blood flow measurements with thermistor, thermography, and laser Doppler	Comparison of skin temperature of involved extremity to asymptomatic extremity	Sympathetic postganglionic vasoconstrictor axons	Early, warmer skin on involved side from vasodilatation; later, cooler skin from vasoconstriction

by psychosocial factors, such as emotional state, previous experience, secondary gain, and expectations. Untreated chronic neuropathic pain can result in needless personal suffering for the patient; excess disability; comorbid emotional problems, including increased risk of suicide; overuse or misuse of psychoactive medications; increased medical care utilization; iatrogenic complications secondary to inappropriate procedures, interventions, and surgeries; and increased economic and social costs. Complex, intractable neuropathic pain clearly requires an interdisciplinary approach that addresses psychosocial as well as biologic factors and that focuses on functional restoration in all areas of life.

Role of Physicians & Nurses

The physician often coordinates patient care, determines diagnoses, identifies patient needs for the team members, and supervises overall patient needs and treatment strategies, either on a team or in a single provider practice. If also acting as a team leader, the physician ensures that the team remains focused on the patient's global level of functioning.

The physician and the nurse must provide reassurance regarding the safety and efficacy of physical and occupational therapy intervention. This is perhaps the most important role the physician and the nurse play for both staff and patient. Their reassurance is particularly important for patients with chronic neuropathic pain. These patients, being very somatically focused as a result of their chronic pain, may react with substantial apprehension to minor changes in physical sensations and patterns. The reassurance of physician and nurse can both inspire the patient to continue with the appropriate care of their pain management regimen and protect the patient from needless diagnostic work-ups and medical interventions.

Psychotherapy

Either in the context of a team or in private practice, a working relationship with a cognitive-behavioral psychologist is essential. Neuropathic pain creates stress; it can also be aggravated by stress as well as other psychological factors. Pain psychologists can ascertain whether or not psychological factors are contributing to excess pain and disability. Because certain coping strategies are more effective than others in managing pain, they can determine the type of coping strategies best suited for each patient and offer reliable forecasts for each strategy's efficacy.

Psychologists can also provide education, counseling, and training in cognitive-behavioral pain management techniques. Because depression and anxiety levels are high among patients with chronic pain, psycholog-

ical evaluation and therapy should be a component of any comprehensive neuropathic pain treatment program. Increasing patient awareness about the stress model of chronic pain (eg, how stress, emotional distress, muscle tension, and deconditioning can increase pain) can be an effective motivator for getting patients to invest in the treatment process.

To achieve effective pain management, securing the patient's understanding and acceptance of the self-management approach is a paramount step in psychological pain management. Patient assent to such a model typically leads to increased motivation, increased dedication to pain management techniques, and an increased expectation of pain management success. Without acceptance of self-management principles, minimal progress is to be expected.

Several relaxation techniques have been shown to be useful in helping patients manage neuropathic pain, including progressive muscle relaxation, controlled (or diaphragmatic) breathing, imagery, autogenic training, biofeedback-assisted relaxation, and hypnosis. Progressive muscle relaxation is a technique that involves the methodical tension and relaxation of sets of voluntary muscles that travel through the body until the patient's whole body is relaxed. It is easily adapted for patients who are unable to tense certain muscle groups. Controlled breathing, often combined with progressive muscle relaxation, involves measured (8 breaths per minute) diaphragmatic breathing to stimulate a relaxation response.

Biofeedback-assisted relaxation provides the patient with feedback about physiologic responses that indicate a relaxed state while the patient uses both progressive muscle relaxation and controlled breathing. Feedback included data about such physiologic responses as galvanic skin response, fingertip surface temperature, muscle tension (with surface electromyography [EMG] biofeedback), heart rate, breathing rate, or electroencephalogram (EEG) responses. Biofeedback has been shown to be effective in a wide range of pain conditions, including neuropathic pain.

Hypnosis can be considered a combination of relaxation, distraction (see below), and suggestion (or placebo effect). It is "highly focused attention during which the alteration of sensations, awareness, and perceptions can occur." Many studies indicate that hypnotic techniques assist in reducing both acute and chronic pain, including neuropathic pain. Because many patients object to hypnotic techniques on religious grounds or because they stand opposed to what they consider a loss of control, some clinicians prefer to use the term "imagery."

Cognitive thinking techniques can aid patients who react to pain episodes with intense anxiety and episodes of catastrophizing. Some patients entertain catastrophic thoughts such as the worry that the pain will never cease, that it will worsen, that they cannot withstand it, that they will have a stroke or heart attack because of the pain, and other such fears. Catastrophic thinking has demonstrated links to increased pain and decreased coping. Psychologists can assist patients in identifying their catastrophic thoughts and coach them in the use of techniques like thought-stopping and cognitive restructuring. These techniques help stem the flow of catastrophic thoughts, and patients can subsequently be taught how to replace them with more adaptive ways of thinking. Cognitive thinking techniques have been shown to be effective in helping patients manage their pain.

Other studies have shown that distraction is another valuable technique for pain management. Distracting activities, such as music and sensory techniques, can all be helpful in the short term.

Emotional distress techniques, including treatment of anger, anxiety, and cognitive-behavioral treatment of depression, are used in conjunction with antidepressants to break the pain-distress-pain cycle. Some antidepressants also have a well-known analgesic effect, particularly for neuropathic pain. Stress management training is another essential element of pain management programs, because many patients lack fundamental proficiency in problem solving, communication, and assertiveness, skills that they will need to return to full functioning. Deficiencies in these areas may be a risk factor for job dissatisfaction and a major risk factor for chronicity.

Family and friends sometimes reinforce pain behaviors and activity avoidance by discouraging a return to functioning and encouraging the sick role, most often in the belief that they are acting in the patient's best interest. Family counseling sessions endeavor to assist family reduction of reinforcement for pain behaviors. Through counseling, the family learns to encourage and buttress a patient's constructive pain management coping techniques and discourage detrimental behaviors.

Depression, anxiety, stress, and other psychological factors have been shown to aggravate some types of neuropathic pain, including phantom limb pain. Some patients state that stimuli that remind them of their injury or loss can trigger pain episodes; other triggers include emotional distress and stress in general. Also, patients who endure a traumatic injury are susceptible to posttraumatic stress disorder and persistent pain.

Treatments for stress and emotional distress may possibly assist in patient pain modulation, but research results are inconclusive. One patient survey indicated that psychological interventions, including antidepressants, did not reduce pain, whereas other studies reported that distraction and relaxation did relieve phantom pain in some patients.

In particular cases where psychiatric diagnoses are ubiquitous, such as multiple sclerosis, psychological interventions can help improve emotional functioning substantially. Two studies report that cognitive-behavioral therapy reduced depression and anxiety when compared with a standard treatment control group. One case study reported that hypnosis resulted in less pain.

Gonzales, in a review of the pathophysiology and treatment of central pain including poststroke pain, stresses the importance of providing psychological intervention in cases in which the pain is resistant to pharmacologic treatment. In the review, Gonzales points out that this population has a high incidence of depression and an increased risk of suicide.

Physical Therapy

Training in both active and passive modalities focused on correcting or modulating the factors that may be contributing to neuropathic pain, such as poor posture, spasm, contractures, or bony ankylosis, is provided by the physical therapist. The goal of physical therapy is to teach the patient stretching and strengthening exercises that enhance flexibility in those muscle groups that would tend to compress the nerve and to simultaneously strengthen the muscle groups that would tend to relieve the compression. For example, the physical therapist working with a patient who has low-back radiculopathy and hyperlordosis might introduce suitable stretching and lumbosacral stabilization exercises; under such instruction, the patient might be able to sustain improved posture and keep the foramen in a more open arrangement, thereby relieving radicular compression. The physical therapist enhances stretching programs by training the patient to apply heat before sustained stretching and ice afterward. Strengthening typically consists of a regimen of active and passive range of motion exercises, eventually progressing to isometric exercises. Later, isotonic exercise and, ideally, supervised weight training may be useful, provided they do not aggravate the compression.

Thermotherapies, ultrasound, and other passive therapies are of limited usefulness in treatment of neuropathic pain. Neuromuscular facilitation and other manipulation therapies can be particularly valuable, primarily in assuaging pressure on a compressed nerve. Physical therapists should be consulted in decision-making when orthotics are indicated. Although bracing may be indicated in the initial stages of rehabilitation, it is not commonly useful as a long-term modality because it creates dependency and causes atrophy in supporting muscles.

Even though they are commonly used in the management of painful neuropathies, electrostimulation methods have not been sufficiently investigated. It remains to be seen whether recent techniques (burst technologies, strength duration variation modalities, or high-frequency, low-amplitude stimulation) improve upon traditional square-wave transcutaneous electrical nerve stimulation. Optimal electrode placement (eg, over a motor point, along the course of nerves, at acupuncture points) remains similarly unresolved. Until the results of more comprehensive studies are available, a patient, flexible, and pragmatic methodology developed by an experienced physical therapist, will provide the best outcome.

A fear of general or specific movements may have developed in some patients with neuropathic pain, who expect motion to be painful. These fears may create patient noncompliance with physical therapy recommendations. The physical therapist can work with the psychologist to identify any such barriers to compliance and provide appropriate psychological treatment.

Occupational Therapy

Workstation assessment, ergonomic correction, and orthotics form the core of neuropathic occupational therapy. In addition, assessment and modification of sleep postures, activities of daily living, and recreational activities are equally important. The identification and application of specific workplace modifications can be very advantageous in some cases, such as wrist padding for keyboard operators. Common sense modification of the existing workplace may be sufficient, but special equipment must sometimes be identified, adjusted, and installed. A work site visit is commonly necessary to suitably evaluate job tasks, to devise a work simulation regimen, and to ensure that all modifications and devices are properly applied.

Occupational therapy should be the principal method for treating compressive-type neuropathies, particularly in a vocational setting. Poor ergonomic work environments may create or aggravate problems like carpal tunnel and repetitive motion or occupational microtrauma-type neuropathies.

The occupational therapist also teaches the patient exercise and flexibility procedures to treat contractures in more serious neuropathic lesions, and prevent their development in other lesions. The occupational therapist should work in conjunction with the orthotist to augment functional recovery, particularly in the context of vocational rehabilitation. Specific braces and tensioning appliances and sometimes serial casting may help prevent or treat contractures in certain patients.

The occupational therapist's role in the treatment of CRPS/reflex sympathetic dystrophy is pivotal. Patients who have this challenging syndrome identify optimal functional restoration as their primary goal, occupational therapies are often fundamental. Scrubbing and stress loading in particular seem to be crucial to optimal outcome, although it is still not known whether the normalized proprioceptive input or the motor output is most beneficial; it is probable that some measure of both are required. Desensitization using a range of textured surfaces or textiles (ie, going from light brushes to silk cloths

to rough toweling) can be vital in conditioning patients for other aspects of therapy and functional rehabilitation. Hydrotherapy and contrast baths may also be essential. In addition, the occupational therapist is able to recommend specialized garments, especially those for edema control. Edema measurement by volumetrics as an indication of improvement and specialized methods of manual lymph drainage have been used effectively.

Vocation Counseling

The vocational counselor intervenes in cases where the patient is unable to return to previous employment. In some cases, job dissatisfaction and anger may be so considerable that the best resolution for patient and employer may be in helping the patient (and employer) acknowledge the need to locate alternative employment and develop methods for doing so. Practical case management can help avoid expensive and extended efforts to return the patient to work that he or she may only be able to handle physically but not emotionally.

2. Pharmacotherapy

The best clinical approach to applied pharmacology currently incorporates empiric observation and identification of possible mechanisms of the neuropathic lesion ("targets"), and then uses the best available pharmacologic information to match these potential disease mechanisms with putative drug mechanisms. Although monotherapy is the ideal approach, rational polypharmacy is often pragmatically used. Rational polypharmacy requires an informed conjecture regarding the underlying pain mechanisms, and a rational combination of drugs that act at different sites in the neuroaxis to interfere and modulate the diagnosed mechanisms. Two basic classes of medications should be considered: prophylactic drugs (used on a regular basis) to manage pain and other symptoms, and abortive drugs (used as needed) for pain or symptom flares. The prophylactic drugs will often be selected by the presentation of the patient's symptoms. For example, if a patient is extremely depressed or anxious and has insomnia, the clinician may choose a tricyclic antidepressant with significant analgesic, sedative, and anxiolytic properties.

Antidepressants

A. TRICYCLIC ANTIDEPRESSANTS

Drugs that are thought of traditionally as antidepressants may be used to treat neuropathic pain because they are analgesic as well. It should be noted, however, that randomized controlled trials evaluating the efficacy of these drugs in alleviating neuropathic pain or reducing specific neuropathic pain symptoms are currently limited. Drugs that have been shown in clinical trials to have a

Table 10–5. Drugs that have Shown Efficacy in Certain Neuropathic Pain Symptoms.

Symptom	Drug
Allodynia	Gabapentin Ketamine IV or IM Lidocaine IV Morphine IV Tramadol
Burning pain	Amitriptyline Gabapentin Phenytoin IV
Hyperalgesia	EMLA cream Gabapentin Lidocaine IV
Shooting, lancinating pain	Amitriptyline Carbamazepine Gabapentin Imipramine Lamotrigine Phenytoin IV Venlafaxine

beneficial impact on specific neuropathic pain symptoms are listed in Table 10–5 and dosages for selected agents are presented in Table 10–6.

Tricyclic antidepressants are accepted choices in neuropathic conditions and a meta-analysis of randomized clinical trials indicate their efficacy in treating neuropathic pain. One of these studies reported that 30 of

Table 10–6. Dosing for Selected Medications.

Drug	Total daily dose	Frequency
Anticonvulsants		
Carbamazepine	100–1000 mg/d	bid to qid
Gabapentin	900–3600 mg/d	tid
Lamotrigine	150–500 mg/d	bid
Antidepressants		
Amitriptyline	10–200 mg/d	qd
Imipramine	10–200 mg/d	qd to bid
Venlafaxine	37.5–340 mg/d	bid to tid
Other		
Lidocaine	0.25–2 mg/kg/d	Continuous IV
Ketamine	0.25–0.5 mg/kg/ dose	q3h (IV or IM)

every 100 patients with neuropathic pain who received antidepressants obtained at least a 50% pain relief.

The antihyperalgesic effects of tricyclic antidepressants may be related to enhancement of noradrenergic descending inhibitory pathways and partial sodium channel blockade, mechanisms that are independent of their antidepressant effects. Moreover, the sodium blocking effect may be the more potent mechanism in this class (which technically includes carbamazepine). When pain is independent of a stimulus, central mechanisms can be reasonably targeted, because these mechanisms cause sensitization of primary somatosensory afferents. Tricyclic antidepressants that cause a balanced inhibition of reuptake of both serotonin and noradrenaline (eg, imipramine, amitriptyline) may be more effective for painful polyneuropathy than those with relative selectivity for noradrenaline reuptake (eg, desipramine).

The responsible clinician must have a repertoire of several tricyclic/quadricyclic drugs, because specific drugs have specific side effects associated with them, and these may sometimes be used to the patients' advantage. For instance, a patient who is in moderate pain, depressed, overweight, and hypersomnolent with psychomotor retardation could be prescribed a tricyclic antidepressant with more noradrenergic selectivity (eg, desipramine), which may be activating and can cause some anorexia, rather than a sedative agent associated with weight gain.

B. SELECTIVE SEROTONIN REUPTAKE INHIBITORS

The performance of selective serotonin reuptake inhibitors for neuropathic pain is not impressive. Certain newer antidepressant agents, including venlafaxine and mirtazepine, show some promise in clinics and have the advantage of a different, more benign side effect and toxicity profile.

Anticonvulsants

The anticonvulsant compounds are some of the best-studied drugs for neuropathic pain, and there is substantial evidence for their efficacy based on meta-analyses and randomized clinical trials. Many of the newer anticonvulsants block sodium and calcium channels, which produces a decrease in neuronal excitability.

A. GABAPENTIN

In fact, gabapentin, widely used for neuropathic pain, first drew the attention of the research community when its successful use in the treatment of CRPS was published in an anecdotal report. The mechanism of action of gabapentin (and now pregabalin) was thought to work primarily through enhancement of endogenous GABA systems that function in pain modulation (but it is not a GABA agonist). New evidence suggests this may not be a primary mechanism, and current theory focuses on "synaptosomes" in the presynapse. In addition, gabapentin may have some effect on the suppression of excitatory amino acids, such as glutamate. In several large randomized clinical trials, gabapentin and pregabalin have demonstrated significant efficacy in postherpetic neuralgia and diabetic peripheral neuropathy.

B. MEMBRANE STABILIZERS

Phenytoin and other membrane-stabilizing antiepileptic drugs (sodium channel blockers) may have some use in neuropathic pain, particularly in cases where there is a potential role for ectopic activity in the generation of pain. Carbamazepine is a membrane stabilizer and has a traditional and perhaps clinically important place in the treatment of neuropathic pain, especially trigeminal neuralgia. Oxcarbazepine may be as effective as carbamazepine and has fewer side effects, according to the results of an open-label trial of patients with painful diabetic neuropathy, but this was not borne out in the pivotal trial.

C. OTHER ANTICONVULSANTS

Many other anticonvulsants such as levetiracetam, topiramate, lamotrigine, and zonisamide have modestly compelling evidence suggesting they may be useful in neuropathic pain, and several large pivotal trials are now in progress.

Anti-Inflammatory Drugs

NSAIDs, corticosteroids, and free-radical scavengers are infrequently used in some neuropathic pain conditions, particularly those associated with considerable inflammation. In neuropathic pain, neuroimmune interactions may occur and provide the rationale for immunosuppressive therapy. Animal studies with cyclosporine, thalidomide, and methotrexate support this premise. NSAIDs inhibit cyclooxygenase (COX) and prevent the synthesis of prostaglandins, which induce inflammation and perhaps peripheral hyperalgesia. In addition to the peripheral anti-inflammatory action of NSAIDs, another proposed mechanism is the blockade of spinal nociceptive processing. However, in several clinical trials of neuropathic pain, NSAIDs have shown mixed results. Ketoprofen has detectable antibradykinin effects as well as the standard antiprostaglandin effect. Randomized clinical trials for COX-2 inhibitors have not been conducted. Corticosteroids can be particularly useful in the early/acute phases of certain types of neuropathic pain (such as radiculopathy) in which significant inflammation exists. A short course of corticosteroids may be indicated, but longer courses have a questionable risk-benefit ratio and numerous contraindications.

Free-radical scavengers (ie, dimethylsulfoxide [DMSO] and vitamin C; see below) may reduce the concentration of reactive oxygen species, which are an acknowledged agent in inflammatory processes that may be involved specifically in neurogenic inflammation.

Opioids

Opioids may be useful, especially in acute stages, but their use for chronic pain management remains somewhat controversial. Several studies of opioids for neuropathic pain suggest their efficacy. In general, neuropathic pain appears to be less responsive to opioids than nociceptive pain; neuropathic pain thus requires higher doses, leading to an increased risk of side effects. To avoid these complications, a strategy that entails the use of nonopioid medications for prophylaxis and reserves the use of opioids for crisis management is indicated. The use of opioid therapy can be linked to increased function, and the use of an acute or subacute opioid protocol is therefore often used to allow the patient to begin to progress in nonpharmacologic therapies.

NMDA Receptor Antagonists

A. KETAMINE AND AMANTADINE

NMDA receptor antagonists (eg, MK-801, ketamine, amantadine) have been considered for management of windup, sensitization, and tolerance to opioids but have been proven too toxic at effective dose levels for regular use. Ketamine has been evaluated in a small study of cancer patients with neuropathic pain who are unresponsive to morphine, and there is considerable ongoing interest in high-dose inpatient protocols of ketamine for CRPS, as well as interest in lower dose inpatient or outpatient protocols. Several delivery systems are also being studied. Amantadine has been evaluated in cancer patients with neuropathic pain and in patients with chronic neuropathic pain, with some support.

B. DEXTROMETHORPHAN

Plain dextromethorphan in pill form may be better tolerated than some of the other NMDA antagonists and may enhance the effect of other medications, specifically opioids. A study in rats demonstrated that combined oral administration of morphine sulfate and dextromethorphan can prevent the development of tolerance to the antinociceptive effects of morphine sulfate. However, dextromethorphan is not effective in low doses, is toxic in doses that are high enough to exhibit efficacy, and so far ineffective when taken on its own.

Other Drugs

Clonidine has been evaluated in its various forms: orally for postherpetic neuralgia, intrathecally in a rat neuropathic pain model, and as a transdermal patch for diabetic polyneuropathy. Unfortunately, a large, randomized clinical trial for neuropathic pain conditions showed no overall efficacy. According to a recent systematic review, data regarding clonidine is not convincing.

Mexiletine, an orally administered antiarrhythmic drug with local anesthetic properties, has been used in some clinics to treat neuropathic pain, but results of a randomized trial in HIV-associated neuropathy exhibited no efficacy. In addition, mexiletine has many problematic side effects.

Systemic lidocaine, administered either intravenously or subcutaneously, may be effective for neuropathic pain but only provides temporary improvement in most trials.

Topical Treatments

Topical treatments for neuropathic pain differ from transdermal medications (eg, the fentanyl patch, transdermal clonidine). Topical treatments deliver medication locally to the affected skin and soft tissues. Topical treatments for neuropathic pain include the lidocaine patch 5%, eutectic mixture of local anesthetics (EMLA) cream, capsaicin, and DMSO.

The lidocaine patch is a non-woven patch containing 5% lidocaine. It is FDA-approved for the treatment of postherpetic neuralgia, and is used increasingly for other neuropathic pain conditions. The lidocaine patch may be useful in some very local or focal neuropathic pain phenomena, including allodynia.

Capsaicin, a vanilloid compound found in chili peppers, causes activation and the dying-back of nociceptive nerve endings by allowing unchecked cation influx. At the site of application, it often induces a painful burning sensation. In a randomized clinical trial, topical capsaicin was effective for the treatment of postherpetic neuralgia. In our experience, however, topical capsaicin has proven to be intolerably painful early on, messy, and associated with very poor compliance.

DMSO is a free radical-scavenging agent. In a high-quality study evaluated in a systematic review, DMSO (50% cream for 2 months) did not show significant pain reduction in persons with CRPS compared with placebo.

Interventional Treatments

Although nerve blocks have been used by physicians for generations for the treatment of neuropathic pain, there is actually very little evidence to support this approach. It also is counterintuitive in the treatment of chronic pain of any sort. Certainly, the transmission of pain can be stopped by local anesthetics, but they all have relatively short half-lives, and any beneficial effect soon wears off.

Regional corticosteroid injection can be very helpful in inflammatory conditions and may be of some use in neurogenic inflammation but are not helpful per se in neuropathic pain. The principal utility of blocks is diagnostic, and the specific nerve involved in generating the neuropathic pain can be identified. They may also have some use in providing a pain free "window of opportunity," so that patients can vest in uncomfortable nonpharmacologic therapy, such as physical therapy.

MANAGING SPECIFIC PAIN SYNDROMES

Hyperalgesia & Allodynia

Because hyperalgesia probably depends on peripheral as well as central mechanisms, treatment can logically be initiated with local therapy. These therapies (ice, sodium ion block) include topical anesthetic agents, such as EMLA cream or lidocaine impregnated patches. Topical agents have been used with variable success in patients with neuropathic pain; however, these results include treatment of a variety of additional conditions besides hyperalgesia. One study monitored the impact of topical EMLA on patients with only hyperalgesia and reported significant efficacy. Moreover, some studies have found that a lidocaine patch has demonstrated efficacy in patients with postherpetic neuralgia, but these studies were not specifically designed to assess hyperalgesia. The 5% lidocaine patch has been approved by the FDA for the treatment of neuropathic pain in patients with postherpetic neuralgia.

The putative mechanism for the efficacy of capsaicin is the selective stimulation of unmyelinated C fiber afferent neurons, which causes the release of substance P. Prolonged application is thought to deplete substance P stores (see above) from sensory nerve endings; this eventually prevents or reduces the transmission of pain. However, repeated applications of capsaicin (3 to 4 times daily for 4 to 8 weeks) are required before clinical effectiveness can be assessed, and it is not always well tolerated.

Many centrally acting medications have been recommended for the management of allodynia. Local anesthetic blocks are effective in temporarily eliminating thermal and sometimes mechanical allodynia; part of this success may result from their ability to inhibit the continued nociceptive input that initiates and maintains central sensitization—one of the causes of allodynia. Topical lidocaine has been used successfully to treat patients with postherpetic neuralgia experiencing allodynia. The use of lidocaine gel or a 5% patch were both significantly more effective than placebo in relieving pain with only minimal increases in lidocaine serum concentrations.

Clinical trials in patients with painful diabetic peripheral neuropathy and postherpetic neuralgia have demonstrated that tricyclic antidepressants are effective in relieving neuropathic pain, but these studies do not differentiate between allodynia and stimulus-independent symptoms such as burning and electrical pain. In addition to being excellent sodium channel blockers (peripheral), the tricyclic antidepressants are known to inhibit the reuptake of serotonin and norepinephrine (central). The analgesic properties of these drugs may be related at least partially to the restoration of inhibitory controls.

Although its mechanism of analgesic effect has not been specifically determined, experimental data suggest that gabapentin acts at multiple central sites. Gabapentin binds with high affinity to a unique site in the brain that is associated with an auxiliary subunit of calcium channels. Gabapentin most likely modifies and modulates first- and second-messenger calcium currents and ultimately may cause a decrease in firing of the transmission cell or a decrease in the release of certain monoamine neurotransmitters. These observed and hypothesized mechanisms might underlie the effect of gabapentin on allodynia. Gabapentin likely also works presynaptically to block synaptosome function, as has been demonstrated in the related drug pregabalin. In a pilot study of patients with various peripheral and central neuropathic pain syndromes, Attal and colleagues demonstrated that gabapentin (up to 2400 mg/d) was effective in reducing tactile and cold allodynia. Gabapentin had no effect on normal mechanical and thermal pain thresholds, suggesting a lack of direct antinociceptive effect. Other GABA-enhancing drugs, including baclofen (a GABA$_B$ agonist), have been shown to be effective in reducing tactile allodynia in rat models.

Traditionally, clinicians have been reluctant to treat pain with opioid analgesics because of multiple concerns, including the threat of diversion, psychological dependency, and cognitive impairment. These fears are variably overestimated in usual clinical practice and the approach has been changing; the clinical use of opioids is becoming more acceptable and perhaps they are now overprescribed. Although opioids may not be as effective in neuropathic pain as in nociceptive conditions, certain evidence supports the short-term use of opioids in patients with allodynia. In a randomized, double-blind, placebo-controlled trial, high-dose morphine (mean 19.2 mg infused over 1 hour) was effective in relieving allodynia in 11 of 19 patients with postherpetic neuralgia. Although adverse effects were common, respiratory depression and excessive sedation were not observed. When therapeutic response to opioids is suboptimal, other routes of administration should be undertaken or combination therapy with other analgesics, such as tricyclic antidepressants, should be considered. No trials of sufficient length allow comment on the comprehensive ramifications of long-term opioid therapy for central sensitization.

Allodynia may also be treated with drugs that antagonize the NMDA receptors responsible for central sensitization. The NMDA antagonist ketamine has demonstrated effectiveness in alleviating allodynia in patients with postherpetic neuralgia, chronic posttraumatic pain, and chronic neuropathic pain. NMDA antagonists have also been used in patients with phantom limb pain (ketamine), orofacial pain (ketamine), surgical neuropathic pain (amantadine), diabetic neuropathy (dextromethorphan), and postherpetic neuralgia (dextromethorphan), though effects on allodynia were not specifically evaluated.

Ectopic Activity at a Neuroma

Theoretically, the effects of the "neuroma sign" (Tinel sign) can be at least partially ameliorated by drugs that block ectopic firing secondary to accumulation of dysfunctional ("leaky") pathologic sodium channels and dysfunctional sodium pumps. To date, supporting data are limited to animal studies. These data show that intravenous lidocaine, tocainide, and mexiletine given in subanesthetic concentrations stop the firing of spontaneously active fibers in the neuroma without blocking conduction. Carbamazepine and phenytoin may also be effective. Some studies suggest that, theoretically, other sodium channel blockers (such as lamotrigine or topiramate) could be useful, but the data are currently inconclusive. All of these drugs have additional and potentially salient effects.

There is some evidence from the rehabilitation literature to support the use of these agents for dramatic neuroma/ectopic activity in such diagnoses as postamputation pain.

Treatment of Stimulus-Independent Pain

Sodium channel blockers are the mainstay of treatment for chronic neuropathic pain syndromes arising from ectopic discharges in nociceptive fibers. Carbamazepine is traditionally the treatment of choice for the shooting pain of trigeminal neuralgia, and it was first proven effective for this condition in the early 1960s. There are many side effects, such as hematopoietic and hepatic toxicity and rash. When skin rash develops, oxcarbazepine can often adequately substitute for carbamazepine, or patients could simply begin with oxcarbazepine, which appears to have a lower incidence of skin rashes than carbamazepine. This is an example of a newer, second-generation drug that has a much improved risk-benefit ratio because the new compound is not metabolized to the toxic epoxide.

Like carbamazepine, lamotrigine has demonstrated higher efficacy than placebo in alleviating the sharp, shooting, or stabbing pain of trigeminal neuralgia when administered in conjunction with phenytoin or carbamazepine to treat refractory cases. However, in a separate placebo-controlled study, lamotrigine (200 mg daily) showed no effect on pain in 100 patients with neuropathic pain of various causes. In still another placebo-controlled trial, a single dose of phenytoin

(15 mg/kg infused intravenously over 2 hours) significantly relieved shooting pain in patients experiencing acute flares of neuropathic pain. In addition, tricyclic antidepressants may be effective for treating shooting pain, possibly because of their sodium channel blocking properties.

Several trials have demonstrated that tricyclic antidepressants are also effective in alleviating burning pain. Drugs evaluated include amitriptyline (2.5 to 150 mg/d), desipramine (12.5 to 250 mg/d), and imipramine (25 to 350 mg/d). However, side effects of tricyclic antidepressants include sedation and anticholinergic effects, which limit their usefulness. Gabapentin generated a moderate but significant relief of both continuous burning pain and paroxysmal (lancinating/shooting) pain.

Attal N et al. Effects of gabapentin on the different components of peripheral and central neuropathic pain syndromes: a pilot study. *Eur. J. Neurol.* 1998;40:191. [PMID: 9813401]

Harden RN. Chronic opioid therapy: another reappraisal. *APS Bull.* 2002;12:1.

McQuay H et al. Anticonvulsant drugs for management of pain: a systematic review. *BMJ.* 1995;311:1047. [PMID: 7580659]

Visceral Pain

Timothy J. Ness, MD, PhD

ESSENTIALS OF DIAGNOSIS

- *The hallmark feature is poor localization in the chest, abdomen, or pelvis.*
- *May be perceived as located within somatic structures (referred pain).*
- *May sensitize somatic structures (secondary hyperalgesia).*
- *Often associated with a visceral function, such as eating, voiding, or defecating.*
- *May represent a neoplastic or a benign process.*
- *Often associated with strong emotional and autonomic responses.*

General Considerations

A. NONSPECIFICITY OF SYMPTOMS

Chronic pain localized to the chest, abdomen, or pelvis can have multiple etiologies ranging from focal sites of inflammation to idiopathic systemic diseases to processes secondary to cancer. These pains fall within the practice of virtually every medical specialty and are some of the most common presenting symptoms for the primary care physician. When the internal organs of the body are the site of origin of pain sensation, the pain is defined as **visceral.**

Because of the diffuse nature of the organization of visceral sensory pathways, visceral sensations may be perceived as located within general body regions or within nonvisceral structures (referred pain). Visceral stimuli can evoke stronger than usual emotional responses, but psychological disturbance may also manifest as complaints of abdominal or chest discomfort. Often, organ-specific localization occurs only with direct stimulation of the organ by physical examination. Indirect evidence for an organ's involvement is an association of the pain with a bodily function, such as urination.

The disease states leading to visceral pain are numerous and discussion of all possibilities is beyond the scope of this chapter. Pains due to cancer and ischemic cardiac disease form special cases due to their profound clinical significance and so are discussed more extensively in Chapters 8 and 18. Likewise, gynecologic pains are also unique and are discussed in Chapter 17. Hence, the scope of this chapter will be to focus on pain arising in organs inhabiting the peritoneal cavity, with discussions related to the more common disease states such as kidney stones, chronic pancreatitis, irritable bowel syndrome (IBS), and interstitial cystitis (IC) as well as a cursory description of less common disorders.

B. STIMULI PRODUCING VISCERAL PAIN

The visceral stimuli that produce reports of pain fall into four main groupings:

1. Chemical stimuli that are secondary to local inflammatory processes.
2. Chemical stimuli that are secondary to ischemia.
3. Mechanical stimuli that are secondary to compressive and obstructive processes and may be modified by inflammation or ischemia.
4. "Functional" stimuli, which are mechanical or chemical stimuli that occur naturally and are typically within physiologic ranges when measured but, for undetermined reasons, lead to profound discomfort.

Cancer, with its diffuse disruption of physiologic processes can produce chemical or mechanical stimuli and be mistaken as functional stimuli. Ischemic stimuli, particularly when recognized as present in cardiac or mesenteric sites, prompt immediate treatment to either reduce metabolic demand or to improve blood and oxygen delivery.

When evaluating symptoms, determining whether the primary pathologic process is potentially life- or tissue-threatening or whether the symptoms indicate syndromes that merely reduce the patient's quality of life is crucial. Symptoms alone cannot distinguish between these differing stimuli that produce visceral pain (Tables 11–1 and 11–2). Many visceral pains are syndromes rather than defined pathophysiologic diseases, so treatments may often be empiric. Hence, evaluation of the distressed patient with chronic visceral pain needs to take into account whether an appropriate, but not necessarily exhaustive, neoplastic work-up has been performed and then perform system-appropriate evaluations to rule

Table 11–1. Life- or Tissue-Threatening Sources of Visceral Pain.

I. DUE TO CANCER
  A. Symptoms in chest, upper abdomen, and back
    1. Esophagus
    2. Stomach
    3. Duodenal
    4. Pancreas
    5. Liver or biliary system
  B. Symptoms in abdomen, flank, and back
    1. Small intestine
    2. Kidney
    3. Ovarian
    4. Testicular
    5. Spinal metastatic involvement
    6. Other metastatic (including carcinomatosis)
  C. Symptoms in lower abdomen, pelvis, and perineum
    1. Uterine and cervical
    2. Colorectal
    3. Urinary bladder
    4. Prostate
II. INFECTIOUS-INFLAMMATORY PAIN STATES
  A. Symptoms in chest, upper abdomen, and back
    1. Esophagitis
    2. Gastritis and duodenitis
    3. Chronic gastric ulcer
    4. Chronic duodenal ulcer
    5. Chronic pancreatitis
    6. Subphrenic abscess
    7. Gallbladder disease
    8. Pericarditis
  B. Symptoms in abdomen, flank, and back
    1. Radiation enterocolitis
    2. Crohn's disease
    3. Ulcerative colitis and other colitis/ulcer
    4. Diverticular disease of the colon
    5. Kidney stones, hydronephrosis
    6. Tuberculous peritonitis

  C. Symptoms in lower abdomen, pelvis, and perineum
    1. Pelvic inflammatory disease
    2. Ulceration of anus or rectum
    3. Posterior parametritis
    4. Tuberculous salpingitis
    5. Urinary bladder distention
III. ISCHEMIA-RELATED ORIGIN
  A. Cardiac ischemia
  B. Acute and chronic mesenteric ischemia
  C. Ischemic colitis
IV. OTHER PAIN STATES
  A. Herniated abdominal organs
  B. Aneurysm of the aorta
  C. Hepatic capsule distention secondary to cardiac failure
  D. Injury of external genitalia
  E. Pain due to hemorrhoids
  F. Familial Mediterranean fever
  G. Porphyria
  H. Lead poisoning
  I. Adrenal insufficiency
  J. Acute herpes zoster
  K. Guillain-Barré syndrome
  L. Fecal impaction

out the presence of readily treatable sources of the pain. A systematic trial of therapeutic options then becomes appropriate.

C. GENERAL EVALUATION OF ABDOMINAL AND PELVIC PAIN

Abdominal pain is a common presenting symptom for the primary care clinician. Initial evaluation includes an interview to assess the acute versus chronic nature of the complaints, exacerbating and ameliorating factors, and history of coexisting disease. Long-term use of medications that alter bowel motility is meaningful. A functionally accurate diagnosis may be determined, based on clinical history, in 75% of patients. Palpation of the abdomen can identify abdominal wall rigidity, suggesting a peritoneal process; distended bowel or underlying masses, suggesting a neoplastic, infectious, or obstructive processes; and localized tenderness, which may suggest a particular organ system. Auscultation of bowel sounds assesses gastrointestinal motility and gives evidence of obstruction.

Rectal and pelvic examinations may give additional information related to local disease. Neurologic examination may demonstrate evidence of neuropathy or localized radiculopathy. Testing for fecal blood, urinalysis, blood cell count with white cell differential, serum amylase and lipase levels, electrolytes, and liver function tests all are considered routine. Determining if performing other tests, such as radiographic evaluations, endoscopic evaluations, ultrasonography, paracentesis or advanced imaging studies, would be helpful depends on the persistence or progression of complaints.

Table 11–2. Quality-of-Life–Related Chronic Visceral Pain Disorders.

I. GASTROINTESTINAL PAIN STATES
  A. Postgastric surgery syndrome (dumping)
  B. Postcholecystectomy syndrome
  C. Dyspepsia, functional disorders of the stomach
  D. Irritable bowel syndrome
  E. Chronic constipation
  F. Proctalgia fugax
  G. Esophageal spasm
II. UROGENITAL PAIN STATES
  A. Urologic disorders
    1. Interstitial cystitis
    2. Urethral syndrome
    3. Loin-pain hematuria
  B. Gynecologic disorders
  C. Male urogenital disorders
    1. Prostatodynia (male chronic pelvic pain disorder)
    2. Orchialgia
III. NONVISCERAL SOURCES OF PAIN
  A. Musculoskeletal
    1. Thoracic, lumbar, and sacral spinal disease
    2. Slipping rib syndrome
    3. Abdominal muscle wall
    4. Fibromyalgia, chronic fatigue syndrome
    5. Generalized rheumatologic disorders
  B. Neurologic
    1. Postherpetic neuralgia
    2. Peripheral neuropathy
    3. Spinal cord injury-related pain
    4. Poststroke pain
    5. Segmental or intercostal neuralgia
    6. 12th rib syndrome
    7. Abdominal cutaneous nerve entrapment syndrome
    8. Abdominal migraine
    9. Postsurgical neuroma
    10. Painful scar
    11. Neuralgias of iliohypogastric, ilioinguinal, genitofemoral nerves
  C. Psychological

■ LIFE- OR TISSUE-THREATENING DISORDERS

CANCER

Clinical Findings

Neoplasms can arise in any visceral structure. Symptoms related to these cancers are similar for all sites, with dull and constant pain a common "early" symptom. Pain is generally localized to the chest or upper abdomen for upper gastrointestinal tract lesions and organs located in the upper abdomen. It is generally localized to lower abdomen and perineum for lower gastrointestinal tract lesions and pelvic organs.

Unfortunately, no symptoms or location is pathognomonic for any specific disease site due to the potential presence of metastatic extension prior to diagnosis. Visceral cancers are frequently asymptomatic until obstruction or invasion of other structures occurs. Anorexia, weight loss, fatigue, nausea, and virtually every other nonspecific symptom can be noted at presentation. Anemia, hematemesis, melena, hematuria, and palpable masses on physical examination may direct further investigation. Appropriate imaging and surgical exploration or biopsy are the definitive diagnostic modalities. Sources of cancer-related pain can be multifactorial (Table 11–3) with components due to local tumor effects or more generalized somatic or neuropathic components due to local involvement and metastases.

Treatment

Treating the cancer may also be pain-producing. Patterns of tumor spread differ between types of tumors, and so general patterns of symptoms related to metastases

Table 11–3. Cancer Pain Syndromes.

I. DUE TO DIRECT TUMOR INVOLVEMENT
  A. Visceral pain
    1. Infiltration of viscus or neighboring viscus
    2. Liver metastases: capsule distention, diaphragmatic irritation
    3. Biliary tree distention-obstruction
    4. Bowel obstruction
    5. Ischemic pain due to mesenteric vessel involvement
  B. Somatic pain
    1. Retroperitoneal involvement (including lymph nodes)
    2. Parietal peritoneum involvement
    3. Abdominal wall involvement
    4. Abdominal distention due to ascites
    5. Bone metastases
  C. Neuropathic pain
    1. Radiculopathy from retroperitoneal spread
    2. Radiculopathy from metastases
    3. Lumbosacral plexopathy
    4. Epidural spinal cord compression
II. DUE TO CANCER THERAPIES
  A. Postoperative pain syndromes
  B. Stent-related complications
  C. Postchemotherapy pain syndromes
  D. Postradiation pain syndromes

also differ. Tumors of the gastrointestinal tract tend to spread through the lymphatics toward the liver and may present with diffuse abdominal complaints. In contrast, prostatic tumors frequently involve the lumbar spine and may present as back pain.

Treatment of the cancer (eg, surgery, chemotherapy, radiotherapy) whether it is curative or palliative is considered a primary treatment for pain. Nerve-killing procedures are an option with the particular site of treatment determined by the site of the symptomatic cancer. For example, celiac plexus blocks may be of benefit for tumors in the upper abdomen, superior hypogastric blocks for tumors in the pelvis, and ganglion of Impar blocks for perirectal and perineal symptoms.

Because various urologic or gastrointestinal structures may become obstructed by neighboring or infiltrating tumor, stenting or diversion of obstructed ureters or bowel segments may be necessary.

Medical treatments are often empirically driven with the aggressive use of opioids, anti-inflammatories, antiemetics, and adjuvant medications.

It is notable that when the cancer has responded to treatment but the treatment itself has proved to be pain-producing, there is frequently reticence on the part of clinicians to provide continued aggressive management of symptoms. Neuropathies, radiation enteritis and colitis, postsurgical phantom pain, neuroma formation, altered biomechanics, adhesions and strictures as well as other effects of "scarring" can all act as pain generators or modulators that may require reinvestigation of the primary metastatic process.

Mercadante S et al. Celiac plexus block for pancreatic cancer pain: factors influencing pain, symptoms, and quality of life. *J Pain Symptom Manage.* 2003;26:1140. [PMID: 14654266]

Van Heek NT et al. Palliative treatment in "peri"-pancreatic carcinoma: stenting or surgical therapy? *Acta Gastroenterol Belg.* 2002;65:171. [PMID: 12420610]

CHRONIC MESENTERIC ISCHEMIA & ISCHEMIC COLITIS

General Considerations

Inadequate blood supply to meet the energy demands of abdominal viscera can lead to reports of pain in a way similar to cardiac angina. When ischemia is present in the gastrointestinal system, severe abdominal pain may be precipitated by the ingestion of a meal. As a consequence, a fear of eating with subsequent weight loss and poor nutritional status may further compromise patients already suffering from atherosclerotic disease. Necrosis of gut wall with subsequent perforation and peritonitis are end-stage manifestations with high mortality. More frequent is compromise of the mucosal barrier to absorption of the bacterial endotoxins held within the gastrointestinal tract and the systemic effects of its absorption.

Clinical Findings

Poor peripheral pulses, abdominal bruits, and arteriographic evidence of stenosis or occlusion in the three main mesenteric arteries are all consistent with the diagnosis of **abdominal angina.** Similar to cardiac disease, abdominal angina may precede infarction, which has devastating life-threatening consequences. Arterial thrombosis, embolic events, venous occlusion, and low-flow states due to poor cardiac output may all lead to the same disastrous results. Ischemic colitis represents approximately half of the cases of morbidity due to mesenteric vascular disease. Evidence of peritonitis develops in 20% of patients with ischemic colitis; surgical exploration is required in these cases.

Initial presentation of ischemic colitis may be persistent diarrhea, rectal bleeding, or weight loss. Vascular comorbidities increase surgical risks and jeopardize outcome. In addition, angioplasties in this region are technically difficult.

Oldenburg WA et al. Acute mesenteric ischemia: a clinical review. *Arch Intern Med.* 2004;164:1054. [PMID: 15159262]

Sreenarasimhaiah J. Diagnosis and management of intestinal ischaemic disorders. *BMJ.* 2003;326:1372. [PMID: 12816826]

CHRONIC PANCREATITIS

General Considerations

Pancreatitis is life- or tissue-threatening because of nutritional disruption, dehydration due to prolonged nausea and vomiting, and altered electrolyte and peripancreatic environment. The general phenomenon of pancreatitis is divided into **acute** (isolated episodes with serum amylase and lipase elevations) and **chronic** (identical symptoms as acute but may lack measurable laboratory abnormalities). Recurrent acute episodes are common early in the development of chronic pancreatitis.

Pathogenesis

The symptoms of pancreatitis can be associated with pancreatic cell death and with ductal fibrosis and calcification. Whereas acute pancreatitis generally resolves without permanent structural abnormalities, most forms of chronic pancreatitis are associated with permanent abnormalities. However, acute-on-chronic episodes in which an acute necrotic episode may occur in a patient with known chronic changes may be seen. Alcohol abuse is the primary cause in 70 to 80% of chronic pancreatitis cases in developed nations. Since symptomatic chronic pancreatitis develops in only 5 to 10% of heavy drinkers, there are likely genetic, infectious, and nutritional factors that also contribute to its development. A person with chronic pancreatitis who continues to abuse alcohol has a 50% mortality rate at 5-years' follow-up (versus a 25-year 50% survivability rate if they abstain from drinking). Chronic pancreatitis may also be idiopathic, although other causes include a pancreas divisum, genetic causes (hereditary-type), previous trauma, previous obstructive episodes, hyperparathyroidism, hyperlipidemia, and a_1-antitrypsin deficiency. Identifiable disease does not firmly correlate with reports of pain.

Clinical Findings

A. SYMPTOMS AND SIGNS

The primary presenting complaint for chronic pancreatitis is deep, boring pain that is located in the epigastric region with frequent radiation through to the back. At onset, it may be episodic but may advance until it is continuous. Any eating, but particularly consumption of fatty foods, may precipitate pain. Positioning, such as sitting upright or leaning forward, may decrease the pain. It may be coupled with nausea and vomiting, so dehydration, malnutrition, and an inability to take oral analgesics may all become problematic. There are no definitive findings on physical examination. Persons with alcoholic chronic pancreatitis may be cachetic and may have stigmata associated with extensive alcohol use and associated liver failure. It may be possible to palpate an inflammatory mass, but abdominal guarding typically precludes adequate examination.

B. LABORATORY FINDINGS

Steatorrhea due to pancreatic insufficiency may be present in advanced disease as may glucose intolerance secondary to developing diabetes mellitus. Elevated serum amylase and lipase levels indicate a pancreatic exocrine cell damaging process, but these blood tests are used less frequently since the sensitivity of other diagnostic modalities such as endoscopic retrograde cholangiopancreatography (ERCP) and computed tomography (CT) have improved. Diffuse intraductal calcium deposition is pathognomonic of chronic pancreatitis.

C. IMAGING STUDIES

Simple abdominal radiographs will support the diagnosis in 30% of cases. A higher sensitivity (60 to 70% sensitive for intraductal abnormalities) is gained by ultrasonographic evaluation. CT is 90% sensitive. ERCP is the gold standard for chronic pancreatitis based on ductal abnormalities that are graded by severity. A system of

stratification or subgroupings of patients by morphologic or functional criteria is still a matter of debate.

Differential Diagnosis

Pancreatic cancer must be considered and is not an uncommon incidental finding during surgical treatment of chronic pancreatitis. Peptic ulcer disease, IBS, gallstones, endometriosis, and all other sources of abdominal pain are also possibilities. A first step in the management of an acute increase in pain in patients with chronic pancreatitis is to exclude such complications as pseudocysts or compression of adjacent visceral structures.

Treatment

A. GENERAL

Some guidelines do exist for the treatment of pain due to chronic pancreatitis. Unfortunately, most published treatment options are only validated by case reports and retrospective series of patients who underwent treatments assessing a particular method. Few studies of chronic pancreatitis pain have used placebo-controlled methods, and of those, even fewer demonstrated robust effects of the studied treatment. Procedural studies have generally not had controls performed. The symptoms of chronic pancreatitis are episodic with frequent exacerbations and spontaneous resolution. Hence, any "open" study that is initiated during an exacerbation is likely to be deemed effective in some patients due to the natural course of the disease. Therapeutic options for chronic pancreatitis are listed in Table 11–4.

For alcoholic chronic pancreatitis, the initial treatment is abstinence from alcohol. As stated before, if the patient continues to drink, he or she has a high mortality rate. It has been commonly reported that total abstinence from alcohol achieves pain relief in up to 50% of

Table 11–4. Treatment Options for Chronic Pancreatitis Pain.

- Abstinence from alcohol
- Opioids
- Anti-inflammatory medications
- Antioxidants and micronutrients
- Endoscopic management (stents, sphincterotomy, stone removal)
- Oral pancreatic enzyme treatment
- Neurolysis
- Intraceliac corticosteroid injections
- Surgical diversion or resection
- Pseudocystic drainage (percutaneous, endoscopic, surgical)

patients, particularly those with mild to moderate disease. Psychological therapies directed toward developing alternative coping mechanisms and abstaining from alcohol are considered vitally necessary, but outcomes related to substance abuse treatment are mixed and not limited to this specific population.

B. MEDICATIONS

Opioids, the primary analgesic therapy of advanced chronic pancreatitis, can be supplemented with adjuvant agents such as antidepressants. It is an unfortunate but common experience of clinicians who treat patients with alcoholic pancreatitis that persons who were dependent on alcohol may become dependent on opioids. Therefore, involvement of behavioral medicine specialists with experience in both pain management and substance abuse is of particular benefit in the monitoring and appropriate treatment of these patients. Anti-inflammatory drugs, such as corticosteroids or non-steroidal anti-inflammatory drugs (NSAIDs), would seem logical choices in the treatment of a chronic inflammatory process. However, case reports of pancreatitis induced by these agents has temporized their use.

Placebo-controlled medical trials of antioxidants and micronutrients, such as vitamins C and E, beta-carotene, S-adenosylmethionine, and selenium, have produced favorable results. Oral pancreatic enzyme treatments have been used as inhibitors of pancreatic enzyme secretion with a resultant decrease in intraductal pressure. This negative feedback strategy has been effective at reducing pain in some studies, but four of six randomized, prospective, placebo-controlled, double-blind studies failed to observe any effect of this treatment. Inhibition of pancreatic secretion, produced by somatostatin or its analogue octreotide, has been reported to reduce pain but two randomized, prospective, double-blind, placebo-controlled studies failed to see any statistically significant improvement in pain.

C. PROCEDURAL THERAPIES

Celiac plexus blocks with local anesthetics have been used for diagnostic purposes but also as primary therapies for chronic pancreatic pain when coupled with corticosteroids. Neurolytic celiac plexus blocks have been performed using alcohol or phenol. Neurolytic celiac plexus blocks for the treatment of nonmalignant pancreatic pain is controversial. Enthusiasm for neurolytic celiac plexus blocks for chronic pancreatitis has been tempered by the apparent limited duration of effect, requiring either retreatment every 2 to 6 months or acceptance of another alternative for care. Sequelae such as chronic diarrhea and the occurrence of uncommon but catastrophic neurologic deficits have also reduced enthusiasm for repeated therapy. Visceral neurolysis via surgical splanchnicectomy or celiac ganglionectomy has been reported.

Thoracoscopic splanchnic nerve resections have been reported.

Surgical diversion or resection is often viewed as the definitive treatment of chronic pancreatitis despite the absence of prospective randomized studies.

Relief of ductal hypertension or obstruction by surgical means via pancreaticojejunostomy is reported as effective in relieving pain for at least 5 years in 70 to 93% of appropriately selected patients who had dilated pancreatic ducts as demonstrated by ERCP and in 40% of patients with nondilated ducts. Partial or total resection of the pancreas leads to pain relief for at least 5 years in 54 to 95% of patients with 0 to 5% morbidity and mortality. Following total resection, the loss of the endocrine function of the pancreas leads to diabetes mellitus with its own associated morbidity and mortality.

Pancreatic pseudocysts are nonepithelialized sacs of pancreatic fluids, blood, and necrotic debris with apparently inadequate drainage. They enlarge, are frequently painful, and risk rupture of their contents into the peritoneal cavity. Treatments have been predominantly procedural with open or percutaneous drainage, followed by marsupialization (connection of the cyst to nearby gastrointestinal structure) if recurrent. Following surgical drainage of pseudocysts, it has been reported that 96% of patients report short-term relief of pain and 53% remain pain free for many years.

The endoscopic placement of stents, sphincterotomy, dilatation, or stone removal are well-established alternatives to surgery in the treatment of biliary tract diseases, and similar techniques for the relief of chronic pancreatic pain have developed. Ultrasound-guided endoscopic drainage of pseudocysts or performance of neurolytic celiac plexus injections have reported benefit. Extracorporeal shock-wave lithotripsy has been coupled with endoscopic procedures to remove stones from the main pancreatic duct with reported pain reduction in some patients.

Prognosis

It has been proposed that the pain of chronic pancreatitis will eventually "burn out" and subside as the disease process progresses to total organ failure. This process occurs at a variable rate and effectively, for some, does not occur. Hence, delay of treatment in the hopes of disease resolution is neither realistic nor ethical.

Andren-Sandberg A et al. Pain management in chronic pancreatitis. *Eur J Gastroenterol Hepatol.* 2002;14:957. [PMID: 12352215]

Cunha JE et al. Surgical and interventional treatment of chronic pancreatitis. *Pancreatology.* 2004;4:540. [PMID: 15486450]

Stevens T et al. Pathogenesis of chronic pancreatitis: an evidence-based review of past theories and recent developments. *Am J Gastroenterol.* 2004;99:2256. [PMID: 15555009]

Pancreatitis Association International http://pancassociation.org

INFLAMMATORY BOWEL DISEASE

General Considerations

Ulcerative colitis (UC) and Crohn's disease (CD) are two recurrent gastrointestinal inflammatory disorders with many similarities in symptoms and histopathology; however, they also have significant differences in extent of the disease process, relapse incidence, and associated complications (such as fistula formation). These disorders can be life- and tissue-threatening due to local spread of infection and the severe alterations in nutrient, fluid, and electrolyte levels. The precise causes of inflammatory bowel disease are unknown, but genetic mechanisms are suspected. Inflammatory bowel disease is more common in whites than blacks or Asians and 3 to 6 times more common in Jews than nonJews. UC is 3 to 5 times more common than CD, but recurrent exacerbations are much less frequent. In UC, the gastrointestinal component of the disease process is restricted to the colon; whereas in CD, there is involvement in all portions of the gastrointestinal tract.

Clinical Findings

Common presenting symptoms include abdominal pain, fever, and altered bowel habits (such as bloody diarrhea). The diagnosis of inflammatory bowel disease is based on biopsy, colonoscopic or endoscopic appearances, or surgical evaluation. Other causes of inflammatory changes such as radiation enteritis or local infection (eg, *Shigella, Salmonella, Amoeba, Clostridium difficile*) must be ruled out. Local complications of inflammatory bowel disease include the formation of fistulas, abscesses, strictures, perforation, and toxic dilation, all of which are more common in CD than UC. Extracolonic features of inflammatory bowel disease include arthritis, skin changes, and evidence of liver disease.

Treatment

Dietary alterations may have some acute effects during a "flare" but have not been demonstrated to alter overall disease progression. Neurolysis is typically avoided since symptoms may act as early indicators of life-threatening complications. Although regional anesthetic techniques have possible short-term benefit during a flare, they have the same risks as neurolysis in that they may mask disease complications. Surgery has remained an integral component in the management of inflammatory bowel disease. Pain treatment related to inflammatory bowel disease forms a limited-choice corollary to chronic pancreatitis. Since reports of pain may be associated with life-threatening complications, these patients may have frequent hospitalizations. The use of motility-altering drugs, such as opioids, may be associated with an increased risk of toxic dilation and subsequently an increase in morbidity and mortality. Similar to other diseases with unknown etiologies, genetic influences, immunologic abnormalities, and infectious organisms have all been implicated and used as rationales for treatment. Primary treatment for exacerbations is typically bowel rest; anti-inflammatories (eg, oral sulfasalazine, possible corticosteroids); nutritional, fluid, and electrolyte management; and treatment of complications. No universal consensus appears to exist in relation to preventative treatment. Multiple therapies, such as oral sulfasalazine, oral olsalazine, oral metronidazole, systemic corticosteroids, and mesalamine enemas or suppositories, have been used not only as reactive treatments for exacerbations but as prophylactic measures. Although results related to use of these agents are encouraging for UC, a multicenter study failed to observe any decrease in the recurrence of CD exacerbations even with sulfasalazine. Immunosuppressants such as azothioprine and cyclosporine have been used for a presumed immunologic etiology. Psychological treatments are justified by the presence of a lifelong, recurrent disease process.

Prognosis

With a prolonged clinical course, there is a potential for the development of carcinoma. There is a stated incidence of colon cancer of 0.5 to 1% per year for every year after the initial 10 years of active inflammatory bowel disease. Surgical treatment of inflammatory bowel disease is normally reserved for the treatment of complications, with 20 to 25% of patients with UC and 70% of patients with CD requiring colectomy. Colectomy presumably resolves UC but does not resolve all of the symptoms of CD since the disease process is panenteric.

American Gastroenterological Association Clinical Practice Committee. American Gastroenterological Association medical position statement: perianal Crohn's disease. *Gastroenterology.* 2003;125:1503. [PMID: 14598267]

Carter MJ et al. Guidelines for the management of inflammatory bowel disease in adults. *Gut.* 2004;53(Suppl 5):V1. [PMID: 15306569]

DIVERTICULAR DISEASE

General Considerations

A diverticulum is a sac or pouch opening from a tubular organ such as the gut. Diverticuli can occur throughout the gastrointestinal tract but prove to be most common in the colon where they occur typically at the site of penetrating blood vessels, but hypopharyngeal (termed "Zenker diverticulum"), duodenal, jejunal, and ileal diverticuli are possible. Meckel diverticuli, the remains of the omphalomesenteric duct of the embryo, is a congenital abnormality present in 2% of the population and located on the ileum close to its connection to the cecum. They are notable since they may contain acid-producing gastric mucosa, which may lead to enteral ulcer formation and associated bleeding. Colonic diverticuli are generally pain free; however, severe abdominal pain and infection may result with the development of inflammation and obstruction of the mouth. The condition is then termed "diverticulitis" and may be associated with abscess formation, obstruction, colonic distention, bleeding, and altered bowel habit (ie, diarrhea, constipation). Painful diverticulosis classically presents as recurrent left lower quadrant colicky pain without evidence of inflammation. Like chronic pancreatitis, diverticular disease can produce pain that is episodic and that can have life-threatening consequences if ignored. A bleeding colonic diverticulum is the most common source of lower gastrointestinal tract bleeding, and segmental colonic resection has the highest success rate at stopping bleeding. However, effects on pain are unclear. Reports of pain do not always correlate with observable disease and symptoms can be nonspecific. Consensus panels have not been able to definitively state when surgery was indicated for symptomatic reasons.

Kohler L et al. Diagnosis and treatment of diverticular disease: results of a consensus development conference. The Scientific Committee of the European Association for Endoscopic Surgery. *Surg Endosc.* 1999;13:430. [PMID: 10094765]

FAMILIAL MEDITERRANEAN FEVER

General Considerations

An autosomal recessive genetic disease linked to chromosome 16, this disorder begins between the ages 5 to 15 and has an increased incidence in Sephardic Jews, Armenians, Turks, Arabs, and other Mediterranean populations.

Clinical Findings

Features include periodic febrile episodes without other cause, serous peritonitis, pleuritis, synovitis, and an erysipelas-like rash. Abdominal pain and arthralgias occur in greater than 95% of the episodes, which vary in frequency from twice per week to once per year; the most common variant occurs in 2 to 4 week intervals with acute episodes typically lasting 1 to 3 days. Amyloidosis with associated kidney failure and arthralgia are the most severe associated sequelae. Leukocytosis and elevated sedimentation rate may be present on laboratory examination.

Treatment

Typical treatment is symptom-driven with the use of systemic analgesics. In controlled studies, colchicine has been demonstrated to decrease the frequency of attacks and risks of amyloidosis. Multiple other prophylactic therapies have been tried without success.

Medlej-Hashim M et al. Familial Mediterranean Fever (FMF): from diagnosis to treatment. *Sante.* 2004;14:261. Review French. [PMID: 15745878]

PORPHYRIA

General Considerations

The increased formation of porphyrins, or their precursors, occurs in several related autosomal dominant genetic disorders with incomplete penetrance, all characterized by the term "porphyria." Three subgroups that all have similar symptoms have been identified: acute intermittent porphyria, hereditary coproporphyria, and variegate porphyria.

Clinical Findings

Acute intermittent porphyria is the most frequently encountered subgroup, with attacks of colicky abdominal pain that are intermittent, may be associated with environmental exposures, and can last for days to months. Certain drugs such as barbiturates, benzodiazepines, alcohol, phenytoin, ketamine, etomidate, meprobamate, and corticosteroids have been particularly implicated as "triggers," although use of many of these agents without the precipitation of a crisis has been reported.

Vomiting, constipation, and abdominal distention are not uncommon. Neurologic dysfunction may occur principally due to demyelination effects with emotional disturbance a nonspecific symptom. Urine and blood tests related to porphyria may only be diagnostic during crises.

Treatment

Treatment involves avoiding known triggers. Crises are treated with intravenous fluids, hematin, and increased carbohydrate intake; pain and nausea are managed with safe analgesics and antiemetics. Most opioids are alleged to be nontriggering; a notable exception is the mixed agonist-antagonist pentazocine. Chlorpromazine, promethazine, and droperidol have all been reported to be safe as antiemetics.

UROLITHIASIS

General Considerations

Movement of stones within the urinary system (ie, renal pelvis and calices, ureters, bladder, urethra) can produce severe pain (renal colic). If urine flow is sufficiently obstructed, kidney function can be destroyed. Urolithiasis may be frequently recurrent in "stone-formers" and may be continuous when numerous or large renal pelvic (staghorn) calculi are present. Diagnosis is based on history of stone formation or imaging studies (ie, intravenous pyelogram or CT scanning).

Treatment

The definitive treatment is the removal of the stone by spontaneous passage, which may be assisted by fragmentation using lithotripsy or surgical removal. Drugs producing a relaxation effect in the ureters include NSAIDs, nifedipine, and tamsulosin. Pain treatments used for renal colic are intended to be "temporizing" until stone removal occurs. As such, narcotics and NSAIDs are the mainstay of treatment. As noted above, there may be particular benefit to using NSAIDs because they may produce ureteral relaxation in addition to analgesia.

UROGENITAL PAIN

Conditions other than urolithiasis that may produce lower abdominal or pelvic pain of visceral origin include chronic or recurrent bacterial infections of the bladder, urethra, vagina, prostate, epididymis, or other associated urogenital structures (eg, pelvic inflammatory disease) and anatomic abnormalities, such as asymptomatic urinary tract diverticuli. Similar to treatments for symptomatic urolithiasis, pain-related treatments are temporizing, with the primary goal being resolution of the underlying pathophysiology by surgical, behavioral, or pharmacologic means.

POLYCYSTIC KIDNEY DISEASE

An autosomal-dominant disease that eventually leads to polycystic kidney disease can also be a cause of visceral pain. Cyst formation, rupture, infection, and secondary compression or traction of neighboring structures can all lead to abdominal, flank, and back pain. Renal stone formation and liver cyst formation are both common comorbidities, and so reports of pain may require an assessment of those etiologies. A general progression from nonpharmacologic methods to non-narcotic analgesics, minimally invasive procedures to progressively more invasive procedures, and use of opioids have been advocated by some clinicians. Procedures unique to polycystic kidney disease include surgical or percutaneous drainage of the cysts with marsupialization to avoid fluid reaccumulation.

Bajwa ZH et al. Pain management in polycystic kidney disease. *Kidney Int.* 2001;60:1631. [PMID: 11703580]

LOIN PAIN–HEMATURIA SYNDROME

This is a descriptive diagnosis with the primary symptom of severe flank pain and the laboratory finding of hematuria. It is of obscure etiology and is associated with inconsistent pathology. Loin pain–hematuria syndrome is more common in women than men, and it is predominantly a diagnosis of exclusion. Accepted by some clinicians as a diagnosis that justifies aggressive interventions, including nephrectomy or renal autotransplantation, its very existence as a discrete clinicopathologic entity has been questioned. Recurrence of pain following surgical procedures including extensive surgical sympathectomy of the kidney has been common except in cases where there was meticulous screening of patients for other urologic, nephrologic, or psychiatric etiologies of the pain. Injection therapies have been normally viewed as short-lived. Transcutaneous electrical nerve stimulation has been reported to result in partial pain relief. Due to the limited success of other modalities of treatment, use of narcotic analgesics may be considered.

Pukenas BA et al. Loin pain hematuria syndrome: case series. *W V Med J.* 2003;99:192. [PMID: 14959511]

ADHESIONS

Laparoscopy may demonstrate adhesions in postabdominal surgery patients with new onset of abdominal or pelvic pain, but the role of these adhesions in producing pain is a matter of debate. It would appear that unless adhesions are producing bowel obstruction, adhesiolysis appears unlikely to produce reliable benefit. Treatment is episodic and symptomatic, but use of narcotic analgesics may lead to further bowel dysfunction and so may be viewed as a late option.

■ QUALITY-OF-LIFE DISORDERS

POSTCHOLECYSTECTOMY SYNDROME

General Considerations

Gallbladder inflammation, gallstones, and associated diseases of the biliary tract are known sources of acute pain that is typically coupled with dyspepsia and occasionally jaundice (when obstruction is present). However, even after surgical resection of the gallbladder, pain may continue; this is called postcholecystectomy syndrome.

Clinical Findings

Typically, the symptoms of postcholecystectomy syndrome are similar to those of cholecystitis: located in the right upper quadrant; associated with nausea; exacerbated by eating; and pain is described as continuous during the day, dull, and frequently colicky. Appropriate work-up will rule out definable disease, such as a retained bile duct stone or secondary pancreatitis. Postcholecystectomy syndrome is a correlate to chronic pancreatitis in that there may be abnormal pressures or motility within the biliary duct. Endoscopic demonstration of elevated sphincter of Oddi pressures suggest sphincter dysfunction as the cause of the syndrome. During ERCP, it may be possible to reproduce the pain by producing intraductal distention.

Treatment

Endoscopic or surgical sphincterotomy or sphincteroplasty have been beneficial in series reports and calcium channel blockers or long-acting nitrates have been proposed as therapeutic. Other treatment options are dietary alterations, surgical reexplorations, focal injections or neurolysis, and traditional analgesics. In many cases, there is no objective identification of a site of pain generation, so treatment is empiric. Furthermore, the cholecystectomy that presumably started the disorder may also have been an empiric treatment.

INTERSTITIAL CYSTITIS & PAINFUL BLADDER SYNDROME

General Considerations

Painful bladder syndrome is a term that has been recently advocated for use on a national level to describe a complex of urologic complaints, including pain, that may have a common etiology. Painful bladder syndrome may possibly be an early form of IC, but it has no agreed upon etiology, pathophysiology, or treatment. IC, which has a similarly undefined list of etiologies and treatments, does have a defining pathology; according to a study group of the National Institute of Diabetes, Digestive and Kidney Diseases, IC is either the presence of mucosal ulcers (a Hunner patch) or "glomerulations," which are small submucosal petechial hemorrhages viewed cystoscopically after sustained distention of the bladder (hydrodistention). Glomerulations are not unique to IC but occur in other forms of cystitis (eg, radiation cystitis) and may be a normal variant, so IC is also a diagnosis of exclusion for those other disorders. There is good evidence that there is a disruption of the normal urothelial barrier

in most (if not all) patients with IC. Prevalence of IC is estimated to be 2 in 10,000, with a female to male ratio of 10:1. The frequent association of IC with other chronic diseases and pain syndromes, such as inflammatory bowel disease, systemic lupus erythematosus, IBS, "sensitive" skin, fibromyalgia, and allergies speaks to the fact there may be multiple different pathophysiologies grouped together under one diagnosis.

Pathogenesis

The etiology of the breakdown in the urothelial barrier in IC and the consequences of this breakdown are as yet unknown. One theory proposes that the breakdown of the urothelial barrier is a failure to maintain adequate formation of glycosaminoglycans, which provide a protective coating to the urothelium. Another theory proposes that IC is a systemic autoimmune disease presenting as a local manifestation with associated abnormal mast cell activity in the bladder, leading to local tissue and neurologic effects. The most mechanistic theory to date relates the breakdown of the urothelial barrier to the presence of a specific peptide present within the urine of patients with IC that impairs urothelial regrowth. The antiproliferative factor is a low-molecular-weight peptide that is present in bladder urine but not renal pelvis urine of patients with IC, is present in over 90% of patients in whom IC has been clinically diagnosed, is not present in other disorders, and is therefore viewed as the best laboratory diagnostic test for IC. The test itself is not currently available but will likely become available pending further validation as a diagnostic test. Whether antiproliferative factor is present due to rheumatologic, immunologic, infectious, genetic, or neurologic causes has not been determined, but it has been demonstrated to produce a downregulation of genes that stimulate epithelial proliferation and upregulates genes that inhibit cell growth. Independent of the specific reason for a urothelial disruption, the simplest explanation of the consequences of this breakdown is that it allows an exposure of urinary constituents, bacterial products, and cell death products to bladder sensory nerves that normally are protected by an intact barrier. This "toxic urine" exposure produces either direct activation or sensitization of peripheral and central nervous system structures.

Clinical Findings

A. SYMPTOMS AND SIGNS

Urgency, frequency, nocturia, and associated pain are the primary symptoms of IC. Pain may be localized to the lower abdomen, pelvis, groin, and perineum. The onset of the disease is normally abrupt, with rapid progression of symptoms often following an "event" such as a prolonged episode of severe urgency while searching for a lavatory. Anxiety and depression are frequent comorbidities. Suprapubic tenderness to palpation may accompany a diagnosis of IC. Patients with IC are 10 to 12 times more likely to report childhood bladder problems than the general population. Although a history of frequent urinary tract infection is twice as common in patients with IC than those without IC, most report infrequent urinary tract infections (fewer than 1 per year) prior to the onset of IC symptoms.

B. SPECIAL TESTS

A cystoscopic examination of the bladder wall for a Hunner patch or the development of glomerulations after hydrodistention is necessary to meet the research definition of IC. However, recently the intravesical potassium sensitivity test has been used as an alternative diagnostic procedure. In this test, 40 mL of a potassium chloride solution (40 mEq in 100 mL water) is administered into the bladder by a catheter and responses observed 3 to 5 minutes later. A positive test is pain and urgency evoked by the potassium solution, but minimal if any symptoms from water instilled into the bladder. As a provocative diagnostic test for IC, the potassium test has good sensitivity (70 to 90%) but may lack specificity; so, at present, this test serves to demonstrate increased urothelial permeability that may accompany multiple painful conditions.

Treatment

The ultimate goal of therapy is to neutralize the factor or factors responsible for a disease process. In the absence of any known causative factors, the treatments for IC have been guided by prudence, and a given patient's therapy typically progresses from the least invasive treatments to the more invasive. A listing of treatments for IC is given in Table 11–5. Most of these treatments were either identified serendipitously or were "theory-driven" by a presumed mechanism of pathophysiology. For example, dietary modification to avoid foods that exacerbate symptoms (eg, acidic foods such as cranberry juice) has much anecdotal support and goes with the toxic urine mechanism. The working assumption of this therapeutic approach is that certain chemicals from foods are excreted into urine and thereby elicit pain. For the same reason, alkalinization of the urine has been used as an early therapeutic approach. As part of the diagnostic process, hydrodistention is normally performed, and this procedure often proves to be therapeutic with short-term reductions in frequency and pain in more than 50% of patients. Patients with symptomatic improvement for 6 months or more are considered candidates for repeat hydrodistention.

Open trials of tricyclic antidepressants, thought to act upon central neural mechanisms that have been sensi-

Table 11–5. Treatment Options for Interstitial Cystitis.

- Dietary modification
- Hydrodistention (with or without intravesical treatments)
  - Dimethylsulfoxide
  - Heparin
  - Corticosteroids
  - Bicarbonate
  - Clorpactin
  - Bacillus Calmette-Guérin
- Botulinum toxin injections
- Antidepressants
- Antihistamines
- Cyclosporine
- Opioids
- Nonsteroidal anti-inflammatory drugs
- Transcutaneous electrical nerve stimulation
- Pentosan polysulfate
- Epidural local anesthetics
- Neurolysis
- Surgical resection or diversion
- Behavioral therapies

tized, have produced reported success rates of 64 to 90%, and oral antihistamines that would counteract histamine released by mast cells have been reported to produce a reduction in symptoms. The oral, renally excreted heparinoid pentosan polysulfate is thought to supplement or replace missing protective glycosaminoglycans on the urothelial surface. The following medications, alone or in combination, have been proposed as possible therapies: intravesical therapy with dimethylsulfoxide, heparin, corticosteroids, bicarbonate, and oxychlorosene (a derivative of hypochlorous acid). The success rates in open trials range from 50% to greater than 90%. Based on the hypothesis that IC is a local manifestation of a systemic autoimmune disease, immunosuppressant therapies such as systemic cyclosporine and intravesical bacillus Calmette-Guérin immunotherapy have been used in open trials with nearly 100% success rates.

Neuromodulation via direct sacral (S3) nerve root stimulation has demonstrated benefit on urgency and frequency but has mixed benefits in relation to pain control. Transcutaneous electrical nerve stimulation has been used in open trials and demonstrated to produce good results or remission in 26 to 54% of patients. Behavioral therapies and self-care strategies such as timed voiding have proved valuable in some persons. Series and case reports suggest that sympathectomy produced by lumbar sympathetic or epidural local anesthetic blocks may have short-term efficacy in up to 75% of patients. Long-term treatment with opioids is an option in patients with IC, but this treatment remains controversial for all nonmalignant processes. Often considered a last resort, surgery in the form of supravesical diversions or cystectomy has also received mixed reports of efficacy.

Prognosis

Epidemiologically, IC is most prevalent in young to middle-age females implying that there may be a resolution of symptoms that occurs with time. It has been reported that up to 50% of patients in whom IC has been diagnosed have spontaneous remissions, with durations of 1 to 80 months. There have been reports of patients with continued bladder pain despite the surgical resection of the bladder.

Chancellor MB et al. Treatment of interstitial cystitis. *Urology.* 2004;63(3 Suppl 1):85. [PMID: 15013658]

URETHRAL SYNDROME

This syndrome is characterized by pain with urination that is coupled typically with urinary urgency, increased frequency, suprapubic or back pain, and an absence of laboratory evidence of infection or inflammation. Urodynamic studies may demonstrate a pulsatile (staccato) or prolonged flow phase and increased external sphincter tone. An absence of other causes of symptoms (including local anatomic causes) is required for the diagnosis. Urethral syndrome is most common in women in their reproductive years and has a high rate of spontaneous remission. Conservative therapy using muscle relaxants, electrostimulation, and behavioral techniques have also been reported to be successful.

IRRITABLE BOWEL SYNDROME (FUNCTIONAL BOWEL DISORDERS)

General Considerations

Like other functional bowel disorders (eg, noncardiac chest pain and functional dyspepsia), IBS is a diagnosis of exclusion that is based on symptoms. It is associated with abnormalities of motility and sensation in different subpopulations. IBS is a common diagnosis and is the reason for 40 to 70% of referrals to gastroenterologists. IBS frequently accompanies other disorders without identifiable histopathology, such as fibromyalgia, noncardiac chest pain, functional dyspepsia, IC, and mixed headaches. It has been associated with significant neuroses and psychoses such as anxiety and depression.

Pathogenesis

There are many diverse hypotheses related to the etiology of IBS including: pain may be psychosocial in origin, pain may be due to motility dysfunction at one or multiple sites in the gut, or pain is a neuropathic process with associated visceral hypersensitivity (the equivalents of somatic hyperalgesia and allodynia). Alternatively, hypersensitivity could be due to peripheral sensitizers such as those contained within and released by mast cells. Like many diagnoses of exclusion, it is likely that multiple pathophysiologies are present in different subgroups and that all of these hypotheses may be correct for different subgroups.

Clinical Findings

A. SYMPTOMS AND SIGNS

IBS typically presents in the third or fourth decades of life and has a female to male ratio of 2:1. There are at least three different clinical presentations of IBS, two of which have no pain or pain as a minor component: (1) watery diarrhea group and (2) alternating constipation-diarrhea group. The third subgroup has abdominal pain as the primary symptom and altered bowel movements as a secondary or exacerbating complaint. In this group, pain is typically in the left lower quadrant or in the suprapubic region and may be precipitated by food ingestion and a need to defecate. Bloating, mucus in the stools, and flatulence are often prominent; anxiety may exacerbate symptoms. Although there is great variation between patients, the particular symptom complex for a given patient generally remains constant. Generalized abdominal tenderness to palpation is common. The classic physical finding is a tender, palpable mass (the sigmoid colon) in the left lower quadrant.

B. SPECIAL TESTS

As a diagnosis of exclusion, imaging and laboratory findings should show no evidence of neoplasm, inflammatory bowel disease, infection, diverticulosis, or other intra-abdominal process. Colonoscopy and barium enema radiography should not demonstrate focal lesions. Stool samples should not have occult blood or infectious organisms present. It is generally agreed that the colons of most patients with IBS are exceptionally reactive to physiologic stimuli such as eating. Unfortunately, the finding is not pathognomonic, and so acts only as supportive evidence for the diagnosis. Although there are no absolute criteria for the diagnosis of IBS except for a report of abdominal pain and altered bowel habit in the absence of identifiable pathology, the ROME criteria have been proposed to facilitate a "positive" diagnosis (Table 11–6). Motility studies and sensation evocation with a

Table 11–6. Diagnostic Criteria for Irritable Bowel Syndrome.

- No identifiable neoplastic, infectious, or inflammatory etiology for symptoms
- Continuous or recurrent symptoms of abdominal pain lasting at least 3 months that is
  Relieved by defecation
    or
  Associated with a change in stool consistency
    or
  Associated with a change in stool frequency with two of the following:
  1. Altered stool frequency (>3/d or <3/wk)
  2. Altered stool form
  3. Altered stool passage (straining, urgency, incomplete evacuation)
  4. Passage of mucus
  5. Abdominal bloating

Table 11–7. Treatment Options for Irritable Bowel Syndrome.

- Dietary modification
  - Food avoidance (eg, caffeine, milk products, legumes)
  - Addition of fiber, bran, or bulking agents
- Behavioral therapies
- Antidepressants
- Anticholinergics, antispasmotics
- Serotonergic antagonists (eg, alosetron for diarrhea predominant irritable bowel syndrome)
- Serotonergic agonists (eg, tegaserod for constipation predominant irritable bowel syndrome)

distending balloon in the rectum or sigmoid colon may prove valuable in the identification of patients as members of different subgroups.

Treatment

IBS has exacerbations and spontaneous resolution of pains, so open trials are of limited value due to placebo rates of 40 to 70%. Procedural treatments have not been a major component of therapy because there is no structural disease to treat. Life-threatening disease may be simply ruled out without an exhaustive investigation, and the patient needs to be assured that their symptoms are believed.

Therapeutic options for IBS are listed in Table 11–7. As part of a diagnostic and therapeutic trial, patients are generally advised to engage in dietary modifications, such as avoiding milk products, avoiding excessive legume consumption (associated with gas production), increasing fiber and bran in cases of constipation, avoiding caffeine- or sorbitol-containing foods, and establishing a stable dietary pattern in hopes of establishing a stable evacuation routine. Anticholinergics and antidiarrheals have been extensively studied and used clinically, but unfortunately their benefit is anecdotal. Traditional advice has been to keep analgesic therapy to a minimum; the use of opioids is particularly discouraged because of concerns related to altered motility.

Tricyclic antidepressants have been shown in controlled studies to be effective, but whether the efficacy is due to their antidepressant, sedative, anticholinergic, or analgesic effects is unclear. Gastrokinetic agents, antidiarrheals, osmotic laxatives, opioid antagonists, chole-

cystokinin antagonists, and peppermint oil have all been proposed as effective. Injection therapies have not been generally used in the treatment of IBS. The newest pharmacotherapy is the use of drugs acting as serotonin receptors such as alosetron ($5-HT_3$-receptor antagonist used for diarrhea predominant IBS) and tegaserod ($5-HT_4$-receptor agonist used for constipation predominant IBS). Behavioral treatments such as hypnotism, cognitive therapy, and supportive psychotherapy have proved valuable, especially if pain is intermittent and a psychiatric comorbidity (such as anxiety or depression) has been identified.

Prognosis

Due to the typically stable nature of a patient's symptom complex, once significant disease has been ruled out, additional or repeat investigation is not necessary unless the symptom complex were to change.

Drossman DA. The functional gastrointestinal disorders and the ROME II process. *Gut.* 1999;45 Suppl 2:II1. [PMID: 10457038]

Spiller R. ROME II: the functional gastrointestinal disorders. Diagnosis, pathophysiology and treatment: a multinational consensus. *Gut.* 2000;46:741B. [PMID: 10764725]

ORCHIALGIA

Pain localized to the testes has a wide differential diagnosis. Possible causes include local processes, such as tumor; infection, such as epididymitis; varicocele, hydrocele, spermatocele; and testicular torsion, which are all potentially acute and chronic sources of pain. Although trauma (including iatrogenic types such as inguinal hernia repair, vasectomy) can lead to chronic inflammatory processes, most causes of altered sensation and pain are idiopathic. Neuropathic etiologies ranging from diabetic neuropathy and entrapment neuropathies to spinal disc disease may all present with testicular pain. Scrotal pain should be differentiated from testicular pain since the nerve supplies differ and may represent differing sites of disease along sacral versus thoracolumbar pathways. Due to the "personal" nature of the site of pain, concerns related to psychological etiologies or sequelae of this chronic pain are maintained.

Treatment of chronic orchialgia has traditionally started with anti-inflammatories or antibiotics. Surgical procedures including epididymectomy, orchiectomy, or denervation procedures have been recommended; however, long-term outcomes are unknown, and retrospective series have suggested limited benefit, particularly in subsets of patients with other pain disorders. There may be benefit from the use of antidepressants, anticonvulsants, membrane-stabilizing agents, opiates and, in some patients, sympatholytic treatments. Because of the wide differential diagnosis of testicular pain, no specific treatment will be universally effective.

Ness TJ. Chronic urologic pain syndromes. *Curr Pain Headache Rep* 2001;5:27. [PMID: 11252135]

PROCTALGIA FUGAX

Defined as episodic spasms of pain localized to the rectum and anus occurring at irregular intervals and without identifiable cause, proctalgia fugax is highly prevalent, occurring in 14 to 19% of healthy persons. Episodes are normally brief (seconds to minutes) and infrequent (normally fewer than 6 per year). They may be precipitated by bowel movements, sexual activity, stress, and temperature changes and may lead to avoidance behavior on the part of the patient. No cause or method of treating or preventing proctalgia fugax has been universally accepted, although spasm of the sigmoid colon, levator ani, and pelvic floor musculature have been postulated as sources of the pain. Local anorectal disease, such as fissures or abscesses, are typically ruled out as alternate sources of pain and spasm. Most reactive pharmacologic treatments have usually proved inadequate due to the brief nature of most episodes. However, clonidine, nitroglycerin, antispasmodics, and calcium channel blockers have all been reported as effective, and inhaled salbutamol was reported to shorten the duration of severe pain. Heat or pressure applied to the perineum, consumption of food or liquids, dilation of the anal sphincter, and assumption of a knee-chest position have been anecdotally reported as beneficial.

PROSTATODYNIA

This disorder is defined as pain attributed to the prostate in the absence of identifiable disease. Also termed "nonbacterial chronic prostatitis" or "male chronic pelvic pain syndrome," it has the hallmark symptoms of dysuria, urinary urgency, poor urinary flow, and perineal discomfort. Laboratory findings should not show evidence of bacteria or white blood cells in prostatic fluids. No strikingly successful treatment options have been described, and so treatments may be empiric trials of medications used in the treatment of chronic pain. Antibiotics are commonly prescribed despite the absence of evidence for a microbiologic infection. If urodynamic measures indicate abnormalities, α-adrenergic-blocking agents (eg, tamsulosin) have been suggested as therapeutic.

Headaches

12

Michel Volcy Gomez, MD & Stewart J. Tepper, MD

Headache disorders constitute a major public health problem. In the United States, the annual expense due to migraine-related loss of productivity is estimated between $5.6 billion and $17.2 billion. Migraines are responsible for approximately 36 million days of bed rest per year and an additional 21.5 million days of restricted activity. Direct costs to the medical system are also high; the total health care cost for patients with migraine averages of $145 per month, compared with $89 per month for persons who do not have migraine. Persons with migraine use 2.5 times the prescription drugs and 6 times the diagnostic services of persons without migraine. Nationally, direct costs are estimated to be as high as $9.5 billion, with $2.7 billion spent for prescription drugs and $730 million for hospital care. Headache represents the fourth most common cause of emergency department visits.

The International Headache Society (IHS) classifies headache into 13 main groups. The second International Classification of Headache Disorders (ICHD-II) recognizes two basic subgroups: primary headache syndromes and secondary headache syndromes (Tables 12–1 and 12–2). Primary headaches are those without any intracranial structural pathology. The primary headaches can be divided into three main groups: migraine, tension-type headache, and trigeminal autonomic cephalalgias. The secondary headaches are symptoms of an identifiable disorder.

MIGRAINE

ESSENTIALS OF DIAGNOSIS

- *At least five attacks, each lasting between 4 and 72 hours.*
- *Pain has at least two of the following: unilateral location, throbbing quality, moderate to severe intensity, or aggravation by routine physical activity.*
- *Associated symptoms include nausea and/or photophobia and phonophobia.*

General Considerations

A. EPIDEMIOLOGY

The prevalence of migraine is age and gender dependent. It is estimated that the 1-year migraine prevalence in Western countries is around 10 to 12%, 6% in men and 15 to 18% in women. Age at onset of migraine is earlier in boys than in girls, but prevalence quickly equalizes until menarche, when female predominance begins. Migraine is two to three times more common in women than in men, with peak prevalence occurring during midlife in both sexes. Migraine prevalence is higher in whites than in blacks or Asians. Significant associations (comorbidities) have been reported between migraine and certain psychiatric disorders (anxiety, depression), stroke in women under the age of 45 years, and epilepsy.

B. DIAGNOSTIC CRITERIA

Successful treatment begins with accurate diagnosis. Well-defined criteria for diagnosing headache published by the IHS have been available for nearly 20 years. The classification scheme has been well suited for research. However, clinically, the criteria are not always used or are misapplied. Many clinicians mistakenly define migraine by a single feature, such as unilaterality or throbbing quality or by the presence or absence of aura. Less than 20% of patients with migraine demonstrate typical aura, a reversible neurologic event lasting longer than 5 minutes but less than 1 hour and followed within 1 hour by the headache.

It has been suggested that the IHS migraine criteria lack accurate sensitivity and specificity. The most sensitive and specific symptom for diagnosis is nausea (sensitivity 82%, specificity 96%), then photophobia (sensitivity 79%, specificity 87%), phonophobia (sensitivity 69%, specificity 87%), and worsening with physical activity (sensitivity 81%, specificity 78%), with approximately 66% of migraine headaches described as unilateral (specificity 78%), and 76% as throbbing (specificity 77%). Recently, osmophobia and taste abnormalities were demonstrated to be very specific (86.7% and 90.2%, respectively) in diagnosing migraine but very insensitive (around 20%).

Table 12–1. Diagnostic Characteristics of Primary Headaches.

Characteristics	Type of headache			
	Migraine without aura	Tension-type headache	Cluster headache	Paroxysmal hemicrania[a]
Number of attacks	At least 5	At least 10 previous attacks with frequency of 12–15 days/month	At least 5	At least 20
Duration	4–72 hours	30 minutes to 7 days	15–180 minutes Frequency: 1–2 per day to 8 per day	2–30 minutes Frequency: > 5 per day ≥ 50% of the time
Description of pain	Unilateral Throbbing Moderate to severe Increases with physical activity	Bilateral Nonthrobbing Mild to moderate Does not increase with physical activity	Severe or very severe Unilateral Orbital, supraorbital, or temporal	Severe or very severe Unilateral Orbital, supraorbital, or temporal
Associated symptoms	At least 1 of following: Nausea or vomiting and/or photophobia *and* phonophobia	No more than 1 of the following: Mild photophobia, mild phono-phobia, mild nausea No nausea or vomiting	At least 1 ipsilateral: Conjunctival injection or lacrimation, nasal congestion or rhinorrhea, eyelid edema, forehead and facial sweating, miosis or ptosis, sense of restlessness	At least 1 ipsilateral: Conjunctival injection or lacrimation, nasal congestion or rhinorrhea, eyelid edema, miosis or ptosis

[a]Responds to indomethacin.

Modified from Headache Classification Subcommittee of the International Headache Society (ICHD-2). *Cephalalgia.* 2004;24(Suppl 1):9.

Table 12–2. Causes of Secondary Headaches.

- Head or neck trauma
- Cranial or cervical vascular disorder
- Nonvascular intracranial disorder
- Substance abuse or its withdrawal
- Infection
- Disorder of homeostasis or regulatory control
- Disorder of cranium, neck, eyes, ears, nose, sinuses, teeth, mouth, or other facial or cranial structures
- Psychiatric disorder
- Cranial neuralgias and central causes of facial pain

Headache experts consider that a stable pattern (>6 months) of episodic, disabling headaches with a normal physical examination is likely to be migraine. Ninety-four percent of patients with a physician diagnosis of nonmigraine primary headache or a new physician diagnosis of migraine at a primary care clinic were determined on the basis of longitudinal diary data to have migraine-type headaches. However, the diagnosis of nonmigraine headache made at a clinic visit is usually inaccurate: 82% of patients with a clinic diagnosis of nonmigraine primary headache were found to have migraine-type headaches when they kept diaries for six attacks, which were reviewed for ICHD diagnoses.

In order to avoid migraine misdiagnosis, it is important to gather information about multiple attacks. Misdiagnosis of migraine is frequently related to (1) a patient's failure to report typical features during a single encounter, (2) self-assigned diagnoses (that is, the patient reports what he or she thinks the diagnosis is), or (3) multiple headache attack types over time. Location of pain, which is not considered in the IHS criteria, often leads to misdiagnosis; most of what is diagnosed as sinus headache is actually migraine. Patients with migraine manifest a wide variety of headache attack types over time, including migraine (with or without aura) and tension-type headaches, often masking proper diagnosis.

The ICHD-II criteria still require separate diagnosis of every headache type in any patient. However, evidence exists that tension-type headache is different in patients with migraine than in those who never manifest migraine; in patients with migraine, the triptans relieve every headache type, including those that look like tension-type headaches. For persons with only episodic tension headache, the triptans are not effective.

In the revision of the ICHD published in 2004, the term "probable migraine" now replaces "migrainous disorder" to describe headache that is missing one criterion for migraine. Migraine or probable migraine occurring on at least 8 days per month in a patient with at least 15 days of headache per month for at least 3 months is chronic migraine. In the new headache classification, the diagnosis of chronic migraine should not be made when medications for acute headaches are overused. For these patients, the diagnosis of medication overuse headache is more appropriate.

Pathophysiology

Migraine may be initiated in an upper brainstem migraine generator (periaqueductal gray, dorsal raphe nucleus) that activates trigeminal efferents to the meninges where inflammation and vasodilation occur. This neurogenic sterile meningitis in turn sensitizes pain afferents, also trigeminal, which convey the nociceptive signal back to the lower brainstem (trigeminal nucleus caudalis) where it is integrated. Following the return of the pain signal centrally, there is activation of adjacent autonomic nuclei (eg, nucleus tractus solitarius) to account for nausea, and then an ascent up to thalamus and cortex. The putative migraine generator in the midbrain periaqueductal gray region has been imaged in functional imaging studies. During migraine, compared with a headache-free period, blood flow increased in the contralateral periaqueductal gray/dorsal raphe nucleus region of the brainstem, even after complete headache relief with a triptan. Iron homeostasis abnormalities have also been found in this region, with increased levels of nonheme iron in tissue from patients with episodic and chronic migraine compared with age-matched, headache-free controls. Thus, the periaqueductal gray/dorsal raphe nucleus, a major source of serotonergic input to the brainstem that also projects to the cortex and is an integral part of the endogenous pain modulatory system, may be the site of migraine generation.

There is also evidence that cortical function is different in persons with migraine. Patients with migraine have reduced habituation to different sensory modalities, they perform tasks that require low-level visual processing faster, and the threshold to produce phosphenes with transcranial magnetic stimulation is lower in those with migraine with aura.

The aura of migraine has been hypothesized to reflect a process related to cortical spreading depression. Cortical spreading depression is misnamed; it is a process in which the cortex is activated, with intense hyperemia, and the activation spreads forward at a rate of 3 to 4 mm/min. The wave of neuronal activation is associated with the aura symptoms and is followed by quiescent neurons analogous to postictal neurons. During this quiescent period, there is associated oligemia, without ischemia. Thus, aura is neuronal, not vascular.

Aura, when it occurs, is anatomically linked to the activation of the trigeminovascular system and the migraine generator. One concept that explains how an aura can occur in the absence of pain, or with a lesser headache than migraine, is that the aura reaches a variable threshold, necessary to trigger the generator and associated pain.

The phenomenon of sensitization on primary pain afferents refers to the presence of enhanced responses to stimuli. The meningeal primary afferents become hypersensitive to mechanical stimulation so that those stimuli normally producing little or no activity now evoke much larger responses. Peripheral sensitization is proposed to underlie the throbbing pain of headache. In addition, second-order neurons receiving input from sensitized primary afferents and skin also become sensitized. This alteration of central neuronal response is called central sensitization and provides a physiologic basis for scalp tenderness and other migraine symptoms (allodynia).

Cutaneous allodynia, the experience of touch as painful, is a marker of central sensitization, and can be demonstrated easily in patients with migraine. It has been found that ipsilateral allodynia develops, especially at the headache peak, in almost 75% of persons with migraine who were tested. The presence of allodynia correlates with illness duration and attack frequency. Reduced efficacy of triptan therapy occurs in the presence of cutaneous allodynia, suggesting the need for early treatment in migraine before central sensitization develops.

Treatment

A. ABORTIVE THERAPY

The objective of treating an acute migraine is to restore normal function by rapidly and consistently alleviating the patient's head pain and the associated symptoms of nausea, vomiting, and sensory phobias without side effects and without attack recurrence. Several drug options and different formulations are available to treat acute migraine. From the medical point of view, the choice of a specific medication type has depended on individual characteristics such as headache intensity, time-to-peak intensity, speed of onset of action of medication, presence of associated symptoms, degree of incapacitation, and patient response. For patients, the most desired qualities for treatment are pain freedom, speed of onset, no headache recurrence, tolerability, medication availability, cost, and overall satisfaction or well-being after taking the medication.

The nonspecific treatments for migraine attacks are aspirin, acetaminophen (and other simple analgesics), nonsteroidal anti-inflammatory drugs (NSAIDs), neuroleptics, opioids, combination analgesics, and short-acting barbiturates. Triptans and ergots are considered the specific migraine treatments. Monotherapy using serotonin (5-HT) subreceptor agonists (5-HT$_{1B}$/5-HT$_{1D}$), especially when administered orally, does not always result in rapid, consistent, and complete relief of all migraine attacks as desired by patients. In addition, the efficacy of some nonspecific migraine agents, such as various NSAIDs, has been shown in many trials and cannot be called into question (Table 12–3).

The paradigm for treating an acute migraine is to start therapy early in its onset. This may prevent the pain from becoming moderate or severe. Migraine progresses on a time and intensity continuum, and more than 70% of untreated, mild migraines eventually become moderate or severe in patients with histories of recurrent disabling migraine. As pain builds, there is increased central trigeminal neuronal sensitivity. In addition, gastroparesis, which is associated with migraine, is thought to impair absorption of oral medication. Thus, the earlier mild migraine pain is treated with an oral triptan, before gastroparesis is established, the more complete the absorption and the greater the probability of response will be.

The occurrence of adverse events associated with triptans in general, and central nervous system side effects in particular, may lead to a delay in initiating or even avoiding an otherwise effective treatment. These side effects are lessened by early administration of the triptans, another reason for early treatment. Finally, there is evidence linking a pain-free response (that is, zero pain, as opposed to just pain relief) with a reduced recurrence of headache and therefore a reduced number of treatments in a given attack. Early treatment is linked to higher pain-free response as well.

1. Triptans—Drugs in this class are the treatment of choice for acute disabling migraine, in the absence of vascular disease. The decision about which triptan to prescribe is often based on the relative need for speed, the formulation needed, and the formulary availability for a given patient. If oral treatment is to be used, it is clear that while seemingly a homogenous group of drugs, there are significant differences in speed of onset, efficacy, recurrence rates, and tolerability among oral triptans.

Triptans relieve migraine symptoms via three possible mechanisms of action: (1) selective intracranial/extracerebral meningeal vasoconstriction; (2) presynaptic inhibition of vasoactive inflammatory neuropeptides release in the meninges; (3) inhibition of the return of pain signals to the trigeminal-cervical complex neurons in the brainstem and upper cervical column. Triptans stimulate 5-HT$_{1B}$ receptors, located predominantly on cranial blood vessels, causing vasoconstriction counteracting neurogenic vasodilation. Triptans also stimulate 5-HT$_{1D}$ receptors located on peripheral and central trigeminal nociceptive nerve terminals, inhibiting nociceptive transmission from pain-sensitive meningeal structures.

In addition, triptans block vasoactive and proinflammatory neuropeptide release through peripheral meningeal 5-HT$_{1D}$-receptor stimulation and may also interact with 5-HT$_{1B\ 1D\ 1F}$ receptors on central neurons, although this remains to be defined.

Headache recurrence can occur with any type of urgent antimigraine treatment and is defined as the return of a headache after successful treatment, generally within 24 hours. When recurrence occurs, the recurrence time for the triptans is generally around 12 hours. The incidence of headache recurrence varies among drugs in the triptan class. Migraine recurrence does not appear to be related to initial clinical efficacy but is influenced by the pharmacologic and pharmacokinetic properties of the individual triptans (Table 12–4). The triptans with longer half-life and greater 5-HT$_{1B}$-receptor potency may have the lowest rates of headache recurrence, although this remains relatively unproven and controversial. One explanation for recurrence might be that the migraine generator is still active in spite of apparent symptomatic relief.

The most common central nervous system treatment-related side effects with triptans are fatigue and somnolence, dizziness, and asthenia. These side effects are rare and may be related to dosage. Eletriptan, rizatriptan, and zolmitriptan have active metabolites, while lipophilicity is lowest for almotriptan and sumatriptan; however, it is not clear that these differences have played out in clear clinical differences in large populations. While population differences are small when triptans are compared, individual preferences for particular triptans can be large.

Triptans are not widely used in clinical practice despite their well-established efficacy. Although the relatively restricted use of triptans may be attributed to several factors, the most important concern has been cardiovascular safety. Triptans all bind to 5-HT$_{1B}$ receptors, causing vasoconstriction, and most people have some 5-HT$_{1B}$ receptors on coronary arteries, although far fewer than on

Table 12–3. Abortive Medications for Migraine.[a]

Drug	Evidence level	Clinical effects	Side effects
NSAIDs, Combination Analgesics, and Nonopiate Analgesics			
Acetaminophen	B	+	Infrequent
Ketorolac IM	B	++	Infrequent
Aspirin	A	++	Occasional
Diclofenac	B	++	Occasional
Flurbiprofen	B	++	Occasional
Ketoprofen	B	+	Occasional
Ibuprofen	A	++	Occasional
Naproxen sodium	A	++	Occasional
Piroxicam	B	+	Occasional
NSAID + caffeine	A	++	Infrequent
Aspirin + acetaminophen + caffeine	A	++	Infrequent
Ergots			
Dihydroergotamine (IV, IM, SC)	B	+++	Frequent
Dihydroergotamine (nasal)	A	+++	Occasional
Ergotamine	B	++	Frequent
Ergotamine + caffeine	B	++	Frequent
Antiemetics			
Metoclopramide	B	+	Occasional
Prochlorperazine	B	++	Occasional
Corticosteroids			
Dexamethasone	C	++	Infrequent
Hydrocortisone	C	++	Infrequent
Opiate Analgesics			
Meperidine	B	++	Frequent
Acetaminophen + codeine	A	++	Occasional
Barbiturate Hypnotics			
Butalbital + aspirin + caffeine	C	+++	Occasional
Butalbital + aspirin + caffeine + codeine	B	+++	Occasional
Miscellaneous			
Isometheptene	B	++	Infrequent
Lidocaine IN	B	+	Infrequent

[a]Table includes nontriptans only.
NSAID, nonsteroidal anti-inflammatory drugs.

Matchar et al. http://www.aan.com; 2000.

Table 12–4. Pharmacologic Characteristics of Triptans.

| Drug | T_{max} (h) | Half-life (h) | Excretion pathway | Characteristics | | | Therapeutic gain at 2 hours (%)[a,b] | Recurrence (%) |
				CNS side effects (%)	Chest side effects (%)			
Sumatriptan	2.0–3.0	2	MAO	1.7–6.3	4–5		6 mg SC 51 20 mg NS 28–55 100 mg 20–40	6 mg SC 34–38 20 mg NS 32–34 100 mg 30
Zolmitriptan	1.5–2.0	3	CYP450/MAO	9.9–11.5	1–6		2.5 mg PO 34 5 mg PO 37 5.0 NS 40	2.5 mg PO 22–37 5.0 mg PO 32 5.0 mg NS 26
Rizatriptan	1.0–1.5	2	MAO	6.1–9.4	1.5–3		10 mg PO 27–40 10 mg ODT 19–46	10 mg PO 30–47
Eletriptan	1.0–1.5	4	CYP3A4	2.6–14.6	4–7		40 mg PO 22–41 80 mg PO 30–53	40 mg PO 19–23
Almotriptan	1.5–2.0	3	CYP450/MAO	1.5	1		12.5 mg PO 26–32	12.5 mg Or 18–29
Naratriptan	2.0–3.0	6	Renal/CYP450	1.9	2–4		2.5.mg PO 22	17–28
Frovatriptan	2.0–3.0	26	Renal	6.0	2–3		2.5 mg PO 16–19	7–25

[a]Represent the mean value.
[b]Defined as the difference in headache response at 2-hours postadministration between placebo and drug-treated patients.
t_{max}, time to peak plasma concentration; CNS, central nervous system; MAO, monoamine oxidase A; SC, subcutaneous; NS, nasal spray; PO, oral; ODT, orally disintegrating tablet; ND, no data.

Rapoport et al. *CNS Drugs.* 2003;17:431.

meningeal arteries. The average incidence of coronary vasoconstriction due to triptans is 10 to 20%, generally not clinically significant in the absence of atherosclerotic coronary artery disease. Triptans cannot be easily differentiated with respect to their effects on human isolated coronary arteries; clinical doses all drugs in this class contract arteries to about the same extent, and the US Food and Drug Administration has placed identical template warnings in the prescribing information for all seven triptans contraindicating their use in patients with vascular disease.

It has been suggested that while caution is advisable for patients with two or more cardiac risk factors (ie, hypertension, diabetes, obesity, age over 40 years in men, postmenopausal women, premature family history of vascular disease, or smoking), triptans can be prescribed without concern among low-risk patients, probably the majority of patients with migraine. Triptans should not be withheld from patients who have either no risk factors or only one risk factor.

The incidence of triptan-associated serious cardiovascular adverse events in both clinical trials and clinical practice appears to be extremely low. Patients with a family history of early atherosclerosis or patients with multiple risk factors are more likely to have endothelial changes predisposing to vasospasm, and initial treatment should be monitored. Obviously, triptan therapy should be withheld from patients with symptomatic or known obstructive coronary disease, and patients at intermediate or high risk should be evaluated prior to treatment. A functional evaluation to exclude coronary disease would suffice in most cases, with further diagnostic investigations only in those patients with positive findings.

Chest symptoms are a rare adverse effect (1 to 4%) unrelated to coronary vasoconstriction in most patients. Although the etiology of chest symptoms remains to be fully elucidated, they could be related to pulmonary vasoconstriction, esophageal abnormalities (increased amplitude and duration of esophageal contractions, abnormal esophageal motility), triptan-associated reductions in the oxygen stores of skeletal muscles, or heightened sensory sensitivity. Overall, the incidence of these symptoms also appears to be dose-related.

Triptans can be divided into fast onset and slow onset (Table 12–5). The fast onset triptans are sumatriptan, zolmitriptan, rizatriptan, almotriptan, and eletriptan. The slow onset triptans are naratriptan and frovatriptan. The slow onset oral triptans take twice as long to work as the fast onset triptans, showing responses at 4 hours comparable to what the fast onset triptans show at 2 hours. Accordingly, the slow onset triptans work on fewer patients, but in general are associated with greater tolerability.

Triptans can be divided by formulation as well. Sumatriptan is available as a subcutaneous injection, nasal

Table 12–5. Formulations of Fast- and Slow-acting Triptans.

Drug	Formulation
Fast-acting	
Sumatriptan	Rapid releasing tablet 25 mg, 50 mg, 100 mg Subcutaneous injection 6 mg Nasal spray 20 mg
Zolmitriptan	Conventional and ODT 2.5 mg, 5 mg Nasal spray 5 mg
Rizatriptan	Conventional tablet and ODT 5 mg, 10 mg
Almotriptan	Conventional tablet 12.5 mg
Eletriptan	Conventional tablet 40 mg, 80 mg
Slow-acting	
Naratriptan	Conventional tablet 1 mg, 2.5 mg
Frovatriptan	Conventional tablet 2.5 mg

ODT, orally dissolvable tablet.

spray, and rapid release tablet. Zolmitriptan is available as a conventional tablet, orally dissolvable tablet, and nasal spray. Rizatriptan is available as a conventional and orally dissolvable tablet. The other 4 triptans are available only as conventional tablets.

Metabolic degradation pathways can also distinguish triptans, which can predict potential drug-drug interactions (see Table 12–4). Triptans with predominantly monoamine oxidase (MAO) degradation pathways (sumatriptan, rizatriptan, almotriptan, and zolmitriptan) should not be used in patients taking MAO inhibitors. Eletriptan, with predominant cytochrome P450 3A4 degradation, should not be used with potent inhibitors of that system (eg, erythromycin, clarithromycin, fluconazole, ketoconazole, verapamil, ritonavir and other similar AIDS drugs).

There is an interaction between propranolol and rizatriptan in which the propranolol raises the rizatriptan serum level. Thus, only the 5-mg dose of rizatriptan should be used with propranolol. The same interaction does not occur between rizatriptan and other β-blockers, or between other triptans and propranolol.

2. Ergotamine and dihydroergotamine—These medications have a high affinity for $5\text{-}HT_{1A}$, $5\text{-}HT_{1B}$, $5\text{-}HT_{1D}$, and $5\text{-}HT_{1F}$, $5\text{-}HT_{2A}$, $5\text{-}HT_{2C}$, and $5\text{-}HT_4$ receptor subtypes, and low affinity for the $5\text{-}HT_{1E}$ receptor. In addition, they bind to receptors in the adrenergic and dopaminergic systems. It is likely that the beneficial effects of ergotamine and dihydroergotamine arise from their agonist properties at $5\text{-}HT_{1B}$, $5\text{-}HT_{1D}$, and perhaps $5\text{-}HT_{1F}$ receptors that, as with the triptans, lead to meningeal vasoconstriction and trigeminal inhibition.

The unwanted side effects of ergotamine and dihydroergotamine probably arise from actions at central $5\text{-}HT_{1A}$ receptors (nausea and dysphoria) and dopamine D_2 receptors (nausea and vomiting). Both dihydroergotamine and ergotamine can cause vasoconstriction and venoconstriction by stimulating α-adrenergic and $5\text{-}HT_{2A}$ receptors. These peripheral vascular effects are more pronounced with ergotamine than with the triptans, since the triptans do not have activity at adrenergic and $5\text{-}HT_{2A}$ receptors. Ergotamine and dihydroergotamine can also constrict coronary blood vessels through actions at coronary artery smooth muscle $5\text{-}HT_{1B}$ and $5\text{-}HT_{2A}$ receptors. The contractile response in coronary arteries is more prolonged with ergots than with triptans.

Ergotamine (orally/rectally, and caffeine combination) may be considered in the treatment of selected patients with moderate to severe migraine. Nausea and vomiting are the most commonly observed short-term adverse effects associated with ergot use. The combination of ergotamine plus metoclopramide reduces the incidence of nausea and vomiting compared with ergotamine alone. Patients with very long attacks or with frequent headache recurrence may be especially suited for treatment with ergotamine because headache recurrence is probably less likely with ergotamine.

Dihydroergotamine SC/IV/IM and nasal spray may be given to patients with nausea and vomiting and can be a reasonable initial treatment choice when the headache is moderate to severe, or in migraine of any severity when nonspecific medication has failed. Parenteral antinauseants are often used with it as adjunctive symptomatic treatments. Clinical opinion suggests that subcutaneous dihydroergotamine is relatively safe and effective when compared with other migraine therapies, and subcutaneous dihydroergotamine has fewer adverse events than when delivered intravenously. Dihydroergotamine can also be used parenterally for menstrual migraine prophylaxis and can be used for cluster headache prevention. Several of the metabolites of ergotamine and dihydroergotamine have biologic activity similar to the parent drugs and are often present in concentrations several times higher. Also, ergotamine and dihydroergotamine are strongly sequestered in tissues, which could contribute to the persistence of their biologic effects.

3. Nonspecific versus specific treatments—The decision about whether to use a nonspecific treatment or a selective $5\text{-}HT_{1B\ 1D}$ agonist, the specific therapies for acute migraine, despite clinical practice experience supporting the better effectiveness of the triptans, remains controversial. Clinical trials do not always reflect the favorable clinical experience with triptans, and direct comparisons made between triptans and some nonspecific treatments (such as NSAIDs) do not always favor triptans. Nevertheless, headache-experienced physicians have found that, in general, triptans provide vastly superior efficacy in comparison to nonspecific agents. Combining specific and nonspecific therapies, in at least a subset of patients, provides additional benefit, including greater efficacy and reduced recurrence when NSAIDs are taken with triptans.

Daily scheduled opioids have been used in some instances to treat intractable headache. However, a long-term study of their effectiveness found a lack of benefit in over 75% of patients with chronic headache who received opioids. Seventy-four percent of those treated either did not show significant improvement or were discontinued from the program for clinical reasons. The relatively low percentage of patients with demonstrated efficacy and unexpectedly high prevalence of misuse (50%) due to dose violations, lost prescriptions, and multisourcing discourage use of opioids in chronic headache patients.

B. PREVENTIVE THERAPY

The purpose of migraine prevention is to reduce the frequency of attacks, modify their severity and impact, and improve the efficacy of abortive therapy. The ultimate goal of migraine prophylaxis is to improve sufferers' quality of life and ameliorate their migraine-related disability. Consequently, migraine preventive strategies should be efficacious, safe, and well tolerated.

Daily migraine preventive therapy is indicated when the following circumstances are present:

1. Migraine recurs despite migraine-specific immediate treatment.

2. Therapy for acute headaches has failed, is contraindicated, or patient experienced significant side effects.

3. Patient preference.

4. Overuse of medications for acute headaches.

5. Special circumstances such as hemiplegic or basilar-type migraine or attacks with a risk of permanent neurologic injury.

Also, daily drug therapy is often recommended in the setting of very frequent headaches or a pattern of increasing attacks over time, with the risk of developing transformation into daily headache with medication overuse.

An effective preventive treatment plan can be achieved by establishing a correct diagnosis; assessing the overall impact of the attacks; creating the plan with the patient in a therapeutic alliance; emphasizing drug dosage, therapeutic effects, and side effects; and describing expectations explicitly. As much as possible, patients should be empowered with their own care.

The preventive medications for migraine can be divided into five major categories:

1. Drugs with high efficacy and mild to moderate adverse events.

2. Drugs that have lower documented efficacy and mild to moderate adverse events.

3. Drugs used based on opinion with either mild to moderate adverse events or major adverse events or complex management.

4. Drugs that have documented high efficacy but significant adverse events or are difficult to use.

5. Drugs that have been found to have limited or no efficacy (Table 12–6).

It is preferable, when possible, to select a particular prophylactic drug based on evidence-based principles, with a balance between therapeutic effects and side effect potential (therapies may lose their effectiveness when poorly tolerated because patients may become noncompliant), and guided by comorbid conditions when present. By carefully selecting preventive medication, potential drug-drug interactions will be minimized and the rate and extent of side effects will be decreased.

1. β-Adrenergic blockers—β-Blockers, the most widely used prophylactic class of drugs in migraine prevention, are up to 60 to 80% effective in producing at least a 50% reduction in attack frequency. Propranolol, the most frequently used β-blocker, has multiple actions contributing to its effectiveness. First, it inhibits norepinephrine release through a β_1-mediated agonist action, reducing central catecholaminergic hyperactivity. Second, propranolol antagonizes 5-HT_{1A} and 5-HT_{2B} receptors, reducing neuronal excitability. Third, propranolol inhibits nitric oxide production by blocking inducible nitric oxide synthase, through β_2-agonist action. Nitric oxide is believed to be the common final pathway for vasodilation in migraine. Fourth, propranolol inhibits excitatory glutamate receptors, decreasing neuronal activity. Finally, propranolol has membrane-stabilizing properties. β-blockers with intrinsic sympathomimetic activity (acebutolol, alprenolol, oxprenolol, pindolol) have not been found to be effective for migraine prevention.

The usual dose of propranolol is 160 mg/d. There are randomized controlled studies establishing the effectiveness for timolol (dose range 20 to 40 mg/d), metoprolol (50 to 100 mg/d), and nadolol (40 to 80 mg/d). Both propranolol and timolol are approved by the US Food and Drug Administration in the prevention of migraine.

The relative efficacy of the different β-blockers has not been clearly established, and most studies show no significant difference between drugs. One trial comparing propranolol to amitriptyline suggested that propranolol is more effective in migraine alone, and amitriptyline is superior for patients with both migraine and tension-type headache.

All β-blockers can produce central nervous system side effects, such as fatigue, sleep disorders, and depression. Another common side effect is decreased exercise tolerance. Less common are orthostatic hypotension, significant bradycardia, and impotence. Congestive heart failure, asthma, and insulin-dependent diabetes are contraindications to the use of nonselective β-blockers.

2. Antidepressants—Amitriptyline, a tricyclic antidepressant (TCA), is a mixed serotonin-norepinephrine reuptake inhibitor (SNRI). In addition, amitriptyline is a sodium channel blocker. Others SNRI antidepressants (eg, imipramine, venlafaxine, duloxetine) may have a potential role in migraine prevention, although they have not been extensively studied. Side effects are common with TCA use. The anticholinergic antimuscarinic adverse effects are most common; however, overdose adverse effects are related to antihistaminic and α-adrenergic overactivity and cardiac toxicity, and orthostatic hypotension can occur. Anticholinergic side effects include dry mouth, constipation, dizziness, mental confusion, tachycardia, blurred vision, and urinary retention. Antihistaminic activity may be responsible for weight gain. Any antidepressant treatment may change depression to hypomania or frank mania in patients with bipolar disorder. Older patients are more vulnerable to anticholinergic side effects.

The dose range for amitriptyline in migraine prevention is 25 to 100 mg. Consensus also suggests effectiveness for nortriptyline in the same dose range.

Evidence for the use of selective serotonin reuptake inhibitors (SSRIs) is poor. They may be helpful in patients with comorbid depression because of their better tolerability profile, but their efficacy in reducing the frequency of episodic migraines is not established. The most common side effects for SSRIs include insomnia, sweating, and sexual dysfunction. The combination of an SSRI and a TCA can be beneficial in treating refractory depression but may require downward dose adjustment of the TCA because levels may significantly increase.

MAO inhibitors are believed to be effective in migraine prevention by expert consensus opinion, but there are no randomized controlled trials. The difficulties in using MAO inhibitors are the requirement for a special exclusion diet and the need for medication restrictions to avoid tyramine-containing products or adrenergic drugs, both of which can precipitate a so-called "cheese effect" or hypertensive crisis. For this reason, MAO inhibitor use in migraine prevention is infrequent. The most common side effects of MAO inhibitors include insomnia, orthostatic hypotension, constipation, increased perspiration, weight gain, peripheral edema. Less common side effects

Table 12–6. Preventive Medications for Migraines.

Drug	Evidence level[a]	Scientific effect	Clinical effect	Therapeutic group	Efficacy (%)
Antiepileptic Drugs					
Divalproex Sodium	A	+++	+++	1	50–75
Gabapentin	B	++	++	2	46–60
Topiramate	A	+++	+++	1	40–70
Zonisamide	C	+	+	3a	40–60
Levetiracetam	C	?	?	3a	36–52
Antidepressants					
Amitriptyline	A	+++	+++	1	50–75
Nortriptyline	C	?	+++	3a	50–75
Fluoxetine	B	+	+	2	50–69
SSRIs	C	?	+	3a	50
Phenelzine	C	?	+++	3b	
β-blockers					
Metoprolol	B	++	+++	2	60–80
Propranolol	A	++	+++	1	60–80
Timolol	A	+++	++	1	
Calcium Channel Blockers					
Verapamil	B	+	++	2	50
Nimodipine	B	+	+	2	
Flunarizine	B	+++	?	4	53–82
Other Antihypertensives					
Lisinopril	C	?	?	3a	30
Candesartan	C	?	?	3a	46
5-HT$_2$ Antagonists					
Cyproheptadine	C	?	+	3a	50
Methysergide	A	+++	+++	4	50
Pizotifen	A	+++	?	4	43
Miscellaneous					
Magnesium	B	++	+	2	60
Vitamin B$_2$	B	++	++	2	59
Feverfew	B	++	+	2	37
Botulinum toxin A	C	+	+	3a	45–80

[a]The levels of evidence per the US Headache Consortium and the Evidence Based Medicine standards follow:
Level A: Established as effective, ineffective, or harmful for the given condition in the specified population.
Level B: Probably effective, ineffective, or harmful for the given condition in the specified population.
Level C: Possibly effective, ineffective, or harmful for the given condition in the specified population.
SSRIs, selective serotonin reuptake inhibitors.
Ramadan et al. http://www.neurology.org; 2000.

include inhibition of ejaculation, anorgasmia, or reduced libido. The dose range for phenelzine is 45 to 60 mg/d.

3. Calcium channel blockers—The mechanism of action of these drugs in migraine prevention is uncertain. Probably, they block 5-HT release, interfere with neurovascular inflammation, or interfere with the initiation and propagation of the cortical spreading depression of aura. Certain forms of aura are associated with inherited calcium channelopathies (eg, familial hemiplegic migraine). These rare forms of migraine respond well to calcium channel antagonist prophylaxis. The evidence for their effectiveness in conventional migraine is not robust. Side effects of the calcium channel antagonists depend on the drug and include dizziness and headache (particularly with nifedipine), depression, vasomotor changes, tremor, gastrointestinal complaints (including constipation), peripheral edema, orthostatic hypotension, and bradycardia with other types. The dose range for verapamil in migraine prevention is 240 to 480 mg/d and for amlodipine, it is 5 to 10 mg/d.

4. Anticonvulsants or neuromodulators—Anticonvulsants or antiepilepsy drugs (AEDs) suppress neuronal activity through different mechanisms. Several neuromodulators possess antimigraine and antipain properties, including valproate, topiramate, gabapentin, levetiracetam, and zonisamide.

a. Valproate—Valproate was the first AED approved by the US Food and Drug Administration for migraine prevention. It may raise inhibitory tone in the hyperexcitable migraine brain via GABA. The usual effective dose of divalproex sodium is 500 to 1000 mg/d of the extended release formulation.

The most frequently reported adverse events are nausea (42%), infection (39%), alopecia (31%), tremor (28%), asthenia (25%), dyspepsia (25%), somnolence (25%) as well as occasional weight loss or gain. Valproate has little effect on cognitive functions and rarely causes sedation. On rare occasions, valproate administration is associated with severe adverse reactions, such as hepatitis or pancreatitis, hyperandrogenism, ovarian cysts, and thrombocytopenia. Valproate is severely teratogenic and should not be used as a first line preventive medication in women of child-bearing age.

b. Topiramate—Topiramate is a neuromodulator agent that was approved by the US Food and Drug Administration for migraine prophylaxis in 2004. Topiramate has a variety of actions that may prevent migraine, including increasing inhibitory GABA activity, blocking calcium channels, and inhibiting carbonic anhydrase.

Topiramate is well tolerated when started at a low dose, usually 15 or 25 mg, and increased weekly up to 100 mg, which is the recommended dose. Topiramate is associated with weight loss (3.3 to 4.1%). It causes transient distal paresthesias in the extremities. Less common side effects are cognitive dysfunction, acute angle-closure glaucoma, both of which are reversible with therapy discontinuation, and kidney stones (1.5%). Very rarely, oligohydrosis and hyperthermia have been described, especially in adolescents.

c. Gabapentinoids—Gabapentin and pregabalin modulate glutamate and GABA function, as well as regulating intracellular calcium influx (see Chapter 3). Gabapentin has been studied in one large randomized controlled study and was effective in reducing migraine frequency with an average effective dose of 2400 mg/d.

The most common adverse events reported in association with gabapentin are dizziness and drowsiness.

d. Levetiracetam—Levetiracetam is a new anticonvulsant with an unknown mechanism of action. It has not proved effective in two small proof of concept trials for episodic migraine prevention, but it shows promise in treatment of chronic daily headache.

Minimally effective doses appear to be 1500 mg and most patients need 2000 to 2500 mg daily, with few adverse events. The most frequent side effects reported (in at least 3% of the patients) have been fatigue or tiredness, somnolence, and dizziness. Rarely, behavioral disturbance develops in patients.

e. Zonisamide—Zonisamide is a sulfonamide derivative, chemically and structurally unrelated to other AEDs. Anecdotally, it has been reported helpful in episodic migraine prevention, but no randomized controlled studies have been completed. Zonisamide has similar mechanism and dosing to topiramate and is sometimes used in patients who responded to but could not tolerate therapy with topiramate. The reported side effects of zonisamide have been paresthesias, fatigue, anxiety, and weight loss. Agitated dysphoria and difficulty concentrating have also been observed.

AEDs have proven effective in migraine prophylaxis. However, in patients responsive to other medications for acute migraine, the AEDs are most cost-effective for those with a high migraine frequency and those with comorbid diseases.

5. Magnesium—This divalent cation is an essential cofactor in more than 350 enzymes. Magnesium may have a role in migraine prevention because low magnesium in the brain appears to destabilize neuronal membranes, resulting in calcium influx and aura initiation. At least 400 to 600 mg of chelated magnesium is necessary for up to 3 months of supplementation in migraine prevention and may be most appropriate for patients with migraine with aura.

6. Riboflavin and Coenzyme Q_{10}—An additional proposed mechanism for migraine brain hyperactivity is a defect in energy generation in the mitochondria. Vitamin

B_2 or riboflavin is required for the electron transport chain. Coenzyme Q_{10}, like riboflavin, participates in the electron transport chain in the mitochondria, although it is not a cofactor but rather transfers electrons. Both have been tested in very small randomized controlled trials and have shown efficacy. The dose of riboflavin may be as low as 25 mg/d, and the dose of coenzyme Q_{10} is 300 mg/d.

7. Feverfew—The evidence for the antimigraine efficacy of feverfew, a dried leaf preparation of the weed Tanacetum pathenium, is not fully established. Feverfew's side effects include mouth ulceration and a more widespread oral inflammation associated with loss of taste. Feverfew's mechanism of action is uncertain.

8. Lisinopril—Lisinopril is an angiotensin-converting enzyme (ACE) inhibitor frequently used to treat hypertension and heart failure. It does not have an indication for the prevention of migraine, although it possesses various pharmacologic effects that may be relevant in the pathophysiology of migraine and was found effective in one small randomized controlled trial. It blocks the conversion of angiotensin I to angiotensin II, and blocks degradation of bradykinin, enkephalin, and substance P. Lisinopril has a clear potential for migraine prophylaxis because patients with migraine more commonly have the ACE DD gene, which codes for a higher ACE activity. The main side effects are cough, hypotension, and fatigue. A dose of 10 mg/d was tested in migraine patients.

9. Candesartan—Angiotensin II type 1 receptors (AT1) are presynaptic inhibitors of GABA release. Candesartan, an angiotensin II-receptor blocker, was also tested in one small randomized controlled trial for migraine prevention at a dose of 16 mg and was effective. Side effects were minimal, except for decreased blood pressure.

10. Serotonin antagonists—The anti-serotonin migraine-preventive drugs are potent $5\text{-}HT_{2B}$- and $5\text{-}HT_{2C}$-receptor antagonists, and these serotonin receptors are believed excitatory to migraine. Methysergide (no longer available in the United States), methylergonovine, cyproheptadine, and pizotifen (not available in the United States) are effective migraine prophylactic drugs and are $5\text{-}HT_{2B}$- and $5\text{-}HT_{2C}$-receptor antagonists. Methysergide breaks down to methylergonovine, and both have side effects including nausea, vomiting, abdominal pain, and diarrhea. Also frequently reported are leg symptoms (restlessness or pain), dizziness, and drowsiness. The major (albeit rare) complication of methysergide, which may also occur with methylergonovine, is the development of retroperitoneal, pulmonary, or endocardial fibrosis (1/1500 to 1/5000). Because methysergide and methylergonovine are ergots and can narrow vessels, they are contraindicated for use with triptans. The dose of methylergonovine in migraine prevention is 0.2 mg three times daily.

Cyproheptadine is an old-fashioned antihistamine which is also a $5\text{-}HT_2$ antagonist. Its effectiveness in migraine is established by consensus only. Common side effects are sedation, weight gain, and dry mouth. The dose of cyproheptadine that works in migraine prevention is 4 to 8 mg each night at bedtime, and it is usually used as adjunctive treatment rather than as primary treatment.

Pizotifen is a similar medication to cyproheptadine, licensed for migraine preventive use in the United Kingdom. It can also cause substantial weight gain and drowsiness.

11. Botulinum toxin—Botulinum neurotoxin type-A (BTX-A) has been approved in the United States for blepharospasm and for forehead wrinkles. BTX-A inhibits the release of the neurotransmitter acetylcholine at the neuromuscular junction, inhibiting striatal muscle contractions. However, BTX-A can also reduce pain in various pain syndromes independent of its muscle paralyzing effects, probably related to decreasing calcitonin gene-related peptide release and reducing the inflammatory and vasodilating components of migraine.

A typical treatment protocol is to inject 100 units of BTX-A symmetrically into glabellar, frontalis, temporalis, trapezius, and other neck muscles. The side effects are transient and can include frontal weakness, ptosis, and local pain. Injections can be repeated every 3 to 6 months if patients have a beneficial effect, which wears off 3 to 6 months after treatment. The efficacy of BTX-A in migraine prevention is not fully established, and large international randomized controlled trials are underway.

12. Tizanidine—Tizanidine is a centrally acting, presynaptic α_2-adrenergic agonist. Its mechanism of action is thought to be through a decrease of norepinephrine release from the upper dorsal brainstem. Thus, its effect in headache prevention may be due to its reducing central excitability. One randomized controlled study of tizanidine found efficacy in preventing chronic daily headache. The most frequent side effects described are somnolence, asthenia, dizziness, and dry mouth in less than 10% of the patients. It is so sedating that tiny doses of 2 to 4 mg are necessary initially, with a gradual ascent (range, 2 to 24 mg). Since therapy with tizanidine may rarely result in liver toxicity, patients should have blood levels monitored.

13. Petasites—Petasites is an extract from the plant Petasites hybridus (butterbur), which grows throughout Europe and parts of Asia. This compound has been marketed in Germany for migraine and seems to act through calcium channel regulation and inhibition of inflammation. Although the butterbur root is toxic, the Petadolex extraction has been followed by German regulatory authorities and appears safe. Two randomized controlled studies suggest efficacy in episodic migraine prevention, with the larger study finding an optimal dose of 150 mg/d.

C. TREATMENT FAILURE

Treatment failures can be grouped into the following five categories:

1. Incomplete or incorrect diagnosis.
2. Inadequate detection of important exacerbating factors (examples of this would include underlying secondary diseases, or medication overuse).
3. Inadequate pharmacotherapy.
4. Inadequate nonpharmacologic treatment.
5. Existence of other factors, including unrealistic expectations and comorbidity.

Migraine is optimally managed with migraine-specific abortive medications if there is significant disability. If frequency of migraine is high, preventive agents should be introduced, selecting the medication based on the patient's medical and psychiatric comorbidity.

Headache Classification Subcommittee of the International Headache Society. The International Classification of Headache Disorders: 2nd ed. *Cephalalgia.* 2004;24(suppl 1):9. [PMID: 14979299]

Lipton RB et al. Prevalence and burden of migraine in the United States: data from the American Migraine Study II. *Headache.* 2001;41:646. [PMID: 11554952]

Lipton RB et al. Why headache treatment fails. *Neurology.* 2003;60:1064. [PMID: 12682307]

Matchar DB et al; US Headache Consortium. Evidence-Based Guidelines for Migraine Headache in the Primary Care Setting: Pharmacological Management of Acute Attacks. American Academy of Neurology; 2000. Available at: http://www.aan.com/professionals/practice/pdfs/gl0087.pdf Last accessed: September 19, 2005.

Rapoport AM et al. The triptan formulations: how to match patients and products. *CNS Drugs.* 2003;17:431. [PMID: 12697002]

Silberstein SD et al. Migraine: preventive treatment. *Cephalalgia.* 2002;22:491. [PMID: 12230591]

Silberstein SD et al. Multispecialty consensus on diagnosis and treatment of headache. *Neurology.* 2000;54:1553. [PMID: 10762491]

TENSION-TYPE HEADACHE

 ## ESSENTIALS OF DIAGNOSIS

- *The headache is often bilateral and has either mild or no nausea, and no more than one of mild nausea, photophobia, or phonophobia.*
- *Pain is characterized as pressing or tightening, mild to moderate, and it occurs in short episodes of variable duration (episodic) or is continuous (chronic).*

Episodic

- *At least 10 previous episodes presenting between 12 and 15 days per month, lasting from 30 minutes to 7 days.*
- *Pain is described as bilateral, nonthrobbing, mild to moderate, and it does not increase with physical activity.*
- *Associated symptoms include: no nausea, and no more than one of photophobia or phonophobia.*

Chronic

- *Typical tension-type headaches on at least 15 days per month for at least 3 months or at least 180 days per year.*
- *Associated symptoms must include no more than one of the following: mild nausea photophobia or phonophobia. Neither moderate to severe nausea nor vomiting are allowed for the diagnosis.*

General Considerations

Tension-type headache is best defined as "not migraine." It is not unilateral, not severe, not throbbing, not worsened by routine physical activity, and not associated with nausea. Patients with tension-type headache do not usually complain about it in the office.

Because of the lack of positive specific symptoms, investigations to exclude other organic diseases are performed more frequently in tension-type headache than in other headaches. A careful history to uncover coexisting depression, anxiety, and other disorders is also extremely important.

In a clinical 10-year follow-up study of episodic tension-type headache, 75% of patients continued to have episodic headaches, but the chronic form developed in 25%. In those persons with initial chronic tension-type headache, 31% remained chronic, medication overuse headache developed in 21%, and the remaining 48% had reversed to the episodic form with or without prophylactic treatment. Depression, anxiety, and medication overuse were predictors for a poor outcome.

It is important to detail the relation of tension-type headache to migraine. The Spectrum Study has shown that there are really two types of phenotypic episodic tension-type headache. Patients with migraine have attacks of what appear to be episodic tension-type headaches clinically but which respond like migraine to triptans when compared with placebo. It is believed that the attacks of episodic tension-type headaches in patients with migraine are phenotypic episodic tension-type headaches, but are genotypic migraine; in other words, those patients with migraine get low-level migraine attacks that look like tension but behave like migraine.

Patients with episodic tension-type headaches who never get migraines do not respond to triptans any better than placebo. They have different, "pure" episodic tension-type headaches not linked to migraine by continuum.

Chronic tension-type headache is chronic, low-level tension headache. Chronic migraine is migraine or probable migraine on at least 8 days per month in patients with headaches at least 15 days per month. The intensity of the daily symptoms and the associated migraine phenomena distinguish the two disorders, and, as noted, medication overuse headache is characterized by ingestion of acute, abortive medications at least 10 to 15 days per month and can appear clinically like chronic tension-type headache or chronic migraine.

Epidemiology

Tension-type headache varies widely in frequency, duration, and severity. In a Danish population-based study, it was found that 59% of persons experiencing tension-type headache had it 1 day a month or less, and 37% had it several times a month. In the total population, 3% had chronic tension-type headache. The tension-type headache male to female ratio is 4:5, indicating that, unlike migraine headache, women are affected only slightly more frequently. In both sexes, the prevalence seems to peak between the ages of 30 and 39 years and then declines with increasing age. The average age of onset of tension-type headache is 25 to 30 years, and the mean tension-type headache duration has been reported to be 10.3 to 19.9 years.

Although tension-type headache is the most prevalent headache and affects 78% of the general population, the substantial societal and individual burden associated with tension-type headache has been overlooked. Most patients with chronic tension-type headache are left with virtually no specific treatment. Daily or near daily headaches constitute a major diagnostic and therapeutic problem, and distinguishing chronic tension-type headache from migraine headache and from medication overuse headache is a substantial diagnostic challenge because management strategies are completely different. Obviously, in medication overuse headache, detoxification is the most important intervention.

Because of its high prevalence, tension-type headache has a greater socioeconomic impact than any other headache type. The direct costs include medical costs and social services; indirect costs stem from lost production in the economy because of morbidity. Indirect costs include reduced quality of life and reduced work capability. Because of the headache attacks, the socioeconomic costs from absenteeism among patients with tension-type headache are quite substantial.

Pathophysiology

The most prominent clinical finding in patients with tension-type headache is considerably increased pericranial myofascial tissue tenderness to palpation. In addition, it has been demonstrated that the pericranial tenderness is associated with the intensity and the frequency of tension-type headache. It is unknown for certain whether the increased tenderness in tension-type headache is a primary or a secondary phenomenon. It has been suggested that increased presence of muscle activity is a normal protective adaptation to pain, muscle ischemia, and abnormal blood flow. The release of neuropeptides (eg, substance P and calcitonin gene-related peptide) from muscle afferents may play a role in myofascial pain. The mode of action of the various mediators is complex and poorly understood.

The increased myofascial pain sensitivity in tension-type headache could be caused by central factors, such as sensitization of second-order neurons at the level of the spinal dorsal horn/trigeminal nucleus and above. It has been suggested that myofascial tenderness may be the result of a lowered pressure pain threshold, central sensitization, or a combination of both.

Treatment

A. Immediate Therapy

Simple analgesics and NSAIDs are used widely to treat acute tension-type headaches. Unfortunately, there is no selective or specific therapy.

As in migraine treatment, simple analgesics, such as aspirin and acetaminophen;, nonopioid analgesics; and antipyretics, such as dipyrone (not available in the United States); NSAIDs; or combination analgesics can be used. Muscle relaxants are not considered to be effective in treating acute episodes of tension-type headache because the few studies done have not shown efficacy, and there is risk of habituation.

B. Preventive Therapy

Preventive treatment is considered if the patient experiences a headache on more than 15 days each month (ie, chronic tension-type headache) or has very frequent episodic tension-type headache. See Preventive Therapy for migraine for medications that can prevent tension-type headache. Randomized controlled studies show amitriptyline, fluoxetine, and tizanidine are specifically beneficial in patients with tension-type headache.

Ashina M. Neurobiology of chronic tension-type headache. *Cephalalgia.* 2004;24:161. [PMID: 15009009]

Ashina S et al. Current and potential future drug therapies for tension-type headache. *Curr Pain Headache Rep.* 2003;7:466. [PMID: 14604506]

Bendtsen L. Central and peripheral sensitization in tension-type headache. *Curr Pain Headache Rep.* 2003;7:460. [PMID: 14604505]

Jensen R. Diagnosis, epidemiology, and impact of tension-type headache. *Curr Pain Headache Rep.* 2003;7:455. [PMID: 14604504]

TRIGEMINAL AUTONOMIC CEPHALALGIAS

The headache syndromes in this category are characterized by trigeminal pain associated with autonomic parasympathetic features that include alterations in sweating, ptosis, miosis, scleral and conjunctival injection, nasal stuffiness, and/or rhinorrhea. The presumed mechanism is V1 trigeminal nerve stimulation that produces activation of cranial parasympathetic reflexes; the presumed pathway involves outflow through the superior salivatory nucleus and the pterygopalatine ganglion.

1. Cluster Headache

 ESSENTIALS OF DIAGNOSIS

- The attack begins abruptly, intensifies rapidly (peaking within 5 to 15 minutes), and ceases suddenly.
- Pain is usually in or around the orbit and temporal locations and may radiate into the ipsilateral neck, ear, cheek, jaw, upper and lower teeth, and nose.
- The pain is severe and described as boring, tearing, stabbing, or burning.
- The attacks are short, lasting, 15 to 180 minutes untreated and occur every other day to eight times per day with alarm clock rhythmicity, occuring more frequently in men.
- The headaches are accompanied by at least one ipsilateral sign: conjunctival injection or tearing, nasal congestion or rhinorrhea eyelid edema, ptosis or miosis, forehead or facial sweatings or intense testlessness or agitation.

General Considerations

Cluster headache is the most common trigeminal autonomic cephalalgia. In its primary form, cluster headache occurs in 0.02 to 0.06% of the population and has incidence rates of 9.8/100.000 inhabitants per year (15.6 males, 4.0 females). The male/female ratio ranges from 4:1 to 12:1.

Pathophysiology

Recent research points to the hypothalamus as the probable generator of cluster headache. The suprachiasmatic nucleus in the hypothalamic gray is a pacemaker region involved in neuroendocrine hypothalamic regulation. Low testosterone levels as well as abnormal secretory circadian rhythms of luteinizing hormone, cortisol, prolactin, growth hormone, follicle-stimulating hormone, and thyroid-stimulating hormone have been found during cluster cycles and interictally. In addition, melatonin is chronically reduced during the cluster phase and interictally.

Positron emission tomography and functional magnetic resonance imaging (MRI) have demonstrated increased ipsilateral hypothalamic gray activity during attacks. More recently, the insertion of stimulating electrodes into this hypothalamic gray area in 15 patients with cluster headache in Italy and Belgium inhibited further attacks.

Clinical Findings

The pain of cluster headache is invariably unilateral, and the side affected is generally consistent for every attack and every cluster period. Very occasionally, the pain may affect the contralateral side, but cluster switching sides during a cluster period is rare enough to warrant a look for secondary causes. Predominantly, the pain is in or around the orbit (92% of cases) and temporal locations (70% of cases) and may radiate into the ipsilateral neck, ear, cheek, jaw, upper and lower teeth, and nose. The pain is described as boring, tearing, stabbing, or burning.

Autonomic features occur in 70 to 90% of patients. During the attack there is at least one autonomic ipsilateral symptom of lacrimation (91% of cases), conjunctival injection (77%), nasal congestion (75%), ptosis or eyelid swelling (74%), or rhinorrhea (72%). Other autonomic features include forehead and facial sweating and miosis. The autonomic features are short-lived, lasting only for the attack duration. Rarely, a partial Horner syndrome (ptosis or miosis) may persist after an acute attack.

The attack begins abruptly and rapidly intensifies, reaching a peak within 5 to 15 minutes. The attack also ceases suddenly, and the patient is often left feeling exhausted. The untreated attack typically lasts from 15 to 180 minutes (75% of attacks last less than 60 minutes). The attack frequency is around one to eight daily. The daily attacks usually last for 2 to 3 months (the cluster period), and the remission period (absence of attacks) can last for months to years.

In cluster headache, there is a remarkable timing predictability with a circadian or circannual periodicity; there is a nightly periodicity with attacks most frequently awakening the patient 90 minutes after falling asleep, corresponding to the onset of the first period of rapid eye movement (REM) sleep. Clinically, cluster headache can present in an episodic form or chronic pattern. In the chronic form, the patient continues to have daily attacks without remission and never has 1 month of no headache/year.

In contrast to migraine, oral contraceptive use, menses, menopause, and hormone replacement therapy do not trigger cluster headache in women. Alcoholic beverages and vasodilator medications, such as nitroglycerin, usually trigger an attack during the cluster period. Unlike persons with migraine, patients with cluster headache are agitated and restless and prefer to be upright and to move about. The pain intensity may cause some patients to wail loudly, and others may engage in destructive activities, such as banging their heads or actually attempting suicide due to the severity of pain. Cluster headache is frequently misdiagnosed, mainly in younger patients, as sinus headache or migraine.

Treatment

Cluster treatment is based on the implementation of immediate, transitional, and prophylactic treatment.

A. ABORTIVE THERAPY

The two most effective abortive treatments are oxygen 100% at a flow rate of 7 to 15 L/min or sumatriptan SC 6 mg. Because of the sudden onset and severity of a cluster headache attack, most oral abortive treatments lack enough speed to be effective. Zolmitriptan (10 mg) was found to be superior to placebo in decreasing pain intensity by two points at 30 minutes, which is too slow for most patients with cluster to tolerate. Sumatriptan (20 mg) and zolmitriptan (5 mg nasal sprays), and dihydroergotamine (1 mg SC and 2 to 4 mg nasal spray) have been recommended as optional abortive therapies. Other alternative abortive therapies studied include 4 to 6% lidocaine, 100 mcL of 0.025% civamide (25 mcg) (capsaicin isomer) nasal drops, and 5 to 10 mg of olanzapine.

B. TRANSITIONAL THERAPY

Transitional therapy is used to offer pain relief as preventive medications are added. Most commonly, corticosteroids are used, such as prednisone 1 mg/kg for 2 to 3 weeks. Other alternatives are methylergonovine 0.6 mg/d, daily ergotamine 1 to 2 mg, naratriptan 2.5 mg twice daily, or greater occipital nerve block.

C. PREVENTIVE THERAPY

Preventive treatment must be used in all patients with cluster. Verapamil, 240 mg to >480 mg, is the preferred treatment. Other prophylactic treatments are lithium, 600 to 1200 mg; valproic acid, 500 to 2500 mg; and topiramate, 25 to 125 mg. Gabapentin has also been suggested as preventive treatment. Usually at least two preventive medications are used together. Optional suggested therapies in refractory cases include methylergonovine, 0.6 mg/day; daily ergotamine; melatonin, 3 to 12 mg; and daily therapy with triptans that have a long half-life, such as naratriptan.

D. SURGICAL THERAPY

When preventive treatment fails, surgical treatment is suggested for refractory cases. A surgical treatment can be recommended for patients with 100% one-sided pain in the first trigeminal division and without psychiatric disease or history of drug abuse. The most frequently used surgical treatment is radiofrequency trigeminal gangliorhizolysis, effective in up to 70% of patients, with recurrence rates of 20% and failure rates around 30%.

Recently, the implantation of hypothalamic stimulators has shown promise but has not yet been tried in North America.

Prognosis

The natural history of cluster headache is related to the clinical presentation. Episodic cluster headache continues to be episodic in 53.2 to 67.1% of cases, becomes chronic in 2.4 to 12.9%, or can go into a prolonged remission period in 13.6 to 38.7%. Chronic cluster headache becomes episodic in 20 to 32.6% of cases, continues as chronic in 48 to 53.1%, or goes into a prolonged remission period in 12%. The factors that portend a bad prognosis are onset after 30 years of age (especially in females), long cluster periods (lasting longer than 8 weeks) with sporadic attacks in between, more than four associated symptoms, and short remission periods (lasting less than 6 months).

2. Paroxysmal Hemicranias

 ESSENTIALS OF DIAGNOSIS

- *Attacks more frequent than cluster attacks: more than five per day for greater than 50% of the time.*
- *No predilection for nocturnal headaches.*
- *Duration of attacks is from 2 and 45 minutes.*
- *Associated symptoms are characterized by the same autonomic phenomena as in cluster headaches.*
- *Absolute responsiveness to indomethacin 75 to at least 150 mg/d.*

General Considerations

Episodic paroxysmal hemicrania and chronic paroxysmal hemicrania are rare syndromes characterized by headaches of short duration, high attack frequency, and associated autonomic symptoms. Clinically, the paroxysmal hemicrania attacks look like short cluster attacks occurring at higher frequency per day. Unlike cluster, with its male predominance, paroxysmal hemicrania appears to be more common in women with a female to male ratio of 3:1. As with cluster, paroxysmal hemicrania that occurs daily for months with periods of remission is considered the episodic form; patients who do not remit over 1 year for at least 1 month have chronic paroxysmal hemicrania.

Clinical Findings

The most important feature that distinguishes paroxysmal hemicrania from cluster is the frequency of attacks per day. Persons with paroxysmal hemicrania have more than five attacks per day for >50% of the time. The pain is severe in intensity and, like cluster headache, has been described as boring or clawlike. Normal headache duration is between 2 and 30 minutes. Associated symptoms are characterized by the same autonomic phenomena as cluster headache. Most patients with chronic paroxysmal hemicrania exhibit lacrimation (62%), nasal congestion (42%), conjunctival injection and rhinorrhea (36%), or ptosis (33%).

Treatment

Paroxysmal hemicrania is one of the rare headache disorders that by definition is totally responsive to indomethacin. The normal starting dose of indomethacin is one 25 mg tablet three times daily for 3 days; this dose can be increased to 2 tablets (50 mg) three times daily if there is no total relief of pain. Most patients respond to 150 mg daily, and the response can be dramatic, with quick and complete dissipation of headache symptoms. A beneficial effect is normally seen within 48 hours after the correct dose is administered. If the patient does not respond to 75 mg three times daily, an alternative diagnosis should be considered. The gastrointestinal side effects normally can be controlled with proton pump inhibitors. Symptoms usually recur within several days after discontinuing indomethacin.

3. Hemicrania Continua

ESSENTIALS OF DIAGNOSIS

- *Primary headache syndrome characterized by a continuous unilateral headache that fluctuates in intensity and is accompanied by autonomic features and jabs and jolts, particularly during painful exacerbations.*
- *Pain is moderate, persistent, daily and continuous, strictly unilateral without side-shift for more than 3 months, without pain-free periods, but with exacerbations of severe pain and associated with at least one ipsilateral autonomic symptom.*
- *Complete response to therapeutic doses of indomethacin.*

General Considerations

Although the pathophysiology of hemicrania continua is still unknown, contralateral posterior hypothalamus and ipsilateral dorsal rostral pons activation have been demonstrated on functional MRI. If posterior hypothalamic and brainstem activation are considered as markers of trigeminal autonomic headaches and migrainous syndromes, respectively, then the activation pattern demonstrated in hemicrania continua overlaps with trigeminal autonomic headaches and migraine.

Clinical Findings

The revised IHS classification defines hemicrania continua as a persistent, daily and continuous headache of moderate intensity that is strictly unilateral without side-shift for more than 3 months, without pain-free periods but with exacerbations of severe pain and associated with at least one ipsilateral autonomic symptom. Other clinical characteristics described are the presence of migrainous features during exacerbation periods, icepick–like pains (jabs and jolts or primary stabbing headaches), or a foreign body sensation in the eye. Hemicrania continua can present as a remitting form (11.8% of cases), as a continuous pattern evolving from a remitting variety (35.3%), or as a chronic disorder from the onset (52.9%).

Treatment

Hemicrania continua responds exclusively to indomethacin treatment. For cases that are refractory to indomethacin therapy, alternatives include other NSAIDs, cyclooxygenase-2 inhibitors, topiramate, lamotrigine, or gabapentin.

Aurora SK. Etiology and pathogenesis of cluster headache. *Curr Pain Headache Rep.* 2002;6:71. [PMID: 11749881]

Bahra A et al. Cluster headache: a prospective clinical study with diagnostic implications. *Neurology.* 2002;58:354. [PMID: 11839832]

Geweke LO. Misdiagnosis of cluster headache. *Curr Pain Headache Rep.* 2002;6:76. [PMID: 11749882]

Matharu MS et al. Trigeminal autonomic cephalgias. *J Neurol Neurosurg Psychiatry.* 2002;72(Suppl II):ii19. [PMID: 12122199]

Rozen TD. Short-lasting headache syndromes and treatment options. *Curr Pain Headache Rep.* 2004;8:268. [PMID: 15228884]

CHRONIC DAILY HEADACHE

Daily or near-daily headache is a widespread problem in clinical practice. The general term of "chronic daily headache" encompasses primary headaches presenting more than 15 days per month and lasting more than 4 hours per day. Chronic daily headache includes chronic migraine, transformed migraine, chronic tension-type headache, new daily persistent headache, and hemicrania continua (Table 12–7). At least 40% of patients who seek medical attention at a specialized headache clinic meet diagnostic criteria for chronic daily headache, of which 80% are women. Of those, 60% suffer transformed migraine, 20% chronic tension-type headache, 20% meet new daily persistent headache criteria, and up to 80% of patients overuse symptomatic medications (medication overuse headache).

Chronic daily headache prevalence in the general population is 4 to 5% (up to 8 to 9% for women). New daily persistent headache is rare (0.1%), chronic migraine is intermediate (1.5 to 2%), and chronic tension-type headache is most common (2.5 to 3%). In contrast to data from specialized clinics, only around 25% of persons with chronic daily headache in the general population overuse analgesics.

Comorbid factors may be significant contributors to the development and maintenance of chronic daily headache, but a causal relationship does not necessarily exist. In addition to medication overuse, the following associations occur commonly in persons with chronic daily headache: hypothyroidism, obesity, snoring, asthma, hypertension, and daily consumption of caffeine.

1. Medication Overuse Headache

 ESSENTIALS OF DIAGNOSIS

- *Headache is present for more than 15 days each month and should develop or markedly worsen during medication overuse.*
- *Headache resolves or reverts to its previous pattern within 2 months after discontinuation of medication.*
- *Medications may include ergotamine, triptans, opioids, combination medications (eg, butalbital mixtures), or simple analgesics for at least 10 days per month for more than 3 months.*

General Considerations

Patients with chronic headaches and medication overuse headaches are particularly difficult to treat because prophylactic medications lack efficacy in this setting, and because discontinuation of the offending medication can lead to a severe withdrawal headache, resembling an acute migraine attack. Withdrawal headache, rebound headache, or medication overuse headache is often accompanied by vegetative symptoms. In addition, patients often show signs of physical and emotional dependence and psychological involvement. A successful treatment has wide-ranging positive benefits reducing both headache and associated disability.

Clinical Findings

Many drugs are known to cause medication overuse headache. The diagnosis of medication overuse headache requires that the headache be present for more than 15 days each month, and the headache should develop or markedly worsen during medication overuse. The headache resolves or reverts to its previous pattern within 2 months after discontinuation of medication.

Medication use needs to occur several times a week to cause medication overuse headache. This syndrome is less likely to develop in patients who intersperse consecutive days of medication use (eg, with menstrual migraine) with long drug-free periods. Headache characteristics associated with overuse vary and may be tension-like or migraine-like, frequently waxing and waning and also varying in location, but neck pain is frequent. There is a circadian rhythmicity to medication overuse headache, with morning headache common, since withdrawal occurs through the night.

Screening questions for drug overuse should always be asked of patients with chronic daily headache. The overused medication may provide information about the patient's neuropsychological condition. Type I patients prefer over-the-counter analgesics or nonsedating prescription medication. Their response to treatment is usually good. Type II or "beaten down" patients are more depressed and limited by headache disability. These patients prefer multiple medications and often use opioids. Psychotherapy and antidepressant medication helps their recovery. Type III patients show drug-seeking and compulsive behavior toward opioids and similar habituating medications. Treatment outcome in this group is poor, and an approach for primary substance abuse may be helpful.

Treatment

A. OUTPATIENT

The initial approach is to discontinue the overused medications. There are two general outpatient strategies. One

Table 12–7. Diagnostic Characteristics of Chronic Daily Headache.

Features	Type of headache				
	Chronic migraine (New 2006 criteria)	***Chronic tension-type headache***	***Hemicrania continua***[a]	***New daily persistent headache (NDPH) (ICHD-II criteria, 2004)***	***New daily persistent headache (NDPH) (Silberstein-Lipton criteria)***
Frequency	$\geq$ 15 days of HA/month	$\geq$ 15 days/month	$\geq$ 15 days/month	$\geq$ 15 days/month $\geq$ 3 months	$\geq$ 15 days/month $\geq$ 1 month
Duration	$\geq$ 4 hours/day untreated	$\geq$ 3 months	$\geq$ 3 months	Daily without remission or $<$ 3 days from beginning	$\geq$ 4 hours (without treatment) Constant
Description of pain	Meets criteria for migraine or probable migraine at least 8 days/month	Bilateral Nonthrobbing Mild to moderate Does not increase with physical activity	Unilateral without side shift Daily and continuous, no pain-free periods Moderate intensity with exacerbations of severe pain	Bilateral Nonthrobbing Mild to moderate Does not increase with physical activity	Abrupt onset of any daily headache
Associated symptoms	Meet criteria for migraine or probable migraine $\geq$ 50% of the headache days/month	No more than one of the following: Mild photophobia Mild phonophobia Mild nausea and no severe nausea or vomiting	At least one ipsilateral: Conjunctival injection or lacrimation, nasal congestion or rhinorrhea, eyelid edema, miosis or ptosis	No more than one of the following: Mild photophobia Mild phonophobia Mild nausea and no severe nausea or vomiting	Sudden onset $<$3 days
	No need for previous history of episodic migraine or transformation		Absolute responsiveness to indomethacin		No secondary cause and no transformation from preexisting headache No response to indomethicin
	Does not meet criteria for new daily persistent headache, chronic tension-type headache, Hypnic headache				

[a]Complete response to indomethacin.
[b]No medication overuse.

Modified from Headache Classification Subcommittee of the International Headache Society (ICHD-2). *Cephalalgia.* 2004;24 (suppl 1):9.

approach is to taper the overused medication, gradually establishing effective preventive therapy as the taper progresses. The second strategy is to abruptly discontinue the overused drug when safe, use a bridge or transitional medication to ease the withdrawal temporarily, and rapidly add preventive treatment at the same time. Drugs used for the bridge include NSAIDs, corticosteroids, ergots, and triptans.

During the washout period, typical withdrawal symptoms can occur (eg, headache exacerbation, nausea, restlessness, and sleep disorder). Typically, the intensity of the headache increases 2 days into the withdrawal period and declines by the end of the week. Once the withdrawal period is over, which may last 1 to 6 weeks without treatment, there is frequently considerable headache improvement, with gradual cessation of daily headache, and reestablishment of an episodic migraine pattern.

B. INPATIENT

Hospital admission should be considered when patients meet the following criteria:

1. Presence of severe intractable headache.
2. Presence of refractory headache or status migrainosus.
3. Multiple visits to emergency department.
4. Requirement of repetitive sustained parenteral treatment.
5. Presence of nausea, vomiting, or diarrhea.
6. Need to detoxify and treat toxicity, dependency, or rebound phenomena, and monitor protectively against withdrawal symptoms.
7. Presence of unstable vital signs.
8. Presence of dehydration, electrolyte imbalance, and prostration that requires monitoring and intravenous fluids.
9. Likely presence of serious disease.

The treatment process can be enhanced and shortened and the patient's symptoms made more tolerable by administering repetitive intravenous dihydroergotamine with an antiemetic, such as metoclopramide. It has been reported that up to 92% of patients became headache-free usually within 2 to 3 days with an average hospital stay of 4 to 7 days. Patients who are not candidates for or do not respond to dihydroergotamine can be treated with repetitive intravenous valproate, ketorolac, other neuroleptics, ondansetron, or corticosteroids. These agents may also supplement repetitive intravenous dihydroergotamine in refractory cases (Table 12–8).

If patients with medication overuse headache do not respond to potentially effective preventive therapies, another trial of previously used preventive medications may be successful after the patient has been detoxified and

has recovered from rebound headache. The patient and the treating physician must understand that a given preventive medication may not become fully effective until the overused medication is eliminated and the washout period complete. Patients suffering from drug-induced headache often exhibit depression, low frustration tolerance, and physical and emotional dependency. Hospitalization can provide patient education and behavior modification and can initiate an outpatient program of preventive and immediate therapy.

Prognosis

As noted above, after the offending agents have been withdrawn, the headache pattern usually becomes episodic. This generally takes weeks, although some reports suggest that the change from daily to episodic headache may take as long as 6 months. At least 60% of these patients no longer have daily headache, and approximately 40% still have migraine attacks. There are no literature reports of spontaneous improvement from rebound headache without detoxification. The relapse rate within 6 months after withdrawal therapy is approximately 30% and increases steadily to 50% after 5 years, without close follow-up.

2. Chronic Migraine

Chronic migraine is the most common type of chronic daily headache in specialty care. Persons with transformed migraine usually report a process of transformation over months or years, and as headache increases in frequency, associated symptoms become less severe and frequent. The process of transformation frequently ends in a pattern of daily or nearly daily headache that resembles chronic tension-type headache, with some attacks of full-blown migraine superimposed. In the original proposal for this disorder, subsequently validated, chronic migraine could occur with or without medication overuse.

Many patients with primary chronic migraine no longer have daily headache after undergoing withdrawal of medication overuse; however, a significant subgroup still has episodic migraine. Nevertheless, regular use of analgesics with an existing history of headache, in particular migraine, is not always the sole factor responsible for the development of chronic daily headache, and complex genetic factors may also play a role. It has also become clear that analgesics per se do not cause the development of daily headache de novo in persons with no previous headache history.

Bigal ME et al. Chronic daily headache: identification of factors associated with induction and transformation. *Headache.* 2002;42:575. [PMID: 12482208]

Table 12–8. Pharmacologic Treatments for Refractory Cases.

Treatment	Efficacy	Dosage	Adverse effects
Dihydroergotamine	Total 72–87% Excellent 23–31% Good 21–28% Fair 28% Poor 13%	0.5–1 mg/8 hours IV	Nausea, dizziness, paresthesias, abdominal pain, chest pressure, arterial or coronary vasospasm
Corticosteroids	Total 75%	Varies	Insomnia, mood changes
Prochlorperazine	Total 75–90% Excellent 63% Reduction 69–75% Worsening 8–10%	5–10 mg/8 hours IV (average 98 mg)	Somnolence, dizziness, parkinsonism, abdominal upset, dystonic reactions, alcathisia
Naproxen	Headache index reduction 40% ($P < .001$) and analgesic intake 46–53% ($P < .001$)	500 mg PO tid 2 mg IV each	Dyspepsia
Lidocaine	Fair 70–90% Pain-free 50–60%	2 mg/kg initially Infusion 2 mg/minute	Local pain, local infection, IV obstruction, anaphylaxis
Histamine	Total 40% Good 70%	2 mcg/kg–70 mcg/kg	None reported
Chlorpromazine	Excellent 63% Poor 9%	12.5 mg/8 hours	Hypotension, nausea, nasal congestion, QT prolongation
Valproic acid	Total 63–80% Good 10–40% Excellent 21–40%	15 mg/kg IV Initially 5 mg/kg every 8 hours	Dizziness, pseudoseizures, dysarthria, dysmetria, dystonic reactions, alcathisia, nystagmus

Total: Average patients with headache reduction > 50% in frequency and severity; **Excellent:** Reduction > 90% in frequency or severity or > 75% if both; **Good:** Reduction > 75% in frequency or severity or > 50% if both; **Fair:** Reduction > 50% in frequency or severity; **Poor:** Reduction < 50% in frequency or severity. **Headache Index:** Days with headache over follow-up days.

Freitag et al. *Headache.* 2004;44:342.

Bigal ME et al. Transformed migraine and medication overuse in a tertiary headache center–clinical characteristics and treatment outcomes. *Cephalalgia.* 2004;24:483. [PMID: 15154848]

Freitag FG et al. US Headache Guidelines Consortium, Section on Inpatient Treatment Chairpersons. Inpatient treatment of headache: an evidence-based assessment. *Headache.* 2004;44:342. [PMID: 15109359]

Krymchantowski AV et al. Out-patient detoxification in chronic migraine: comparison of strategies. *Cephalalgia.* 2003;23:982. [PMID: 14984232]

Levin M. Chronic daily headache and the revised international headache society classification. *Curr Pain Headache Rep.* 2004;8:59. [PMID: 14731384]

Limmroth V et al. Features of medication overuse headache following overuse of different acute headache drugs. *Neurology.* 2002;59:1011. [PMID: 12370454]

Srikiatkhachorn A. Pathophysiology of chronic daily headache. *Curr Pain Headache Rep.* 2001;5:537. [PMID: 11676888]

NEUROIMAGING IN PRIMARY HEADACHES

The primary reason to obtain a neuroimaging study in a headache sufferer is to rule out significant and treatable disease. Secondary indications include relieving patient anxiety as well as avoiding litigation concerns responding to a family request. The threshold for investigating headache decreases in patients with red flags or atypical signs. Red flags include sudden severe headache; change in headache pattern, such as rapid increasing headache frequency or severity; changes in headache characteristics; 100% one-sided headaches; or headache in special populations, such as the elderly and persons with HIV or cancer.

Imaging studies should always be considered in patients with focal neurologic signs or atypical symptoms, such as seizures. The prevalence of neuroimaging abnormalities in patients who have episodic migraine with normal neurologic examination is around 0.18%. In chronic daily headache sufferers without red flags, abnormalities are found in 0.67%. Nonspecific brain abnormalities have been reported in 12 to 46% of migraine sufferers; however, in the population as a whole, there is not enough evidence to demonstrate that migraine is an independent risk factor for cerebrovascular disorders. The potential discovery of serious treatable lesions is about 0.4% in migraine using computed tomography or MRI scans, and the side effects related to the use of these diagnostic tools can be as high as 10% due to iodine reaction and claustrophobia.

The US Headache Consortium Guidelines identified four consensus-based recommendations for imaging:

1. Testing should be avoided if it will not lead to a change in management.

2. Testing is not recommended if the person is not significantly more likely than anyone else in the general population to have significant abnormality.

3. Testing should be done in patients when suspicion of a serious problem is high, even in the absence of known predictors of abnormalities (red flags).

4. Neuroimaging studies should be considered in patients with unexplained abnormal neurologic findings.

Evans RW. Diagnostic testing for headache. *Med Clin North Am.* 2001;85:865. [PMID: 11480262]

Frishberg B et al. US Headache Consortium. Evidenced-Based Guidelines in the Primary Care Setting: Neuroimaging in Patients with Nonacute Headache. American Academy of Neurology; 2000. Available at: http://www.aan.com/professionals/ practice/pdfs/gl0088.pdf Last accessed: September 19, 2005.

Jamieson DG et al. The role of neuroimaging in headache. *J Neuroimaging.* 2002;12:42. [PMID: 11826596]

Back Pain

Edgar Ross, MD

13

Back pain is the most common cause of chronic pain in the United States, yet the most effective treatment of low back pain remains elusive. There is no general consensus on best practices for either diagnosis or treatment of back pain. Because of the high incidence in the work force, disability from back pain is very high and costly. Because of the lack of consensus, the cost of diagnosis and treatment remain very high. The high costs of back pain come not just from the pain but also from the disability secondary to the pain, needless diagnostic tests, and ineffective treatment.

Most of the diagnostic testing that is ordered is not needed. Even the most sophisticated diagnostic testing often cannot objectively validate most of the spinal pain that is reported by patients. Numerous guidelines have been published that attempt to clarify this problem. For example, the nationally recognized guidelines published by the Agency for Healthcare Research and Quality can assist clinicians in deciding which diagnostic tests are appropriate and which treatment approaches are effective. Diagnosing and treating low back pain efficiently, avoiding ineffective procedures, and minimizing the harmful effects of a sedentary lifestyle can have a substantial impact on patient suffering, lost income, disability, and health care costs.

Deyo RA. Low back pain. *N Engl J Med.* 2001;344:363. [PMID: 11172169]

Susman J. The care of low back problems: less is more. *Am Fam Physician.* 2002;65:2217. [PMID: 12074523]

Van Tulder M et al. Low back pain (chronic). *Clin Evid.* 2004;12:1659. [PMID: 15865740]

ESSENTIAL CRITERIA

- *Most spinal pain is self-limited.*
- *A definitive diagnosis cannot be made in upward of 85% of patients, primarily because of the multiple etiologies of back pain and nonspecific nature of diagnostic tests.*
- *Low back pain accounts for 40 to 50% of patient visits to pain clinics.*

- *Back pain can be categorized as acute (lasting <6 weeks), subacute (lasting 6 to 12 weeks), or chronic (lasting 12 weeks or longer).*
- *Treatment usually consists of appropriate medications for both the neuropathic and nociceptive complaints.*

GENERAL CONSIDERATIONS

Incidence

Back pain is the second leading reason for physician office visits in the United States today. The prevalence of spinal pain in the United States has been reported as up to 37%, and the peak incidence is found between 45 to 60 years of age. This incidence translates into the fact that 80% of all Americans will seek care at some point in their lives for acute back pain. Notably the age range of 45 to 60 is usually the most productive time period for most workers. This observation is most likely the reason that back pain is responsible for more than one-third of the total disability payments in the United States. The indirect costs of lost earnings are even higher.

Natural History of Back Pain

Table 13–1 presents the duration of symptoms and the prognosis for acute, subacute, and chronic pain. In general, treatment in the good prognosis groups should be supportive with avoidance of interventional therapies (such as surgical procedures), which could carry more risk than benefit. On the other hand, patients who are not improving as expected should be reexamined, and further diagnostic testing performed to rule out potentially serious occult conditions. With persistent pain, referrals to chronic pain programs should be made promptly. This proactive approach can be helpful in avoiding the consequences of deconditioning and resultant long-term disability.

Classification

The following classification categories are based on the presenting symptoms and are very useful for determining prognosis, planning treatment, and diagnostic testing:

Table 13–1. Duration of Symptoms and Prognosis of Acute, Subacute, and Chronic Pain.

Type of pain	Duration of symptoms	Prognosis
Acute	Less than 6 weeks	60% of patients return to function within 1 month
Subacute	6–12 weeks	90% of patients return to function within 3 months
Chronic	12 weeks or longer	Much less likely to resolve

1. Nonspecific spinal pain
2. Radicular symptoms
3. Potential serious spinal condition (Table 13–2)

The most common diagnosis is nonspecific spinal pain. Although many theories have been suggested to explain this type of pain, none have been conclusively validated. Despite the many diseases that are known to be associated with back pain, the pathophysiology of the most common diagnostic group remains unknown. Nonspecific spinal pain is generally thought to be secondary to musculoskeletal dysfunction, but no consistent and specific finding has ever been found. For the rest of the potential diagnoses, the pathophysiology of back pain depends on the disease process underlying the patient's complaints.

Radicular back pain is usually associated with spinal nerve irritation or compression. Table 13–3 outlines the differential diagnosis of back pain and includes potentially serious spinal conditions—the last classification.

Etiology of Benign Back Pain

At present, the evolution of chronic back pain is thought to begin with end plate damage. The disk receives most of its blood supply from the end plate. Disk degeneration begins with this compromise in blood supply first near the end plate and later in the disk nucleus. In support of this mechanism, arteriosclerosis of the vascular tree leading to lumbar segmental arteries is also associated with increased incidence of disk degeneration and back pain complaints. Considerable evidence now suggests that the healthy lumbar disk is primarily innervated in the annulus and to a limited extent in the pulposis. With degenerative changes, innervation progresses and extends deeper into the nucleus pulposus. Inflammatory mediators have also been identified inside the disk during discography in patients who report concordant pain. Along with the pathologic process described, the loss of disk height has important consequences on spinal dynamics. The vertebral body has a three-joint articulating relationship with its adjoining vertebral bodies. The change in dynamics, and structural relationships stresses the synovial facet joints, which leads to osteoarthritis, with the potential of subluxation, segmental instability, and chronic pain. The paradoxical reports of patients with advanced radiographic degenerative findings and little discomfort could be explained by the conclusion of this process through complete loss of mobility in the spinal segment by autofusion. Genetics is also thought to play a role in the susceptibility to back pain. A particular person's susceptibility is determined by the reaction to an injury as initiated by inflammatory mediators that are released and expressed along with differences in the underlying structural composition of the disk. Genetics appear to be significant early in a person's life; other risk factors, such as injury, lifestyle and nutrition, have a more important role after the second decade.

Hurri H et al. Discogenic pain. *Pain.* 2004;112:225. [PMID: 15561376]

Mahmud MA et al. Clinical management and the duration of disability for work-related low back pain. *J Occup Environ Med.* 2000;42:1178. [PMID: 11125681]

Table 13–2. Back Pain Classification Based on Pathophysiology.

Classification	Description of presenting symptoms	Pathophysiology
Nonspecific spinal pain	Localized pain Usually minimal or no physical findings	Unknown Could be secondary to change in the dynamics of the spinal elements
Radicular symptoms	Radiating pain usually dermatomal	Usually spinal nerve compression or irritation, or both
Potential serious spinal condition	See Tables 13–3 and 13–4	Depends on diagnosis

Table 13–3. Overview of Differential Diagnosis of Back Pain.

    I. **Rheumatologic conditions**
        A. Seronegative spondyloarthropathies
            1. Ankylosing spondylitis
            2. Psoriatic arthritis
            3. Reactive spondyloarthropathy, including Reiter syndrome and enteropathic arthritis
        B. Rheumatoid arthritis
        C. Polymyalgia rheumatica
        D. Nonarticular rheumatic disorders (eg, myofascial pain)
   II. **Cancer**
        A. Primary tumors of the spine
            1. Multiple myeloma
            2. Other bone or cartilage tumors, such as osteoid osteoma
        B. Metastatic spinal disease
  III. **Infections**
        A. Osteomyelitis
        B. Discitis
        C. Epidural abscess
        D. Herpes zoster
  IV. **Vascular conditions**
        A. Abdominal aortic aneurysm causes pain by rupture, erosion of adjacent structures, or dissection
        B. Epidural hematoma
        C. Hemoglobinopathy (eg, sickle cell disease)
   V. **Metabolic disorders**
        A. Osteoporosis (primary or secondary)
        B. Paget disease
  VI. **Referred pain**
        A. Pelvic disorders
            1. Endometriosis
            2. Torsion of organ or structure
            3. Pelvic inflammatory disease
            4. Prostatitis
            5. Cystitis
        B. Abdominal disorders
            1. Pancreatitis or cancer of the pancreas
            2. Duodenal ulcers
            3. Renal pathology or stones
  VII. **Spine structure problems**
        A. Facet joints
        B. Spinal stenosis
        C. Paraspinal muscles
        D. Sacroiliac joint
        E. Spondylolysis or spondylolisthesis
        F. Nonspecific back pain
 VIII. **Other causes**
        A. Hip joint
        B. Shoulder joints
        C. Costovertebral joints
        D. Trochanteric bursa
        E. Guillain-Barré syndrome
        F. Meningeal irritation
        G. Fibromyalgia syndrom
  IX. **Psychological factors (myriad of different diagnoses)**

Table 13–4. A Methodical Approach to Rule Out Serious Causes (Red Flags) of Back Pain.

Evaluation	Features	Comments
Obtain a comprehensive history	A new onset of back pain and history of cancer Predilection toward infections New onset of back pain in patients older than 50 years of age Metabolic bone disorder Unintended weight loss	Even if there is no history of metastatic disease Patients using immunosuppressive medications Benign back pain usually presents in younger patients Osteoporosis or hyperparathyroidism Atypical in uncomplicated back pain
Determine the patient's chief complaint	History of significant trauma Pain worse at night Pain not relieved by any position Change in bladder or bowel function Bilateral radicular pain Extreme pain unrelieved by any therapy Numbness or paresthesia in the perianal region Unexplained limb weakness Progressive neurologic changes	Atypical for uncomplicated back pain Atypical for uncomplicated back pain Single dermatomal neurologic defect is usually benign
Perform a physical examination	Pulsatile abdominal mass Fever with back pain Pattern of physical findings not compatible with benign mechanical disease	Also look for enlarged aorta on flat plate of abdomen or other radiographic studies Consider infection
Obtain laboratory tests	Elevated sedimentation rate Elevated white count	Elevated in many conditions including metastatic disease, infection and rheumatic conditions May be the only laboratory indicator in discitis or epidural abscess
Evaluate treatment response	Lack of response to conservative therapies	Reevaluate for other causes

ASSESSMENT

Initial Evaluation

The evaluation of a patient with back pain is often not a straightforward process. The true cause of back pain is found in only 20% of cases. Despite this, the need to rule out serious illnesses that present as back pain requires a thorough evaluation of the patient in a methodical and cost-effect approach (Table 13–4). Usually, the initial history and physical examination along with basic laboratory tests are sufficient to identify patients who are at risk for serious disease or who have "red flags" (see Table 13–4) or who require further workup. Notice that obtaining radiographic films is not part of the initial evaluation.

Diagnostic Testing

Because of the long-term nature of low back pain, patients often request additional diagnostic testing; the temptation is to respond to patient's concerns even when no clear-cut reason exists. Understanding key points of a patient's history and the pathophysiology of spinal pain can be helpful in providing the appropriate care for these difficult cases. Patients who are not responding to treatment as expected should be reevaluated with consideration given to a potential alternate diagnosis. Table 13–5 outlines disease categories, differential diagnosis along with key points, and the presumed underlying pathophysiology.

Despite the myriad of conditions that can cause back pain as listed in Table 13–5, discogenic back pain is

Table 13–5. Key Points for Spinal Pain.

Disease category	Key points	Pathophysiology	Comments
Rheumatologic conditions	Occurs in 1.9% of the white population If patient is HLA-B27 positive, susceptibility is increased 20-fold The SI joint is the most commonly involved joint and affected in 50% of cases	Genetic predisposition with environmental triggers	The most common spine manifestations in this class is Reiter syndrome and ankylosing spondylitis
Neoplasm (primary or metastatic)	Metastatic disease is 25% more common than primary tumors Spinal metastasis is found in 70% of patients with primary tumors The most common tumors that metastasize to the spine are breast, lung, prostate, kidney, lymphoma, melanoma, and the GI tract	Metastatic disease is spread by the venous channels in the epidural space (Batson plexus)	Multiple myeloma is the most common primary spinal malignancy Rare below 40 years of age
Infections	General incidence is unknown for bacterial and fungal infections Presence should be suspected in patients with localized pain to percussion and reports of fever Spine infections are frequently misdiagnosed on initial presentation Consider herpes zoster infection	May be acute or chronic Causes vary from postspinal surgery infections to local seeding from deep tissue infections to remote seeding Herpes zoster causes dermatomal neuropathic pain	Acute infections are usually associated with pyogenic organisms With chronic infections, consider fungal infection or TB Herpes zoster can mimic radicular symptoms
Vascular, hematologic	Half of all patients with ruptured abdominal aortic aneurysm complained of back pain first Rarely, back pain can be caused by epidural hematomas Inherited hematolgic diseases, such as thalassemia or sickle cell disease, are commonly associated with spinal pain	Pain caused by compression of adjacent structure by rapid enlargement of vessel Sickle cell disease or thalassemia cause pain through bony infarcts	Epidural hematomas are associated with anticoagulation therapy, trauma, or recent spinal procedure (such as epidural)
Endocrine or metabolic osteoporosis	Osteoporosis is most common and often seen in older women	Risk factors include thin, white, postmenopausal women; smoking; alcohol intake; and sedentary lifestyle Pain caused by compression fractures or microfactures of affected bone Up to 50% of fractures are painless	Other risk factors include nutritional disorders, drug effects, genetics, and endocrine disorders
Paget disease	Paget disease contributes to pain directly about 2% of time	Unknown how Paget disease contributes to pain	Treatment of Paget disease often improves pain

Continued

Table 13–5. Key Points for Spinal Pain. (*Continued*)

Disease category	Key points	Pathophysiology	Comments
Referred pain	Incidence as cause of back pain is unknown	Pain referred to the back from other disease is common with visceral pathology, such as endometriosis, pulmonary embolism, and ulcer disease	Abdominal and retroperitoneal disease most commonly referred to as lumbar spine Other areas, such as chest, are less common
Mechanical causes of spinal pain	98% of all causes of spinal pain are from this category	These pains have much in common for presentation Pain is primarily caused by inflammatory factors followed by mechanical derangement Pain persisting after previous spinal surgery is not uncommon A complete understanding of the cause is unknown	Structures that can originate pain include muscle, disk, facet joint and capsule, ventral dura, anterior posterior ligaments, and dural root sleeves
Other sources of spine pain 　Hip pathology	Hip pathology is an unusual cause for back pain	Pain is rarely referred to the buttocks, most common to the groin	Check range of motion hip
Guillain-Barré syndrome	Rare cause of back pain	Inflammation of the spinal meninges and stretching of them cause the pain	Distinguish from bacterial infections or neoplastic infiltration
Meningitis	May be acute or chronic	Inflammation of the spinal meninges and stretching of them cause the pain	Lumbar puncture definitive
Psychological causes	Unknown incidence Studies show that true psychological causes are very rare	Unknown	Psychological stressors can contribute to pain

SI, sacroiliac; GI, gastrointestinal; TB, tuberculosis.

thought to be the most common source of pain for non-specific back pain. The evolution process begins with disk degeneration. As the process continues, secondary deterioration of facet joints, ligaments, and muscles follows, leading to a change in movement dynamics. Despite the temptation to associate structural changes seen on radiographic imaging of the spine with the cause of a person's pain, no such correlation has ever been proven. In addition, degenerative spinal conditions, which are asymptomatic but can be seen radiographically, do not necessarily predict future back pain complaints.

Evaluation of Musculoskeletal Back Pain

Estimates have suggested that as much as 98% of back pain arises from the disruption of the musculoskele-

tal system supporting the back. Despite this high incidence, finding the pain generator that explains the source of back pain is often elusive. This is in part secondary to the many different components of the spine that are pain sensitive. In addition, any particular injury may effect one or more painful components of the spine. Pain sensitive structures of the spine include:

1. Outer annular fibers of the intervertebral disk.

2. The anterior and posterior longitudinal ligaments surrounding the disk.

3. The facet joint capsules.

4. Paraspinal muscles.

5. Ventral side of the dura mater.

6. Dural root sleeves.

7. The spinal nerves themselves, when irritated.

These pain sensitive structures—separately or in combination—form many of the common clinical diagnoses that are thought to underlie mechanical back pain.

Carragee EJ. Clinical practice. Persistent low back pain. *N Engl J Med.* 2005;352:1891. [PMID: 15872204]

Cherniack M et al. Clinical and psychological correlates of lumbar motion abnormalities in low back disorders. *Spine J.* 2001;1:290. [PMID: 14588334]

Cohen R et al. Primary care work-up of acute and chronic symptoms. *Geriatrics.* 2001;56:26. [PMID: 11710812]

Devereaux MW. Neck and low back pain. *Med Clin North Am.* 2003;87:643. [PMID: 12812407]

Pennekamp W et al. Feasibilities and bounds of diagnostic radiology in case of back pain. *Schmerz.* 2005;12:117.

DIFFERENTIAL DIAGNOSIS

Table 13–3 presents an overview of a differential diagnosis of back pain that include less benign causes of back pain. Rheumatic conditions often present with significant morning stiffness. With light exertion, the pain commonly improves; later in the day with sustained activity the pain begins to increase again. Typically, the spine is more generally affected in rheumatic conditions. In some instances, the disease is confined to a discrete area; the diagnostic approach for discrete areas of pain is covered in the mechanical spinal pain section. Although helpful, a complete history and physical examination are rarely diagnostic. A specific history of symptoms involving the eyes, skin, and gastrointestinal tract can be very helpful for some of these diagnoses. Laboratory tests and radiologic imaging are frequently necessary for definitive diagnosis. Table 13–6 presents a diagnostic approach to the rheumatic pain conditions.

There are a couple of characteristic findings that differentiates neoplastic spinal pain from benign spinal pain. First, pain that wakes a patient up at night typically indicates neoplastic pain. Second, percussion of the spine is often painful with neoplastic disease but not benign spinal pathology.

Table 13–7 lists nonmechanical causes of spinal pain, clinical findings, and potentially helpful diagnostic approaches.

STRUCTURAL PATHOLOGIES OF BACK PAIN

Discogenic Back Pain

The disk is the largest avascular structure found in the body. Back pain, which arises from this structure, is known as discogenic back pain. Degeneration of the disk results from desiccation of the disk secondary to the breakdown of nucleus pulposis constituents, including proteoglycans and loss of collagen protein crosslinking. Repetitive daily activities, such as chronic axial and rotational forces, can lead to a weakened disk causing the development of microtears of the annulus and healing with fibrosis formation. This eventually leads to diminishing of the blood supply and further degeneration. Periodic complaints of back pain with resolution are thought to be secondary to this process. Acute annular tears may be the most common cause of back pain. Patients often report a feeling of a pop, which began with a flexion motion while lifting an object. Pain associated with this injury is increased by flexion and sitting (especially in a car). Unless the spinal nerve is compromised, the pain is nonradicular, with the physical examination revealing paraspinal muscle spasm but no neurologic deficits. Straight leg-raising test is negative, but patients sometimes report increased back pain. Flexion of the spine is limited. Internal disk disruption is a similar condition that is also associated with back pain. The frequency of leg pain is more common. Magnetic resonance imaging (MRI) studies often show a desiccated disk seen as dark shading in the involved level. The pain is thought to be from annulus tears leading to inflammation and abnormal movement of the spinal segment. Provocative discography followed by computed tomography (CT) scan showing leakage of contrast into the epidural space is confirmatory. Further injury to the disk, which includes progressive annular disruption, can lead to the protrusion of nucleus pulposis into the outer annulus seen as a bulging disk. At first, the posterior longitudinal ligament contains the disk material. If the posterior longitudinal ligament weakens, the nucleus pulposis may herniate and lead to either nerve root inflammation or frank compression, or both. Nociceptors found in the dural sleeve, dura, and posterior and anterior longitudinal ligaments contribute to the back and leg pain commonly found in these patients. Midline herniation of the disk can leave the patient only with back pain and little or no leg pain. Herniated disks are often associated with a flexion-type of injury associated with lifting and twisting. Patients may report a snap or pop at the time of injury. Severe pain is not always reported immediately but may worsen over several days. Large disk herniations can cause significant spinal stenosis with neurologic compromise, leading to cauda equina syndromes. These conditions must be looked for because they could require emergent surgeries to avoid irreversible neurologic injury. In these conditions, the patient may have a history of muscle weakness and the loss of bowel or bladder control. Physical examination reveals ipsilateral or bilateral positive straight leg-raising. True bilateral positive straight leg-raising is considered to be nearly confirmatory for spinal nerve root irritation.

Table 13–6. Diagnostic Approaches in Evaluating Rheumatologic Conditions Causing Back Pain.

Diagnosis	Clinical findings	Laboratory tests	Imaging studies	Comments
Ankylosing spondylitis	Usually affects patients between ages of 30–40 years More common in males than females; can be confused with seronegative RA. Dull, diffuse low back pain with referral to the legs and buttocks is common Later, extreme morning stiffness and severe night pain Patient is in a slightly flexed trunk position	90% of patients are HLA-B27 positive Note: test is not specific due to high prevalence (10%) of HLA-B27 positive in general population	X-ray films show definitive sacroiliitis CT scans of SI joint more sensitive, but less discriminating Bone scans somewhat helpful SPECT and MRI about 50% accurate only Later in the course, "bamboo" appearance on plain x-rays	Most common of the seronegative spondylo-arthropathies Occasionally, symptoms include peripheral joints Late presentation includes respiratory compromise and unmovable back
Psoriatic arthritis	Usually seen in older patients with skin changes typical of psoriasis over elbow or knees	No specific laboratory tests Can find increase in ESR levels and anemia	Look for peripheral joint involvement Findings similar to Reiter syndrome	Found in 5–7% of patients with psoriasis
Reactive spondyloarthropathies				
Reiter syndrome	Reiter is very common in males Usually, pain is located in lumbar spine, and legs Look for mucocutaneous lesions of the mouth, genitals, palms, soles, and nails	ESR can be elevated but variable Synovial fluid analysis shows elevated WBC count	SI joint inflammation on CT scan	SI joint is the most common site of pain
Enteropathic arthritis	Symptoms of reactive arthritis associated with inflammatory bowel disease	No specific laboratory tests	No specific radiographic tests	Enteropathic arthritis is a form of reactive spondylitis and sacroiliitis
RA	Symptoms can affect the entire spine because of spondyloarthropathy Cervical area is most commonly affected Typical patient is female, young to middle age Patient usually has morning stiffness, weight loss, fatigue, and low-grade fever	Anemia Elevated ESR levels 80% of patients have a positive rheumatoid factor Synovial fluid analysis shows elevated WBC counts, decreased viscosity, low glucose	Plain x-ray films of peripheral joints Periarticular joint swelling Osteopenia In the cervical spine, late findings include atlantoaxial subluxation and multiarticular changes	See text Peripheral joints affected first, which are swollen, tender to palpation, joints boggy to palpation Course of RA is highly variable
Myofascial pain	Regional or localized muscle or ligament pain Often associated with history of trauma Loss of range of motion in the extremity is an important finding	No specific laboratory tests	No specific radiographic tests	See Chapter 15 Presence of trigger points is diagnostic

CT, computed tomography; ESR, erythrocyte sedimentation rate; MRI, magnetic resonance imaging; RA, rheumatoid arthritis; SI, sacroiliac; SPECT, single photon emission computed tomography; WBC, white blood cell.

Table 13-7. Nonmechanical Conditions That Cause Spinal Pain.

Diagnosis	Clinical findings	Laboratory tests	Imaging studies	Comments
Fibromyalgia	Diffuse myofascial-like pain	No specific findings	Not helpful No specific findings	See Chapter 15 for further information
Neoplastic disease	Back pain is the presenting symptom in 90% of patients Pain is often indolent and unresponsive to rest Pain most severe at night Later in course, neurologic findings become common History of recent weight loss	Elevated ESR, WBC counts, serum calcium and uric acid levels Serum or urine electrophoresis for paraproteins diagnostic for multiple myeloma	Early-on metastasis may not be seen with plain films Bone scans positive in 85% of patients MRI can be diagnostic even when bone scans or plain films are normal	Presence of neoplastic disease is correlated with low back pain lasting longer than 1 month, history of cancer, age older than 50 years, failure to improve with conservative therapy, elevated ESR level, and anemia
Spinal infections	New onset of acute back pain in patients with history of recent infection, fever or severe pain at rest	Obtain an ESR level if patient has possible history, even if patient does not have a fever	Plain film findings lag significantly behind initial presentation MRI or CT scanning is imaging of choice Look for disk collapse	Osteomyelitis and discitis produce radiographic changes Epidural infections are sometimes difficult to diagnose Epidural abscess is a surgical emergency
Vascular problems, such as aneurysm, epidural hematoma, psoas muscle bleeds	50% of patients with abdominal aortic aneurysm complain of acute pain Pain may radiate to hips Look for hemodynamic instability Mass may be palpable Consider epidural hematoma with a history of trauma, anticoagulation therapy, or spinal block; focal spinal pain that is not relieved by rest Psoas muscle bleed associated with pain on extension of the hip	No specific laboratory tests	Outline of aneurysm may be seen on plain films CT scan is often definitive For epidural hematomas, MRI is definitive	Epidural hematomas are rare causes of back pain If not diagnosed promptly, irreversible neurologic injury can occur

(Continued)

Table 13–7. Nonmechanical Conditions That Cause Spinal Pain. (*Continued*)

Diagnosis	Clinical findings	Laboratory tests	Imaging studies	Comments
Hematologic inherited hemoglobin-opathies	History of these conditions	Hemoglobin electrophoresis proving presence	Possible confirmation of bony infarcts Presence does not prove or disprove presence of pain	Often very few objective findings with acute pain episode
Endocrine or metabolic				
Osteoporosis	Pain often has acute onset and is very severe, gradually diminishing over a few months Spontaneous 46% of time Trivial trauma in 36% of patients Found in postmenopausal women and in persons with genetic disorders	No specific blood tests	Radiographic imaging for fractures Bone scan for determining age of fractures Various approaches to determine presence of osteoporosis	Patient demographics for risk factors include, history of smoking, alcohol intake, nutrition history, and medication history
Paget disease	Rarely has pain	Elevated alkaline phosphatase	Characteristic finding on plain x-ray films of skull or long bones	May be familial Treatment may include calcitonin or bisphosphonates in symptomatic disease
Referred pain	History specific for conditions Consider if colicky pain, periodicity with menstrual cycle, atypical presentations Histories of visceral problems are helpful	Laboratory testing for diagnosing specific conditions	Radiographic imaging for diagnosing specific conditions	Colicky type of pain very uncommon from back
Mechanical causes of spinal pain	Increase of pain with postures that increase pressure on spine, such as sitting, maintaining a posture for a long time, stretching of injured tissues Look for increase of pain with specific movements	Laboratory tests usually not helpful Helpful to rule out other causes	Plain radiographs are not very helpful MRI and other testing may show changes, but poor correlation with etiology of pain	See Figure 13–1

[a]Examples include sickle cell anemia, sickle cell hemoglobin-c disease, and sickle cell β-thalassemia.
CT, computed tomography; ESR, erythrocyte sedimentation rate; MRI, magnetic resonance imaging; WBC, white blood cell.

MRI or CT scan is confirmatory. Myofascial pain, degenerative spine disease, foraminal stenosis, epidural fibrosis, and even peripheral neuropathies should also be part of the differential diagnosis for this type of clinical presentation.

Spinal Stenosis

The long-term degenerative changes of the intervertebral disks leads to significant changes in the loading and stress of movement in the facet joints, postural muscles, and ligaments of the spine. Once begun, these processes can lead to spine instability and further mechanical disruption, which also eventually extends to neighboring vertebral bodies. Early in the course of spinal stenosis, the neuroforamen remain open with extension but narrow with flexion. At this stage, patients will only report pain with flexion. The continued trauma can lead to spinal nerve adhesions causing traction on the nerve root resulting in pain. Reparative processes lead to new bone growth resulting in spurring, calcification of ligaments, narrowing of the spinal canal and the neuroforamen. If the narrowing continues, the spinal stenosis can become critical, which leads to neurogenic claudication. Congenital spinal stenosis that is rarely significant at a younger age places a patient at higher risk for developing clinical significant symptoms later in life. Patients often report low back pain, either intermittent or constant, that may radiate to one or both legs. Pain is increased with ambulation and decreased by rest. Pain is relieved by rest or lying down. Critical spinal stenosis leads to a feeling of leg heaviness and diffuse anterior thigh numbness and occasional pain. The classic description of neurogenic claudication by a patient is calf pain relieved by rest and ambulation distance improved by a hunched forward gait facilitated by a cane, walker or grocery cart. The disease may or may not be progressive. On physical examination, neurologic changes may or may not be present. CT and MRI scans confirm the diagnosis; CT scanning shows the bony elements best, and MRI visualizes the microelements better. Significant spinal stenosis can also be caused by spondylolisthesis. The pain arises from either disk pathology or the posterior longitudinal ligament through shearing forces because of abnormal movement. Instability of the vertebral body only worsens the clinical picture. Flexion and extension films showing the pathologic movement confirms this diagnosis.

Facet Joint Pain

The dual facet joints found superior and inferior on each vertebral body form the basic articulation surface along with the intervertebral disk that allows spinal column movement. The facet joint is a true diarthroidal joint with articular cartilage and a synovial capsule that is richly innervated with nociceptors. Thus, the facet joint has the potential of significant pain, although making a clinical diagnosis remains very difficult and controversial. Despite the importance of the facet joint in spinal mechanics, the true incidence of pain from this structure remains unknown. As with all synovial joints, chronic inflammation and stresses that come from change in articulation forces as seen with disk degeneration lead to loss of articular surface and potentially chronic pain. Further deterioration leads to abnormal motion, subluxation and increased instability, eventually evolving into spondylolisthesis. Synovial cysts with nerve irritation or compression can also lead to radicular pain. In addition, the sclerosis induced by this process can lead to foraminal stenosis and or even spinal canal stenosis. Because of the proximity to the spinal foramen, inflammation, instability, and stenosis can lead to either local or radicular pain patterns. Patients with facet joint pain often report nonspecific back pain radiating at times to buttocks and even down the legs stopping at the knees. Pain is increased with rotation of the back, standing erect, spine extension, and lying prone. Neurologic examination is normal. Paravertebral muscle tenderness can also be elicited by palpation. Radiographic examination is not diagnostic. Single photon emission computed tomography (SPECT) scanning may be helpful for detecting inflammation involving the joints. The only definitive way to diagnose facet joint pain is selective joint injection using local anesthetic and radiographic guidance.

Postspinal Surgery Pain

Persistent pain after back surgery is commonly seen in pain management centers. This diagnosis applies to those patients in whom an appropriate diagnostic workup has been done and no other new or recurrent disease can be identified. The etiology of postspinal surgery pain remains unknown, but proposed causes include the following:

1. Continued degenerative process from the altered surgical anatomy
2. Surgical nerve trauma
3. Traction on neural elements from scar tissue
4. Persistent pain secondary to central sensitization

Patients presenting with this syndrome often give a history of short-term relief from the original surgery followed by reoccurrence. Patients also report multiple surgical procedures because of failed fusions and persistent or recurrent disk pathology. The pain is often described in terms that suggest a neuropathic component. Since the clinical picture is often one of longstanding pain, severe deconditioning and psychological comorbidities are commonly seen. Pain is continuous and seems to be independent of activity. MRI with gadolinium enhancement usually confirms the presence of epidural scarring. Whether the epidural scarring and the persistent pain are causally related remains unproven.

Myofascial Back Pain

Low back pain from a primary injury to the back muscles and ligaments is thought to be a very common cause of back pain. Patients usually report localized symptoms caused by either an associated increase in activity from their usual norm or from acute injury. On examination, muscle tenderness and spasm are usually noted with decreased range of motion. Trigger points may also be palpable. No neurologic changes are noted. The patient with involvement of the piriformis muscle may report radicular symptoms. Patients with a history of diminished activity are at higher risk for this type of injury. However, when no clear cause can be found, nonspecific back pain is often the diagnosis in many patients.

Table 13–8 summarizes the different mechanical causes of spinal pain as well as the clinical presentation and imaging findings that can be used to further confirm the diagnosis.

Hip & Sacroiliac Joint Pathology

Both the hip and sacroiliac (SI) joints are often an unrecognized source of pain attributed to the back pain. Table 13–9 describes clinical considerations useful in the diagnosis.

Psychological Aspects of Back Pain

Longstanding chronic back pain often has a significant psychological component, which can impact the diagnostic workup, prognosis, and treatment. A chronic back pain history should also include a patient's mood, work history (if relevant), family dynamics, and any potential for secondary gain. Because of the nonspecific nature of back pain, a patient's level of pain is often called into question. Waddell signs have often been used to verify a patient's back pain complaints. The presence of Waddell signs should not interfere with the therapeutic relationship between physician and patient. The presence of three or more Waddell signs can be indicative of significant psychological distress. The five Waddell criteria follow:

1. Abnormal tenderness on patient evaluation, such as subcutaneous tenderness.
2. Abnormal results after performing orthopedic maneuvers, such as rotation of the shoulder reproduces sciatica, pressure on head producing back pain.
3. Evidence of distractibility (eg, ability to perform a specific maneuver without pain when position

changes; positive straight leg-raising test, but the patient is able to sit on the side of the bed with legs dangling).
4. Nonphysiologic weakness or sensory disturbance or give way weakness on muscle strength testing.
5. Overall patient reaction to physical examination of painful areas with embellishment of their symptoms.

Carragee EJ et al. Diagnostic evaluation of low back pain. *Orthop Clin North Am.* 2004;35:7. [PMID: 15062713]

Klauser A et al. Inflammatory low back pain: high negative predictive value of contrast-enhanced color Doppler ultrasound in the detection of inflamed sacroiliac joints. *Arthritis Rheum.* 2005;53:440. [PMID: 15934066]

Onesti ST. Failed back syndrome. *Neurologist.* 2004;10:259. [PMID: 15335443]

Waddell G. Subgroups within "nonspecific" low back pain. *J Rheumatol.* 2005;32:395. [PMID: 15742427]

Waddell G et al. Observation of overt pain behaviour by physicians during routine clinical examination of patients with low back pain. *J Psychosom Res.* 1992;36:77. [PMID: 1531680]

DIAGNOSTIC APPROACH TO BACK PAIN

In general, mechanical back pain located in the lumbar and lower thoracic regions is associated with a change in posture. In higher areas of the back, movement or traction on the involved area induces pain. Commonly, mechanical pain is increased with loading of the back. Usually, postures such as sitting are more painful than standing. Lying down typically improves the pain in mechanical spine disorders. Figure 13–1 presents a stepwise diagnostic approach to mechanical back pain. This diagnostic algorithm (see end of chapter) can be very helpful in determining most causes of back pain. Because of the presence of multiple different causes or nondiagnostic clinical histories, physical examinations, or radiographic imaging, some back pain needs to be investigated further. Diagnostic procedures can be helpful in these situations to further refine the diagnosis and focus therapy that is likely to be more effective. Occasionally, diagnostic procedures can serve a dual purpose of providing therapy as well (see Treatment section below).

Diagnostic Procedures

Because of the difficulty in diagnosing the source of a patient's back pain, considerable interest has always been expressed in selective neural blockade for more definitive diagnosis. Typically, a diagnostic procedure (with the exception of discography) consists of inserting a needle that is guided radiographically to the area believed to be responsible for the patient's pain; local anesthetic and corticosteroid (to enhance the analgesia and potentially provide long-term relief) are then injected. Using

Table 13–8. Mechanical Causes of Back Pain.

Source of pain	Clinical presentation	Imaging studies	Comments
Intervertebral disk	Pain can be sudden or gradual, often associated with an inciting event Patient may report an audible noise with onset of pain Pain is central and often radiates in the involved dermatome Loading and maintenance of posture increases pain, flexion limited by pain Internal disk disruption is thought to be a cause of nonradiating back pain	In the absence of "red flags," imaging is usually not required Disk degeneration and protrusion is found in 64% of the general population without pain Provocative discography with or without CT scan be useful for diagnosing internal disk disruption	Acute episodes usually improve over several weeks Often there are recurrences. 90% of patients improve; 10% become chronic
Facet joint	Cannot be reliably diagnosed clinically Pain is usually lateralized to the paraspinal areas, increased by extension, lateral flexion, or rotation to the painful side Pain is increased with posture changes	Facet joint changes seen on imaging have no meaningful correlation with patient's pain complaints Bone or SPECT scan may be more helpful Diagnosis can only be made with fluoroscopic-controlled facet injections	Difficult to make a diagnosis Accounts for pain in 15–20% of patients
Spinal stenosis	Generally affects older population History of recurrent or chronic pain Pain aching, paresthesias, heaviness in the legs with walking Rapid improvement in symptoms with sitting, stooping, or flexion of back	Plain films show spinal stenosis Differential with vascular claudication by angiograms or other noninvasive vascular testing	Improved walking tolerance with uphill incline, pushing a grocery cart, or using a walker.
Paraspinal muscles	Pain vague or diffuse, aching quality Muscles may have palpable tenderness, presence of trigger points Muscles exhibit loss of flexibility	Not helpful	Pain often improved by rest and standing Clear role of paraspinal muscles in spinal pain is unknown
Spondylolysis and spondylolisthesis	History and physical examination is not very helpful for a specific diagnosis Pain increased by extension and improved with flexion	Necessary for diagnosis	In young patient, may be secondary to acute stress fracture
Adhesive arachnoiditis	History of spinal surgery, trauma, spinal infection, disk herniation or spinal bleeds Pain often has elements of both neuropathic and musculoskeletal pain May have varying degrees of numbness, which is nondermatomal and patchy	MRI may show clumping of nerve fibers or adhesive arachnoiditis or both	Presence of arachnoiditis does not prove patient has pain
Other sources of spinal pain	Joint pathology and bursitis in areas near the spine can mimic spinal pain Physical examination findings include localized tenderness and restriction of range of motion in shoulder or hip joints Bilateral symptoms are a "red flag" and should be more thoroughly investigated	Radiographic findings show joint pathology, which should suggest the possibility of arthritis. Not as helpful for bursitis or myofascial pain	In patients with degenerative arthritis of the spine it is not uncommon to have hip or shoulder pathology as well Myofascial pains such as piriformis syndrome can simulate radiculopathy

CT, computed tomography; MRI, magnetic resonance imaging; SPECT, single photon emission computed tomography.

Table 13–9. Clinical Considerations for SI and Hip Joint Pain.

Source of pain	Clinical presentation	Imaging studies	Comments
SI joint	Radiates pain often into ipsilateral buttock, posterior thigh, and groin Pain is reproduced by pressure over joint, forced flexion on the involved side along with the extension and abduction of the contralateral side Despite this, physical examination is not very reliable for this diagnosis	Often not helpful Poor correlation with radiographic findings and pain Pain is often not from joint but from ligaments and tissues stabilizing the joint	Often unrecognized source of low back pain
Hip joint pathology	Usually pain radiates to the groin or to the knee May produce an antalgic gait sufficient to produce back pain, and in later stages causes dysfunction of the joints of the back	Plain films or MRI of joint usually definitive Bone scan may be confirmatory	Internal and external rotation of the joint may reproduce the pain

MRI, magnetic resonance imaging; SI, sacroiliac.

the patient's report of pain relief as a guide, a diagnosis is then made that would allow more specific treatment or help plan a surgical procedure, if needed. Although this idea is very attractive, a consensus on the reliability and specificity of these procedures remain illusive. Several factors may be present that call into question the diagnostic validity of these procedures:

1. Pain is a subjective complaint. Many different factors in a patient's background can influence reporting relief. In addition, these procedures are rarely placebo-controlled. Physician misperception of what the patient is reporting may also contribute to the unreliability of the diagnostic procedure.

2. Pain may be episodic, and therefore, the nerve block may be falsely reported as helpful when it is not.

3. There have been suggestions that local anesthetic deposited distally to the pain generator may also provide analgesia via antidromic spread.

4. Despite radiographic control with the use of contrast, there still is potential of spread to surrounding areas affected by the pathologic process, leading to false-positive results.

5. Pain pathways are not necessarily hard-wired; the nervous system is capable of central sensitization and forming new pathways for nociception. Diagnostic neural blockade in this situation leads to an incomplete understanding of the neural anatomy.

These caveats should not lead to the conclusion that diagnostic nerve blocks have no usefulness. Caution should be used in interpreting the results, as with any diagnostic test. Most procedures used for treatment of back pain have a dual use, with the exception of discography (see Treatment section below).

Discography

Because of the poor correlation of radiographic imaging for discogenic pain, discography has been advocated as the definitive test. Radiographic guidance along with contrast can define a painful disk and provide information regarding abnormal structural anatomy. Changes in contrast spread along with the patient's pain report can be used to identify a diseased disk. In addition, discography may be used to complement other tests, such as myelogram or event MRI. Discography can also be used to define a painful disk when other imaging options, such as MRI in failed spinal surgery, are nonspecific. Multilevel positive discography can be suggestive of poor outcomes for fusion surgery as well. Injection of the disk with a corticosteroid has also been noted to have therapeutic value, although with an increased risk of disk infection.

The components of the normal lumbar disk are made of gelatinous nucleus pulposis and outer dense laminated fibroelastic layer known as the annulus fibrosis. Unlike the cervical area, the facet joints in the lumbar area do not protect the nerve roots. Therefore, a posterior and lateral herniation of the disk with impingement of the spinal nerves is not uncommon. Discography is indicated when traditional diagnostic approaches, such as imaging studies and electromyography, have failed to determine

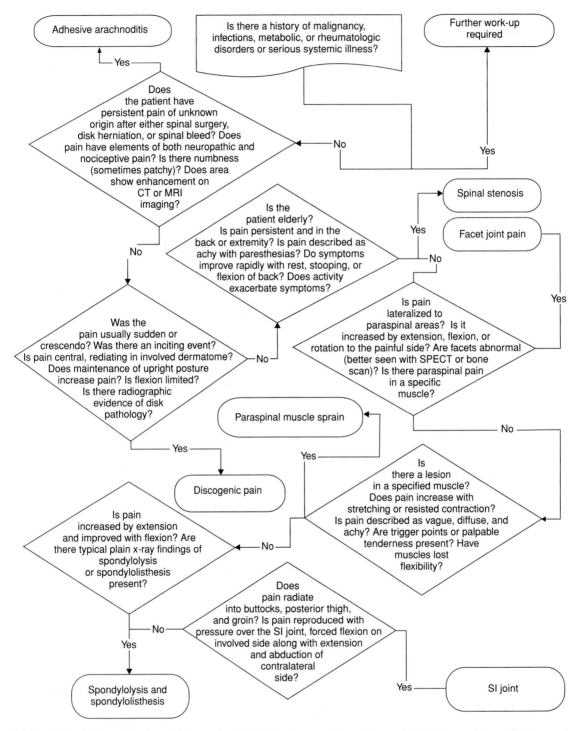

Figure 13–1. Diagnostic approach to mechanical back pain. Complete history and physical examination fail to reveal "red flags". CT, computed tomography; MRI, magnetic resonance imaging; SPECT, single photon emission computed tomography.

a cause of persistent pain. Discography seeks to provoke pain that reproduces the patient's pain complaint; this is known as concordant pain. Discordant pain is pain that does not simulate the patient's pain. The procedure should be done on at least three levels, including an asymptomatic level for a control. For the procedure, water-soluble contrast is used to identify the appropriate needle location. Resistance to injection is noted, along with any pain that the patient reports. A healthy disk is not painful, and some resistance is normal.

A syringe attached to a pressure manometer is often used to avoid over pressurization of the disk. The limit should be 100 mm Hg. Based on the patient's pain report, a second control disk is injected. If failure to elicit pain or discordant pain is reported, other levels may be done to identify the painful disk. Postprocedure CT scan can detect extravasation of contrast indicating a torn annulus. Although there are many variations of this procedure, the patient is placed in a prone oblique position. Under radiographic guidance, a 7-inch 22-gauge needle is inserted 1.5 inches from the midline and just below the level of the spinous process. Care should be taken to avoid advancement through the disk. Anteroposterior and lateral views are continuously obtained to ensure appropriate placement. A more lateral approach can facilitate the procedure in patients with extensive facet joint arthritic changes or significant disk degeneration. The L5–S1 disk is sometimes difficult to reach especially in females. If necessary, a paramedian or transthecal approach can be used at this level.

Antibiotic prophylaxis is mandatory for this procedure. Some experienced practitioners suggest intradiscal antibiotic either in addition to or instead of intravenous prophylaxis. In patients who are not allergic, cefoxitin is the preferred antibiotic because of its ability to penetrate the disk and its coverage of *Staphylococcus epidermidis*.

Pain secondary to the procedure is the most common complication and is usually self-limited. Other, more significant complications include discitis, trauma to the nerve roots, local damage to blood vessels, and even epidural hematoma.

Selective Nerve Root Injections

Selective nerve root injections have been used for a long time for both therapeutic and diagnostic goals (see Treatment section below).

Facet Joint Injections

Facet joint injections have been advocated as a significant treatment of mechanical back pain (see Treatment section below). Guided injections into facet joints with or without placebo injections have been suggested as a diagnostic tool. Minimal support for this approach for surgical decisions is found in the literature. As a diagnos-

tic tool for radiofrequency procedures, this procedure has considerably more support.

Atlas SJ et al. Evaluation and treatment of low back pain: an evidence-based approach to clinical care. *Muscle Nerve.* 2003;27:265. [PMID: 12635113]

Cohen SP et al. Lumbar discography: a comprehensive review of outcome studies, diagnostic accuracy, and principles. *Reg Anesth Pain Med.* 2005;30:163. [PMID: 15765459]

Onesti ST. Failed back syndrome. *Neurologist.* 2004;10:259. [PMID: 15335443]

Pang WW et al. Selective lumbar spinal nerve block, a review. *Acta Anaesthesiol Sin.* 1999;37:21. [PMID: 10407523]

Tuite MJ. Facet joint and sacroiliac joint injection. *Semin Roentgenol.* 2004;39:37. [PMID: 14976836]

Yuan PS et al. Nonsurgical and surgical management of lumbar spinal stenosis. *Instr Course Lect.* 2005;54:303. [PMID: 15948458]

TREATMENT

Despite reports of severe pain, most spinal pain is self-limited. In the absence of "red flags," treatment should consist of appropriate medications for both neuropathic and nociceptive elements. Consensus recommendations based on the guidelines published by the Agency for Healthcare Research and Quality suggest a limited role for bed rest. Prolonged bed rest has no place in the treatment of spinal pain. Disuse muscle atrophy and generalized deconditioning can quickly develop, making treatment much more difficult.

Patient activity is often limited because of pain, so sufficient analgesia becomes extremely important to maintain appropriate activity. The management of chronic back pain treatment is based on the following three principles:

1. **Management of the nociception.** Sufficient analgesia using medications, procedures, or both is fundamental for improving a patient's rehabilitative potential and restoration of activity. A general consensus exists regarding the use of a treatment continuum for back pain. In general, medication is tried first (Table 13–10), with procedures reserved for nonresponsive patients. Interventional therapies are generally considered prior to irreversible neurolytic procedures.

2. **Psychological and behavioral therapies.** Chronic pain with all of its losses is commonly associated with comorbid disorders of depression and anxiety. In addition, premorbid psychological diagnosis that is inhibiting return to function also should be treated. See Table 13–11 for an overview.

3. **Rehabilitation.** Longstanding pain is commonly associated with deconditioning. A comprehensive rehabilitation program that does more than just focus on a specific site of pain is extremely important for restoration of function. See Table 13–12 for selected rehabilitative therapies.

Table 13–10. Pharmacologic Management of Back Pain.

Drug class	Examples	Mechanism of action	Uses for pain management	Discussion
Opioids	Multiple different compounds, such as morphine, fentanyl, hydromorphone, hydrocodone, oxycodone	Primary analgesic action is on the μ receptor	Primary role in acute cancer pain Adjuvant role in neuropathic pain	Dependence liability with long-term use Careful patient selection is needed
Nonopioids	Acetaminophen	Possible COX-3 receptor effect	As primary analgesic or in combination with opioids	Concerns about liver toxicity in long-term use and interactions with alcohol
NSAIDs	Both mixed NSAIDs and selective COX-2 inhibitor	Both a peripheral and central effect to varying degrees	Nociceptive pain, possible use in neuropathic pain	Caution in patients with cardiovascular disease
Psychotropics	Psychostimulants Antipsychotics Benzodiazepines	Different mechanisms	Adjuvant role as antiemetic Helpful for sedation and delirium	Little use in mechanical low back pain
Anticonvulsants	Most useful first-generation includes carbamazepine Second-generation includes gabapentin, pregabalin, lamotrigine, topiramate, and oxcarbazazepine	Increase in inhibitory transmitters, sodium channel blockade, and others	Neuropathic pain Possible role as adjuvant in acute pain	50% of patients with back pain are estimated to have a neuropathic component
Membrane stabilizing agents	Local anesthetics Mexiletine	Sodium channel blockade	Neuropathic pain	Not effective for radiculopathies
Topical medications	Various OTC drugs Lidocaine patch Doxepin Capsaicin TCAs Compounded drugs	Topical anesthetics Substance P depletion	Localized hyperalgesia	Anecdotal evidence for back pain
NMDA antagonists	Ketamine Dextromethorphan Memantine	NMDA receptor	Potential opioid analgesia Neuropathic pain Modulate opioid tolerance	Anecdotal evidence for back pain
Muscle relaxants	Baclofen Diazepam and other benzodiazepines Carisoprodol Chlorzoxazone Metaxalone Methocarbamol Orphenadrine Clonidine Tizanidine Cyclobenzaprine	Various mechanisms Usually attributed to a central effect	Acute myofascial pain syndromes	Anecdotal evidence for chronic back pain Carisoprodol may have dependence liability
α-Agonists	Clonidine Tizanidine	Enhance opioid analgesia Helpful for withdrawal symptoms	Headache and neuropathic pain	Tizanidine has muscle relaxant abilities in chronic back pain
Antidepressants	TCAs SNRIs SSRIs	Blockade of norepinephrine and serotonin reuptake. They each have demonstrated analgesic effect.	Generalized analgesic, specifically helpful with neuropathic pain	Potentially helpful for psychological comorbidities

COX, cyclooxygenase; NMDA, *N*-methyl-D-aspartate; NSAIDs, nonsteroidal anti-inflammatory drugs; OTC, over-the-counter; SNRI, serotonin–norepinephrine reuptake inhibitors; SSRIs, selective serotonin reuptake inhibitors; TCA, tricyclic antidepressants.

Table 13–11. Overview of Psychological Therapies.

Therapy	Description
Hypnosis and visualization	The patient is taught to visualize relaxing mental images, such as a secluded beach or peaceful meadow This helps decrease anxiety and facilitates deep relaxation
Guided imagery	Directed visualization focusing on specific psychological issues using pain-decreasing images
Biofeedback	Relaxation technique to measure a physiologic phenomenon, such as muscle tension, and to provide an audible or visual feedback indicating a state of relaxation
Cognitive-behavioral therapy	This teaches various techniques, such as distraction training, cognitive restructuring, role-playing, or mental imagery
Group therapies	When well-planned and with appropriate patient dynamics, group therapy is very helpful The interaction is planned to share important breakthroughs in insight, discuss progress with treatment, and different strategies for overcoming everyday obstacles to improvement
Family therapy	Patients and their families often feel angry with each other The family can be a significant stressor but is an important source of support that is needed for progress This approach attempts to bring insight on how to provide support without enabling continued disability

Table 13–12. Rehabilitative Therapies Useful for Back Pain.

Rehabilitative therapy	Description of treatment and goals
Modalities, such as heat, ice, ultrasound	These are temporary short-lasting therapies and therefore should only be used as adjuvant to an active rehabilitation
Stretching	Mild and controlled stretching prepares the patient for further activity Care should be taken to avoid injuring tight muscles that have not been active for a long time
Cardiovascular exercise	Patients with chronic pain are very often deconditioned. A general aerobic program can increase endurance and activity tolerance. Aerobic exercise has antidepressant effects.
Work conditioning	This is a specific program that is used to prepare patient for return to work A job description is obtained, and the goals of therapy should lead to the physical demands of that type of work
Strength training	This is usually focused on the site that was significantly weakened by the original insult This approach is also used to train alternate muscle to supplement the site of original injury Care should be taken to keep the goals realistic and avoid further injury
Orthotics and prosthetics	Adaptive aids are often very useful for return to function The benefits of truly understanding a patient's impairments and creatively designing adaptive aids can be very helpful in enhancing function

Table 13–13. Procedure Efficacy and Diagnosis.

Diagnosis	Epidural steroid injection	Facet joint or medial bundle branch injection	Spinal cord stimulation
Discogenic pain	++		
Herniated disk	+++		
Spinal stenosis	+++	+	+
Foraminal stenosis	+	++	+
Facet arthropathy	++	+++	
Myofasical pain			
Failed spinal surgery			++

Key: +, minimal effectiveness and diagnostic usefulness; ++, moderate effectiveness and diagnostic usefulness; +++, very effective and diagnostically useful.

1. Therapeutic Procedures

Multiple different procedures are known to be effective in mechanical back pain. Because of the overlap of pathology that is commonly seen in patients with mechanical back pain, efficacy of a procedure is sometimes used to establish a diagnosis (Table 13–13).

Procedures are often used to treat back pain. As both the structural and neuroanatomy have become better understood, many new procedures have been developed to treat back pain. Considerable controversy exists regarding how and when to use many of these procedures. Procedures are often introduced for widespread use before they have been sufficiently studied. In addition, because of the significant variability in presentation, studies of outcomes of treatment approaches in the medical literature are often difficult to interpret. When to use a procedure and what symptoms respond the best as well as the efficacy in various conditions remain unclear. In a recent review of 15,000 studies and 150 expert reviews using criteria that controlled for methodologic quality, only two procedures had enough literature support to definitively determine whether benefit was obtained. This review showed that epidural steroid injections showed short-term benefit, and spinal cord stimulation had a lack of overall benefit despite many studies showing that 50% improvement was noted in 50% of patients at 5 years. Yet, all pain practitioners know patients who have derived long-term benefits from the large variety of procedures. This discrepancy can only be explained by what has been known for a long time. As the specificity and selectivity of available procedures increase, the need to understand the patient and make an accurate diagnosis is paramount. The key points in using procedures to treat pain are patient selection; making an accurate diagnosis along with determining what the pain generator is in each patient; and avoidance of repeated procedures, which provide little or no long-term response.

Epidural Steroid Injections

A. Indications

Administration of a combination of depot steroid injections and local anesthetic is helpful in a variety of conditions including radiculopathies, localized nonradiating spine pain, spondylosis, vertebral compression fractures, postherpetic neuralgias, and malignant pain syndromes secondary to localized metastasis.

Usually, a series of three injections are performed 1 month apart. For patients with partial relief, an evaluation should be undertaken before each injection to determine whether additional injections are needed. There is no evidence to suggest that more than three injections are of additional benefit within a 6-month period. For patients reporting continued pain, a comprehensive evaluation should be undertaken with reevaluation of the treatment plan.

B. Complications

Epidural steroid injections should not be performed in the presence of local or systemic infections. Coagulation status must be normal to avoid epidural hematoma. Despite these precautions, epidural infection and hematoma can still occur. Other serious complications can include spinal cord injury and total spinal anesthesia with resultant respiratory depression, hypotension, and cardiovascular collapse. Unrecognized intravenous injections leading to local anesthetic toxicity of the central nervous system, heart arrhythmias, and even complete atony have occurred. Less serious complications include persistent paresthesia and worsened of the pain from needle trauma. Inadvertent dural puncture is a common complication with an incidence of at least 1% in experienced hands. Concerns have been expressed periodically regarding potential detrimental effects of corticosteroids on the meninges leading to arachnoiditis. Despite many years of experience, no association has been documented.

Systemic corticosteroid absorption can have detrimental effects on patients with diabetic tendency. In addition, the potential of adrenal gland suppression should also be kept in mind. Adrenocortical suppression is certainly possible and is one of the limiting factors for repeating this procedure.

C. Evidence for Efficacy

Epidural steroid injection is one of the most common procedures done for back pain. There is substantial evidence for at least short-term efficacy in the treatment of radiculopathies. Other nonmalignant conditions have less support, with mainly expert opinion and case series found in the literature. For malignant pain syndromes, epidural injections have been shown to be effective in cohort studies and case series. Patients with subacute back and leg pain are thought to be the ideal candidates. Efficacy is also better in patients without previous surgery. Patients with leg pain only have the best long-term outcomes. Patients with spinal stenosis usually have a less favorable prognosis, unless there is an acute increase in recent pain. Patients with preexisting psychosocial issues may have a less favorable outcome.

Caudal Epidural Injection

The entrance to the caudal canal is found through the sacral hiatus. This hiatus is formed in the midline by the incomplete fusion of the posterior elements of S4 and S5. The sacrococcygeal ligament covers this U-shaped area and is a landmark guiding needle placement.

Lumbar Selective Nerve Root Injection

A. Anatomy

The lumbar nerves exit the intraspinal canal through their respective foramen, which are located immediately below the transverse process. The nerve divides almost immediately and gives off a branch to the adjacent facet joint. The paravertebral nerve also gives off branches to the sympathetic chain. The spinal nerve is accessible for blockade just distal to the spinal foramen.

B. Indications

Neuropathic pain syndromes with etiologies such as herniated disk or malignant tumors will respond to this block. In addition, this procedure is used to diagnose pain conditions of the chest wall and lower abdominal area.

C. Complications

Complications are usually rare. Intracord injections are rare. Occasionally, persistent paresthesias have been reported. Other complications include nerve root injury and intrathecal injection by errant needle placement or through a larger than expected dural cuff.

D. Evidence for Efficacy

There is substantial evidence for short-term efficacy for treatment of radiculopathies. Other nonmalignant conditions have less support, with mainly expert opinion and case series found in the literature. For malignant pain syndromes, epidural injections have been shown to have efficacy with cohort studies and case series published. The selective nature and radiographic guidance used in this procedure may improve response and efficacy rates. This procedure is also used as part of the presurgical evaluation of radiculopathy.

Sacral Nerve Root Injections

A. Anatomy

The sacrum is the terminal portion of the spine. It has a very irregular surface with four paired sacral foramina nerves. The five sacral nerves exit the spinal canal via the sacral hiatus. The sacral nerves provide sensation and motor innervation to the external anal sphincter and levator ani muscles. The second through the fourth sacral nerves provide the majority of sensation to pelvic viscera and external genitalia.

B. Indications

Sacral nerve root injections can be used to diagnose neuropathic conditions of the sacral nerves and treat pelvic pain syndromes as well as radiculopathies.

C. Technique

The sacral nerves can be blocked using a transforaminal approach with radiographic guidance; the beam is angled to visualize the approach through the posterior foramen. The needle is then inserted through the identified angle. A nonradiographic approach can also be used after identifying standard bony landmarks.

D. Evidence for Efficacy

Nerve root injections have been shown in case series to be effective for nerve compression symptoms involving the sacrum. This procedure can also be used as part of a diagnostic workup for back, SI joint pain, or hip joint pain.

Lumbar Facet Joint Injection

A. Anatomy

The facet joints are formed by the articulations of the superior and inferior articular facets of the lamina of the adjacent vertebrae. The joints are true synovial joints and extensively innervated. Each joint receives innervation from above and below as well as the level at which it is located.

B. INDICATIONS

Lumbar facet joint injection is indicated for paraspinal thoracic pain secondary to trauma from twisting, acceleration-deceleration injuries, fractures, and neoplasm.

C. TECHNIQUE

Lumbar facet joint injection must be done under fluoroscopic guidance. Two approaches are described, either injection into the capsule of the joint known as a medial bundle branch block (MBB) or intra-articular joint injection. Depending on the procedure, the fluoroscopic beam must be aligned obliquely to visualize the joint or be in the anteroposterior position for the MBB. The needle is advanced to the middle of the articular pillar where the medial branch passes. With the intra-articular procedure, the joint surfaces are visualized by an oblique position of the fluoroscopic camera.

D. EVIDENCE FOR EFFICACY

Numerous studies have shown efficacy for these procedures. No differences in outcomes have been documented for facet joint injections or MBBs. These injections have also been used to predict response to radiofrequency lesioning of MBB at the same levels.

Facet Joint Denervation

A. ANATOMY

The approach for facet joint denervation is essentially the same as the approach for an MBB.

B. INDICATIONS

Facet denervation is indicated for patients who have reported short-term pain relief with a local anesthetic injection using the procedure as described for an MBB. Using RFL or other denervation techniques, longer-term relief can be obtained.

C. TECHNIQUE

For all procedures, the needle is advanced under radiographic guidance. For lumbar denervation procedures, a needle is advanced to the junction of the superior articular and transverse process. Sensory testing to determine appropriate location of the needle as well as anteroposterior and lateral views of the needle are required. Denervation is usually done after injection of a small amount of local anesthetic.

D. EVIDENCE FOR EFFICACY

Many cohort studies and some randomized trials have provided evidence for efficacy.

Ablative Procedures for Discogenic Pain

Intradiscal electrothermaplasty (IDET), nucleoplasty, percutaneous disk decompression, and radiofrequency lesioning are all newly described procedures for discogenic back pain. Each procedure has different physiologic effects on the structure of the disk. In contrast to IDET, nucleoplasty as well as percutaneous decompression procedures improve radicular symptoms.

A. INDICATIONS

Ablative procedures are indicated for chronic discogenic back pain that has lasted for at least 6 months and for patients who have not had satisfactory improvement after an aggressive exercise program. The patient should have a complete examination of the source of pain, including MRI without nerve compression, as well as normal findings on neurologic examination. The patient should have proven concordant pain as determined by discography, ideally at one level only. These procedures are most often used for a single painful disk with a minimum of 50% preservation of normal height. Contraindications include inflammatory arthritis, anticoagulation therapy, advanced spinal disease, and segmental instability.

B. TECHNIQUE

The approach is essentially the same as discography. A 17-gauge needle is inserted to guide placement of a probe, which is placed into the nucleus pulposis. Occasionally, bilateral approaches are needed to cover the entire disk. Using either radiofrequency or a heating element, the collagen and nociceptors are denatured after careful placement. Company-specific equipment is required to perform IDET, with defined protocols on the length and level of energy programmed into the energy source. With the disk decompression procedure, a battery-operated device is inserted through the introducer needle that has been placed into the disk. The procedure is completed by turning on the device, which then mechanically decompresses the disk. Postprocedure rehabilitation is thought to be extremely important in successful outcomes.

C. COMPLICATIONS

The complications are similar to discography, with the additional risk of thermal damage to the spinal cord and the spinal nerves. Several cases have been reported where the catheter has broken inside the confines of the disk. No long-term complications have been reported by leaving the broken portion of the catheter in place.

D. EVIDENCE FOR EFFICACY

Several randomized studies and a number of short-term nonrandomized studies have shown efficacy. Long-term outcomes >1 year in patients receiving these procedures remain unknown. Some studies have shown that outcomes compare favorably to spinal fusion.

Vertebroplasty

A. ANATOMY

The relevant anatomy consists of the vertebral body, which is located between the disk spaces of the lumbar and thoracic spine. Little information exists regarding using this procedure in the cervical area.

B. INDICATIONS

Vertebroplasty is performed for compression fractures with loss of height in the vertebral column secondary to osteoporosis or malignancies.

C. TECHNIQUE

Vertebroplasty must be done under radiographic guidance. Often monitored anesthesia care or conscious sedation is required. There are two different types of vertebroplasty, using methyl-methacrylate alone or a balloon filled with methyl-methacrylate. The approach of this procedure depends on the location of the fracture. The usual approach in the thoracic spine involves placement through the vertebral lamina. In the lumbar area, the approach is paravertebrally directly into the body. A 17-gauge needle is inserted through the lamina into the vertebral body bilaterally. The needle then serves as a guide for the cannula, which is then inserted into the fracture. The cement is usually mixed with radio-opaque materials, such as barium, to allow for visualization. Cement volume is usually equally divided into bilateral injection sites, which prevents unequal height restoration. Cement volume can vary from 0.5 mL to 4.0 mL. Care should be taken to avoid increased injection pressures, which can lead to extrusion of the cement, which could lead to complications. Postprocedure CT scan is undertaken for verification of appropriate cement placement.

D. COMPLICATIONS

Many serious but rare complications have been reported for the methyl-methacrylate, including cement embolism, spinal cord injury by unrecognized injection into the epidural space, and somatic nerve injury from placement of the cannula.

E. EVIDENCE FOR EFFICACY

Many case series have reported efficacy for this procedure with long-term follow-up.

Intraspinal Neurolytic Procedures

A. ANATOMY

See description under nerve root injections, above.

B. INDICATIONS

Intraspinal neurolytic procedures are indicated for malignant conditions in patients with limited life-expectancy.

Care must be taken to carefully select patients in whom loss of motor function and loss of bowel or bladder control would not adversely affect their quality of life. This procedure has little place in the treatment of noncancer pain. Some investigators are advocating the use of pulse radiofrequency lesioning of the dorsal root ganglion in chronic radicular neuropathic pain syndromes.

C. TECHNIQUE

Neurolytic procedures on selected nerve roots can be done in patients with malignancies. Approaches include selective rhizotomies or neurolysis of the involved nerve root using either extradural or intradural techniques, most often done with radiographic guidance. Usually, the nerve root is first blocked with local anesthetic to determine pain relief potential and possible loss of function. The neurolytic procedure is then scheduled at a different time. For selective intrathecal rhizotomies, the patient is placed in a lateral position. When alcohol is used, the patient is positioned with the painful side up to allow for the hypobaric nature of alcohol. The volume of fluid used is specifically tailored to the levels required to achieve analgesia. High volumes can be used for patients in sitting positions to treat sacral nerve roots. Smaller volumes are needed for individual nerve root rhizotomies. These procedures should only be performed in extreme circumstances when adjacent to nerves controlling bowel, bladder, or limb function or in the upper cervical levels. For epidural procedures, the patient is often prone, and a catheter is placed at the appropriate level. Phenol is the preferred epidural neurolytic agent.

D. COMPLICATIONS

Unintended loss of function is the primary complication that may be minimized by using small volumes and carefully selecting patients. Proximity to areas of the spinal cord controlling limb function increases risk.

E. EVIDENCE FOR EFFICACY

There is substantial case experience in the literature to support use in cancer pain. There is very little evidence supporting the use of these procedures for chronic noncancer pain.

Epiduroscopy

A. ANATOMY

The most common entry point is the caudal canal. Please see caudal steroid injections for more details regarding the anatomy and technique.

B. INDICATIONS

Proponents of epiduroscopy suggest that direct visualization of the spinal canal can add an extra dimension to diagnosing spinal disease. The promise of a visually guided procedure would potentially increase the efficacy rates. In addition, spinal adhesions that are not able to be diagnosed by any other method could be seen and lysed by direct visualization.

C. Technique

The scope is inserted into the epidural space often using radiographic guidance through a previously placed cannula. Irrigation is used to improve visualization.

D. Complications

Complications are similar to other catheter procedures in the epidural space and include infection; bleeding, potentially leading to epidural hematomas and nerve compression; and nerve damage with permanent impairment of function. In addition to visualization of spinal pathology, a specialized technique using a wire reinforced catheter known as epidural lysis of adhesions has been described. This catheter can be placed either with an epidural needle or the epidural scope.

E. Evidence for Efficacy

There are no randomized prospective clinical trials available to verify the increased efficacy that proponents of this procedure suggest. With further development, this procedure and appropriate instruments hold the promise of a whole new approach to the treatment of difficult to manage chronic back pain.

Epidural Decompressive Neuroplasty

A. Anatomy

The relevant anatomy is the same for epidural catheter placement.

B. Indications

The procedure is indicated when adhesions of the epidural space are suspected, which can restrict movement or cause traction on the neural elements. Adhesions are thought to underlie some intractable chronic back pain. Previous surgery, trauma, or infection is thought to cause adhesions that are amenable to this procedure.

C. Technique

This procedure requires radiographic guidance, a specialized wire-wound epidural catheter, and contrast. With the patient typically under conscious sedation, the catheter is inserted into the epidural space at a location several vertebral bodies below the area of suspected disease. For lumbar procedures, the caudal canal is used. Corticosteroids, local anesthetics, and mild neurolytic solutions (such as hypertonic saline) have been advocated for this procedure.

D. Complications

Complications are similar to those described for epidural catheters. Neurolytic solutions and aggressive technique can damage the spinal cord and nerve roots.

E. Evidence for Efficacy

Large case series have reported improvement.

Sacroiliac Joint Injections

A. Anatomy

The SI joint is a synovial joint that forms the articular surface of the sacrum and ilium on either sides of the sacrum. This joint is irregular in contour and is matched on the ilium side with reciprocal irregularities. An articular capsule covers the joint and attaches to the periphery of the articular surfaces.

B. Indications

Injections are indicated for SI joint pain that is determined on physical examination. This procedure is also indicated as a diagnostic procedure for surgical intervention. The incidence of SI joint pain may be as high as 30% in patients reporting chronic low back pain.

C. Technique

Using radiographic guidance, the SI joint is identified. A 22-gauge needle is introduced about 2 cm medial at an angle into the joint. Placement can be confirmed by the use of contrast and anteroposterior and lateral views. Alternatively, CT scan can be used for confirmation of needle placement.

D. Complications

An increase in local pain is not uncommon. Local anesthetic can leak through the joint and anesthetize both sacral and lumbar somatic nerves.

E. Evidence for Efficacy

Numerous case series have confirmed short-term efficacy for the corticosteroid injection procedure. Radiofrequency lesioning of the joint has shown prolonged improvement in one case series.

Spinal Cord Stimulation

A. Anatomy

The bounds of the epidural space have been described above. Location of involved spinal nerves determines location of the stimulating electrodes in the epidural space.

B. Indications

Electrical stimulation of the central nervous system has long been used for analgesia in neuropathic pain states. Although many theories exist as to the mechanism of analgesia, frequency modulation of the central nervous system masking the neuropathic sensation is the leading explanation. Epidural placement of multielectrode arrays can be effective for a variety of conditions and are helpful for a diverse number of neuropathic pain conditions, including failed spinal surgery. Screening trials showing at least 50% efficacy is a very important prognostic factor for long-term efficacy. Preprocedure psychological evaluation is also considered to be helpful in screening of potential candidates.

C. TECHNIQUE

Epidural placement of the electrode is similar to the placement of epidural catheters. Trial stimulation determines efficacy prior to implantation of the system. Fastidious attention to the fixation of the electrode is important to avoid movement and to achieve long-term efficacy. Two types of pulse generators exist: an external system that relies on radiofrequency current for power and a battery-operated implantable pulse generator (IPG). The IPG portion of the device can be implanted either in the buttock (over the greater trochanter) or in the abdominal wall (most common).

D. COMPLICATIONS

Complications are very similar to epidural catheter placement. In addition, because of the presence of a foreign body, surgical infections commonly lead to explantation of the device. MRI imaging is contraindicated in patients with spinal cord stimulation. The battery life of an IPG is limited and requires replacement on exhaustion. Battery life depends on the current use, number of active electrodes, and both rate and pulse width settings of each patient. Superficial skin irritation can limit therapy in patients with radiofrequency devices. Other complications unique to this procedure include electrode migration or fracture with consequent loss of analgesia. Patients walking through some theft detectors have reported IPG interference.

E. EVIDENCE FOR EFFICACY

Patients who are candidates for this procedure often have not responded to other therapies. The increased sophistication of these devices with multiple electrode arrays and patient-programming options have continued to improve efficacy in well-selected patients who have realistic treatment goals.

Neuroaxial Infusion Systems

A. ANATOMY

Epidural infusion systems are generally used only for short-term relief. Intrathecal catheters and fully implanted pumps are generally used for long-term therapy. Intrathecal catheters can be directed toward the appropriate level within the spinal canal. Care must be taken to avoid damage to the spinal cord. Commonly these catheters are inserted using a modified epidural needle that should be placed below the level of termination of the spinal cord, which is at L1. Special circumstances can exist when this is not feasible, such as previous fusion surgery or other anatomic abnormalities.

B. INDICATIONS

Neuroaxial infusion systems are indicated for chronic intractable pain, which cannot be managed by more conventional means in a patient who is not a candidate for a surgical approach and who has responded poorly to oral medications. For noncancer pain, the most common indication is failed spinal surgery. As with spinal cord stimulation, patient selection is the key to long-term efficacy. Patients should have both a psychological screening test and neuroaxial medication trial. No clear consensus exists whether this trial should be an epidural or intrathecal catheter trial. Single shot trials are also considered predictive of success, although most experienced clinicians believe that catheter trials are a better predictor of success. Various medications and combinations are used to provide analgesia. These include opioids, local anesthetic solutions, baclofen, and clonidine.

C. TECHNIQUE

The procedure is similar to that for epidural placement, except the needle is advanced into the intrathecal space. The presence of cerebrospinal fluid confirms placement. The intrathecal catheter is then advanced to the desired level. For back and leg pain, the catheter is typically advanced to the T12–T10 level. For the pump implantation, an incision and dissection is used to create a pocket sufficient in size to hold the pump. This pocket is usually located in the anterior abdominal wall; care must be taken so that the pump does not rub against the ribs and that its placement is away from a belt and elastic waistbands of a patient's undergarments. After the creation of the subcutaneous pocket, the spinal catheter is then tunneled from the posterior incision site to the pump pocket and attached to the pump.

There are two types of pumps: fixed flow and programmable. Fixed flow pumps are usually less costly and can hold more drug volume, but dosing changes require pump refills, which can become expensive with higher cost drugs and multiple dose changes. Programmable pumps can provide various programming options including complex infusion programs. Dosing changes are easily done, with programmed increase in the pumps infusion rate. Intrathecal administration is preferred over epidural for long-term therapy because of the greater potency of medications infused into the cerebrospinal fluid and the epidural fibrosis that is often found in patients with spinal surgery.

D. COMPLICATIONS

There is a 1 to 5% reported risk of infection. Other complications are nerve injury, persistent paresthesias, and even paraplegia. Minor complications include pocket seromas, hygromas, and spinal headaches from cerebrospinal fluid leaks. Complications associated with refilling the pump include inadvertent side port injections especially in older pumps which lack safety screens. This mistake may deliver an intrathecal injection of months' worth of medication and provoke respiratory and cardiovascular collapse, even death. Programming errors are also potential complications, which can lead to death from drug overdoses.

Complications from spinal opioids include nausea and vomiting, urinary retention, and respiratory depression. Respiratory depression is unlikely in patients who are already tolerant to the effects of systemic opioids except when other systemic problems, such as pneumonia, occur; the respiratory depressant effects of opioids may become addictive with the development of such systemic problems.

Spinal opioid therapy can apparently be continued for years without significant complications. Recently, concerns about catheter granulomas have been raised. The mechanism of development is still being debated, but a noninfectious inflammatory response to the intraspinal opioid may be the cause. Severe neurologic compromise can occur when these granulomas enlarge and remain undiagnosed.

E. EVIDENCE FOR EFFICACY

In most situations, no single medication can be effective for both neuropathic and nociceptive pain. Because of this observation, most experienced clinicians who implant neuroaxial systems choose medication combinations to provide optimal analgesia while diminishing side effects. There is substantial literature documenting case series and expert experience suggesting long-term efficacy in well-selected patients.

Trigger Point Injections

A. ANATOMY

Trigger points are characterized by areas of tender nodules or distinct bands of muscle, palpation of which can reliably refer pain to consistent locations on the trunk or extremities. Trigger points are identified by applying pressure over the presumed location until the patient's pain is replicated.

B. INDICATION

Injection of trigger points may improve both the range of motion and the function of the affected area. This procedure may play a useful role in conjunction with a rehabilitation program.

C. TECHNIQUE

A trigger point can be injected either with a dry acupuncture needle or a needle filled with saline or local anesthetic with or without a corticosteroid. This procedure is often repeated during the rehabilitation program in order to treat recurrences. Recently, botulism toxin has been advocated for use during trigger point injections in order to treat resistant myofascial pain secondary to recurrent trigger points.

D. COMPLICATIONS

Following the procedure, the pain elicited from the trigger point area may temporarily worsen. Misdirected needles may puncture adjacent organs and blood vessels. Inadvertent intravascular injection of local anesthetic may precipitate seizures or systemic toxicity. Botulism toxin injections can lead to systemic effects, such as widespread muscle weakness or even anaphylaxis in allergic patients.

E. EVIDENCE FOR EFFICACY

Well-controlled outcome studies are limited, in part due to the lack of consistent criteria for the diagnosis of trigger points. Case series and small controlled studies have demonstrated short-term improvement. Case series suggest that botulinum toxin is efficacious. Multiple and repeated trigger point injections do not have any support for efficacy. Trigger point injections without rehabilitation are often ineffective as well.

Psoas Muscle Injection

A. ANATOMY

The psoas muscle lies deep to the transverse process of the lumbar spine. It originates at multiple levels from the transverse processes of each lumbar vertebra and typically courses below the inguinal ligament to insert with the iliacus muscle as a conjoint tendon onto the lesser trochanter.

B. INDICATIONS

Treatment of deep, ill-defined back pain with occasional coincident groin pain may indicate psoas muscle spasm.

C. TECHNIQUE

With the patient prone, using either fluoroscopy with contrast or CT scan for radiographic guidance, two needles are inserted using a "loss of resistance" technique into the psoas compartment.

D. COMPLICATIONS

Following injection of local anesthetic, the branches of the lumbar plexus, which traverse the psoas muscle, may be temporarily affected. Poor aseptic technique has led to infection of the psoas compartment.

Table 13–14. Low Back Pain Diagnosis and Treatment Approaches.

Diagnostic categories	Treatment approaches
Rheumatologic	Refer to specialty care for primary treatment of disease Use analgesic approaches as needed to maintain activity levels
Cancer	Refer to specialty care for primary treatment of disease
Infections of the spine	Refer to specialty care for primary treatment See Figure 13–7
Vascular	Refer to specialty care for treatment of primary pathology.
Metabolic	Refer to specialty care for primary treatment of disease See Figure 13–8
Referred pain (eg, pelvic and abdominal disorders)	Refer to specialty care Refer to specialty care
Mechanical spine pain	
Discogenic back pain	See Figure 13–2
Facet joints	See Figure 13–3
Spinal stenosis	See Figure 13–4
Adhesive arachnoiditis	Direct spinal cord stimulation Microlysis
Spondylolysis/spondylolisthesis	See Figure 13–5
Paraspinal muscles	Trigger point injections Massage Physical therapy
Nonspecific back pain	Limited rest, analgesics, antispasmodics, then resumption of normal activities to tolerance
SI joint	See Figure 13–6
Myofascial pain	Massage Corticosteroid or anesthetic injections (or both)
Other causes of back pain	
Guillain-Barré syndrome	Refer for specialty care
Herpes zoster	Look for rash and treat as a neuropathic pain problem
Meningeal irritation	Refer for specialty care
Fibromyalgia syndrome	See Chapter 15
Hip joints	See treatment of osteoarthritides in Chapter 14
Trochanteric bursa	See treatment of osteoarthritides in Chapter 14
Psychological factors	Refer for cognitive-behavioral therapy or other therapies as required after evaluation

E. EVIDENCE FOR EFFICACY

Several cohort series suggest efficacy. Injection of botulinum toxin into the psoas muscle has been reported to decrease the duration of pain originating from persistent muscle spasm.

Piriformis Muscle Injection

A. ANATOMY

This muscle arises from the pelvic surface of the sacrum, the sacrotuberous ligament and the posterior portion of the ilium. The muscle then courses through the sciatic foramen to insert into the upper border of the greater trochanter.

B. INDICATIONS

Injection of this muscle is indicated for assessment and treatment of piriformis syndrome. Patients presenting with this syndrome often complain of radiculopathy-like symptoms, which can be confused with lumbar radiculopathy.

C. TECHNIQUE

The muscle in thin persons can often be palpated; pressure on the muscle reproduces the symptoms. The muscle is approached in a similar fashion as the posterior approach to the sciatic nerve. A nerve stimulator or electromyography can be used to increase accuracy.

D. COMPLICATIONS

With the sciatic nerve in the immediate vicinity, anesthesia and paresthesia can occur. Local pain and irritation is the most frequent complication.

E. EVIDENCE FOR EFFICACY

Piriformis syndrome is a well-known syndrome and several case series have shown improvement with this procedure.

2. Noninvasive Therapies

Table 13–14 divides the causes of low back pain into nine categories:

1. Rheumatologic
2. Cancer
3. Infections of the spine
4. Vascular
5. Metabolic
6. Referred pain
7. Mechanical spinal pain
8. Other causes
9. Psychological factors

Figure 13–1 shows the diagnostic approach to mechanical pain. There are six treatment algorithms that demonstrate the approach to managing the various types of mechanical back pain, including discogenic spinal pain, facet joint pain, spinal stenosis, spondylolysis or spondylolisthesis, and SI joint pain. Other treatment algorithms outline the approach to managing spinal infection, metabolic bone disease, and failed spinal surgery.

Alvarez DJ et al. Trigger points: diagnosis and management. *Am Fam Physician.* 2002;65:653. [PMID: 11871683]

Amoretti N et al. Percutaneous nucleotomy: preliminary communication on a decompression probe (Dekompressor) in percutaneous discectomy. Ten case reports. *Clin Imaging.* 2005;29:98. [PMID: 15752964]

Broadhurst NA. Piriformis syndrome: Correlation of muscle morphology with symptoms and signs. *Arch Phys Med Rehabil.* 2004;85:2036. [PMID: 15605344]

Cohen SP et al. Nucleoplasty with or without intradiscal electrothermal therapy (IDET) as a treatment for lumbar herniated disc. *J Spinal Disord Tech.* 2005;18 Suppl:S119. [PMID: 15699797]

Davis MP et al. Palliative care: a long-term solution for long-term care. Part 3: analgesic therapy. *Home Care Provid.* 2001;6:164. [PMID: 11581590]

Fine PG et al. Meeting the challenges in cancer pain management. *J Support Oncol.* 2004;2:5. [PMID: 15605922]

Garcia Ruiz PJ et al. Posterior CT guided approach for botulinum toxin injection into spinal psoas. *J Neurol.* 2003;250:617. [PMID: 12814112]

Harris GR et al. Managing musculoskeletal complaints with rehabilitation therapy: summary of the Philadelphia Panel evidence-based clinical practice guidelines on musculoskeletal rehabilitation interventions. *J Fam Pract.* 2002;51:1042. [PMID: 12540330]

Igarashi T et al. Lysis of adhesions and epidural injection of steroid/local anaesthetic during epiduroscopy potentially alleviate low back and leg pain in elderly patients with lumbar spinal stenosis. *Br J Anaesth.* 2004;93:181. [PMID: 15194631]

Kim SI et al. Caudal-epidural corticosteroids in post-laminectomy syndrome: treatment for low-back pain. *Compr Ther.* 1975;1:57. [PMID: 130222]

Lang E et al. Multidisciplinary rehabilitation versus usual care for chronic low back pain in the community: effects on quality of life. *Spine J.* 2003;3:270. [PMID: 14589185]

McLain RF et al. Epidural steroid therapy for back and leg pain: mechanisms of action and efficacy. *Spine J.* 2005;5:191. [PMID: 15749619]

Muto M et al. Vertebroplasty in the treatment of back pain. *Radiol Med (Torino).* 2005;109:208. [PMID: 15775889]

Nash TP. Epiduroscopy for lumbar spinal stenosis. *Br J Anaesth.* 2005;94:250. [PMID: 15629909]

Nguyen H et al. Spinal analgesics. *Anesthesiol Clin North America.* 2003;21:805. [PMID: 14719721]

Ohnmeiss DD et al. Patient satisfaction with spinal cord stimulation for predominant complaints of chronic, intractable low back pain. *Spine J.* 2001;1:358. [PMID: 14588316]

Pincus T et al. Cognitive-behavioral therapy and psychosocial factors in low back pain: directions for the future. *Spine.* 2002;27:E133. [PMID: 11880850]

Slipman CW. A critical review of the evidence for the use of zygapophysial injections and radiofrequency denervation in the treatment of low back pain. *Spine J.* 2003;3:310. [PMID: 14589192]

Tuite MJ. Facet joint and sacroiliac joint injection. *Semin Roentgenol.* 2004;39:37. [PMID: 14976836]

Vad VB et al. Transforaminal epidural steroid injections in lumbosacral radiculopathy: a prospective randomized study. *Spine.* 2002;27:11. [PMID: 11805628]

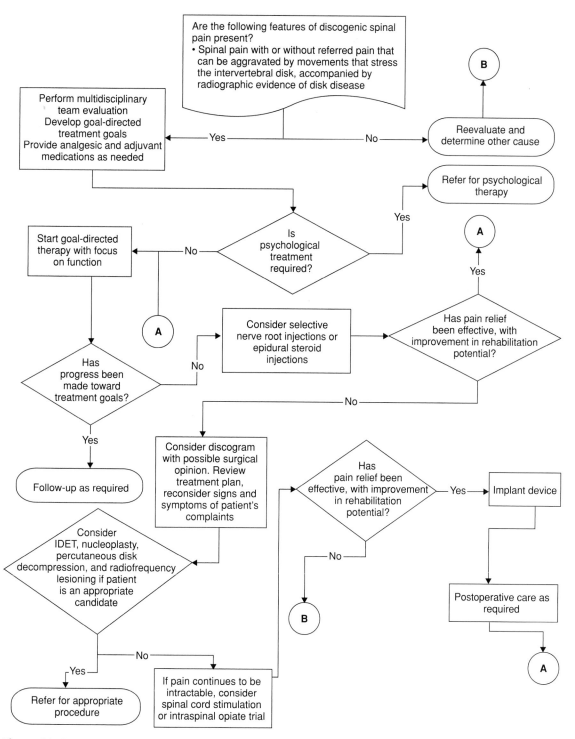

Figure 13–2. Treatment of discogenic spinal pain. Spinal pain due to torn annulus, internal disruption, or prolapsed intervertebral disk. IDET, intradiscal electrothermoplasty. A and B = Go to corresponding letter within algorithm.

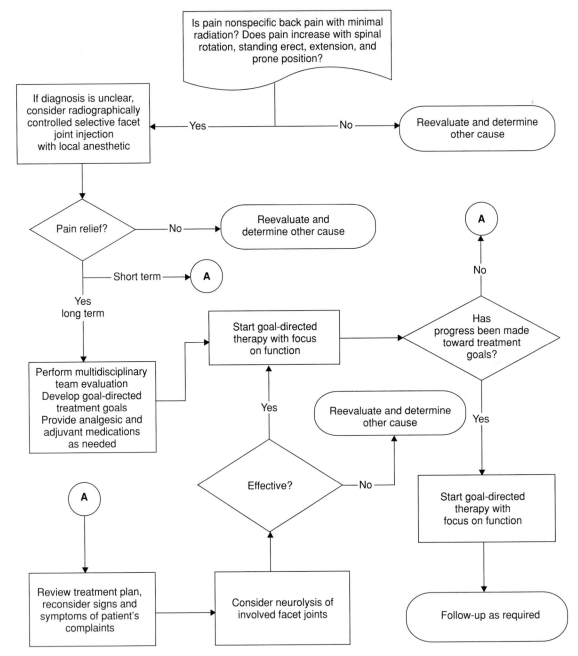

Figure 13–3. Treatment of facet joint pain. Pain, with or without referred pain, stemming from one or more facet joints; pain due to sprains or other injuries to the capsule of facet joints or arthritic changes. A = Go to corresponding letter within algorithm.

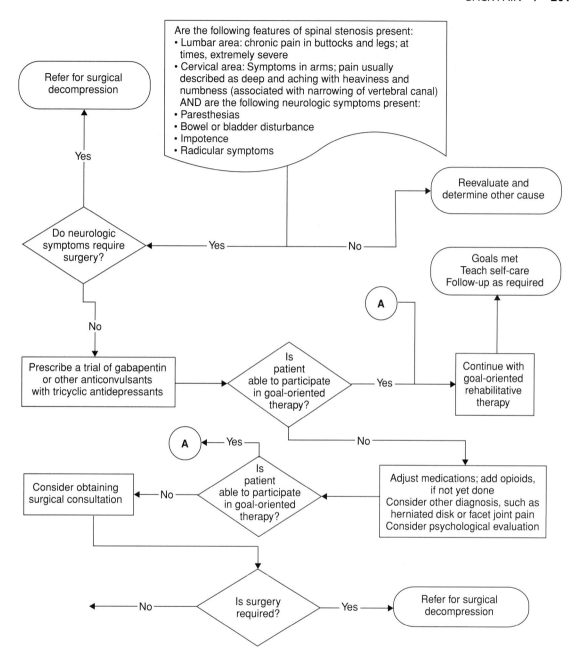

Figure 13–4. Treatment of spinal stenosis pain. Pain due to narrowing of the vertebral canal at multiple levels, usually of the cervical or lumbar vertebrae. A = Go to corresponding letter within algorithm.

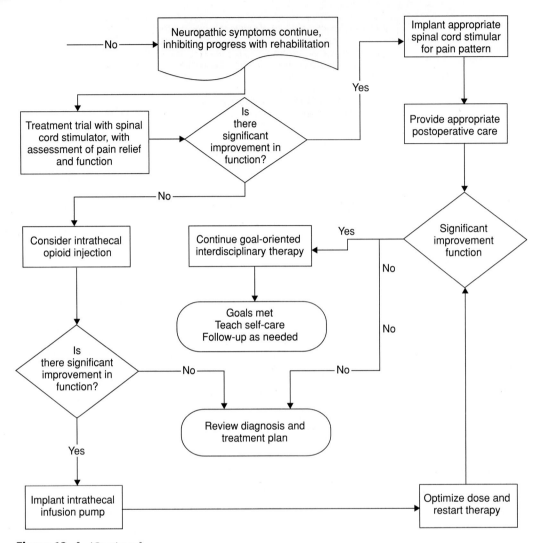

Figure 13–4. (*Continued*)

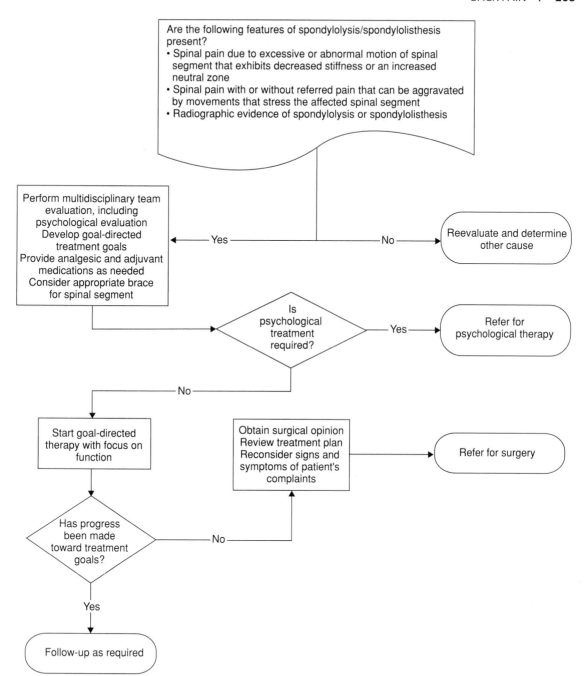

Figure 13–5. Treatment of spondylolysis or spondylolisthesis.

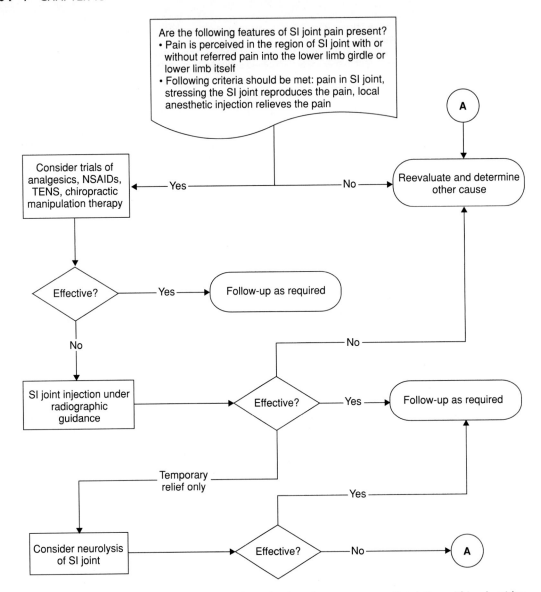

Figure 13–6. Treatment of sacroiliac (SI) joint pain. A = Go to corresponding letter within algorithm. NSAIDs, nonsteroidal anti-inflammatory drugs; TENS, transcutaneous electrical nerve stimulation.

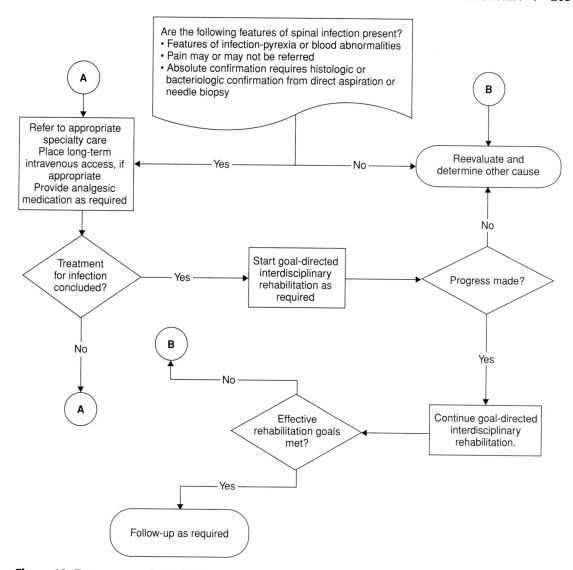

Figure 13–7. Treatment of spinal infection. Spinal pain in the context of specified infection or likely infection. A and B = Go to corresponding letter within algorithm.

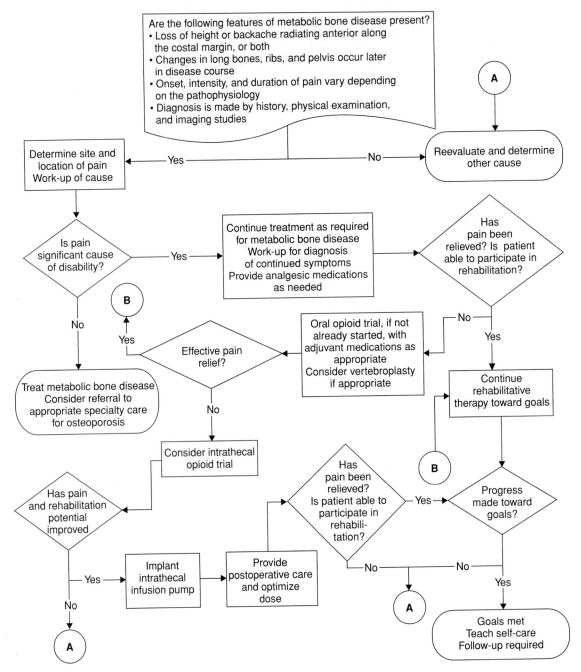

Figure 13–8. Treatment of metabolic bone disease. A and B = Go to corresponding letter within algorithm.

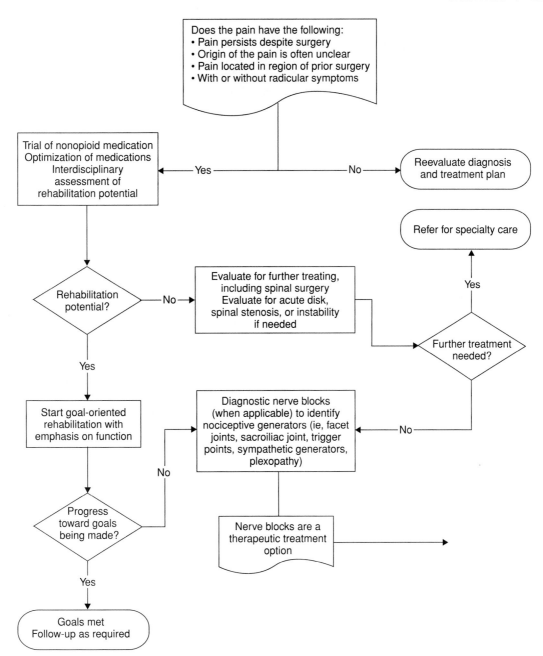

Figure 13–9. Treatment of failed spinal surgery. A and B and C = Go to corresponding letter within algorithm.

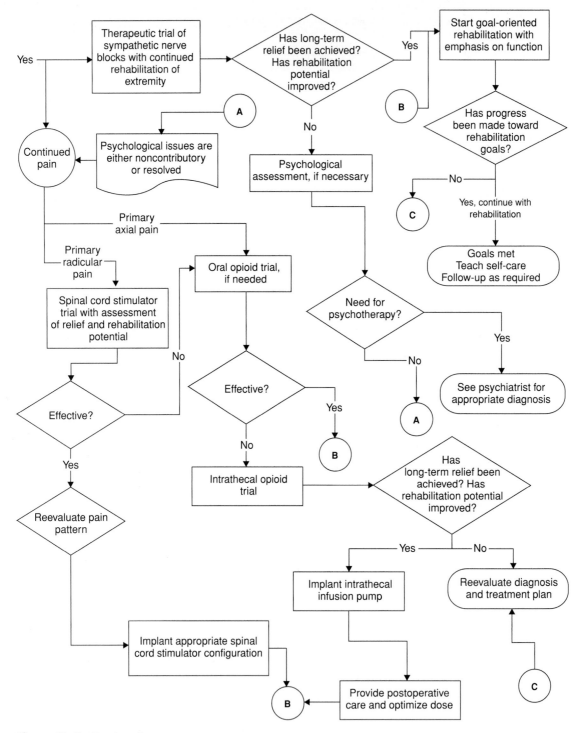

Figure 13–9. (Continued)

Osteoarthritis & Rheumatoid Arthritis

14

Daniel J. Mazanec, MD, Russell C. DeMicco, DO, & Edwin L. Capulong, MD

OSTEOARTHRITIS

ESSENTIALS OF DIAGNOSIS

- *A monoarticular or oligoarticular disorder that is asymmetric with minimal inflammatory findings.*
- *No systemic manifestations.*
- *Morning stiffness lasting less than 1 hour; pain relieved by rest.*
- *Radiographic changes showing joint space narrowing, osteophytes, bony cysts, and subchondral sclerosis.*
- *Laboratory findings are normal.*

General Considerations

Osteoarthritis (OA) is one of the most common musculoskeletal disorders and has a significant impact on functional activities. In the absence of a congenital joint deformity or serious trauma, OA is rare before 40 years of age. Prevalence increases with advanced age. Current data suggest that there are approximately 41 million Americans suffering from symptomatic OA. Men have a higher incidence and prevalence under the age of 50. This difference diminishes after the age of menopause. African Americans have a higher incidence of OA than whites.

Pathogenesis

OA is a multifactorial disorder resulting from a complex interplay of age, genetic, and environmental factors. Risk factors range from nonmodifiable to modifiable. Nonmodifiable risk factors include age, genetic predisposition, and congenital joint anomalies. Modifiable risk factors include diet, physical activity, obesity, and some metabolic disorders.

Joint trauma increases the risk of OA, particularly in the presence of joint malalignment, such as knee valgus deformity, leg length discrepancy, and joint instability brought about by quadriceps weakness or atrophy. In addition, strenuous physical activity and repetitive or mechanical stress (dystonia or spasticity) may hasten the development of arthritic changes in affected joints.

In the case of spasticity or dystonia, arthritic changes depend on the sites of involvement. In the neck, dystonia may produce cervical spondylosis, and in the hip, it may increase the risk of hip OA. In both cases, dystonia may develop at a younger than expected age because of persistent mechanical stress. In patients with prior trauma (eg, meniscal tear or hip injury), the risk of knee OA increases by five to six times, and hip OA by four times, respectively.

Age-related changes in the musculoskeletal tissues include calcification of joint cartilage, increased joint laxity due to muscle weakness and diminished joint proprioception. Overall, these factors may lead to increase propensity to arthritic changes and increase risk of falls in the elderly.

Increased concordance rates of clinical OA between monozygotic versus dizygotic twins support the notion of genetic predisposition to the disease. Clinical manifestations that may be suggestive of genetic predisposition include early age of onset, location (hands and hips) and family history.

Prevention

Primary prevention of OA entails risk factor modification. Weight reduction, work environment modification for occupation-related disorders (cumulative trauma or repetitive stress disorders), and appropriate physical activity may reduce the risk of OA. Proper training, warmups, stretching exercises prior to physical activity, and maintenance of muscle strength may diminish trauma to the knees or hips, reducing the risk of OA.

Oxygen radicals have been associated with aging and variety of disorders, including OA, coronary artery disease, cataracts, and cancer. Nutritional factors play a major role in modulating oxygen radicals. In the joint, free oxygen radicals can cause damage to cartilage. Vitamin C, a potent antioxidant, may reduce the cartilage loss and retard progression of degenerative disease. In the Framingham study, persons with lower consumption of vitamin C had an increased fourfold risk of OA. Other antioxidants, including vitamins A and E did not show the same efficacy as vitamin C. In fact, in recent studies, vitamin E did not demonstrate any effect on pain modulation. Vitamin A supplementation may increase risk of fragility fracture among males by a factor of seven.

Vitamin D may have a favorable effect on chondrocytes and may play a role in preventing arthritic changes, particularly in the knees. Suboptimal levels of vitamin D affect calcium metabolism and osteoblast activity affecting bone mineral density. Risk of knee OA may be increased as much as threefold in vitamin D–deficient patients.

Estrogen deficiency may play a role in progression of OA via stiffening of the bone, transmitting force to the overlying cartilage. In the Framingham study, estrogen replacement therapy has a moderate protective effect against worsening radiographic knee OA, although not statistically significant.

Secondary prevention is defined as limiting the progression of established degenerative joint disease and requires specific and prompt rehabilitation of injured joints with proper use of therapeutic exercise for rehabilitation. Education regarding activity modification in workplace or recreational activities may be helpful in retarding progression of degenerative joint disease.

Clinical Findings

A. SYMPTOMS AND SIGNS

OA is readily distinguished from rheumatoid arthritis (RA) and other inflammatory joint disorders by the pattern of joint involvement and the absence of systemic manifestations. In OA, pain is typically worse in the morning, with stiffness lasting a few minutes to less than 1 hour. Joint involvement is frequently asymmetric in a monoarticular to oligoarticular pattern, without evidence of systemic inflammation or extra-articular features (eg, fever, weight loss, rash, and presence of nodules).

In the hands, OA classically affects distal interphalangeal joints and less commonly the proximal interphalangeal joints or metacarpophalangeal joints. Other commonly affected joints include hips and knees as well as the cervical and lumbar spine. In the absence of trauma, elbows, wrists, and shoulders are less often affected (Table 14–1). On physical examination, bony enlargement of the affected joints is noted. Joint effusion may be present, and crepitus may be felt with joint motion.

Table 14–1. Characteristic Findings in Osteoarthritis, Rheumatoid Arthritis, Gout, and Pseudogout.

Characteristics	Osteoarthritis	Rheumatoid arthritis	Gout	Pseudogout
Sites of predilection	DIP, PIP Knees and hips	Polyarticular wrist, MCP, PIP Extraskeletal sites	Usually asymmetric Monoarticular MTP joint, ankles, knees, and feet Tophaceous deposits in ears, elbow joint, hands, knees, feet	Usually polyarticular Knees, wrists, MTPs, hips, and shoulders
Synovial fluid	Normal	>2000 WBC/mcL	Positive urate crystals	Positive calcium pyrophosphate crystals
Laboratory findings	Normal	Positive rheumatoid factor Presence of anti-CCP antibody	Serum uric acid level >7.0	Serum uric acid level normal
Radiographic findings	Joint space narrowing Osteophytes Subchondral sclerosis	Juxta-articular osteoporosis Joint erosions	Normal in early disease Joint space narrowing and erosions with overhanging edge	Punctate and linear densities in the articular hyaline or fibrocartilaginous tissues

Table 14–2. Characteristics of Synovial Fluid in Noninflammatory, Inflammatory, and Septic Arthritis Compared with Normal Findings.

Characteristics	Normal	Noninflammatory arthritis	Inflammatory arthritis	Septic arthritis
Volume	<3 mL	<3 mL	>3.5 mL	>3.5 mL
Color	Clear to light	Light yellow	Yellow-opaque	Greenish yellow
WBC	< 200/mcL	200–300/mcL	3000–50,000/mcL	> 50,000/mcL
Polymorphonuclear leukocytes	< 25%	< 25%	50% or more	75% or more
Culture and Gram stain	No growth	No growth	Usually no growth	Usually positive
Glucose (md/dL)	Equal to serum	Equal to serum	Lower than serum	Lower than serum

B. LABORATORY FINDINGS

Laboratory findings in OA are usually normal and are performed to exclude other arthropathies. Laboratory studies indicated in selected patients include measuring uric acid levels, erythrocyte sedimentation rate, rheumatoid factor, antinuclear antibodies (ANA), and synovial fluid analysis. Synovial fluid analysis is helpful if infectious or crystalline arthritis must be excluded. In OA, synovial fluid is characteristically noninflammatory. White blood cell count and differential analysis of synovial fluid is used to differentiate inflammatory versus noninflammatory arthritis. Synovial fluid Gram stain and bacterial culture is helpful when infection is suspected (Table 14–2). Light polarizing microscopy can distinguish monosodium urate crystals, which appear as negatively birefringent versus calcium pyrophosphate crystals, noted as positively birefringent.

C. IMAGING STUDIES

The clinical suspicion of OA is confirmed with plain radiographs of the affected joint. Typical findings include asymmetric joint space narrowing, osteophyte formation, degenerative cysts, and subchondral bone sclerosis. These radiographic changes can help classify the grade of OA (Table 14–3).

Severity of radiographic degenerative changes correlates imperfectly with clinical symptoms. OA is frequently asymptomatic and may coexist with other rheumatic disorders. Careful assessment for other causes of joint pain is required before attributing symptoms to osteoarthritic changes.

Magnetic resonance imaging (MRI) is more sensitive than plain radiographs for demonstrating cartilage loss, subchondral cyst formation, and osteophytes. In addition, MRI is more sensitive in identifying soft tissue injuries, including meniscal and ligamentous abnormalities.

Differential Diagnosis

In most cases, OA is easily distinguished from RA and other inflammatory arthritides by the absence of inflammation and laboratory abnormalities, by the pattern of joint involvement, and by radiographic changes. In contrast to RA and other inflammatory arthritides, OA is characterized by minimal articular inflammation without systemic manifestations. In contrast to OA, joint distribution in RA involves the wrist, proximal interphalangeal joint and metacarpophalangeal joint, sparing the distal interphalangeal joints.

Gouty arthritis is characterized by elevated serum uric acid levels, sudden onset of pain, erythema, and swelling most commonly affecting metatarsophalangeal joint of the big toe (podagra). Other joints may also be affected, including knees, ankles, and feet. Involvement is usually asymmetric (see Table 14–1). On physical examination, there is exquisite tenderness overlying an erythematous and swollen joint. In severe cases, tophaceous deposits can be seen in the ears, elbow joint, hands, knees, and feet. Synovial fluid examination for monosodium urate crystals is the definitive diagnostic test for suspected gouty arthritis. Another crystalline osteopathy, pseudogout (also called calcium pyrophosphate dihydrate deposition

Table 14–3. Kellgren-Lawrence Classification of Radiographic Changes in Osteoarthritis.

Grading	Description
Grade 1 OA	Joint space narrowing Densification of underlying bone
Grade 2 OA	Further aggravation of grade 1.
Grade 3 OA	Grade 1 and 2 plus loss of joint space Start of osteophyte formation
Grade 4 OA	Grade 1, 2, 3 plus bone cysts

[CPPD] disease) may also be identified by examination of synovial fluid. In addition to CPPD, a radiograph may show punctuate or linear densities in the articular hyaline or fibrocartilaginous tissues (see Table 14–1).

Treatment

The treatment of OA emphasizes a multidisciplinary approach, encompassing nonpharmacologic and pharmacologic treatment. The most important nonpharmacologic treatment for OA is exercise. Other options include weight loss, lifestyle modification, use of assistive devices, patient education, and occupational rehabilitation. The following medications may be helpful in treating OA: topical creams, acetaminophen, nonsteroidal anti-inflammatory drugs (NSAIDs), tramadol, opioids, and intra-articular injections.

The primary objectives of treatment are reduction of pain, improvement of function, and preservation of joint structure. Nonpharmacologic and pharmacologic interventions should be exhausted before considering surgical therapy.

Exercise

In general, it is better to rest an acutely painful joint for a few days before starting an active physical therapy or exercise program. The duration of a supervised therapeutic exercise is variable, but the emphasis should be the transition to a long-term home-based exercise maintenance program.

The goals of exercise may be specific to the affected joints. In the knees, for example, isometric strengthening of the quadriceps femoris muscles reduces joint instability and prevents disuse atrophy.

For short-term rehabilitation of the knee, closed kinetic chain exercises (feet are in contact with the floor or a solid surface) produce less stress at the knee joint and simulate functional movements; examples include walking, knee bending, seated leg presses, stair climbing, and stationary bicycling. Open kinetic chain exercises, on the other hand, involve exercises where the feet are not in contact with a solid surface, producing more tension in the soft tissues surrounding the knee joint; examples include knee extension, straight leg raising, and leg adduction in lateral decubitus position.

For short-term rehabilitation of knee OA pain, closed kinetic chain exercises are beneficial, but for long-term therapy (more than 3 months), open kinetic chain exercises may be more effective for pain control.

The use of aquatic therapy is beneficial for patients with lower extremity OA in whom weight-bearing exercise may be difficult.

Studies in people with knee OA have clearly demonstrated clinical benefit to a supervised fitness walking

Table 14–4. Physical Activity Recommendations by the ACR for Persons with OA

Aerobic Exercise for People with Hip or Knee OA
• Accumulate 30 minutes of moderate intensity (50–70% maximal HR) physical activity on at least 3 days a week.
• Tailor the type of aerobic activity and venue to individual needs.
• If overweight, combine physical activity with diet modifications.
• Incorporate self-management education into exercise recommendations and programs.
Neuromuscular Rehabilitation for People with Knee OA
• A lower extremity exercise program should combine strengthening, endurance, coordination, balance, and functional exercise.
• Recommended programs will progress in duration, intensity, and complexity; be tailored to the individual needs, abilities, and preferences; move from clinical supervision to self-directed community setting; and be periodically reviewed, revised, and reinforced.

OA, osteoarthritis; ACR, American College of Rheumatology; HR, heart rate.

program. In one trial, supervised walking plus light stretching and strengthening exercises as well as patient education for up to 30 minutes three times weekly reduced knee osteoarthritic pain by 27% and increased the functional walking distance by 18% compared with baseline. At 1-year follow-up, patients who did not maintain an exercise program showed loss of functional benefits.

Overall, weight loss and a moderate intensity exercise program prove to be beneficial not only in terms of increased cardiovascular endurance but also improving pain perception as reported in the Fitness Arthritis and Senior Trial (FAST). The American College of Rheumatology and American Geriatrics Society have developed guidelines for exercise in OA (Tables 14–4 and 14–5).

Topical Analgesics

Capsaicin is a topical medication available without prescription. It stimulates unmyelinated C fiber afferent neurons causing a release of substance P. With prolonged use, capsaicin reversibly depletes stores of substance P from sensory nerve endings reducing the transmission of painful stimuli from the peripheral nerve fibers to the higher centers. Capsaicin can be an effective treatment of

Table 14–5. Exercise Recommendations by the American Geriatric Society for Persons with Osteoarthritis.[a]

- Warm up: 5 minutes
- Exercise:
  - Isometric strength training: daily
  - Isotonic strength training: 2–3 times per week
  - Flexibility training: daily
  - Aerobic training (endurance): 3–5 times per week
- Cool down: 5 minutes

[a]Many patients need to concentrate on strength and flexibility training first before considering aerobic training. The exercise program should be adapted to the patient's age and functional ability.

Table 14–6. Risk Factors for NSAID Toxicity.

Gastrointestinal
Age >65 years old
Use of oral corticosteroids
History of abdominal pain and ulcer disease
Use of antiplatelet and anticoagulation drugs
Renal
Age >65 years old
Renal insufficiency
Hypertension
Congestive heart failure
Use of diuretics
Use of angiotensin-converting enzyme inhibitors

NSAID, nonsteroidal anti-inflammatory drug.

acute exacerbations of osteoarthritic pain. For maximum benefit, it should be applied to the affected joint three or four times daily. Patients must be instructed to wash their hands carefully after each application as the drug may be very irritating if accidentally brushed into the eyes.

Acetaminophen

The American College of Rheumatology has recommended the use of acetaminophen as the first-line agent for mild symptomatic OA. Clinical trials have demonstrated significant improvement in pain and functional scores of patients with knee and hip OA treated with approximately 4 g of acetaminophen daily, comparable to treatment with naproxen 750 mg daily. In contrast, lower doses of acetaminophen are inadequate and generally inferior to treatment with NSAIDs in OA patients. A major advantage of acetaminophen versus NSAIDs is an excellent safety profile in doses less than 4 g daily. However, side effects may include liver enzyme elevation and drug sensitivity. In patients without underlying liver disease, dosages up to 4 g daily are well tolerated.

Nonsteroidal Anti-Inflammatory Drugs

Nonselective NSAIDs (cyclooxygenase [COX]-1 and COX-2) have been the mainstay in treating moderate to severe OA for many years because of their combined analgesic and anti-inflammatory actions. Risk factor assessment should be done in patients who are being considered for long-term therapy. A need for a gastroprotective agent should be considered in patients at high risk for gastrointestinal toxicity (Table 14–6).

COX-2 selective NSAIDs have been the medication of choice in OA patients at risk for gastrointestinal tox-

icity. However, recent trials suggest a 1.5 to 2.0 times increased risk of cardiovascular events in patients receiving COX-2 selective NSAIDs, particularly rofecoxib and valdecoxib (both now withdrawn from the market), compared with nonselective COX inhibitors (see Chapter 3).

Tramadol

Tramadol is a weak opioid receptor agent and norepinephrine and serotonin reuptake inhibitor. Tramadol is used for moderate to severe OA pain and should be considered in patients who do not respond to acetaminophen or NSAIDs. Tramadol is also used as an adjunctive therapy with NSAIDs. Maximum dosing for younger patients (younger than 65 years of age) is 400 mg/d in four divided doses, and for older patients (older than 65 years of age) is 300 mg/d in four divided doses. Side effects include drowsiness, constipation, and gastrointestinal symptoms (see Chapter 3). Tramadol is rarely associated with seizures but should be used with caution in high-risk patients or patients taking antidepressants. Low risk exists for abuse potential and withdrawal symptoms (see Table 3–2).

Opioids

For patients with significant pain and functional impairment despite maximal nonpharmacologic treatment and nonopioid analgesic or NSAIDs, opioids should be considered. Advantages of opioids include superior analgesic effect for nociceptive pain and lack of significant end organ toxicity. Fears of tolerance and diversion have proved unfounded in recent studies of opioid therapy of nonmalignant musculoskeletal disease. In patients at very high risk for NSAID-related gastrointestinal or renal adverse effects, opioid agents may offer a superior risk benefit profile.

Intra-Articular Injections

A. CORTICOSTEROID INJECTIONS

Intra-articular corticosteroid injections are indicated in some patients with symptomatic OA; it is especially effective as adjunct treatment in patients in whom oral therapy is contraindicated or inadequate. In general, a large weight-bearing joint, such as the knee or hip, should not be injected more than 3 or 4 times per year. The agents most commonly used are methylprednisolone (80 to 120 mg per dose) and triamcinolone (20 to 40 mg per dose). These are usually combined with an anesthetic agent such as lidocaine (0.5 to 1%) or bupivacaine (0.25 to 0.5%). The volume and dose injected varies depending on the size of the joint.

Aseptic technique should be observed for all procedures. Before injecting, aspiration of synovial fluid for gross fluid examination may be performed if infection is a concern. If the fluid appears turbid or greenish-yellowish in color, injection should be aborted and synovial fluid analysis and culture should be performed.

If fewer than four injections are done per year, cartilage damage, pseudo-Charcot arthropathy, and avascular necrosis are rare complications. Patients should be warned of the more common complications, including infection, hemarthrosis, and corticosteroid-induced hyperglycemia in a diabetic patient.

B. VISCOSUPPLEMENTATION

Hyaluronan is a glycosaminoglycan responsible for synovial fluid viscoelasticity, which is reduced in OA joints by catalytic enzymes. Viscosupplementation therapy involves intra-articular injection of a hyaluronan derivative. Preparations available include hylan G-F 20 (administered weekly for 3 consecutive weeks) and sodium hyaluroniate (given as a weekly intra-articular injection for 5 weeks).

Clinical trials have produced conflicting results, but in a recent study, hylan G-F 20 showed significant analgesic effect compared with placebo as early as the third week continuing up to the eighth week following treatment. Previous uncontrolled cohort studies have demonstrated up to 1 year of symptomatic relief.

Experience with viscosupplementation in hip OA is limited, but recent reports suggest symptomatic relief and improvement of function at 3 months following injection. Adverse reactions include acute joint pain with effusion (particularly with hylan G-F 20 preparation), bleeding, and infection.

Surgery

Older patients who have not responded to nonoperative treatment and are suffering from a moderate to severe disability due to pain should be considered for surgery. In younger patients in whom the risk of long-term failure or complication for artificial joints is high, delaying total joint arthroplasty, if possible, is the rule. Appropriate, "lesser" alternative procedures, such as arthroscopic debridement meniscectomy or high tibial meniscectomy for knee OA, should be considered.

Total hip and knee arthroplasty provide significant pain relief that usually translates to functional improvement. Perioperative mortality is below 1%. Early complications include deep venous thrombosis, pulmonary embolism, and infection. Late complications include aseptic loosening brought about by deterioration of cement (methylmethacrylate). Revision arthroplasty may be indicated in such patients.

Alternative Therapy

A. GLUCOSAMINE

The most popular alternative treatment for OA is glucosamine sulfate, which is derived from oyster or crab shells. Glucosamine has been proposed as both a preventive modality and treatment for mild OA. A proposed mechanism of action is stimulation of proteoglycan synthesis, which may either prevent or retard the clinical progression of OA. Preliminary studies suggest a significant analgesic effect in about two-thirds of patients, comparable to NSAID therapy. In addition, a small placebo-controlled trial found reduced progression of radiographic knee OA in persons treated with glucosamine. The recommended therapeutic dose is 1500 mg of glucosamine daily. Glucosamine is well tolerated with few side effects. A combination of glucosamine and chondroitin has not been shown to have significant benefit versus glucosamine alone.

B. S ADENOSYLMETHIONINE

S adenosylmethionine (SAMe) is reported to increase production of proteoglycans, potentially benefiting patients with OA. Randomized trials demonstrating efficacy in OA have not been reported. SAMe is claimed to be as effective as NSAIDs in terms of symptom relief, with fewer side effects. SAMe (800 mg/d orally in two doses) is primarily advocated for mild OA. SAMe may take up to 1 week to produce clinical effects. Side effects include nausea and skin irritation. Other proposed potential indications include fibromyalgia and depression.

C. ACUPUNCTURE

In a recent randomized, controlled trial, acupuncture was demonstrated to be efficacious in treating osteoarthritic knee pain. The basis for the analgesic effect of acupuncture is postulated to be either release of endoge-nous opioids or, alternatively an interference with pain transmission based on the gate theory of pain. In addi-tion, absence of known side effects makes acupuncture an attractive treatment option for patients unresponsive to or intolerant of more traditional therapy, including NSAIDs.

Baldwin CT et al. Absence of linkage or association for osteoarthritis with the vitamin D receptor/type II collagen locus: The Fram-ingham Osteoarthritis Study. *J Rheumatol.* 2002;29:161. [PMID: 11824954]

Berman BM et al. Effectiveness of acupuncture as adjunctive therapy in osteoarthritis of the knee: a randomized, controlled trial. *Ann Intern Med.* 2004;141:901. [PMID: 15611487]

Cicuttini FM et al. Effect of estrogen replacement therapy on patella cartilage in healthy women. *Clin Exp Rheumatol.* 2003;21:79. [PMID: 12673893]

Conrozier T et al. Intra-articular injections of hylan G-F 20 in pa-tients with symptomatic hip osteoarthritis: an open-label, mul-ticentre, pilot study. *Clin Exp Rheumatol.* 2003;21:605. [PMID: 14611109]

Cubukcu D et al. Hylan G-F 20 efficacy on articular cartilage quality in patients with knee osteoarthritis: clinical and MRI assessment. *Clin Rheumatol.* 2005;24:336. [PMID: 15599642]

Emkey R et al. Efficacy and safety of tramadol/acetaminophen tablets (Ultracet) as add-on therapy for osteoarthritis pain in subjects re-ceiving a COX-2 nonsteroidal antiinflammatory drug: a multicen-ter, randomized, double-blind, placebo-controlled trial. *J Rheuma-tol.* 2004;31:150. [PMID: 14705234]

Hannan MT et al. Estrogen use and radiographic osteoarthritis of the knee in women. The Framingham Osteoarthritis Study. *Arthritis Rheum.* 1990;33:525.[PMID: 2328031]

Malonne H et al. Efficacy and tolerability of sustained-release tra-madol in the treatment of symptomatic osteoarthritis of the hip or knee: a multicenter, randomized, double-blind, placebo-controlled study. *Clin Ther.* 2004;26:1774. [PMID: 15639689]

McAlindon T et al. Effectiveness of glucosamine for symptoms of knee osteoarthritis: results from an internet-based randomized double-blind controlled trial. *Am J Med.* 2004;117:643. [PMID: 15501201]

McAlindon TE et al. Efficacy of glucosamine and chondroitin for treatment of osteoarthritis. *JAMA.* 2000;284:1241. [PMID: 10979101]

Messier SP et al. Exercise and dietary weight loss in overweight and obese older adults with knee osteoarthritis: the Arthritis, Diet, and Activity Promotion Trial. *Arthritis Rheum.* 2004;50:1501. [PMID: 15146420]

Michaelsson K et al. Serum retinol levels and the risk of fracture. *N Engl J Med.* 2003;348:287. [PMID: 12540641]

Opotowsky AR et al; NHANES I follow-up study. Serum vitamin A concentration and the risk of hip fracture among women 50 to 74 years old in the United States: a prospective analysis of the NHANES I follow-up study. *Am J Med.* 2004;117:169. [PMID: 15276595]

Raynauld JP et al. Safety and efficacy of long-term intraarticular steroid injections in osteoarthritis of the knee: a randomized, double-blind, placebo-controlled trial. *Arthritis Rheum.* 2003;48: 370. [PMID: 12571845]

Richy F et al. Structural and symptomatic efficacy of glucosamine and chondroitin in knee osteoarthritis: a comprehensive meta-analysis. *Arch Intern Med.* 2003;163:1514. [PMID: 12860572]

Roddy E et al. Evidence-based recommendations for the role of ex-ercise in the management of osteoarthritis of the hip or knee–the MOVE consensus. *Rheumatology (Oxford).* 2005;44:67. [PMID: 15353613]

Solomon DH et al. Relationship between selective cyclooxygenase-2 inhibitors and acute myocardial infarction in older adults. *Circu-lation.* 2004;109:2068. [PMID: 15096449]

Sowers M. Epidemiology of risk factors for osteoarthritis: systemic factors. *Curr Opin Rheumatol.* 2001;13:447. [PMID: 11604603]

White WB et al. Effects of the cyclooxygenase-2 specific in-hibitor valdecoxib versus nonsteroidal antiinflammatory agents and placebo on cardiovascular thrombotic events in patients with arthritis. *Am J Ther.* 2004;11:244. [PMID: 15266215]

Witvrouw E et al. Open versus closed kinetic chain exercises in patellofemoral pain: a 5-year prospective randomized study. *Am J Sports Med.* 2004;32:1122. [PMID: 15262632]

Witvrouw E et al. Open versus closed kinetic chain exercises for patellofemoral pain. A prospective, randomized study. *Am J Sports Med.* 2000;28:687. [PMID: 11032226]

Wluka AE et al. Supplementary vitamin E does not affect the loss of cartilage volume in knee osteoarthritis: a 2 year double blind randomized placebo controlled study. *J Rheumatol.* 2002;29:2585. [PMID: 12465157]

Ytterberg SR et al. Codeine and oxycodone use in patients with chronic rheumatic disease pain. *Arthritis Rheum.* 1998;41:1603. [PMID: 9751092]

RHEUMATOID ARTHRITIS

 ESSENTIALS OF DIAGNOSIS

- RA remains a clinical diagnosis that requires the pres-ence of symmetric, polyarticular, inflammatory arthri-tis for at least 4 to 6 weeks.
- The presence of at least four of the criteria established by The American College of Rheumatology. Criteria 1 through 4 must be present for at least 6 weeks.

General Considerations

RA is a chronic progressive autoimmune disease with varying systemic features that affects 2.1 million peo-ple in the United States. RA causes pain, progressive joint destruction, fatigue, loss of mobility, and inabil-ity to perform activities of daily living. The primary pathology is a hypertrophied inflammatory synovium ultimately leading to erosive joint disease with pain, loss of function, and progressive disability. RA might be better termed "rheumatoid disease" because of its mul-tiple extra-articular manifestations, including pleuritis, pericarditis, vasculitis, and pulmonary nodules among others (Table 14–7).

RA accounts for more than 9 million physician vis-its per year and at least 250,000 hospitalizations. The

Table 14–7. Extra-articular Manifestations of Rheumatoid Arthritis.

System affected	Manifestation
General	Fever Lymphadenopathy Fatigue Weight loss
Cardiac	Pericarditis Myocarditis Coronary vasculitis
Pulmonary	Pleuritis Nodules Interstitial lung disease Bronchiolitis obliterans
Neuromuscular	Entrapment neuropathy Peripheral neuropathy Mononeuritis multiplex
Dermatologic	Subcutaneous nodules Palmar erythema Vasculitis
Ocular	Keratoconjunctivitis sicca Episcleritis Scleritis Choroid and retinal nodules
Hematologic	Felty syndrome Anemia

substantial economic burden of RA is associated with both treatment costs and lost productivity and employment. Furthermore, RA significantly reduces life expectancy; age-adjusted mortality rates are increased by about 50%.

Epidemiologic studies indicate that the prevalence of RA is 0.5 to 1% of the adult populations in the United States and Europe. Certain Native American tribes show prevalence up to 5.3%. Prevalence increases with age and peaks between the ages of 40 and 60 years.

Joint pain and stiffness significantly impact quality of life in people with RA. Many people experience pain that impairs physical and psychological function despite receiving appropriate and aggressive treatment for underlying disease. Pain is sometimes viewed as an indication of disease activity even though disease activity and severity do not predict intensity of pain or level of function of the individual.

Most commonly, RA follows a progressive course punctuated by disease flares. Spontaneous lasting remission is rare, occurring in less than 5% of patients. Specific criteria for defining clinical remission include the following:

1. Duration of morning stiffness lasting 15 minutes or longer
2. No fatigue or joint pain by history
3. No joint pain or tenderness or range of motion
4. No soft tissue swelling in joints or tendon sheaths
5. Erythrocyte sedimentation rate less than 30 mm/h for females or less than 20 mm/h for males
6. C-reactive protein less than 10 mg/L

Early diagnosis and treatment of RA are crucial to maintaining optimal functional status in most patients. Recent studies describe development of erosive disease within the first few months of disease. Early and aggressive treatment may limit joint damage, preserving movement and ability to work while reducing medical costs and potential surgery.

Pathogenesis

RA is a disease of an aberrant immune response in a genetically predisposed host that leads to chronic progressive synovial inflammation and destruction of the joint architecture. The hallmark of RA is the proliferation of inflamed synovium, which spreads over the articular surface as a pannus and damages cartilage, bone, and joint capsule. Although research continues to broaden the understanding of the pathophysiologic mechanisms involved in the development and progression of RA, no clear triggering agent has been identified.

Although the precise cause of RA is unknown, hormonal, genetic, and environmental risk factors have been identified. The incidence of RA increases with age. However, incidence begins to decline when people reach their mid-70s. Females are 2 to 3 times more likely to develop rheumatoid arthritis than males. Genetic factors also play a role in some patients. There is a well-established association between RA and HLA-DR4 with an increased relative risk of in 4 to 5 patients with this allele. Recent research has demonstrated an association between RA and Runt-related transcription factor 1 (RUNX1), organic cation transporter gene SLC22A, and peptidyl-larginine deiminases citrullinating enzyme 4 (PADI4). Of lifestyle factors, only smoking has been associated with an increased risk of developing RA.

Prevention

Since the precise etiology of RA has not been identified, preventing the disease is not possible. However, the destructive capacity, pain and stiffness, and resultant disability of RA may be reduced with appropriate recognition and early treatment.

Many nonspecific approaches have been suggested to prevent or minimize recurrences or flares. These include proper nutrition, relaxation, low-impact exercise, flexibility exercises, yoga, tai chi, counseling, meditation, hydrotherapy, and stress reduction.

Clinical Findings

A. SYMPTOMS AND SIGNS

1. ACR criteria—The 1987 revised criteria of the American College of Rheumatology for RA were developed to aid with clinical assessment and performance of clinical trials. RA is diagnosed in patients who meet at least four of the following criteria (criteria 1 through 4 must be present for at least 6 weeks):

1. Morning stiffness lasting at least 1 hour or longer
2. Presence of 3 or more arthritic joint areas (of 14 possible areas)
3. Arthritis of the hands
4. Symmetric arthritis
5. Rheumatoid (subcutaneous) nodules over bony prominences, extensor surfaces, or juxta-articular regions
6. Serum rheumatoid factor
7. Radiographic changes typical of RA (Table 14–8)

RA manifestations may be articular (joint pain, swelling, and stiffness) or nonarticular (see Table 14–7). Nonarticular findings may be classified as systemic (fever, fatigue) or nonsystemic (pleuritis, vasculitis, Felty syndrome, and Sjögren syndrome).

Articular RA can start in any joint, but it most commonly begins in the smaller joints of the fingers, hands, and wrists. Joint involvement is usually symmetric. Joints typically involved include the metacarpophalangeal, proximal interphalangeal, and wrists with sparing of the distal interphalangeal joints. Carpal tunnel syndrome may be an early manifestation of RA. The temporomandibular joint may also be involved. Joints are painful and typically swollen and warm. Prolonged

---

Table 14–8. Diagnostic Criteria for RA Established by the American College of Rheumatology.

- Morning stiffness or stiffness after rest lasting >1 hour
- Polyarthritis of at least 3 joints in 14 areas
- Arthritis of the hand joints
- Symmetric arthritis
- Rheumatoid nodules
- Serum rheumatoid factor
- Radiographic changes

RA, rheumatoid arthritis.

---

stiffness in the joints in the morning or after prolonged inactivity is characteristic of inflammatory arthritis such as RA.

2. Physical examination—Actively inflamed joints are swollen, warm, and tender to palpation. On palpation of the joint, a boggy sensation results from the combination of synovial proliferation and fluid. Synovial proliferation in the flexor tendons of the fingers fills the palm, giving it a flat appearance. Joint range of motion is initially limited by pain and later by contractures. Grip strength is reduced. Carpal tunnel syndrome and synovitis at the elbow manifested as inability to fully extend may be early indications of presence of RA. Ulnar deviation of the fingers at the metacarpophalangeal joint is a common deformity in established disease that results from radial deviation of the wrist and slippage of the extensor tendons to the ulnar side of the metacarpophalangeal joints. Another deformity of the hand that develops in chronic disease is the swan-neck deformity, which results from the flexion of the distal interphalangeal joint and metacarpophalangeal joint with hyperextension of the proximal interphalangeal joint. The boutonniere deformity is caused by avulsion of the extensor hood over the proximal interphalangeal joint. In advanced disease, subluxation and flexion deformities are common and involve the knees, ankles, elbows, wrists, shoulders, hands, and feet.

B. LABORATORY STUDIES

1. Rheumatoid factor—Rheumatoid factor is found in the serum of about 85% of persons with RA. In the individual patient, rheumatoid factor titer is of limited prognostic value, and serial titers are of no value in following the disease process. Higher rheumatoid factor titers tend to correlate with more severe and unremitting disease, more radiologic abnormalities, nodules, extra-articular lesions, and worse functional ability. Conversely, seronegative patients generally have less destructive disease. Rheumatoid factor may be negative in early stages of disease and is not specific for RA. Rheumatoid factor may be present in other connective tissue disorders such as systemic lupus erythematosus (SLE), Raynaud disease, scleroderma, Sjögren syndrome as well as autoimmune thyroid disease and chronic infections such as tuberculosis and endocarditis.

2. Anticyclic citrullinated peptides—Many patients with RA have IgG antibodies to citrullinated peptides (anti-CCP antibody). Such anti-CCP antibodies appear relatively early in RA, are highly specific for the disease (98%), and can be measured by quite reproducible, readily available assay systems. Several experimental observations suggest that the immune responses to citrulline could play a significant role in the pathogenesis of RA inflammation. In contrast to RF, anti-CCP antibodies fluctuate with activity of the disease.

3. Acute phase reactants—Acute-phase reactants such as the erythrocyte sedimentation rate and C-reactive protein measure the inflammatory response and correlate well with the degree of synovial inflammation. They are useful for following the course of inflammatory activity in an individual patient or monitoring response to treatment. Erythrocyte sedimentation rate is an indirect measure of inflammatory proteins and is not reliable in patients with significant anemia.

Thrombocytosis and eosinophilia occur more often in patients with severe disease, high rheumatoid factor titer, rheumatoid nodules, and extra-articular manifestations. Normochromic normocytic anemia of chronic disease is frequently seen in active RA.

C. DIAGNOSTIC IMAGING

1. Radiography—Early radiographic changes in RA include swelling of the soft tissues and periarticular osteopenia. With progressive disease, erosive changes appear. Baseline radiographs of hands or feet should be obtained within 3 months of diagnosis of RA and every 12 to 24 months thereafter to assess development or progression of destructive erosive change.

Since tenosynovitis of the transverse ligament of C1, which stabilizes the odontoid process of C2, may produce significant C1–2 instability, patients with RA planning surgery with general anesthesia (intubation) should be evaluated with a set of lateral flexion and extension views of the cervical spine.

2. Magnetic resonance imaging—New RA lesions may be detected 1 to 5 years earlier with MRI than with conventional radiography. MRI is particularly useful in identifying synovitis.

D. SPECIAL TESTS

It is important to assess functional status and monitor clinical disease activity during treatment. Traditional historical measures of rheumatoid disease activity include duration of morning stiffness (decreases in response to treatment) and time of onset of systemic fatigue (occurring later with response to treatment). Patient self-assessed pain level using a Visual Analogue Scale is very useful in monitoring disease activity and response to treatment. However, pain levels may be significant due to residual joint destruction even without active disease. Less specific historical indicators include need for supplemental or "rescue" analgesics and lost work days. Clinical measures of disease activity include counting the number of swollen joints or in the absence of fixed deformity, range of motion of involved joints. Several well-validated self-administered instruments are available to monitor functional status in RA patients. These include the Health Assessment Questionnaire and the Arthritis Impact Measurement Scale.

Differential Diagnosis

Table 14–9 outlines the key distinguishing features of the seven conditions discussed in this section, including OA, systemic lupus erythematosus (SLE), polymyalgia rheumatica (PMR), infectious arthritis, crystalline arthritides, seronegative spondyloarthropathies, and

Table 14–9. Key Distinguishing Features.

Condition	Feature
Osteoarthritis	Late age at onset Lack of inflammation and constitutional symptoms DIP and PIP involvement
Systemic lupus erythematosus	Positive antinuclear antibody Typically not erosive
Polymyalgia rheumatica	Predominant hip and shoulder involvement Temporal arteritis symptoms
Infectious arthritis	Duration is key
Crystalline arthritides	Synovial fluid analysis is usually definitive
Seronegative spondyloarthropathies	Back pain Affects more men than women
Fibromyalgia	Absence of swelling, rheumatoid factor, and ESR/CRP elevation

DIP, distal interphalangeal; PIP, proximal interphalangeal; ESR, erythrocyte sedimentation rate; CRP, C-reactive protein.

Table 14–10. Differential Diagnosis of Rheumatoid Arthritis.

Acute Inflammatory Disorders

Crystal-induced arthropathy
   Gout
   Pseudogout

Infectious arthritis
   Gonococcal
   Nongonococcal
   Viral

Connective tissue disease-associated arthritis
   Systemic lupus erythematosus
   Polymyositis
   Dermatomyositis
   Scleroderma

Seronegative spondyloarthropathies
   Reiter syndrome
   Psoriatic arthritis

Chronic Inflammatory Disorders
Osteoarthritis

Connective tissue disease–associated arthritis
   Systemic lupus erythematosus
   Polymyositis
   Dermatomyositis
   Scleroderma

Seronegative spondyloarthropathies
   Ankylosing spondylitis
   Reiter syndrome
   Psoriatic arthritis
   Enteropathic arthropathies

Chronic regional pain syndrome

fibromyalgia. Table 14–10 lists a more detailed differential diagnosis that is divided into acute and chronic inflammatory disorders.

A. OSTEOARTHRITIS

OA is differentiated from RA by onset later in life, pattern of joint involvement (proximal interphalangeal, distal interphalangeal, monoarticular involvement of hip or knee, propensity for neck and low back), and absence of inflammatory signs and symptoms. OA is rarely erosive and lacks the morning gelling and systemic features associated with RA.

B. SYSTEMIC LUPUS ERYTHEMATOSUS

SLE and other connective tissue diseases may mimic RA with symmetric joint inflammation. SLE is not typically erosive. Clinical manifestations of SLE (eg, fever, serositis, dermatitis, nephritis) and serologic findings (eg, cytopenia, ANA seropositivity, anti-DNA seropositivity) assist with making the correct diagnosis.

C. POLYMYALGIA RHEUMATICA

PMR and giant cell arteritis may present with symmetric polyarthritis. RA in the elderly may mimic PMR. The presence of arteritic signs or symptoms such as headache, joint claudication, or visual change with predominant shoulder and hip girdle stiffness support the diagnosis of PMR.

D. INFECTIOUS ARTHRITIS

Infectious arthropathies are an important consideration in the setting of fever and polyarthritis. Joint aspiration as well as synovial fluid cultures and blood cultures are often helpful in establishing the diagnosis of bacterial arthritis. Lyme disease may present with myalgias and arthralgias in the setting of erythema chronicum migrans and history of tick bite. Viral arthritides (parvovirus B19, rubella infection, or immunization) often distinguish themselves by history of exposure, accompanying rash, and self-limited course.

E. CRYSTAL DEPOSITION ARTHRITIS

Polyarticular crystal arthropathies, such as gout and pseudogout, may mimic RA. Synovial fluid analysis is usually definitive in crystalline arthritis if performed early during an acute attack. Erosions may be seen in gouty arthritis but they differ from the marginal erosive changes of RA. Chondrocalcinosis may be apparent with pseudogout.

F. SERONEGATIVE SPONDYLOARTHROPATHIES

The seronegative spondyloarthropathies include enteropathic arthritides, psoriatic arthritis, ankylosing spondylitis, and reactive arthritis. Seronegative spondyloarthropathies characteristically present with asymmetric inflammatory disease of the large joints. Involvement of the lumbosacral spine, absence of small-joint disease, and sausaging of the digits support the diagnosis of seronegative spondyloarthropathies. Coexisting uveitis, urethritis, psoriasis, or inflammatory bowel disease also favor a diagnosis of seronegative spondyloarthropathies.

G. FIBROMYALGIA

Although noninflammatory, fibromyalgia may present with diffuse symmetric arthralgias and stiffness at rest. Normal laboratory and imaging studies with the absence of synovitis help differentiate fibromyalgia from RA. Fibromyalgia coexists in 10 to 15% of the patients in whom rheumatic diseases such as RA and SLE are diagnosed.

Treatment

Medications used in the treatment of RA may be categorized as analgesics, anti-inflammatory agents, or disease-modifying antirheumatic drugs (DMARDs)

Table 14–11. Pharmacologic Treatment for Rheumatoid Arthritis

Analgesics
Opioid
Nonopioid
Anti-inflammatory Agents
NSAIDs
Traditional
Celecoxib
Corticosteroids
Disease-modifying Antirheumatic Drugs
Methotrexate
Sulfasalazine
Immunosuppressive Agents
Azathioprine
Cyclophosphamide
Cyclosporine
Anticytokine Therapy
Anti-TNF agents
Etanercept
Infliximab
Adalimumab
Interleukin receptor antagonists
Anakinra
Other Agents
Gold
Minocycline

NSAIDs, nonsteroidal anti-inflammatory drugs; TNF, tumor necrosis factor.

(Table 14–11). In general, analgesics and anti-inflammatory drugs relieve symptoms but do not retard joint damage. Typically, they are more rapidly acting in providing symptomatic benefit in comparison to DMARDs, though newer anti-tumor necrosis factor (TNF) agents also often provide prompt relief of pain and stiffness.

Most patients are initially treated with a combination of an anti-inflammatory agent and one or more DMARDs. Pure analgesics have an important role in supplementing symptom control, particularly pain, and as substitutes for NSAIDs in patients who are intolerant or who are at high-risk for adverse effects. Intra-articular administration of a corticosteroid is important adjunctive therapy in some patients with active disease in an isolated joint. In patients with a polyarticular flare, systemic corticosteroids, either orally or parenterally may provide acute symptom control.

Immediate therapy with DMARDS not only improves symptom control but more importantly retards the progression of erosive, destructive joint disease at an earlier stage. The American College of Rheumatology currently recommends DMARD therapy within 3 months of disease onset. Hopefully, this more aggressive approach will result in preservation of joint structure and function, reduced long-term disability, reduced health care costs and preservation of economic productivity.

In the management of RA, nonpharmacologic treatment must not be neglected. Patient education, physical and occupational therapy, activity modification, and psychosocial support also play important roles in optimizing patient outcome.

Surgical treatment, particularly joint replacement, has dramatically improved the quality of life of many patients with RA over the past 30 years.

A. NONSTEROIDAL ANTI-INFLAMMATORY DRUGS

NSAIDs have long been used as initial therapeutic agents in RA for rapid symptom control. These agents inhibit to some degree one or both COX enzymes (COX-1 and COX-2). The traditional NSAID adverse effects gastropathy and nephrotoxicity are primarily associated with inhibition of COX-1 synthesis. Older, nonselective NSAIDs affect both enzymes, resulting in greater risk of COX-1 adverse effects.

Gastric or duodenal ulcers that can be seen endoscopically develop in 15 to 20% of persons taking nonselective NSAIDs. More significant symptomatic lesions develop in 2 to 4% with 1 to 2% noting ulcer complications of bleeding or perforation. Risk factors for NSAID gastropathy include older age, higher dose NSAID, previous history of peptic ulcer disease, previous use of antacids or H_2-antagonists, concomitant use of corticosteroids, and more severe inflammatory disease.

Selective COX-2 inhibitors are associated with an approximate 50% reduction in prostaglandin-mediated clinical gastrointestinal toxicity in comparison to nonselective agents. However, accumulating evidence suggests therapy with newer selective COX-2 agents (ie, rofecoxib and valdecoxib, which are no longer available) is associated with a significant increase in cardiovascular adverse events including myocardial infarction and stroke, particularly at higher doses and in higher risk patients. No difference in efficacy between COX-2 inhibitors and nonselective drugs has been demonstrated. In addition, no difference in renal toxicity between the two classes of NSAIDs has been shown.

Based on currently available data, patients with rheumatoid disease who require NSAID therapy but who are at high risk for gastrointestinal adverse effects and who have no history or risk factors for cardiovascular events may be treated with celecoxib. Alternatively, a nonselective NSAID may be combined with a proton pump inhibitor such as omeprazole for gastric protection. In patients with significant cardiovascular risk factors or history, selective COX-2 NSAIDs should be avoided.

Unfortunately, co-therapy with low-dose aspirin for cardiovascular prophylaxis in such patients negates the COX-2 inhibitor's beneficial reduction of gastrointestinal toxicity. Low-dose (<10 mg prednisone equivalent) corticosteroid therapy combined with a pure analgesic such as acetaminophen represents a reasonable alternative to an NSAID for management of inflammatory symptoms.

B. CORTICOSTEROIDS

Corticosteroids may be administered systemically or locally for treatment of RA. Low-dose (<10 mg prednisone equivalent) corticosteroids taken orally are typically combined with other medications in initial management of RA. Corticosteroids provide prompt suppression of inflammation and may be viewed as "bridging therapy" while treatment with more slowly acting DMARDs is being initiated. Many patients remain on long-term corticosteroid therapy, however, posing risk of long-term corticosteroid toxicity, particularly cataracts and bone loss (osteoporosis). In persons in whom longer term use of corticosteroid therapy is anticipated, baseline bone density measurement is recommended and prophylactic treatment with calcium supplementation, vitamin D, and antiresorptive therapy such as diphosphonates should be considered.

For patients experiencing generalized "flares" of disease activity, a short, rapidly tapering course of an oral corticosteroid may provide prompt, short-term relief of severe polyarticular and systemic symptoms. Alternatively, intramuscular injection of a "depo" corticosteroid may provide similar benefit. Use of such "pulse" treatment should be reserved for episodic treatment of severe flares and probably limited to 2 to 3 times yearly. Excessive administration of intramuscular or pulse corticosteroids is associated with risk of iatrogenic Cushing syndrome as well as the full range of corticosteroid toxicity and should prompt reevaluation of the patient's regular rheumatoid therapy.

Intra-articular injection of corticosteroid may effectively reduce inflammatory pain and swelling in joints refractory to systemic therapy. Injection into any single joint should be limited to three or four times within 1 year. Systemic absorption of corticosteroid occurs and diabetic patients should be warned about the possibility of transient hyperglycemia.

C. DISEASE-MODIFYING ANTIRHEUMATIC DRUGS

The defining characteristic of a DMARD is the ability to retard erosive joint damage by controlling synovial inflammation. For most older DMARDs, the precise mechanism of action is unknown.

The American College of Rheumatology currently recommends starting DMARD therapy within 3 months of disease onset. Most patients should be started on DMARD therapy at the time of initial diagnosis. DMARDs may be used as monotherapy or in combinations depending on the disease severity, prognostic features, costs, and comorbidity. In addition to slowing radiographic progression of disease, DMARDs are more effective than NSAIDs in reducing systemic symptoms such as fever or fatigue.

1. Antimalarials—These agents, including hydroxychloroquine and chloroquine, are less potent DMARDs often used to treat early or mild RA in combination with an NSAID. Hydroxychloroquine is well tolerated but slow-acting, which is a characteristic feature of most older DMARDs. Patients may not notice therapeutic effect for 3 to 6 months. If total daily dose is limited to 5.5 mg/kg/d and never exceeds 400 mg/d, serious retinal toxicity is rare. Annual ophthalmologic examination is required in all patients, however, to detect retinopathy.

2. Methotrexate—Methotrexate is a folate analog that blocks DNA synthesis, though its antirheumatic effect may be related to other anti-inflammatory properties of the drug.

For most patients with active RA, methotrexate remains the first-line choice because of its established and sustained efficacy with manageable toxicity as well as a substantial cost advantage over newer biologic agents. Approximately 60% of patients with RA respond to methotrexate, which is comparable to the results seen with newer biologic agents, such as etanercept.

Methotrexate is typically administered in a once weekly oral dose of 7.5 to 15 mg. Escalation of dose by 2.5 to 5.0 mg increments based on clinical response should be considered at 4- to 6-week intervals. In the absence of significant toxicity, the dose of methotrexate may be increased to 20 to 25 mg weekly based on the clinical response. Clinical response to the drug occurs with 4–12 weeks. Clinical indicators of response include reduced morning stiffness and systemic fatigue as well as the number of swollen, tender joints. A significant proportion of patients with early RA can achieve disease control for at least 1 year by taking methotrexate alone.

Methotrexate is excreted by the kidneys and is contraindicated in patients with creatinine levels over 2.0 to 2.5 mg/dL. Patients who consume significant amounts of alcohol on a regular basis should not be treated with methotrexate because of risk of hepatic toxicity. In general, limiting alcohol intake to the equivalent of a glass of wine once or twice weekly is reasonable advice for patients taking methotrexate. Regular monitoring of liver function tests (complete blood count, aspartate aminotransferase, and alanine aminotransferase) is appropriate, but hepatic fibrosis may occur in the face of normal enzymes. Regular liver biopsy to monitor for fibrosis is not routinely recommended at antirheumatic doses of methotrexate.

In patients in whom methotrexate is contraindicated, initial therapeutic alternatives include sulfasalazine, hydroxychloraquine, or even etanercept or adalimumab, depending on the severity of the disease.

Methotrexate may be combined with anti-TNF drug therapy (etanercept, infliximab, or adalimumab). Recent trials suggest combined methotrexate and anti-TNF therapy is more efficacious than monotherapy with either agent. However, long-term toxicity of combined therapy is unknown, (ie, is the risk of lymphoma increased?). Also, cost-benefit analysis of combined versus monotherapy needs further study. Patients with active rheumatoid disease who do not respond to anti-TNF therapy alone or in combination with methotrexate should be considered for treatment with anakinra (see below).

3. Leflunomide—Leflunomide is a pyrimidine synthesis inhibitor with a clinical profile very similar to methotrexate. Efficacy that is similar to methotrexate, including reduction in radiographic erosive disease, has been demonstrated. Like methotrexate, hepatic toxicity occurs, elevating liver enzymes. Diarrhea is a common side effect of the drug, which may require discontinuation of treatment. Leflunomide therapy is initiated with a 3-day loading dose (100 mg/d) and then continued in a single 20-mg daily dose. Like methotrexate, improvement in signs and symptoms occurs within about 6 weeks. Regular monitoring for thrombocytopenia and liver enzyme elevation should be performed.

4. Sulfasalazine—Though initially developed as an anti-inflammatory antirheumatic drug in the precorticosteroid era more than 60 years ago, sulfasalazine has been more widely used to treat inflammatory bowel disease. Sulfasalazine demonstrates modest DMARD qualities including reduction in radiographic erosive disease and improvement in articular inflammatory signs and symptoms. The mechanism of action of the drug in RA is not known, but the metabolites of the drug—sulfapyridine and 5-ASA—have a variety of effects on cellular immune function.

Sulfasalazine is best administered in an enteric-coated form to reduce the risk of gastrointestinal toxicity. Therapy is initiated at a dose of 500 mg/d with escalation over 1 to 2 months to the full antirheumatic dose of 2000 mg/d. Sulfasalazine is slow acting with approximately 3 months of therapy required before clinical improvement occurs. Toxicity of sulfasalazine includes gastrointestinal distress (minimized by the enteric-coated preparation) and, rarely, agranulocytosis. Complete blood count should be performed regularly to monitor for toxicity.

D. Immunosuppressive Agents

Azathioprine, cyclophosphamide, and cyclosporine have largely been replaced as treatment for severe, active RA by newer biologic therapies including anti-TNF agents (etanercept, infliximab, adalimumab) and interleukin receptor antagonists (anakinra). In general, use of these older immunosuppressives is limited primarily by significant toxicity. Cyclosporine commonly causes hypertension and renal impairment, complicating its use with methotrexate in RA. Cyclophosphamide is an alkylating agent with significant toxicity. Hemorrhagic cystitis, bone marrow suppression, and risk of lymphoma are major concerns. Azathioprine is the most commonly used drug in this group, often in combination with methotrexate. Bone marrow suppression and concerns regarding oncogenicity limit its usefulness.

E. Anticytokine Therapy

The newest agents available for treatment of RA are targeted at proinflammatory cytokines, which are central to the pathogenesis of the disease. Sometimes referred to as "biologics" for "biologic response modifiers," these presently include three drugs targeted at TNFα and one interleukin-1b antagonist. TNFα and interleukin-1b are secreted by synovial macrophages and T helper lymphocytes and play a major role in pannus development and joint destruction. They stimulate proliferation of synovial cells and production of collagenase, which degrades cartilage contributing to erosive joint damage.

TNFα also promotes recruitment of other inflammatory cells and increased secretion of interleukins, perpetuating the inflammatory process. By specifically interfering with this inflammatory cascade, the biologics produce prompt and significant clinical effects in patients with RA. The cost of anticytokine therapy is substantial, exceeding $12 000 annually. This represents a significant consideration in choice of first-line therapy for many patients.

1. Etanercept—Etanercept is a TNFα receptor fusion protein that binds soluble TNFα, inhibiting its ability to bind to cellular surface receptors and exert its proinflammatory effects. Etanercept produces comparable clinical improvement to methotrexate (20 mg weekly) in the signs and symptoms of RA but does so much more rapidly, often within 2 weeks of the first dose. Long-term studies comparing methotrexate and etanercept suggest comparable benefits in reducing radiographic damage to joints. Combined therapy with etanercept and methotrexate is more effective than either drug alone. Long-term follow-up studies now beyond 6 years suggest continued efficacy and safety of combined methotrexate and etanercept.

Etanercept is administered by subcutaneous injection, either in a single 50-mg weekly dose or in two 25-mg split weekly doses with comparable efficacy. Mild injection site reactions occur in about one-third of patients, particularly during early therapy. Opportunistic infections, which may be life-threatening rarely occur in patients treated with etanercept.

Reactivation of tuberculosis is a particular concern and patients should be screened for tuberculosis by history and with a purified protein derivative (PPD) skin test before starting therapy. Demyelinating disease and non-Hodgkins lymphomas have rarely been reported in patients using etanercept. The incidence of non-Hodgkins lymphomas in etanercept-treated patients is comparable to the RA population in general. Cytopenias have rarely been reported.

2. Infliximab—Infliximab is a chimeric (murine/human) IgG monoclonal antibody to TNFα which in combination with methotrexate has comparable efficacy to etanercept in the treatment of RA. The drug is administered by intravenous infusion at a dose of 3 to 5 mg/kg at intervals of 4 to 8 weeks. Clinical response is rapid. Antibodies to the drug develop in about 40% of patients but do not appear to affect efficacy or safety.

Infusion reactions characterized by headache, rash, nausea, or hypotension may occur and are usually mild. As with etanercept, serious infections, particularly tuberculosis, have been reported with infliximab therapy. Most cases represent reactivation of dormant disease and occur within 6 months of starting infliximab therapy. Extrapulmonary disease is common. Screening as discussed with etanercept is mandatory in patients before initiating treatment. Anticytokine treatment should be suspended in patients in whom a serious infection is developing. Vaccination with a live vaccine is contraindicated during treatment with all TNF inhibitors. Higher doses of infliximab (10 mg/kg) in patients with heart failure have caused worsening of the failure. As with etanercept therapy, infliximab treatment has been associated with development of autoantibodies, including anti–double-stranded DNA. Rarely, a lupus-like reaction has been seen with either infliximab or etanercept. Since all patients receiving infliximab are also treated with methotrexate, appropriate monitoring for methotrexate adverse effects, as discussed earlier, is required.

3. Adalimumab—Adalimumab is a fully human recombinant IgG antibody to TNFα with similar efficacy and toxicity to etanercept and infliximab. Adalimumab is effective as monotherapy or in combination with methotrexate. Adalimumab provides additional benefit to patients taking a stable dose of methotrexate alone. Adalimumab is administered by subcutaneous injection in a recommended dose of 40 mg every other week.

4. Anakinra—Interleukin-1 receptor antagonist protein (IL-1Ra) is a naturally occurring IL-1 inhibitor that binds to the IL-1 receptor without producing cellular activation, effectively blocking the proinflammatory effects of IL-1. Anakinra is a human recombinant IL-1 receptor antagonist that has demonstrated efficacy in patients with RA. Clinical benefits and radiographic effects are generally fewer than those with anti-TNFα agents. Anakinra is administered daily by subcutaneous injection.

A significantly increased risk of serious infection has been seen when anakinra is combined with anti-TNFα drugs such as etanercept. Combination with older DMARDs such as methotrexate or sulfasalazine appears safe.

F. Analgesics

Pure analgesics play an important role in arthritis pain management. In patients with active RA, inflammatory pain is best managed with NSAIDs, corticosteroids (systemic or intra-articular) and ultimately with control of disease by a DMARD such as methotrexate. The presence of active inflammation is suggested by prolonged morning stiffness, systemic fatigue, and palpable joint swelling (synovitis) and warmth. However, some patients with active disease require additional analgesic treatment during initiation of DMARD therapy or because of toxicity or intolerance to NSAIDs or corticosteroids. For some patients, full dose acetaminophen is adequate adjunctive treatment but many require at least transient or supplemental treatment with an opioid analgesic.

Some patients with RA who have responded well to DMARD therapy still experience significant pain as a consequence of significant joint damage from quiescent prior synovitis. In these patients, inflammatory signs and indicators are absent. These symptoms do not require escalation of anti-inflammatory or DMARD therapy.

Treatment of pain in persons with controlled or "burnt-out" RA is similar to pain management discussed for OA and involves local (topical or intra-articular) modalities, assistive devices, as well as nonopioid and opioid analgesics.

G. Other Therapies

Gold compounds administered parenterally or orally have demonstrated efficacy and a long history of use in RA but are rarely used at this time. Less than 10% of patients continue taking gold 5 years after starting therapy in contrast to much higher rates of patients treated with methotrexate or anticytokine drugs. For similar reasons, D-penicillamine use for RA has declined precipitously as well.

Minocycline is an antibiotic that has been shown to favorably affect signs and symptoms of RA. Its mechanism of action is unknown but the drug has anti-inflammatory properties. No disease-modifying effect has ever been demonstrated.

H. Nonpharmacologic Therapies

A comprehensive approach to treatment of rheumatoid arthritis is required to ensure the efficacy of the management plan, ultimately providing decreased pain, increased mobility, and improved patient satisfaction and quality of life.

1. Education—Patient education is essential early in the disease course and on an ongoing basis. Because RA may make a patient prone to fatigue and muscle weakness, energy conservation and joint protection techniques are important in limiting pain while maintaining function. Education is directed at patients and family members.

2. Exercise—Muscle strengthening or aerobic exercise programs also play an important role in maintenance of function and optimizing outcome. All individuals should be encouraged and supported to participate in the minimum level of physical activity recommended by the US Surgeon General—at least 30 minutes of moderate physical activity on most days of the week. Persons with OA and RA who have difficulty in maintaining minimum levels of physical activity may be referred to physical or occupational therapy to evaluate and reduce impairments in range of motion, flexibility, strength, and endurance as well as receive instruction in joint protection strategies. Therapists will properly prepare an individual for successful participation in a community-based or self-directed exercise program. In addition, modalities such as splinting, ice, heat, paraffin baths (see Chapter 6), and massage have been shown to be useful for pain management in adults with RA. Transcutaneous electrical nerve stimulation (TENS) has been shown to improve wrist function while reducing pain with minimal adverse effects in RA patients.

3. Self-management techniques—A patient's thoughts, feelings, emotions, and behavior, and his or her family's response, can influence the arthritis pain experience. Therefore, education about pain, pain management options, and self-management programs should be communicated to the patient and family as an integral and cost-effective part of treatment. The degree to which RA affects daily activities depends in part on how well the patient can cope with the disease. Cognitive-behavioral therapy may be used to reduce pain and psychological disability and to enhance self-efficacy and pain coping. Use of assistive equipment or devices (Table 14–12) is another adjunctive treatment to help maintain function while minimizing or reducing pain.

4. Alternative therapies—People with arthritis should be advised to maintain an ideal body weight and adhere to a balanced diet containing adequate amounts of

Table 14–12. Assistive and Adaptive Equipment to Help Patients with Rheumatoid Arthritis.

Aimed at Improving Movement or Positioning
Compression gloves
Elastic wrist extensor orthoses
Resting hand splints
Thumb post splints
Dynamic splints
Ankle and foot orthoses
Knee braces
Spinal orthoses
Aimed at Improving Activities of Daily Living
Custom shoes
Canes
Crutches
Walkers
Wheelchair
Scooters
Built-up handles on brushes (tooth and hair) and eating utensils
Button/zipper hook
Velcro fasteners on clothing
Elastic shoe laces
Sock aids
Long handle shoe horn
Jar openers

protein, fat, vitamins, and minerals. Adults should lose weight if their body mass index is greater than 30 and follow a weight management program. Fish oil supplements, fasting, and a vegetarian diet may reduce pain in some patients with RA. Evidence from double-blind, placebo-controlled randomized clinical trials supports dietary omega-3 polyunsaturated fatty acids in reducing morning stiffness and joint tenderness in RA. However, the clinical application of fish oil in the treatment of RA is not well-defined in terms of dose and duration of therapy. Fish oil has not been shown to benefit patients with OA.

Fasting has been shown to reduce pain and stiffness associated with RA. However, most persons relapse as food is reintroduced. Fasting followed by a vegetarian diet for 1 year has shown a reduction in the number of tender joints and duration of morning stiffness. Reduction of joint inflammation and pain was sustained if vegetarian diet was followed. There is insufficient evidence of the benefits of electromagnetic field therapy to recommend its use in the management of pain related to arthritis. Prayer and spirituality may also play a role in reduction of pain in patients with RA.

I. SURGERY

Indications for surgery in RA include loss of function and pain that is refractory to medical management. For optimal functional results, people with disabling arthritis should be referred for surgical care prior to the onset of joint contracture, severe deformity, advanced muscular wasting, and deconditioning rather than as a last resort. If the patient has severe pain in the hips and knees that significantly limits activities despite any drug or nondrug therapies, with significant radiographic damage, orthopedic referral should be considered.

1. Arthroplasty—Joint replacement surgery restores the integrity and functional power of a joint. For many people with RA whose joints are severely damaged, joint replacement surgery can restore joint function, reduce pain, or correct a deformity. Hip and knee total joint arthroplasty provide major improvement in musculoskeletal function and improved quality of life with benefit of complete pain relief in most cases. Because of their documented effectiveness, these procedures should be offered to patients when nonsurgical management becomes less effective and preferably before deconditioning becomes severe and difficult to reverse.

2. Arthrodesis—Arthrodesis is the surgical removal of the articular surface and fixation of the two bones to promote bone fusion at the prior joint. Joints treated with total joint arthroplasty (hip, knee, shoulder, and less frequently the elbow) are rarely treated with arthrodesis because of the likelihood of functional deficit. The most successful arthrodesis is performed on joints where replacement is not an option, such as the subtalar, calcaneocuboid, talonavicular, midfoot joints of the feet, and the lesser joints of the hands and feet.

3. Synovectomy—Synovectomy is sometimes performed to remove inflammatory tissue and retard joint destruction. Synovectomy of selected joints may transiently alleviate symptoms and improve function in the first year after operation. Long-term benefits of synovectomy are less clear and concurrent medical therapy must be maintained. Removal of synovial tissue from the wrist and dorsal tendon sheath and resection of the ulnar head might prevent rupture of extensor tendons in patients at risk.

Table 14–13. Poor Prognostic Indicators for Patients with Rheumatoid Arthritis

More than 10–20 joints involved
Extra-articular manifestations (especially nodules and vasculitis)
Rheumatoid factor–positive
Erosions on radiographs within 2 years of disease onset
HLA-DR4 genetic marker
Education level lower than 11th grade

Prognosis

The course of the disease varies considerably among individuals. Poor prognosis is suggested by earlier age at disease onset, high titer of rheumatoid factor, elevated erythrocyte sedimentation rate, and swelling of more than 20 joints. Extra-articular manifestations of RA, such as rheumatoid nodules, Sjögren syndrome, episcleritis and scleritis, interstitial lung disease, pericardial involvement, systemic vasculitis, and Felty syndrome, may also indicate a worse prognosis (Table 14–13).

Studies have shown that patients with active, polyarticular, rheumatoid factor–positive RA have a greater than 70% probability of joint damage or erosions developing within 2 years of the onset of disease. Since studies have demonstrated that DMARDs may alter the disease course in patients with recent-onset RA, particularly those with unfavorable prognostic factors, aggressive treatment should be initiated as soon as the diagnosis has been established. Frequently, the disease can be controlled with a combination of treatments. Treatment may vary depending on the severity of the symptoms.

Remission is most likely to occur in the first year and the probability decreases as time progresses. About 20% of persons will have experienced remission by 10 to 15 years from diagnosis.

Between 50 and 70% of patients with RA will remain capable of full-time employment. After 15 to 20 years, only 10% of patients are severely disabled, and unable to perform simple activities of daily living (washing, toileting, dressing, eating). The average life expectancy of patients with RA may be shortened by 3 to 7 years. Patients with severe forms of RA may die 10 to 15 years earlier than expected.

American College of Rheumatology Subcommittee on Rheumatoid Arthritis Guidelines. Guidelines for the management of rheumatoid arthritis: *Arthritis Rheum.* 2002;46:328. [PMID: 11840435]

Borchers AT et al. The use of methotrexate in rheumatoid arthritis. *Semin Arthritis Rheum.* 2004;34:465. [PMID: 15305245]

Bukhari MA et al. Influence of disease-modifying therapy on radiographic outcome in inflammatory polyarthritis at five years:

Results from a large observational inception study. *Arthritis Rheum.* 2003;48:46. [PMID: 12528102]

Choi HK. Diet and rheumatoid arthritis: Red meat and beyond. *Arthritis Rheum.* 2004;50:3745. [PMID: 15593227]

Ejbjerg B et al. Low cost, low field dedicated extremity MRI is highly specific and sensitive for synovitis and bone erosions in rheumatoid arthritis wrist and finger joints: A comparison with conventional high-field MRI and radiography. *Ann Rheum Dis.* 2005;64:1280. [PMID: 15650012]

Haraoui B. The anti-tumor necrosis factor agents are a major advance in the treatment of rheumatoid arthritis. *J Rheumatol Suppl.* 2005;72:46. [PMID: 15660467]

Herman CJ et al. Use of complementary therapies among primary care clinic patients with arthritis. *Prev Chronic Dis.* 2004;1:A12. [PMID: 15670444]

Kuritzky L et al. Advances in rheumatology: Coxibs and beyond. *J Pain Symptom Manage.* 2003;25:S6. [PMID: 12604153]

Li LC. What else can I do but take drugs? The future of research in nonpharmacological treatment in early inflammatory arthritis. *J Rheumatol Suppl.* 2005;72:21. [PMID: 15660459]

Maddison P et al. Leflunomide in rheumatoid arthritis: Recommendations through a process of consensus. *Rheumatology (Oxford).* 2005;44:280. [PMID: 15657072]

Maetzel A. Cost-effectiveness estimates reported for tumor necrosis factor blocking agents in rheumatoid arthritis refractory to methotrexate—a brief summary. *J Rheumatol Suppl.* 2005;72:51. [PMID: 15660469]

O'dell J. Rheumatoid arthritis initial therapy: Unanswered questions. *J Rheumatol Suppl.* 2005;72:14. [PMID: 15660457]

Osiri M et al. Leflunomide for treating rheumatoid arthritis. *J Rheumatol.* 2003;6:1182. [PMID: 12784387]

Pincus T et al. Methotrexate as the "anchor drug" for the treatment of early rheumatoid arthritis. *Clin Exp Rheumatol.* 2003;21(Suppl 31):S179. [PMID: 14969073]

Quinn MA et al. Very early treatment with infliximab in addition to methotrexate in early, poor-prognosis rheumatoid arthritis reduces magnetic resonance imaging evidence of synovitis and damage, with sustained benefit after infliximab withdrawal: Results from a twelve-month randomized, double-blind, placebo-controlled trial. *Arthritis Rheum.* 2005;52:27. [PMID: 15641102]

Rantapaa-Dahlqvist S et al. Antibodies against citrullinated peptide and IgA rheumatoid factor predict the development of rheumatoid arthritis. *Arthritis Rheum.* 2003;48:2741. [PMID: 14558078]

Sander O. Long-term use of combination DMARDs did not sustain disease remissions, but delayed joint damage in early rheumatoid arthritis. *ACP J Club.* 2005;142:9. [PMID: 15656250]

Saraux A et al. Value of antibodies to citrulline-containing peptides for diagnosing early rheumatoid arthritis. *J Rheumatol.* 2003;30:2535. [PMID: 14719190]

Schooff M et al. Is leflunomide as safe and effective in the treatment of rheumatoid arthritis as other DMARDs? *Am Fam Physician.* 2003;68:849. [PMID: 13678131]

Stephensen CB. Fish oil and inflammatory disease: Is asthma the next target for n-3 fatty acid supplements? *Nutr Rev.* 2004;62:486. [PMID: 15648824]

Fibromyalgia

15

Roland Staud, MD

ESSENTIALS OF DIAGNOSIS

- *Chronic widespread pain for more than 3 months (upper and lower body and lower back) and mechanical tenderness indicated by ≥ 11 of 18 tender points.*
- *Insomnia, fatigue, and distress.*
- *Abnormal hypothalamic-pituitary axis response to stress.*
- *Coaggregation with major mood disorders.*
- *Coaggregation with other chronic pain syndromes, such as irritable bowel syndrome, chronic fatigue syndrome, migraine, Gulf War syndrome, and lower back pain.*

General Considerations

Fibromyalgia syndrome (FM) is a chronic pain syndrome, characterized by generalized pain, tender points, disturbed sleep, and pronounced fatigue. Pain in FM is consistently felt in the musculature and is related to sensitization of central nervous system (CNS) pain pathways. The pathogenesis of FM is unknown, although abnormal concentration of CNS neuropeptides and alterations of the hypothalamic-pituitary-adrenal axis have been described. There is a large body of evidence for a generalized lowering of pressure pain thresholds in FM patients. Importantly, this mechanical allodynia in patients with FM is not limited to tender points but appears to be widespread. In addition, almost all studies of patients with FM have shown abnormalities of pain sensitivity while using different methods of neurosensory testing.

By definition, FM encompasses the extreme end of chronic widespread pain in the general population and is a chronic illness that disproportionately affects women (9:1). Like many other syndromes, FM has no single specific feature but represents a symptom complex of self-reported or elicited findings. In 1990, the American College of Rheumatology (ACR) published diagnostic criteria for FM that include chronic widespread pain (>3 months) and mechanical allodynia in at least 11 of 18 tender points. Most tender point sites are located at tendon insertion areas and have shown few detectable tissue abnormalities. Besides musculoskeletal pain and mechanical tenderness, most FM patients also complain of insomnia, fatigue, and distress. The familial coaggregation and frequent comorbidity of FM with major mood disorders also suggests a role for neuroendocrine and stress-response abnormalities.

Burckhardt CS et al. *Guideline for the Management of Fibromyalgia Syndrome Pain in Adults and Children*, APS Clinical Practice Guideline Series #4. Glenview, IL: American Pain Society; 2005.

Giesecke T et al. Subgrouping of fibromyalgia patients on the basis of pressure-pain thresholds and psychological factors. *Arthritis Rheum.* 2003;48:2916. [PMID: 14558098]

Maquet D et al. Pressure pain thresholds of tender point sites in patients with fibromyalgia and in healthy controls. *Eur J Pain.* 2004;8:111. [PMID: 14987620]

Neeck G. Neuroendocrine and hormonal perturbations and relations to the serotonergic system in fibromyalgia patients. *Scand J Rheumatol Suppl.* 2000;113:8. [PMID: 11028824]

Petzke F et al. Differences in unpleasantness induced by experimental pressure pain between patients with fibromyalgia and healthy controls. *Eur J Pain.* 2005;9:325. [PMID: 15862482]

Petzke F et al. What do tender points measure? Influence of distress on 4 measures of tenderness. *J Rheumatol.* 2003;30:567. [PMID: 12610818]

Russell IJ. The promise of substance P inhibitors in fibromyalgia. *Rheum Dis Clin North Am.* 2002;28:329. [PMID: 12122921]

Thieme K et al. Predictors of pain behaviors in fibromyalgia syndrome. *Arthritis Rheum.* 2005;53:343. [PMID: 15934120]

Pathogenesis

Patients with FM, which is a pain amplification syndrome, are highly sensitive to painful and nonpainful stimuli, including touch, heat, cold, and chemical stimuli. However, it should be noted that the hypersensitivity of these patients is not limited to pain, but also includes light, sound, and smell. The cause for the heightened sensitivity of patients with FM is unknown, but CNS pain processing abnormalities have been reported in several studies. Most of these studies found evidence of central sensitization indicating lowered nociceptive thresholds at the dorsal horn of the spinal cord and the brain. Although peripheral nociceptive input is required for pain in FM, an important characteristic of central sensitization is that it requires very little sustained nociceptive input from peripheral tissues for the maintenance of the sensitized state and chronic pain.

A. GENETIC OR FAMILIAL PREDISPOSITION

There is increasing evidence of a familial aggregation for FM, although these data often are inferential rather than definitive. Several prospective studies have suggested that relatives of patients with FM display higher than expected rates of FM. Family members of patients with FM also display a high frequency of a number of conditions related to FM, including irritable bowel syndrome, chronic fatigue syndrome, migraine headaches, and mood disorders. Many of these allied conditions, such as migraine headaches and major depression, have also been noted independently to have a familial predilection.

B. TRIGGERING EVENTS

The onset of FM has frequently been associated with certain triggers. Like many illnesses, the start of FM symptoms may occur when genetically predisposed individuals become exposed to certain environmental triggers that can initiate the development of symptoms. Most environmental exposures that have been described as triggers for FM can be categorized as "stressors" including physical trauma; infections; emotional distress; endocrine disorders; and immune activation, which sometimes result in autoimmune disorders.

These stressors seem to result in high degrees of pain, disability, life interference, and affective distress as well as decreasing levels of physical activity. Some of the strongest evidence supporting the association of trauma and FM symptoms was obtained during prospective studies of adults with neck injuries. Compared with adults with lower extremity fractures or ankle injury, neck trauma carried a more than 10-fold increased risk of developing FM within 1 year of injury. Additional evidence supporting such an association include sleep abnormalities postinjury, local injury sites as a source of chronic distal regional pain, and recent evidence of extensive CNS neuroplasticity in FM. Chronic pain after neck injury raises several important questions about the role that injury location plays in long-term outcome. Obviously, there is something different between neck and leg trauma. One important fact may be related to the difference in local pain sensitivity, with neck and upper chest area showing decreased mechanical pain thresholds compared with the lower extremities. Further prospective studies, however, are needed to confirm this association and to identify whether trauma plays a causal role in FM pain.

C. ABNORMAL RESPONSE TO STRESSORS

The biologic response to stressors appears predictable in animals and humans. Particularly, events that are perceived as inescapable or unavoidable, or which appear unpredictable, evoke the strongest adverse biologic responses. This may explain why trauma victims appear to develop much higher rates of FM than injured persons who are responsible for the incident. In addition, early life stressors can have a permanent and profound impact on subsequent biologic responses to stress, which may explain the higher than expected incidence of traumatic childhood events in persons in whom chronic pain later develops.

D. POSTTRAUMATIC STRESS DISORDER IN FM

More than 50% of patients with FM have been found to suffer from posttraumatic stress disorder (PTSD) in the United States and Israel. Compared with the prevalence of PTSD in the general population (6%), patients with FM show a greatly increased rate of PTSD that is similar to Vietnam veterans and victims of natural disasters or motor vehicle accidents. PTSD often occurs after a significant traumatic event and is characterized by behavioral, emotional, functional, and physiologic symptoms.

Relevant traumatic events related to PTSD are usually perceived by the person as threatening his or her life or physical integrity and can lead to emotional responses including horror, helplessness, or intense fear. The psychological symptoms of PTSD include reexperience of the traumatic event, avoidance, and increased arousal. It has been shown that the experience of trauma is associated with increased somatic and physical complaints, including pain. Not surprisingly, the incidence of FM is increased in patients with PTSD (21%); the combination of FM and PTSD is often associated with increased pain ratings, more distress, and higher functional impairment. As with several other disorders, however, it is unclear whether PTSD is the cause or consequence of FM.

E. FM AS AN AFFECTIVE SPECTRUM DISORDER

Numerous studies have reported that FM and major depressive disorder are comorbidities. The outcome of a recent large family study of FM probands was consistent with the hypothesis that FM and major depressive disorder are characterized by shared, genetically mediated risk factors. Although the findings of this study should not be interpreted to mean that major depressive disorder and FM represent different forms of the same syndrome, they strongly suggest that FM and major depressive disorder share important CNS mechanisms.

F. THE ROLE OF CENTRAL SENSITIZATION

Tissue sensitization after injury has long been recognized as an important contribution to pain and may play an important role in FM pain. This form of sensitization is related to changes of the properties of primary nociceptive afferents (peripheral sensitization), whereas

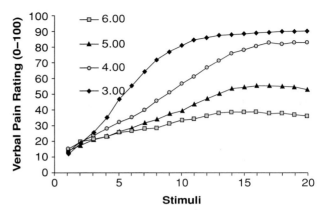

Figure 15–1. Windup of healthy persons. Twenty identical heat stimuli (52°C) were applied to the hand. With increasing stimulus frequency (1 tap every 3–6 seconds), the pain ratings progressively increased.

central sensitization requires functional changes in the CNS (neuroplasticity). Such CNS changes may result in central sensitization, which manifests itself as the following:

1. Increased excitability of spinal cord neurons after an injury.
2. Enlargement of these neurons' receptive fields.
3. Reduction in pain threshold.
4. Recruitment of novel afferent inputs.

Behaviorally, centrally sensitized patients, like FM sufferers, report abnormal or heightened pain sensitivity; this hypersensitivity spreads to uninjured sites and pain is generated by low threshold mechanoreceptors that are normally silent in pain processing. Thus, tissue injury may not only cause pain but also an expansion of dorsal horn receptive fields and central sensitization.

There are several important points that are relevant for clinical practice. When central sensitization has occurred in patients with chronic pain (eg, in those with FM), very little additional nociceptive input is required to maintain the sensitized state. Thus, seemingly innocuous daily activities may contribute to the maintenance of chronic pain states. In addition, the decay of painful sensations is prolonged in FM, and therefore, patients should not expect drastic changes of their pain levels during brief therapeutic interventions. Many analgesic medications do not seem to improve central sensitization, and some medications (including opioids) have been shown to maintain or even worsen this central phenomenon.

G. Temporal Summation of Second Pain (Windup) in FM

The noninvasive method of summation of second pain or windup can be used in FM patients for evaluation of central sensitization. This technique reveals sensitivity to input from unmyelinated (C) afferents and the status of the N-methyl-D-aspartate (NMDA) receptor systems

that are implicated in a variety of chronic pain conditions (Figure 15–1). Thermal, mechanical, or electrical windup stimuli can be easily applied to the skin or musculature of patients. Commercial neurosensory stimulators are readily available that can be used for windup testing. Patients with FM show excessive summation of C-fiber mediated pain. Temporal summation depends on activation of NMDA transmitter systems by C nociceptors, and chronic central pain states like FM can result from excessive temporal summation of pain.

H. Pain Amplification

1. Temporal summation of second pain or windup—Repetitive C-fiber stimulation can result in a progressive increase of electrical discharges from second order neurons in the spinal cord. This important mechanism of pain amplification in the dorsal horn neurons of the spinal cord is related to temporal summation of second pain or windup. **First pain** is conducted by myelinated Aδ pain fibers and is often described as sharp or lancinating and can be readily distinguished from second pain by most persons. **Second pain** (transmitted by unmyelinated C fibers) is strongly related to chronic pain states and is most frequently reported as dull, aching, or burning. Second pain increases in intensity when painful stimuli are applied more often than once every 3 seconds. This progressive increase represents temporal summation (termed "windup") and has been demonstrated to result from CNS rather than peripheral nervous system mechanisms. Importantly, windup and second pain can be inhibited by application of NMDA receptor antagonists, including dextromethorphan and ketamine.

2. Abnormal windup in patients with FM—Abnormal windup and central sensitization may be relevant for FM pain because this chronic pain syndrome is often associated with extensive secondary hyperalgesia and allodynia. Several recent studies have obtained

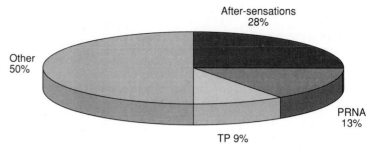

Figure 15–2. Predictors of clinical pain intensity in patients with fibromyalgia. A statistical model consisting of windup aftersensations, pain-related negative affect (PRNA), and tender point (TP) count, accounts for 50% of patients' variance in clinical pain intensity.

psychophysical evidence that input to central nociceptive pathways is abnormally processed in patients with FM.

When windup pain is evoked both in healthy persons and persons with FM, the perceived magnitude of the experimental stimuli (heat, cold, electricity) is greater among persons with FM, as is the amount of temporal summation within a series of stimuli. Following a series of stimuli, after-sensations are greater in magnitude, last longer and are more frequently painful in persons with FM. These results indicate both augmentation and prolonged decay of nociceptive input in patients with FM and provide convincing evidence for the presence of central sensitization.

3. Windup measures as predictors of clinical pain intensity—The important role of central pain mechanisms for clinical pain is also supported by their usefulness as predictors of clinical pain intensity in patients with FM. Thermal windup ratings correlate well with clinical pain intensity (Pearson's r = 0.529), thus emphasizing the important role of these pain mechanisms for FM. In addition, statistical prediction models that include tender point count, pain-related negative affect, and windup ratings have been shown to account for 50% of the variance in FM clinical pain intensity (Figure 15–2).

Arnold LM et al. Family study of fibromyalgia. *Arthritis Rheum.* 2004;50:944. [PMID: 15022338]

Bradley LA. Psychiatric comorbidity in fibromyalgia. *Curr Pain Headache Rep.* 2005;9:79. [PMID: 15745615]

Buskila D et al. Genetic factors in neuromuscular pain. *CNS Spectr.* 2005;10:281. [PMID: 15788956]

Buskila D et al. The development of widespread pain after injuries. *J Musculoskelet Pain.* 2002;10:261.

Carli G. Neuroplasticity and clinical pain. *Prog Brain Res.* 2000;129:325. [PMID: 11098700]

Cohen H et al. Prevalence of post-traumatic stress disorder in fibromyalgia patients: overlapping syndromes or post-traumatic fibromyalgia syndrome? *Semin Arthritis Rheum.* 2002;32:38. [PMID: 12219319]

Price DD et al. Enhanced temporal summation of second pain and its central modulation in fibromyalgia patients. *Pain.* 2002;99:49. [PMID: 12237183]

Raphael KG et al. Comorbidity of fibromyalgia and posttraumatic stress disorder symptoms in a community sample of women. *Pain Med.* 2004;5:33. [PMID: 14996235]

Raphael KG et al. Familial aggregation of depression in fibromyalgia: a community-based test of alternate hypotheses. *Pain.* 2004;110:449. [PMID: 15275798]

Russell MB. Epidemiology and genetics of cluster headache. *Lancet Neurol.* 2004;3:279. [PMID: 15099542]

Sherman JJ et al. Prevalence and impact of posttraumatic stress disorder-like symptoms on patients with fibromyalgia syndrome. *Clin J Pain.* 2000;16:127. [PMID: 10870725]

Staud R. Evidence of involvement of central neural mechanisms in generating fibromyalgia pain. *Curr Rheumatol Rep.* 2002;4:299. [PMID: 12126581]

Staud R. New evidence for central sensitization in patients with fibromyalgia. *Curr Rheumatol Rep.* 2004;6:259. [PMID: 15251072]

Staud R et al. Abnormal sensitization and temporal summation of second pain (wind-up) in patients with fibromyalgia syndrome. *Pain.* 2001;91:165. [PMID: 11240089]

Staud R et al. Evidence for abnormal pain processing in fibromyalgia syndrome. *Pain Med.* 2001;2:208. [PMID: 15102253]

Staud R et al. New insights into the pathogenesis of fibromyalgia syndrome. *Med Aspects Hum Sex.* 2001;1:51.

Staud R et al. Peripheral and central sensitization in fibromyalgia: pathogenetic role. *Curr Pain Headache Rep.* 2002;6:259. [PMID: 12095460]

Staud R et al. Ratings of experimental pain and pain-related negative affect predict clinical pain in patients with fibromyalgia syndrome. *Pain.* 2003;105:215. [PMID: 14499438]

Vierck CJ et al. The effect of maximal exercise on temporal summation of second pain (windup) in patients with fibromyalgia syndrome. *J Pain.* 2001;2:334. [PMID: 14622813]

Clinical Findings

FM is a clinical syndrome that encompasses patients at the extremes of chronic musculoskeletal pain in the general population. Although the 1990 ACR diagnostic criteria for FM have shown 85% specificity for this illness, they do not mean that FM exists only in persons fulfilling these definitions. Similar to systemic lupus or rheumatoid arthritis criteria, FM criteria were narrowly defined for study purposes. For clinical use, FM should be considered in all patients who have widespread pain and tenderness but who do not have structural or inflammatory tissue abnormalities. However like many chronic pain syndromes, FM becomes clinically relevant frequently after significant dysfunction or affective distress has occurred. At this crucial point, FM sufferers often become patients and seek medical care. However, epidemiologic research has clearly shown that secondary gain or malingering do not seem to play a major role for FM patients' health care seeking.

A. Symptoms and Signs

Most important for the diagnosis of FM is widespread chronic musculoskeletal pain of unknown origin that has led to functional impairment or distress. Pain has to be reported in all four quadrants of the body as well as the lower back. However, the pain does not have to be in all body quadrants at the same time. Pain is considered to be chronic when it has been present for at least 3 months. Other physical findings include the following:

1. Insomnia and fatigue.
2. Mechanical allodynia (tender points).
3. Central sensitization (abnormal temporal summation of second pain).
4. Increased activation of pain-related brain areas (functional magnetic resonance imaging [MRI]).
5. Abnormal hypothalamic-pituitary stress response.
6. Dysautonomia (abnormal heart rate variability, neurally mediated hypotension).

Besides chronic widespread pain, patients with FM need to show evidence of widespread mechanical tenderness. So-called tender points are used to evaluate mechanical allodynia. Tender points are located in areas of tendon insertion sites (Figure 15–3) and can be tested with an algometer or by thumb pressure. A tender point is present when pain threshold is detectable at pressures of ≤ 4 kg applied to these sites. Similarly, when thumb pressure is applied to a tender point site and pain threshold is reached at or before the thumb nail blanches, a tender point has been verified. The locations of tender points are listed in Table 15–1.

B. Laboratory Findings

There are no specific laboratory abnormalities detectable in patients with FM. Elevated levels of substance P (more than three times normal) and nerve growth factor in the cerebrospinal fluid of FM patients have been reported in three different studies. Conversely, decreased concentrations of serotonin and noradrenalin have been found in the cerebrospinal fluid of FM patients. Otherwise, patients with FM have normal laboratory examinations.

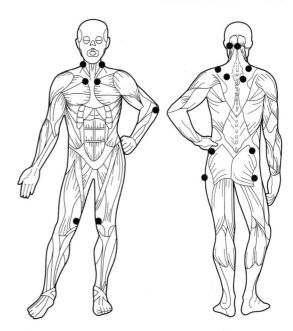

Figure 15–3. Location of 18 tender points.

Elevated erythrocyte sedimentation rates or C-reactive protein concentrations should raise suspicion for chronic inflammatory or neoplastic diseases. Thyroid function studies, including thyroid-stimulating hormone and free T4 levels are helpful in ruling out thyroid dysfunction. Because the differential diagnosis for FM includes inflammatory and metabolic myopathies, screening for elevated creatine kinase levels and aldolase is useful. Chronic infections such as tuberculosis, HIV, or hepatitis B and C should always be excluded in high-risk populations. Laboratory evaluations of unproven value for the diagnosis of FM include autoimmune

Table 15–1. Locations of Tender Points in Patients with Fibromyalgia.

- Occiput, at insertions of the suboccipital muscle
- Lower neck (posterior), at the transverse processes of C5–C7
- Trapezius (anterior), at midpoint of the upper border
- Supraspinatus (anterior), above the scapular spine near the medial border
- Anterior chest, second costochondral junction
- Lateral epicondyle, 2 cm distal to epicondyles
- Gluteal, upper outer quadrants of buttocks
- Greater trochanter, posterior to the trochanteric prominence
- Knees, at medial fat pad proximal to the joint line

antibodies, antipolymer antibodies, Epstein-Barr virus antibodies, Lyme disease antibodies, yeast antibodies, and serotonin antibodies.

C. IMAGING STUDIES

Although brain imaging studies of patients with FM have not identified structural changes, more specific brain imaging protocols using functional MRI can be used to show increased activation of pain-related brain areas in patients with FM. In patients with high likelihood for multiple sclerosis, brain imaging is indicated and necessary for making the diagnosis. Otherwise, radiologic evaluation of the spine and painful joints may help in identifying major pain generators, such as osteoarthritis and inflammatory arthritis.

D. SPECIAL TESTS

Quantitative neurosensory testing with mechanical, thermal, and electrical stimuli to the skin and muscles has shown profound pain processing abnormalities, including hyperalgesia, allodynia, and central sensitization, in patients with FM. Specifically, testing of temporal summation of second pain (windup) and R-III nociceptive reflex measurements have demonstrated abnormalities consistent with central sensitization in FM.

E. SPECIAL EXAMINATIONS

Besides a manual tender point examination, a body pain diagram completed by the patient is clinically useful. The number of pain areas shaded on a body pain diagram shares a linear relationship with clinical pain intensity and can be easily obtained in clinical practice.

Pain can be measured using pain rating scales. Table 15–2 lists the pain rating scales and their useful-

Table 15–2. Pain Rating Scales and Their Usefulness in Evaluating Patients with Fibromyalgia.

Scale	Description and rating
Visual Analogue Scales	Line 10- to 15-cm long is used for pain magnitude matching Best pain scale
Numerical Pain Scales	Pain rated using number from 0 to 100 Useful pain scale
Verbal Descriptor Scale	Verbal pain descriptors linked to numerical scale Useful pain scale
Pain Faces Scale	Shows expressions on faces to describe amount of pain Lacks reliability; not useful

ness in evaluating patients with FM. The Visual Analogue Scale is superior to the Numerical Pain Scale because of its ratio scaling properties. Validated pain scales often use end points such as "no pain at all" and "most intense pain sensation imaginable." However, to obtain clinically relevant pain ratings, pain occurring within a specific time period should be measured (eg, the usual pain during the previous day or the previous week).

In addition, testing for major mood disorders should be obtained using validated questionnaires like the Beck Depression Inventory (a score of ≥ 21 indicates clinical depression).

Staud R et al. Body pain area and pain-related negative affect predict clinical pain intensity in patients with fibromyalgia. *J Pain.* 2004;5:338. [PMID: 15336638]

Differential Diagnosis

Many systemic illnesses can present with diffuse pain similar to FM, including myofascial pain syndrome, polymyalgia rheumatica, rheumatoid arthritis, Sjögren syndrome, inflammatory myopathies, systemic lupus erythematosus, multiple sclerosis, and joint hypermobility syndrome. Furthermore, several infectious diseases, including hepatitis C, Lyme disease, coxsackie B infection, HIV, and parvovirus infection, have been described as a trigger for chronic pain. Although most patients with FM report the insidious onset of pain and fatigue, approximately half of all patients describe the start of chronic pain after a traumatic event. Because a large epidemiologic study provided recent evidence for increased cancer mortality in patients with widespread pain, this differential diagnosis needs to be considered in many patients with FM.

A. MYOFASCIAL PAIN SYNDROME

Myofascial pain or regional musculoskeletal pain is commonly encountered in clinical practice. Myofascial pain syndrome is defined as a chronic pain syndrome accompanied by trigger points in one or more muscles or groups of muscles and is a common cause of neck and shoulder pain, tension headaches, and lower back pain. Similar to FM, it is found more frequently in women than in men and is often associated with limitation of movement, weakness, and autonomic dysfunction as well as the trigger points and referred pain.

B. TRIGGER POINTS

Trigger points represent areas of local mechanical hyperalgesia that can be found in myofascial pain syndrome and several chronic pain conditions, including FM, osteoarthritis, and rheumatoid arthritis. Trigger points are specific areas of hyperirritability in muscle but can also be detected in ligaments, tendons, periosteum, scar tissue, or skin. Trigger points are located in palpable "taut bands" and produce local and referred pain, which is specific for the particular muscle. When trigger points are mechanically stimulated, the "taut bands" within a muscle, rather than the entire muscle, will contract. Trigger points are often associated with a local muscle "twitch response," which can easily be elicited by needling or palpation of the trigger point. Latent trigger points are similar to active trigger points, but they are not associated with spontaneous pain and no referral of pain occurs. However, latent trigger points are painful when palpated.

C. Relationship Between Myofascial Pain and FM

Approximately 70% of patients with FM have trigger points. A tender point is considered to be different than a trigger point because of the absence of referred pain, local twitch response, and a taut band in the muscle. The distinction between a tender point and a trigger point requires careful physical examination. Trigger points, however, are frequently located in areas of muscular tender points of patients with FM suggesting that some muscular tender points in patients with FM may actually be trigger points.

The presence of trigger points in most if not all patients with FM represents evidence for local muscle abnormalities in this chronic musculoskeletal pain syndrome. Although it is unclear whether trigger points are the cause or effect of muscle injury, they represent abnormally contracted muscle fibers. This muscle contraction can lead to accumulation of histamine, serotonin, tachykinins, and prostaglandins, which may result in the activation of local nociceptors. Prolonged muscle contractions may also result in local hypoxemia and energy depletion.

D. Inflammatory Connective Tissue Diseases

Many patients with chronic arthritis (up to 25%) also have chronic widespread pain similar to FM. These patients may also have the following symptoms: chronic fatigue, impaired memory and concentration, and mood abnormalities. However, most of these patients will have findings suggestive of inflammation (including joint pain and swelling, rashes, and muscle weakness) as well as laboratory abnormalities, including elevated erythrocyte sedimentation rate, C-reactive protein, anemia, and autoantibodies (rheumatoid factor, cyclic citrullinated peptide antibodies, antinuclear antibodies).

Thus, a detailed clinical examination and laboratory testing may be necessary to exclude inflammatory connective tissue diseases in chronic pain patients with arthritis or rash.

McBeth J et al. Association of widespread body pain with an increased risk of cancer and reduced cancer survival: a prospective, population-based study. *Arthritis Rheum.* 2003;48:1686. [PMID: 12794837]

Meyer HP. Myofascial pain syndrome and its suggested role in the pathogenesis and treatment of fibromyalgia syndrome. *Curr Pain Headache Rep.* 2002;6:274. [PMID: 12095462]

Treatment

Treatment of patients with chronic widespread pain needs to be individually tailored. This includes the assessment of biopsychosocial abnormalities, which are readily detectable in most patients with FM. Importantly, the identification of pain generators is essential for an effective treatment plan. Thus, patients with arthritis, particularly osteoarthritis of the spine, will benefit from muscle relaxants, physical therapy, and massage. In addition, these patients may respond well to therapy with cyclooxygenase (COX) inhibitors. Identification and treatment of mood abnormalities is crucial because affective spectrum disorders seem to share important mechanisms with FM.

A. Pharmacologic Treatments

Pharmacotherapy for FM has been most successful with antidepressant, muscle relaxant, or anticonvulsant drugs. These drugs affect the release of various neurochemicals (eg, serotonin, norepinephrine, substance P) that have a broad range of activities in the brain and spinal cord, including modulation of pain sensation and tolerance. However, none of these drugs are currently approved by the US Food and Drug Administration for the treatment of FM.

Most patients with FM respond to low-dose tricyclic antidepressants, such as amitriptyline, and to cyclobenzaprine as well as cardiovascular exercise, cognitive-behavioral therapy, patient education, or a combination of these therapies. Also tramadol, selective serotonin reuptake inhibitors, serotonin-norepinephrine reuptake inhibitors, and anticonvulsants have been found to be moderately effective. There is some evidence for the efficacy of strength training exercise, acupuncture, hypnotherapy, biofeedback, massage, and warm water baths. However, many commonly used FM therapies like guaifenesin have been found to be ineffective.

Based on published evidence, a stepwise FM management approach can be recommended. Confirmation of the diagnosis is crucial and relevant FM pain mechanisms, including the important role of pain generators, must be explained to the patient and family. This often

Table 15–3. Medications for Treating Patients with Fibromyalgia.

Drug	Prescribing guidelines
First-line therapy	
Amitriptyline	25–50 mg at bedtime
Cyclobenzaprine	10–30 mg at bedtime
Second-line therapy	
Tramadol	200–300 mg/d
Fluoxetine	20–80 mg
Sertraline	100–300 mg
Venlafaxine	150–300 mg
Duloxetine	60 mg
Pregabalin	450 mg
Gabapentin	800–3600 mg
Third-line therapy	
Growth hormone	Helpful in subset of patients with low growth hormone levels
Opioids	Should be considered only after all other medicinal and nonmedicinal therapies have been exhausted

alleviates concerns about the nature of chronic musculoskeletal pain. Any comorbid illnesses, such as mood disturbances or primary sleep disturbances, need to be identified and treated. It is important to refer patients with high levels of depression or anxiety to a psychologist or psychiatrist. First-line medications for FM pain are low doses of tricyclic antidepressants or cyclobenzaprine (Table 15–3). These medications provide dual benefits including improvement of mood and central sensitization. All patients with FM should begin a cardiovascular exercise program. In addition, treatment often needs to include cognitive-behavioral therapy or stress reduction with relaxation training. A multidisciplinary approach combining each of these modalities may be most beneficial.

Patients with FM not responding to these steps should be referred to a rheumatologist, physiatrist, psychiatrist, or pain management specialist. It is important to remember that FM is not a homogenous illness with several subgroups based on psychosocial status and biological response to pain. The ability of patients with FM to manage their pain seems to correlate with their functional status. Brain imaging and psychological profiles have identified at least three FM subgroups:

1. Patients who are highly dysfunctional.
2. Patients who are interpersonally distressed.
3. Patients who cope effectively.

Such studies provide an explanation why some treatments seem to be differentially effective in individual patients. Thus, optimal FM management will require a combination of pharmacologic and nonpharmacologic therapies with patients and health care professionals working as a team.

1. Antidepressants and muscle relaxants—Several trials have demonstrated effectiveness of amitriptyline (25 to 50 mg) and cyclobenzaprine in trials lasting 6 to 12 weeks. The effective dose of cyclobenzaprine for FM pain has been 10 to 40 mg/d. Tricyclic antidepressants are effective for pain, mood, function, and quality of sleep.

Less strong evidence is available for the effectiveness of selective serotonin reuptake inhibitors, such as fluoxetine, in managing FM pain. Serotonin and norepinephrine reuptake inhibitors, such as venlafaxine (150 to 300 mg/d) and duloxetine (60 mg/d), demonstrated improvement of pain, sleep, and function in FM patients.

2. Analgesics—Tramadol, with or without acetaminophen, has been effective in patients with FM. There is, however, no evidence that nonsteroidal anti-inflammatory drugs (NSAIDs) improve FM pain, although they may be useful when combined with tricyclic antidepressants. There is no good evidence to recommend opioids for FM pain. However, opioid analgesics should be considered after all other medicinal and nonmedicinal therapies have failed.

3. Anticonvulsants—Gabapentin is frequently used for the treatment of chronic pain but has not yet been studied in FM. However, the second-generation anticonvulsant pregabalin (450 mg/d), which has been found to be effective in FM, significantly improves pain, sleep, fatigue, and health-related quality of life.

4. Other medications—Several small trials have shown that tropisetron, a 5-hydroxytryptamine-3 (5HT-3) receptor antagonist, and 5-hydroxytryptophan, an intermediate metabolite of L-tryptophan, are effective for FM pain. Although benzodiazepines or similar sedatives are effective for insomnia and anxiety they do not seem to affect FM pain.

5. Hormones and supplements—A study of corticosteroids showed that prednisone (10 mg/d) was ineffective for FM pain. Growth hormone supplementation moderately improves function of patients with FM who have low hormone levels. At this time the usefulness of thyroid hormone, dehydroepiandrosterone (DHEA), melatonin, or calcitonin is unproven for the treatment of FM. Other treatments, such as dietary modifications, nutritional supplements, magnesium, herbal, and vitamin therapy have not been adequately evaluated in FM. Although frequently used, guaifenesin has shown no significant effects on pain over the long term.

B. NONPHARMACOLOGIC TREATMENTS

1. Physical therapy—Cardiovascular aerobic exercise is one of the most effective treatments for FM. This therapeutic benefit was first recognized 20 years ago and has been subsequently confirmed in multiple trials. Pool exercise is usually well tolerated and especially helpful. In addition, aerobic exercise including cycling, dance, and walking in-doors significantly improves FM pain and function. The combination of aerobic exercise with education can significantly improve physical function, global well-being, fatigue, and sleep.

2. Cognitive-behavioral therapy—There is strong evidence that psychological and behavioral therapy, especially cognitive-behavioral therapy, is effective in managing FM pain. In addition, meditation, relaxation, and stress management seem to be useful. Multidisciplinary treatment including education, cognitive-behavioral therapy, or both, combined with exercise showed beneficial effects on patient self-efficacy, significant decreases in pain, and improvements on a 6-minute walk. Importantly, improvements in the treatment outcomes were maintained over a long time in patients receiving combination therapy.

3. Other treatments—There is some evidence to support the use of acupuncture in patients with FM because it can decrease pain ratings and medication use. Similarly, chiropractic spinal manipulation, soft-tissue massage, ultrasound, and inferential current seem to have positive effects on patients with FM.

Sim J et al. Systematic review of randomized controlled trials of nonpharmacological interventions for fibromyalgia. *Clin J Pain.* 2002;18:324. [PMID: 12218504]

Prognosis

FM can be mild or disabling but often has substantial emotional and social consequences. About 50% of all patients have difficulty with or are unable to perform routine daily activities. Estimates of patients who have had to stop work or change jobs range from 30% to 40%. Patients with FM suffer job losses and social abandonment more often than people with other conditions that cause pain and fatigue. Although FM symptoms seem to remain stable over extended periods of time, several long-term studies indicate that physical function and pain worsen. Significant life stressors often result in a poor outcome, including diminished capacity to work, poor self-efficacy, increased pain sensations, disturbed sleep, fatigue, and depression.

FM, like many other chronic illnesses, is treatable, and remission can occur in many patients who actively participate in effective disease management programs. When FM is perceived to be the consequence of an injury, patients often have a more severe condition than those without a history of injury. A recent study reported higher mortality rates in patients with widespread pain compared with those without chronic pain. Although this study did not specifically look at FM subgroups, the findings may be relevant for patients with chronic pain conditions such as FM. The higher mortality rate was mostly associated with cancer, although the cause for this association is currently unknown.

Sickle Cell Disease

Eufemia Jacob, PhD, RN & Elizabeth Ely, PhD, RN

Sickle cell disease (SCD) is a group of conditions characterized by production of abnormal hemoglobin, with clinical manifestations that vary by genotype and age. The first description of sickle cell disease was made in 1910 by Dr. James B. Herrick who noted that a patient of his from the West Indies had an anemia characterized by unusual red blood cells that were "sickle"-shaped. Sickling of the red blood cells was demonstrated to be related to low oxygen, and the low oxygen altered the structure of the hemoglobin in the molecule. Sequencing the DNA of the sickle hemoglobin showed that a glutamic acid at position 6 of the β-globin chain was replaced by a valine. Using the known information about amino acids and the codons that coded for them made it possible to predict the mutation in sickle cell disease. This made sickle cell disease the first genetic disorder whose molecular basis was known.

ESSENTIALS OF DIAGNOSIS

- *Identified through newborn screening in 48 states.*
- *Confirmatory testing by serum electrophoresis.*
- *Because this is a genetic disorder, the phenotype (disease expression) is extremely variable, though the genotype can somewhat predict disease severity.*
- *There are four principal genotypes: SCD-SS, SCD-SC, SCD-β^0-thalassemia, and SCD-β^+-thalassemia.*
- *Hallmark symptoms of the disease are anemia and vaso-occlusive pain.*
- *Early diagnosis is essential so that prophylaxis with penicillin can be started by 3 months of age.*
- *Pain in SCD often begins as dactylitis (hand/foot syndrome), starting at 6 months of age for some children and continues as the most common disease manifestation throughout life.*

General Considerations

SCD is a chronic disease affecting 1 in 400 black Americans; 1 in 12 is a carrier of the trait. In infants and young children, infection is of greatest concern because it can lead to sepsis, splenic sequestration, silent infarct in the brain or overt stroke, acute chest syndrome, and vaso-occlusive pain. As children reach adolescence and adulthood, risks of stroke, renal disease, pulmonary hypertension, and leg ulcers increase, and the vaso-occlusive pain can become debilitating and chronic (eg, avascular necrosis of the hip or shoulder).

Pathogenesis

Following are the four principal genotypes:

1. **SCD-SS** is the most common and most severe genotype.
2. **SCD-SC** genotype generally causes less severe disease, though patients with this genotype are at higher risk for sickle retinopathy than those with SCD-SS.
3. **SCD-β^0 thalassemia** is considered to cause disease as severe as SCD-SS.
4. **SCD-β^+ thalassemia** causes a milder form of the disease.

Compared with normal red blood cells, which survive 120 days in the bloodstream, sickle hemoglobin S, C, β^0-thalassemia, and β^+-thalassemia, which replace hemoglobin A in SCD, survive only 10 to 30 days, resulting in anemia, reticulocytopenia, and increased workload for the spleen. Under conditions of lower oxygen tension (eg, fever, reactive airway disease, dehydration, stress), hemoglobin becomes elongated in shape "sickled" and clumps together in the microvasculature causing oxygen depletion to tissues and eventual necrosis. The sickling can occur anywhere in the body causing organ damage as well as pain.

Prevention

Early diagnosis is essential so caregivers may be taught how to monitor infants and young children for known complications. Children should be examined in a specialty clinic at least 2 to 3 times a year.

All children 3 to 4 months through 5 years of age are given penicillin prophylaxis (penicillin VK 125 mg twice a day, increased to 250 mg, twice a day at 3–5 years of age). Parents and caregivers of infants with SCD should be taught to palpate the spleen on a daily basis and note any changes in size. Also, caregivers need to know that a fever of 101°F or above is an emergency and needs immediate attention.

Immunizations need to be up-to-date. All patients with SCD need the influenza vaccine yearly beginning in infancy as well as pneumoccocal immunization with PCV7 (Prevnar) in infancy and PPV23 (Pneumovax) at 24 months.

While many complications are difficult to prevent, some basic health maintenance behaviors are important to adopt at a young age and include the following:

1. Decreasing exposure to persons with respiratory infections or illness.
2. Washing hands meticulously.
3. Identifying reactive airway disease and treating it aggressively.
4. Avoiding extreme temperatures and dressing appropriately.
5. Drinking enough fluids to avoid dehydration.
6. Getting adequate sleep to decrease fatigue.
7. Minimizing psychological stressors.
8. Eating a balanced nutritional diet with folic acid and zinc supplementation.
9. Monitoring growth and development closely, both for growth delay and neurocognitive development.
10. Performing transcranial Doppler (TCD) screening, starting at 2–3 years of age for patients with SCD-SS genotype. TCD velocity > 200 cm/sec is an abnormal finding. Continue screening yearly.
11. Tracking school attendance and performance.
12. Avoiding high altitudes, such as mountain climbing and flying in a depressurized airplane.
13. Avoiding reptiles due to increased risk of exposure to *Salmonella.*

Preventing vaso-occlusive pain is difficult because there are few identifiable precipitating events. Viral illness or bacterial infection, dehydration, stress, changes in the weather, menses, and fatigue are all possible causes of vaso-occlusive pain. Perhaps the most frustrating aspect of dealing with vaso-occlusive pain is its variability both in occurrence and morbidity, even when the patient is carefully adhering to guidelines for prevention. The variability in the frequency of pain episodes is generally related to the hemoglobin phenotype, level of fetal hemoglobin, concurrent illness, physical condition, psychological factors, and social variables. Chronic pain syndromes may develop in patients with chronic damage to bones, nerves, and other tissues with inflammation and fibrosis.

Clinical Findings

The clinical manifestations of SCD include hemolytic anemia, increased frequency and severity of infections, tissue and organ damage, and recurrent painful episodes caused by ischemia. Hemolytic anemia causes moderate to severe decrease in the hemoglobin level, increased reticulocytes produced in the bone marrow, jaundice from increased bilirubin, and increased lactic dehydrogenase.

Bacterial infections cause significant morbidity and mortality, and the early loss of splenic function increases the risk of severe infections, such as meningitis, pneumonia, sepsis, osteomyelitis, and salmonellosis.

Tissue and organ damage, reduced delivery of oxygen to tissues and organs that result from increased blood viscosity, adherence of blood cells to vascular walls, and activation of the coagulation system may contribute to such complications as vascular occlusion, infarctions, ischemic necrosis, and hemorrhage. Damage may occur to any organ in the body, including the brain, lungs, liver, spleen, kidneys, bones, and eyes.

Recurrent painful episodes are caused by ischemia due to decreased blood flow, inflammation from bone marrow, and muscle necrosis.

The reason for most emergency department visits and hospitalizations is management of pain associated with an acute vaso-occlusive painful episode, with the average length of stay lasting between 5 and 10 days.

Ballas SK. Sickle cell anaemia: progress in pathogenesis and treatment. *Drugs.* 2002;62:1143. [PMID: 12010077]

Benjamin LJ et al. *Guideline for the Management of Acute and Chronic Pain in Sickle Cell Disease.* Glenview, IL: American Pain Society; 1999.

Dampier C et al. Vaso-occlusion in children with sickle cell disease: clinical characteristics and biologic correlates. *J Pediatr Hematol Oncol.* 2004;26:785. [PMID: 15591896]

Taylor C et al. Clinical presentation of acute chest syndrome in sickle cell disease. *Postgrad Med J.* 2004;80:346. [PMID: 15192168]

Pain Assessment

Because of the unpredictable, recurrent, intense, and frequently persistent pain experiences that occur during the lifetime of persons with SCD, the American Pain Society recommends two categories of assessment: rapid pain assessment and comprehensive pain assessment.

The goal of **rapid pain assessment** during a painful episode is immediate treatment. Pain assessment is relatively brief and easy to perform (Table 16–1). It is important to assess not only pain intensity, using an age-appropriate scale, but also other dimensions such as pain location and pain quality. Measurements need to be repeated over time and supplemented by physical findings, laboratory data, and diagnostic procedures.

Table 16–1. Rapid Pain Assessment during a Painful Episode.

- Use developmentally and cognitively appropriate pain measure
  - FLACC Pain Rating Scale (0 to 2 years)
  - CHEOPS Observational Rating Scale (0 to 2 years)
  - Faces (Wong-Baker, Bieri, Oucher) Pain Rating Scale (3 to 7 years)
  - Adolescent Pediatric Pain Scale (8 years and older)
  - 0 to 10 Numerical Rating Scale (8 years and older; adults)
  - McGill Pain Questionnaire (adults)
- Assess dimensions of sickle cell pain
  - **Intensity:** varies from mild to excruciating both within and between episodes
  - **Location:** the most frequent sites affected are the abdomen, back, chest, and joints
  - **Quality:** described as deep-seated, boring, or like a toothache
  - **Onset:** consider any precipitating events to inform potential prevention strategies
  - **Duration:** severity of pain varies from mild transient attacks of 5–10 minutes in a wrist to a more severe, generalized pains lasting days or weeks and requiring hospital management
  - **Variations/rhythms:** painful episodes develop most frequently in late afternoon and during the night
  - **Frequency:** painful episodes are most frequent between 19 to 39 years of age and increase significantly in males 15 to 25 years of age; painful crises decrease after age 30 and are rare after age 40; in persons over 20 years of age, mortality is highest in those with the most frequent painful episodes.
- Frequency of assessment
  - Before intervention
  - At peak effect
  - At frequent intervals (10–15 minutes) until adequacy and duration's effects are determined (type and route dependent)
- Document interventions and response to facilitate tracking of effectiveness as well as for evaluation of interventions in a timely manner

SOURCE: Data from Benjamin LJ et al. *Guideline for the Management of Acute and Chronic Pain in Sickle Cell Disease.* Glenview, IL: American Pain Society; 1999.

Pain occurs at any location where nociceptors are present. It may be localized, involve several areas, be diffuse, or be migratory. Pains are generally bilateral and symmetric and may move from one joint to another. Tenderness or pressure over affected sites is common. Pain location surface area may decrease dramatically even when pain intensity does not change. Figure 16–1 is an example of body outline drawings that illustrate no change in pain intensity ratings from day 1 to day 3, and a dramatic change in the number and spatial distribution of painful body areas.

The assessment of pain quality may suggest the type of tissue involvement. Pain perceived as constant, gnawing, aching, sharp, or throbbing may be well localized and may involve the musculoskeletal system. Pain perceived as constant, dull, deep, or squeezing, and which is often accompanied by nausea, vomiting, hypertension, tachycardia, tachypnea, and diaphoresis may result from the activation of nociceptors in the thoracic and abdominal viscera. Pain perceived as severe, constant, dull ache, with superimposed paroxysms of burning, shooting, or electric shocklike sensations may result from ischemia, necrosis, inflammation, or infarction to the central or peripheral neural tissues. If these types of pain persist, neuropathic pain may develop and may be more difficult to treat.

Comprehensive pain assessment occurs at the time of admission and at least once or twice a year, and more frequently as needed. The goal of comprehensive clinical assessment is treatment planning that involves the patient, family, and health care team.

Multidimensional assessment is summarized in Table 16–2 and includes physiologic, sensory, affective, cognitive, behavioral, and sociocultural factors. A multidisciplinary approach should include hematologists, pain teams, psychologists, physiotherapists, nurses, pharmacists, and others as warranted.

Differential Diagnosis

During the initial rapid pain assessment, it is vital to detect medical complications requiring specific therapy. The cause of the pain dictates the therapy. Therefore, asking the patient what type of pain he or she typically experiences during an episode is helpful. If the pain episode is typically what the patient experiences, the patient is treated for a routine pain episode. If

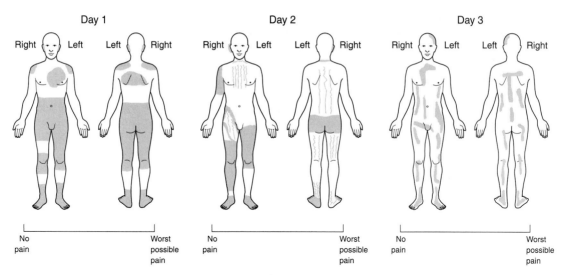

Figure 16–1. Patient markings on body outline diagram of location of pain on days 1, 2, and 3. Pain intensity ratings did not change (9.0 centimeter on the word graphic rating scale). However, the surface area and spatial distribution of the pain changed dramatically. (Adapted, with permission, from Savedra MC et al. Pain location: validity and reliability of body outline markings by hospitalized children and adolescents. *Res Nurs Health.* 1989;12:307.)

the pain is not typical, the cause of pain (Table 16–3) needs to be determined and may include any of the following:

1. Infection
2. Dehydration
3. Acute chest syndrome versus pneumonia (fever, tachypnea, chest pain, hypoxia, chest signs)
4. Severe anemia
5. Cholecystitis
6. Splenic enlargement

Table 16–2. Comprehensive Clinical Assessment of Pain.

Physical factors	Dimensions of pain
Blood pressure	Intensity
Heart rate	0 to 10 numerical rating scale (mild, 0–3; moderate, 4–6;
Respiration	severe, 7–10)
Oxygen saturation level	Location and quality
Chest and abdominal findings	Precipitating factors
Pain sites, tenderness, warmth, swelling	**Impact of pain on functioning**
Laboratory data	Self-care
Radiology data	School/work
Demographic and psychosocial factors	Social activities
Age and developmental level	Relationships
Gender	Parenting ability (adults)
Family factors	
Cultural factors	
Adaptation to sickle cell disease	
Coping styles	
Cognitive abilities	
Mood	
Level of distress	

SOURCE: Data from Benjamin LJ et al. *Guideline for the Management of Acute and Chronic Pain in Sickle Cell Disease.* Glenview, IL: American Pain Society; 1999.

Table 16–3. Complications of Sickle Cell Disease and Their Management.

Complications	Diagnosis/clinical findings	Related information	Management
Acute chest syndrome	Pulmonary infiltrates on chest radiograph Chest pain Fever Reduced oxygen saturation Decreased heart rate and respiratory rate	Bacterial or viral infection Pulmonary fat embolism Pulmonary edema Microvascular/macrovascular lung infarction	Cautious administration of analgesia and IV hydration Oxygen supplementation Empiric antibiotics while awaiting culture results Transfusion in presence of multilobar involvement with anemia, rapidly progressive, and respiratory failure Exchange transfusion if hemoglobin SS concentration needs to be reduced to less than 30%
Aplastic crisis	Transient arrest in erythropoiesis with secondary decreased HgB concentrations, decreased 1 g/dL from baseline	Infection with parvovirus B19, and sometimes *Streptococcus pneumoniae, Salmonella,* or Epstein-Barr virus	Transfusions, which can be intermittently necessary for several weeks IV immune globulin may be administered if patient has refractory parvovirus B19 infection
Splenic se-questration	Splenic enlargement Significant drop in hemoglobin, decreased 1 g/dL from baseline	Vaso-occlusion in the spleen which causes a marked decrease in hemoglobin concentration	Exchange transfusion If recurrent, splenectomy may be indicated after an acute episode
Silent infarct or overt stroke	CT scan to evaluate for hemorrhage followed by MRI; MRA in presence of intracranial hemorrhage TCD flow study to detect subclinical neurologic disease/silent infarct Screening with TCD should be done by 3 years of age or younger for SCD-SS genotype and continued yearly	The following risk factors have been identified: previous transient ischemic attack, low steady-state hemoglobin, increased steady-state leukocyte count, acute chest syndrome within the previous 2 weeks, elevated systolic blood pressure. Intracranial hemorrhage has a very high immediate mortality; peak incidence between ages 20 and 29; presents with headache, increased intracranial pressure, altered level of consciousness, and focal neurologic deficits	Use of exchange transfusion to keep HgbS concentration below 30% during an acute stroke May be prevented with transfusions in children However, prophylactic transfusion for strokes in adults has not been studied and is generally not recommended

Continued

Table 16–3. Complications of Sickle Cell Disease and Their Management. *Continued*

Complications	Diagnosis/clinical findings	Related information	Management
Hypertension	Increased blood pressure	May reflect underlying renal disease	β-Blockers and calcium channel blockers are the mainstays of therapy ACE inhibitors may be useful if patient has proteinuria Diuretics are used with caution so that dehydration and sickling are not precipitated
Gallstones	Abdominal ultrasound for diagnosis Abdominal pain, icteric sclera often present	Increased bilirubin production from chronic hemolysis increases risk of gallstones	Surgical removal
Renal	Renal ultrasound, cystoscopy, and culture Hematuria, proteinuria, nocturnal enuresis	Painless hematuria; proteinuria is present in 25% of adults with sickle cell disease; can progress to nephrotic syndrome from membranopro-liferative glomerulo nephritis	Aggressive hydration to keep urine flow high, alkalinization of urine and bedrest Sickle cell disease is not a contraindication for hemodialysis or renal transplant
Avascular necrosis	MRI of affected joint Joint pain, change in gait if hip is affected	Peak incidence between 25 and 35 years of age	Joint replacement may be necessary to treat pain and improve function. Hip coring to increase blood flow and relieve symptoms. Physical therapy aimed at increasing joint mobility and strength.
Priapism	Failure of an erection to subside spontaneously	Between 30 and 50% of male patients report at least one episode in their lifetime	May subside spontaneously Failure of an erection to subside after several hours is an urologic emergency Management includes aggressive IV hydration, opioids for pain relief, and exchange transfusion if necessary May require penile aspiration

CT, computed tomography; MRI, magnetic resonance imaging; MRA, magnetic resonance angiography; TCD, transcranial Doppler; ACE, angiotensin-converting enzyme.

Table 16–4. Diagnostic Indications.

Indications	Diagnostic procedure
Febrile, breathless, tachypnea, chest pain, chest signs, decreased oxygen saturation levels	Chest radiograph
Oxygen saturation less than 95%; unexpected drowsiness, lethargy	Continuous oxygen saturation monitoring Arterial blood gases
High amylase, increased jaundice, abdominal pain	LFTs
Hemoglobin value normal or lower or falling	CBC with reticulocytes
Abnormal LFTs, abdominal pain, splenomegaly	Ultrasound of abdomen
Febrile, rigors, hypotensive	Blood and urine cultures
Reticulocytopenia	Parvovirus B19 serology
Seizure, transient ischemic attack, stroke, severe headache, weakness	MRI/MRA
History of trauma, persistent unexplained swelling	Limb radiographs

LFT, liver function tests; CBC, complete blood count; CT, computed tomography; MRI, magnetic resonance imaging.

7. Abdominal crisis
8. Neurologic events (cerebral infarct, cerebral hemorrhage, transient ischemic attack, seizure)
9. Priapism.

Investigations should be directed toward specific clinical problems (Table 16–4).

Benjamin LJ et al. *Guideline for the Management of Acute and Chronic Pain in Sickle Cell Disease.* Glenview, IL: American Pain Society; 1999.

Jacob E et al. Changes in intensity, location, and quality of vaso-occlusive pain in children with sickle cell disease. *Pain.* 2003;102:187. [PMID: 12620610]

Moritani T et al. Sickle cell cerebrovascular disease: usual and unusual findings on MR imaging and MR angiography. *Clin Imaging.* 2004;28:173. [PMID: 15158221]

Taylor C et al. Clinical presentation of acute chest syndrome in sickle cell disease. *Postgrad Med J.* 2004;80:346. [PMID: 15192168]

Zar HJ. Etiology of sickle cell chest. *Pediatr Pulmonol Suppl.* 2004;26:188. [PMID: 15029647]

Complications

The severity of symptoms and the occurrence of the various complications caused by SCD (Table 16–3) are variable. Morbidity and mortality of SCD begins in infancy and continues through middle age, the current lifespan for persons with SCD. Persons with the SCD-SS genotype are at greatest risk for most of the complications and for greatest severity of pain. However, clinical phenotypes are not clearly understood and anyone with any form of the disease can experience complications and risks of this disease.

SCD has the potential for multisystem involvement during the patient's lifetime because the sickled hemoglobin can cause decreased blood flow in the microvasculature of any area of the body (Table 16–3).

Treatment of Pain

The lack of consistency in health care professionals in the emergency department and acute care units often results in different approaches to pain management with each visit. According to the American Pain Society, severe pain is a medical emergency and should be treated promptly and aggressively until the patient indicates that the pain is tolerable. Persons who seek medical attention at an emergency department usually have exhausted all homecare options or outpatient therapy. The selection of analgesics and loading dose is based on prior history and current assessment. The patient should be asked what medication and dosage are usually given, what side effects have been experienced in the past, what medication is usually taken at home, and what medication has been taken since the onset of present pain. The patient may be receiving long-term opioid therapy at home, and therefore, some degree of tolerance may have developed. A different potent opioid or a larger dose of the same medication may be indicated. Because mixed opioid-agonist-antagonists (eg, pentazocine, nalbuphine, butorphanol) may precipitate withdrawal syndromes, these should be avoided if the patient was taking opioids chronically at home.

To facilitate initial pain management, patients can be issued cards (serving as a "passport") that they carry with them at all times (Figure 16–2). The diagnosis, baseline

Emergency Department

Alert!

I have sickle cell disease and may have a
severe infection and life-threatening
complications that need immediate attention.

**AAA BBB SICKLE CELL CENTER
CDEF Medical Center, USA**

INFORMATION CARD

**Please call the Hematology/Oncology
Team
Daytime Hours: 123-456-7899
Nights & Weekends: 123-456-9987**

**Hematologist: D. Johnson, MD
Name: Mary Doe
DOB: 12 - 3 - 45
MR#:   123 456 489
Dx: SCD–SS
WT: 59.3 kg
Hx:** Acute chest syndrome, stroke,
multiple vaso-occlusive crisis, on
chronic transfusion for frequent
pain and silent infarct, renal
scarring and hypertension.

Hgb baseline: 8.7 g/dL

Home medications: Enalapril 2.5 mg
PO twice daily; folic acid 1 mg
daily; penicillin VK 250 mg PO bid;
Desferal daily. MS Contin 30 mg
q12h with 15 mg IR q3h prn pain

Pain regimen for severe pain:
PCA basal rate: Morphine 2 mg/h
Interval push: Morphine 3 mg/dose
Lockout interval: 6 minutes
Hourly maximum: 32 mg

Figure 16–2. Example of a "passport" card with individual information about patient's diagnosis, baseline hematologic data, and usual analgesic requirements specified in the back, as well as name and phone number of the primary care provider or hematologist.

hematologic data, and usual analgesic requirements should be specified on these cards. The name and phone number of the primary care provider or hematologist, or both, should also be included on the card in case emergency department physicians have questions or need consultation. An ideal goal is to have analgesics be given within 30 minutes of entering the emergency department, and effective analgesia should be achieved by 60 minutes. Pain, respiratory rate, and sedation should be assessed every 20 minutes until pain is well controlled. Once pain is controlled, the underlying cause should be assessed more comprehensively; carefully investigate those that are not typical pain for patient.

Admission to the hospital is indicated under the following circumstances:

1. The patient is not pain free after 8 hours of outpatient treatment.
2. The patient returns for additional therapy within 48 hours of previous inpatient or outpatient treatment of a pain episode.
3. The patient has a pain episode plus any one of the following: infection, significant hypoxia or acido-

sis, pregnancy, cardiac decompensation, priapism, thromboembolic events in lungs and central nervous system or bone infarctions, aplastic or hyperhemolytic crisis (fall in hemoglobin >1 g/dL over baseline), or hepatic syndromes or cholecystitis.

In the step-wise approach to vaso-occlusive disorders, pain management is warranted. Nonsteroidal antiinflammatory drugs (NSAIDs) and weak opioids are used for mild pain, and opioids are added as needed for moderate to severe pain.

A. NSAIDs AND ACETAMINOPHEN

The management of mild to moderate pain includes the use of NSAIDs or acetaminophen (Table 16–5). NSAIDs are nonsedating and mostly given orally, except for ketorolac, which is also available parenterally. Parenteral ketorolac has been shown to have an equivalent analgesic action to morphine. NSAIDs and acetaminophen have ceiling doses, beyond which no increased analgesia is achieved with increasing doses. Persons with SCD have varying degrees of hepatic impairment, and therefore, acetaminophen may be contraindicated. Also, for persons with gastritis, peptic ulcers, coagulopathies, and renal

Table 16–5. Nonopioids used for mild pain.

Drug	Dosage[a]
Acetaminophen	10–15 mg/kg q4h; 650 mg q4h PO
Ibuprofen	10 mg/kg q6–8; 400–800 mg q4h
Ketoprofen	0.5 mg/kg q6h; 25–75 mg q6–8h
Naproxen	5–7 mg/kg q8–12h; 500 mg initially, then 250 mg q6–8h
Ketorolac	0.5 mg/kg IV q8h; 30 mg IV initially, then 15–30 mg q6h max 5 days or 120 mg/day or 10 mg q4–6h PO; max 40 mg/d

[a]Based on weight of 50 kg or more.
SOURCES: Data from Taketomo C et al. Pediatric Dosage Handbook. Hudson, Ohio: Lexi-Comp; 2004; Benjamin LJ et al. *Guideline for the Management of Acute and Chronic Pain in Sickle Cell Disease.* Glenview, IL: American Pain Society; 1999.

failure, NSAIDs are contraindicated. Clinicians should monitor doses and frequency of treatment. Urinalysis and biochemical measures of renal function should be monitored every 3 to 6 months if NSAIDs are frequently used.

B. OPIOIDS

The American Pain Society recommends the use of opioid or opioid formulations with short duration of action for pain lasting less than 24 hours, for rescue dosing with breakthrough pain, or until the sustained-release opioid preparation reaches steady-state levels. For sickle cell–related pain requiring several days to resolve, sustained-release opioid preparations are more convenient and provide more consistent analgesia. Opioids such as codeine and oxycodone are used orally for mild or moderate pain (Table 16–6). They are often used in combination with nonopioid analgesics (Table 16–7), such as acetaminophen or aspirin. However, the presence of acetaminophen or aspirin limits the amount of opioid that can be administered using these combinations (Table 16–8).

1. Titration—The starting dose of opioids for severe sickle cell pain usually depends on pain intensity, the patient's size, and their previous opioid experience. An initial loading dose equivalent to 5–10 mg of morphine (0.1–0.2 mg/kg for children) is recommended (Table 16–9). An additional smaller rescue dose of 2.5–5.0 mg (0.05–0.10 mg/kg for children) every 30–60 minutes may be given if needed to achieve or maintain adequate analgesia. Ketorolac (15–30 mg IV) or ibuprofen (600 mg PO; 10 mg/kg in children) every 6 hours is added if the patient has no history of renal disease, peptic ulcer disease, or other contraindications.

Table 16–6. Opioids for Moderate to Severe Pain.

Drug	Dosage
Codeine	0.5–1 mg/kg q3–4h PO 15–60 mg q3–6h (50 kg or more)
Morphine (MSIR)	0.3 mg/kg q3–4h PO 10–30 mg q3–4h PO (50 kg or more)
Oxymorphone	0.5–1.5 mg q6h IV
Hydrocodone/ oxycodone	0.15–0.20 mg/kg q3–4h PO 10 mg q3–4h PO (50 kg or more)

SOURCES: Data from Taketomo C et al. Pediatric Dosage Handbook. Hudson, Ohio: Lexi-Comp; 2004; Benjamin LJ et al. *Guideline for the Management of Acute and Chronic Pain in Sickle Cell Disease.* Glenview, IL: American Pain Society; 1999.

Response to therapy should be evaluated 15 to 30 minutes after each dose, and dosages should be titrated to relief. Relief is defined as a score of 2 or greater on a pain relief scale (0 = no relief, 1 = little relief, 2 = moderate relief, 3 = good relief, 4 = complete relief), or a 50% reduction from the upper end of the pain intensity scale. Significant relief has not been achieved if a patient rates 0 or 1 on the above pain relief scale. Titration should

Table 16–7. Combination NSAID and Opioid Therapy for Mild to Moderate Pain.

Drug	Dosage
Hydrocodone + acetaminophen	0.6 mg/kg/d Not to exceed 1.25 mg/dose in children younger than 2 years of age; 5 mg/dose for children 2–12 years of age; or 10 mg/dose for patients older than 12 years of age
Hydrocodone + ibuprofen	1–2 tablets q4–6h Maximum 5 tablets per day
Oxycodone + acetaminophen	0.05–0.15 mg/kg/dose (oxycodone) Maximum 5 mg q4–6h; 1–2 tablets q4–6h
Codeine + acetaminophen	0.5–1 mg/kg/dose (codeine) q6h 15–60 mg q4–6h; usual 30 mg/ dose codeine

SOURCES: Data from Taketomo C et al. Pediatric Dosage Handbook. Hudson, Ohio: Lexi-Comp; 2004; Benjamin LJ et al. *Guideline for the Management of Acute and Chronic Pain in Sickle Cell Disease.* Glenview, IL: American Pain Society; 1999.

Table 16–8. Available Opioid Combination Products.

Drug combination	Dosage and formulation
Acetaminophen + codeine	**Oral** 300 mg of acetaminophen + 7.5 mg, 15 mg, 30 mg, or 60 mg of codeine **Elixir** 120 mg/5 mL of acetaminophen +12 mg/5 mL of codeine
Acetaminophen + oxycodone	**Oral** 325, 500, or 650 mg of acetaminophen + 2.5, 5.0, 7.5, or 10 mg of oxycodone **Elixir** 325 mg/5 mL of acetaminophen +5 mg/mL of oxycodone
Aspirin + oxycodone	325 mg of aspirin + 2.25 or 4.5 mg of oxycodone
Acetaminophen + hydrocodone	**Oral** 325, 400, 500, 650, or 750 mg of acetaminophen +2.5, 5.0, 7.5, or 10 mg of hydrocodone **Elixir** 108 or 167 mg/5 mL of acetaminophen + 2.5 mg/5 mL of hydrocodone
Ibuprofen + hydrocodone	200 mg of ibuprofen + 7.5 mg of hydrocodone

SOURCE: Data from Taketomo C, Hodding J, Kraus D. Pediatric Dosage Handbook. Hudson, Ohio: Lexi-Comp; 2004.

continue until adequate relief scores are achieved, or until side effects become problematic.

There may still be some patients who may request the use of meperidine. However, the patient needs to be informed that it is the least potent and shortest-acting of the synthetic opioids and the least effective in providing analgesia for severe pain. More importantly, it may increase the risk of seizures when administered long-term because of the excitatory effects of its metabolite, normeperidine, on the nervous system. Some authors have argued that the incidence of meperidine-associated seizures is extremely small (0.4% of patients; 0.06% of admissions) and the risk of seizures should not dissuade clinicians from using this drug. However, the American Pain Society recommends that meperidine be reserved for very brief treatment courses for patients who have reported and demonstrated its effectiveness, or who have allergies or uncorrectable intolerances to other opioids. Meperidine should not be used for longer than 48 hours or doses >600 mg/24 hours.

2. Patient controlled analgesia—For severe pain, intravenous administration with bolus dosing and continuous infusion using a patient controlled analgesia (PCA) device may be necessary. For titration using PCA, a loading dose is administered, then, one-third of the estimated 24-hour dosing is administered by continuous infusion (Table 16–9). The other two-thirds is administered by patient or nurse in divided doses per hour on demand, with every 5 to 10 minutes lockout intervals. This may be given every 5 minutes during the first 2 hours to relief, which is the titration phase. A reassessment must be made every 60 minutes to titrate the appropriateness of the interval and dose until adequate relief is achieved.

Approximately 25 to 50% of maintenance dose may be administered for breakthrough pain. PCA settings may be adjusted if the number of rescue doses is increasing and the intervals between doses are too long. Standard orders should provide naloxone and resuscitation equipment in proximity. PCA should be immediately stopped and the physician notified for oversedation and respiratory rate less than 8 breaths per minute. PCA use and degree of pain control should be evaluated frequently and at least every 24 hours. Orders should be rewritten every 48 hours.

3. Weaning—When the patient is no longer experiencing severe pain, the patient requiring more than 5 to 7 days of opioids should have tapering doses to avoid the physiologic symptoms of withdrawal (dysphoria, agitation, nasal congestion, piloerection, diarrhea, sweating, and seizures). Weaning schedules for PCA have not been systematically studied. In general, the continuous infusion rate is progressively reduced prior to discontinuation, while the patient can continue to use demand doses for analgesia. Doses of long-acting oral analgesics, such as sustained-release oral morphine, may be used to replace continuous infusion dosing. The demand doses can be subsequently reduced if analgesia remains adequate. Weaning should not occur if a patient continues to experience severe pain. A patient may be discharged with a morphine equivalent equianalgesic dose (see Table 16–9) obtained by converting the continuous infusion rates to equivalent oral analgesics.

C. ADJUVANT MEDICATIONS

To increase the analgesic effect of opioids, reduce side effects of analgesics, or manage symptoms (eg, anxiety and depression) associated with sickle cell pain, adjuvant medications may be added to the pain management regimen (Table 16–10). Sedatives and anxiolytics are used in combination with a potent opioid. Sedatives and anxiolytics may mask the behavioral response to pain

Table 16–9. Guidelines for Morphine, Hydromorphone, Fentanyl for Moderate to Severe Pain.

Drug	Guidelines
Morphine	IV: 0.1–0.2 mg/kg/dose q2–4h Usual maximum 15 mg/dose 5–20 mg/dose q2–6h; 10 mg/dose q4h prn (for persons weighing more than 50 kg) PO: 0.2–0.5 mg/kg/dose q4–6h, (for persons weighing less than 50 kg) 0.3 to 0.6 mg/kg/dose q12h (controlled-release) 10–30 mg q4h prn; controlled-release 15–30 mg q8–12h (for persons weighing 50 kg)
Morphine (PCA)	*Loading dose:* 0.03 to 0.1 mg/kg *Push dose:* 0.01–0.03 mg/kg *Basal rate:* 0.03 mg/kg/h initially; continuous infusion: 0.025–2.6 mg/kg/h *Lockout interval:* 6–8 minutes *Hourly maximum:* 0.1 mg/kg/h to 6–8 mg/h, initially. For persons weighing more than 50 kg, 0.8–10 mg/h, usual range up to 80 mg/h; increase as needed to an amount that would relieve the pain
Hydromorphone	PO: 0.03–0.08 mg/kg/dose q4–6h prn; maximum, 5 mg/dose 0.06–0.08 mg/kg q3–4h; 7.5 mg q3–4h (for persons weighing 50 kg or more) IV: 0.015 mg/kg/dose q3–6h prn as needed Older children and adults (PO, IV, IM, SQ): 1–6 mg/dose q3–4h prn; usual adult dose 2 mg/dose; 0.015–0.020 mg/kg q3–4h IV 1.5 mg q3–4h IV (for persons weighing 50 kg or more)
Hydromorphone (PCA)	*Loading dose:* 20 mcg/kg (max 1.5 mg) *Push dose:* 5 mcg/kg/dose *Basal rate:* 1.5 mcg/kg/h *Lockout interval:* 6–8 minutes *Hourly maximum:* 20 mcg/kg/h
Fentanyl	IV: 0.5–2 mcg/kg/dose; may repeat at 30–60 minute intervals Adults: 25–50 mcg; may repeat 25 mcg at 5 minute intervals, 4–5 times if needed
Fentanyl (PCA)	*Loading dose:* 1–2 mcg/kg *Push dose:* 0.3–1 mcg/kg/dose *Basal rate:* 0.1–1 mcg/kg/h initially; titrate upward as needed *Lockout interval:* 6–8 minutes *Hourly maximum:* 1.25 mcg/kg/h

IV Morphine Equivalent Equianalgesic Conversions

1 mg IV morphine = 20 mg PO codeine
1 mg IV morphine = 3 mg PO morphine
1 mg IV morphine = 3 mg PO hydrocodone
1 mg IV morphine = 3 mg PO oxycodone
10 mg IV morphine = 1.5 hydromorphone
6.66 mg IV morphine = 1 mg hydromorphone

PCA, patient-controlled analgesia.
SOURCES: Data from Taketomo C, Hodding J, Kraus D. Pediatric Dosage Handbook. Hudson, Ohio: Lexi-Comp; 2004; Benjamin LJ et al. *Guideline for the Management of Acute and Chronic Pain in Sickle Cell Disease.* Glenview, IL: American Pain Society; 1999.

Table 16-10. Adjuvant Medications.

- Antihistamines (eg, hydroxyzine, diphenhydramine)
- Tricyclic antidepressants (eg, amitriptyline, imipramine)
- Benzodiazepines (eg, diazepam, lorazepam, clonazepam)
- Antipsychotics (eg, thioridazine, haloperidol)
- Barbiturates (eg, phenobarbital)
- Anticonvulsants (eg, phenytoin, carbamazepine)

SOURCE: Data from Benjamin LJ et al. *Guideline for the Management of Acute and Chronic Pain in Sickle Cell Disease.* Glenview, IL: American Pain Society; 1999.

Table 16-11. Nonpharmacologic Management of Sickle Cell Pain.

Strategies	Examples
Psychological	Distraction Imagery Education/teaching Hypnotherapy Psychotherapy
Behavioral	Deep breathing Relaxation exercise Self-hypnosis Biofeedback Behavior modification
Physical	Hydration Heat Massage Physical therapy TENS Acupuncture Acupressure

TENS, transcutaneous electrical nerve stimulation.
Adapted, with permission, from Benjamin LJ et al. *Guideline for the Management of Acute and Chronic Pain in Sickle Cell Disease.* Glenview, IL: American Pain Society; 1999.

without providing analgesia when used alone; however, when they are used in combination with opioids, risk for increased sedation is higher. Since sedation precedes opioid-induced respiratory depression, sedation levels should be monitored, and the use of incentive spirometry every 1 to 2 hours is recommended. Dose of opioids may be adjusted, or caffeine or methylphenidate may be added to the regimen as needed. For pruritus, adjunct medications such as diphenhydramine, hydroxyzine, continuous low-dose naloxone infusion, or switching to other opioids, such as hydromorphone or fentanyl have been effective in some cases. The use of opioids increases the risk for constipation, which can be minimized or prevented with the use of a stool softener and an osmotic laxative.

D. NONPHARMACOLOGIC MANAGEMENT

Although analgesic medications are the mainstay of pain management during acute painful episodes, the combination with the use of nonpharmacologic management strategies (Table 16–11) provide additive effects. Their use may increase the effects of analgesics or result in decreased use of pain medications.

Information about pain and treatments should be communicated to the patient and family as an integral part of ongoing treatment. Education about self-care strategies, positive coping strategies, strategies for communicating with health care providers, and the cards that patients can carry at all times (see Figure 16–2) should be provided. Health care providers need not only prepare the patient with the "passport" but also need to communicate with emergency department staff. For example, working with emergency department personnel to develop protocols and establish lines of communication when patients with SCD come to the emergency department.

Cognitive therapies may be used to enhance active coping skills, decrease negative or dysfunctional thinking patterns, and facilitate therapeutic changes in mood. Distraction is very effective and can be done by repeated and prepared inspirational or affirming phrases, singing, talking, doing mental calculations, visualizing images, or engaging in any mental activity that is fully absorbing. Hypnotherapy techniques include hypnosis, meditation, imagery, and relaxation. Acupuncture and acupressure applied by the fingers to trigger points or acupuncture sites are based on the belief that optimal health is directly connected to a balance of flow of the life force along energy pathways called meridians.

E. OTHER TREATMENTS

Hydroxyurea has been demonstrated to significantly reduce the annual rates of acute painful vaso-occlusive episodes and hospitalizations. However, many patients continue to have painful crises, and the response to hydroxyurea is difficult to predict. It is possible that some patients have problems with compliance. Close monitoring is required to prevent myelotoxicity, and there is a low risk for mutagenicity associated with long-term use. The beneficial effects of hydroxyurea may not be manifest for several months, and at least a 6-month trial is recommended. The most common side effect is myelosuppression, which is dose-dependent and is usually transient but may be prolonged. Nausea, vomiting, and skin rashes have also been reported.

Anie KA et al. Psychological therapies for sickle cell disease and pain. *Cochrane Database Syst Rev.* 2000;(3):CD001916. [PMID: 10908516]

Benjamin LJ et al. *Guideline for the Management of Acute and Chronic Pain in Sickle Cell Disease.* Glenview, IL: American Pain Society; 1999.

Benjamin LJ et al. Sickle cell anemia day hospital: an approach for the management of uncomplicated painful crises. *Blood.* 2000;95:1130. [PMID: 10666181]

Bodhise PB et al. Non-pharmacologic management of sickle cell pain. *Hematology.* 2004;9:235. [PMID: 15204105]

Claster S et al. Managing sickle cell disease. *BMJ.* 2003;327:1151. [PMID: 14615343]

Elander J et al. Pain management and symptoms of substance dependence among patients with sickle cell disease. *Soc Sci Med.* 2003;57:1683. [PMID: 12948577]

Maxwell K et al. Experiences of hospital care and treatment seeking for pain from sickle cell disease: qualitative study. *BMJ.* 1999;318:1585. [PMID: 10364116]

Nadvi SZ et al. Low frequency of meperidine-associated seizures in sickle cell disease. *Clin Pediatr (Phila).* 1999;38:459. [PMID: 10456240]

Sumoza A et al. Hydroxyurea (HU) for prevention of recurrent stroke in sickle cell anemia (SCA). *Am J Hematol.* 2002;71:161. [PMID: 12410569]

Barriers to Adequate Pain Management

Patients with SCD often delay seeking treatment for pain until pain is very severe and intolerable. They prefer to treat their pain at home overnight or over the weekend until the Hematology Clinic or Sickle Cell Clinic opens when their primary care hematologist is available. However, the severity of pain compels most patients to go to the emergency department. While the hematologist in the clinic is familiar with the patient's clinical profile and the complications of SCD, the physician in the emergency department is less focused on the special nature of SCD. In 50% of the patients, there are no objective signs of a painful crisis.

The delay in seeking treatment violates a major guiding principle in pain management, which is that prevention of pain is always better than treatment. Pain that is established and severe is often more difficult to control. When pain is untreated, sensory input from injured tissues reaches spinal cord neurons and may cause subsequent pain responses to be enhanced or amplified. Long-lasting changes in cells within spinal cord pain pathways may occur after a brief painful stimulus and may lead to the development of chronic and persistent pain conditions. Recent studies on pain emphasize a distinct neurochemistry of persistent pain, which is not merely a prolonged acute pain symptom of the disease. There are underlying physiologic mechanisms that lead to the persistence of pain if left untreated. Clinicians may, therefore, consider establishing an early intervention or prevention protocol that may be instituted in an emergency department, urgent care, or day hospital, for hydration and early aggressive pain management. Protocols for outpatient management in a day care center have been developed as an alternative to hospital admission. The use of day hospitals and outpatient management protocols have reduced unnecessary hospital admissions.

The use of opioids, whether inpatient or outpatient, is the mainstay of therapy for severe pain. A major barrier to the use of opioids for effective management of sickle cell pain is the confusion between opioid tolerance, physical dependence, and addiction. Tolerance and physical dependence are expected pharmacologic consequences of long-term opioid use. The first signs of tolerance are decreased duration of the action of medication and patients experience pain before the next scheduled dose of opioid. When tolerance develops, larger doses or shorter intervals between doses may be needed to achieve the same analgesic effect. Pain experts question whether tolerance to the analgesic effect of opioids is a significant clinical problem and suggest that requests for higher doses of drug may reflect increasing pain stimuli. Physical dependence develops when opioids are given for more than 5 to 7 days. Withdrawal symptoms, such as dysphoria, nasal congestion, diarrhea, nausea, vomiting, sweating, and seizures may occur when opioids are stopped without weaning. Doses should be tapered to avoid the physiologic symptoms of withdrawal.

Addiction is not physical dependence. Addiction is psychological dependence, which is a very complex phenomenon with genetic, psychological, and social components. The use of opioids for acute pain relief is not addiction, regardless of the dose or duration of time the opioids are administered. Fears related to addiction among patients, family, and health care providers are unwarranted and lead to inadequate treatment.

Addictive disease includes a pattern of compulsive drug-use behaviors characterized by a continued craving for an opioid. Patients with addictive disease have a need to use the opioid for effects other than pain relief. They do not have control over drug use, and they compulsively use drugs despite the harmful effects. The risk for the development of these behaviors in patients with SCD is not any higher than other groups of patients.

The diagnosis and treatment of addiction (see Chapter 7) requires a referral to an addiction medicine specialist. The management of patients with a history of substance abuse is particularly a difficult and challenging problem. For those patients in whom an addictive disorder is suspected, an appropriate referral to an addiction specialist for a complete evaluation, diagnosis, and treatment should be made, rather than imposing judgment and denying the patient adequate pain management.

Some patients whose pain is managed poorly will try to persuade the medical staff to give them more analgesic, engage in clock-watching, and request specific medications or dosages. These patients are often perceived as manipulative and demanding. Because patients with SCD have lifelong experiences with medications that work and do not work, they are very knowledgeable about the medications and doses that are effective. Therefore, their requests for specific medications and doses should be respected and not be interpreted as indications of drug-seeking behavior.

Iatrogenic pseudoaddiction may develop in patients who are given doses of opioids that are inadequate to relieve their pain or in patients whose doses are not tapered after a course of treatment. Pseudoaddiction or clock-watching behavior may be resolved by communicating with the patient to ensure accurate assessment, involving them in decisions about their pain management, and by administering adequate opioid doses.

Benjamin LJ et al. *Guideline for the Management of Acute and Chronic Pain in Sickle Cell Disease.* Glenview, IL: American Pain Society; 1999.

Elander J et al. Understanding the causes of problematic pain management in sickle cell disease: evidence that pseudoaddiction plays a more important role than genuine analgesic dependence. *J Pain Symptom Manage.* 2004;27:156. [PMID: 15157040]

Elander J et al. Pain management and symptoms of substance dependence among patients with sickle cell disease. *Soc Sci Med.* 2003;57:1683. [PMID: 12948577]

Kirsh KL et al. Abuse and addiction issues in medically ill patients with pain: attempts at clarification of terms and empirical study. *Clin J Pain.* 2002;18(4 Suppl):S52. [PMID: 12479254]

Prognosis

The prognosis of sickle cell disease usually refers to the likely outcome of the disease. Sickle cell chronic lung disease is a prime contributor to mortality in young adult patients with SCD, especially those with the SCD-SS genotype. The prognosis of SCD may include the duration and number of complications, prospects for recovery, survival rates, death rates, and other outcome possibilities in the overall prognosis of SCD. Such forecast issues are by their nature unpredictable.

The average lifespan of a patient with SCD is now in the forties and continues to rise due to improved treatment. Some patients suffer only mildly whereas others have severe complications. Among patients with SCD who were older than 20 years of age, those with more frequent pain episodes tended to die earlier than those with less frequent episodes. Increased frequency of pain episodes was associated with a low hemoglobin, low hematocrit, and low fetal hemoglobin levels. The number of pain episodes per year is a measure of clinical severity and correlates with early death in patients with SCD over the age of 20.

In 1984, bone marrow transplantation in a child with SCD produced the first reported cure of the disease. The transplantation was done to treat acute leukemia. The child's SCD was cured as a side event. The procedure nonetheless set the precedence for later transplantation efforts directed specifically at SCD.

Bakanay SM et al. Mortality in sickle cell patients on hydroxyurea therapy. *Blood.* 2005;105:545. [PMID: 15454485]

Chakrabarti S et al. Will developments in allogeneic transplantation influence treatment of adult patients with sickle cell disease? *Biol Blood Marrow Transplant.* 2004;10:23. [PMID: 14752776]

Locatelli F et al; Eurocord Transplant Group. Related umbilical cord blood transplantation in patients with thalassemia and sickle cell disease. *Blood.* 2003;101:2137. [PMID: 12424197]

Prasad R et al. Long-term outcome in patients with sickle cell disease and frequent vaso-occlusive crises. *Am J Med Sci.* 2003;325:107. [PMID: 12640284] http://www.scinfo.org
The Sickle Cell Information Center at the Georgia Comprehensive Sickle Cell center at Emory University provides a monthly update on professional publications about sickle cell disease, new web sites that might be helpful, and conferences of interest for health care professionals and parents as well as educational products and services.

http://www.rhofed.com/sickle/index.htm
This is the web site of the 10 Comprehensive Sickle Cell Disease Centers funded by the National Heart Lung and Blood Institute of the National Institutes of Health. The ongoing research and clinical care focus of these centers is listed along with links to other sites that provide educational resources on sickle cell disease.

http://www.nhlbi.nih.gov/health/prof/blood/sickle/index.htm
At this web site, the fourth edition of *The Management of Sickle Cell Disease* can be viewed and downloaded.

http://is.dal.ca/~pedpain/
This site is dedicated to providing information about up-to-date pain research in children and provides links to web resources for children and families to help them cope with painful procedures and learn how best to tell others about pain.

Chronic Pelvic Pain

17

Fred M. Howard, MS, MD

General Considerations

Chronic pelvic pain (CPP) is nonmenstrual pelvic pain lasting 6 months or more that causes functional disability or requires medical or surgical treatment. The mean age of women with CPP is about 30 years. Its estimated prevalence is 4%, which is similar to the prevalence of migraine headaches, asthma, and low back pain in women. CPP is the indication for 12% of all hysterectomies and for over 40% of gynecologic diagnostic laparoscopies. Direct costs of health care for CPP in the United States are estimated at $880 million per year, and direct and indirect costs may total over $2 billion per year.

On average, women have CPP for 2 to 5 years before they seek medical help. CPP often leads to years of disability and suffering, with loss of employment, marital discord and divorce, as well as numerous visits to physicians with unsuccessful results.

CPP may be due to disorders of the reproductive tract, urologic organs, gastrointestinal system, musculoskeletal system, and psychoneurologic system (Tables 17–1 through 17–5). Occasionally, one of these disorders is the only diagnosis and curative treatment is possible. More often the etiology of CPP is not discernible or it is associated with several diagnoses that contribute to pain ("pain generators"). For example, endometriosis, irritable bowel syndrome (IBS), poor posture, and emotional stress may all be pain generators in a single patient, yet treatment of each of these disorders still may not result in cure of pelvic pain. Thus, a multidisciplinary approach is often ideal.

Clinical Findings

Obtaining a complete history is a crucial component of the clinical evaluation. In addition to a comprehensive pain history (discussed in Chapter 2), a thorough review of symptoms relating to the most commonly involved systems—the gastrointestinal, urologic, reproductive, and musculoskeletal systems—should be done. Intake pain questionnaires greatly facilitate the ability to obtain a detailed history. A useful form is available from the International Pelvic Pain Society (www.pelvicpain.org). Intake questionnaires should be used to supplement—not replace—history-taking, allowing the patient to tell her story. Not only does using intake questionnaires allow the chance to obtain a more detailed history, they also allow the clinician to observe the patient's reaction to critical aspects of the history, thereby enhancing rapport and trust. A patient is often reluctant to talk about bowel, bladder, and sexual functions, so it is important to ask her specific questions about these functions and their relationship to pain.

It is useful to have the patient mark the location of her pain on a pain map (Figure 17–1). Pain of visceral origin is usually not well localized and may be depicted as fairly diffuse. Somatic pain is more likely to show a dermatomal distribution or a myotomal pattern.

Cyclic pain related to menses is often characteristic of gynecologic disorders such as endometriosis, adenomyosis, and pelvic congestion, but such a pattern also may occur with nonreproductive tract disease, such as interstitial cystitis (IC) and IBS. A history of pain or increased pain with coitus (dyspareunia) is frequently interpreted as pathognomonic of psychological or gynecologic disease. In fact, dyspareunia is present in about 50% of women with CPP and occurs as commonly in urologic, gastrointestinal, and musculoskeletal disorders as in psychological and gynecologic disorders.

Obtaining a history regarding pregnancy and delivery is another aspect of pain evaluation. Onset during or immediately after pregnancy may suggest a musculoskeletal disorder, particularly peripartum pelvic pain syndrome. Pregnancy and childbirth are traumatic events to the musculoskeletal system, especially the pelvis and back. In addition, the hormonal changes of pregnancy cause laxity of ligaments, and this may lead to pain. Risk factors associated with pregnancy and pain include lumbar lordosis, delivery of a large infant, muscle weakness and poor physical conditioning, a difficult delivery,

Table 17–1. Gynecologic Diseases That Cause or Are Associated with Chronic Pelvic Pain in Women.

Extrauterine
- Adhesions
- Adnexal cysts
- Chronic ectopic pregnancy
- Chlamydial endometritis or salpingitis
- Endometriosis
- Endosalpingiosis
- Neoplasia of the genital tract
- Ovarian retention syndrome (residual ovary syndrome)
- Ovarian remnant syndrome
- Ovarian dystrophy or ovulatory pain
- Pelvic congestion syndrome
- Pelvic inflammatory disease (PID)
- Postoperative peritoneal cysts
- Residual accessory ovary
- Subacute salpingo-oophoritis (chronic PID)
- Tuberculous salpingitis

Uterine
- Adenomyosis
- Atypical dysmenorrhea or ovulatory pain
- Cervical stenosis
- Chronic endometritis
- Endometrial or cervical polyps
- Intrauterine contraceptive device
- Leiomyomata
- Symptomatic pelvic relaxation (genital prolapse)

Table 17–2. Urologic Diseases That Cause or Are Associated with Chronic Pelvic Pain in Women.

- Bladder neoplasm
- Chronic urinary tract infection
- Interstitial cystitis
- Radiation cystitis
- Recurrent, acute cystitis
- Recurrent, acute urethritis
- Stone/urolithiasis
- Uninhibited bladder contractions (detrusor dyssynergia)
- Urethral diverticulum
- Urethral syndrome
- Urethral caruncle

Table 17–3. Gastroenterologic Diseases That Cause or Are Associated with Chronic Pelvic Pain in Women.

- Carcinoma of the colon
- Chronic intermittent bowel obstruction
- Colitis
- Constipation
- Diverticular disease
- Hernias
- Inflammatory bowel disease
- Irritable bowel syndrome

vacuum or forceps delivery, and use of gynecologic stirrups for delivery.

A thorough physical examination is also essential. Because the physical examination, especially the pelvic examination, is often painful for the woman with CPP, it is essential that the physician go slowly enough to allow her to recover and relax between various portions of the examination. Even a "routine" pelvic examination is emotionally and physically stressful for many patients with CPP.

A major goal of the examination is to detect, in as much as possible, the exact anatomic locations of tenderness and correlate these with areas of pain. This requires a

Table 17–4. Musculoskeletal Diseases That Cause or Are Associated with Chronic Pelvic Pain in Women.

- Abdominal wall myofascial pain (trigger points)
- Chronic coccygeal pain
- Compression of lumbar vertebrae
- Degenerative joint disease
- Disk herniation or rupture
- Faulty or poor posture
- Fibromyalgia
- Fibromyositis
- Hernias: ventral, inguinal, femoral, Spigelian
- Low back pain
- Muscular strains and sprains
- Neoplasia of spinal cord or sacral nerve
- Neuralgia of iliohypogastric, ilioinguinal, and/or genitofemoral nerves
- Pelvic floor myalgia (levator ani spasm)
- Piriformis syndrome
- Rectus tendon strain
- Spondylosis

Table 17–5. Psychoneurologic Disorders That Cause or Are Associated with Chronic Pelvic Pain in Women.

- Abdominal cutaneous nerve entrapment in surgical scar
- Abdominal epilepsy
- Abdominal migraine
- Bipolar personality disorders
- Depression
- Familial Mediterranean fever
- Neurologic dysfunction
- Porphyria
- Shingles
- Sleep disturbances
- Somatic referral

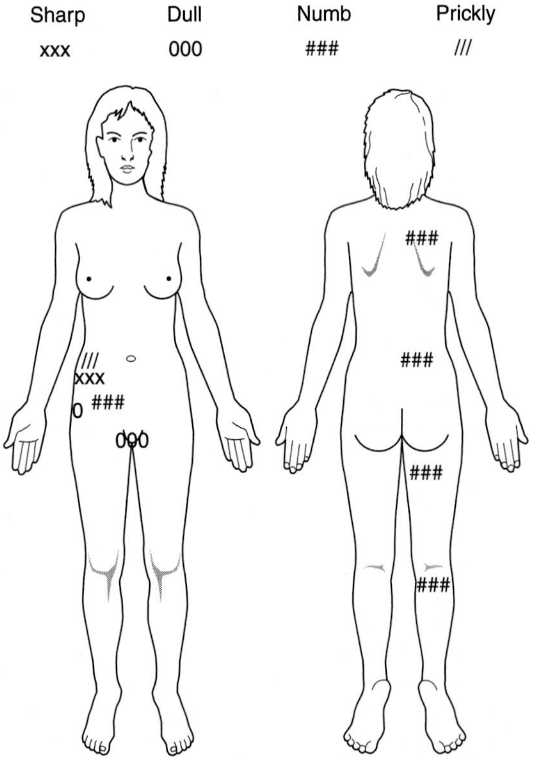

Sharp	Dull	Numb	Prickly
xxx	000	###	///

Figure 17–1. Example of a pain map in a pelvic pain patient.

systematic and methodical attempt to duplicate the pain by palpation or positioning.

Logistically, the examination is facilitated if it is performed in the following order:

1. Standing examination.
2. Sitting examination.
3. Supine examination.
4. Lithotomy examination.

Only the lithotomy portion of the examination is reviewed in this chapter. Once the patient is in the lithotomy position, initially inspect the external genitalia for redness, discharge, abscess formation, excoriation, perineal fistula, ulcerations, pigment changes, condylomata, atrophic changes (thinning, paleness, loss of vaginal rugae, protruding urethral mucosa), or signs of trauma. Look for fistulas and fissures because they may occasionally be the first objective evidence of inflammatory bowel disease.

Perform basic sensory testing to sharpness, dullness, and light touch, and test the bulbocavernosus and anal wink reflexes. Use a cotton-tipped swab to evaluate the vestibule for the localized tenderness of vulvar vestibulitis (localized vulvodynia); hold the labia apart and gently palpate the vestibule, vulva, hymen, and the area of the minor vestibular glands with a cotton-tipped swab. Patients with vulvar vestibulitis demonstrate exquisite tenderness in localized areas at the minor vestibular glands just external to the hymen, with normal sensation in adjacent vulvar areas (Figure 17–2). Use a cotton-tipped applicator or single digit palpation to evaluate the vulva and pubic arch for trigger points and for skin or mucosal lesions that reproduce the patient's symptoms. Pay particular attention to areas of previous vulvar or vaginal trauma and scars from surgeries or deliveries.

Assess the pelvic floor muscles for pain or tension by insertion of a Sims retractor or a single blade of the speculum into the posterior vagina while asking the patient to relax. The resistance to downward or posterior pressure can be evaluated to reveal increased muscle tone, tension, or spasm. This maneuver may also reproduce part of the patient's symptom complex. Single speculum blade or Sims type retractor examination may also reveal evidence of pelvic relaxation, with uterine descensus, cystocele, enterocele, or rectocele.

The traditional speculum examination is done for full visual inspection and to obtain requisite cytologic and bacteriologic specimens. It is reasonable to test for sexually transmitted diseases with cervical cultures or smears for gonorrhea and chlamydia, as well as syphilis serology, hepatitis B surface antigen screening, and HIV testing as deemed appropriate. Note the position of the cervix, as lateral displacement suggests possible ipsilateral

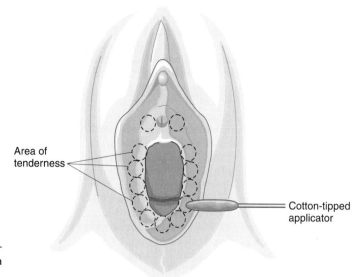

Area of tenderness

Cotton-tipped applicator

Figure 17–2. Areas of tenderness to cotton tip palpation with localized vulvodynia (vulvar vestibulitis).

uterosacral endometriosis. Use a cotton-tipped swab to evaluate the cervical os and the paracervical and cervical tissues for tenderness. In patients who have had a hysterectomy, palpate the full vaginal cuff for tenderness with a cotton-tipped applicator. If localized tender points are elicited, it may be worthwhile to block them with 1% lidocaine and reevaluate for tenderness after 5 minutes.

Always initiate the manual portion of the pelvic examination with a single index finger, first noting any introital tenderness or spasm. Vaginismus can be identified by involuntary introital spasm at this point in the examination. Next, directly palpate the levator ani muscles for tone and tenderness. The levator ani muscles are easily palpated during vaginal examination. They lie adjacent to the lateral vaginal walls just above the hymeneal ring. The medial margins of the muscles are slightly thicker than a standard pencil, running in an anteroposterior direction. Identification may be confirmed by having the patient contract her pelvic muscles. The anus elevates when the levators are contracted. Normally this palpation causes only a pressure sensation, but in patients with pelvic floor myalgia, it may cause pain consistent with at least part of the patient's clinical symptoms. In some patients with pelvic floor myalgia, there will also be tenderness of the coccyx, lateral sacrum, or sacrococcygeal ligaments. Digital pressure on the involved muscle characteristically reproduces or intensifies the patient's pain symptoms. It is not unusual for the tenderness to be unilateral.

Palpate the piriformis, coccygeus, and obturator internus muscles bilaterally seeking tenderness that reproduces the patient's pain. The piriformis muscles are somewhat more difficult to palpate than the levators. Rectal examination may allow an easier evaluation than vaginal examination. Next, the sacrospinous ligament and area of Alcocks canal are palpated to elicit any tenderness suggestive of pudendal neuralgia.

Palpate the anterior vaginal, urethral, and trigonal areas to reveal any areas of tenderness, induration, or thickening. Urethral tenderness with or without discharge is consistent with chronic urethritis or chronic urethral syndrome. Next, evaluate the "gutter" on either side of the urethra for any fullness, fluctuance, or discomfort that might suggest a urethral diverticulum or vaginal wall cyst. Also evaluate the bladder base for tenderness; its presence is consistent with trigonitis or IC.

Next, still using a single digit, palpate the cervix, paracervical areas, and vaginal fornices for tenderness or trigger points. Cervical tenderness may suggest problems such as cervicitis, repeated cervical trauma (usually from intercourse), or pelvic infection. Vaginal forniceal tenderness may suggest problems such as pelvic infection, endometriosis, ureteral tenderness, or trigger points.

Compress the uterus against the sacrum to evaluate uterine tenderness. Uterine tenderness may be consistent with diseases such as adenomyosis, pelvic congestion syndrome, pelvic infection, or premenstrual syndrome. A uterus that is immobile and fixed in position, especially a retroflexed position, may suggest endometriosis or adhesions. Next, palpate the coccyx with the single digit and attempt to move it 30 degrees or less. This part of the examination may also be done during the bimanual or rectovaginal examination. Normally the coccyx moves 30 degrees without eliciting pain, but in patients with coccydynia this movement elicits pain.

Palpate the adnexal areas next, still using a single digit without the use of the abdominal hand. This is often a more accurate manner of assessing intrinsic tenderness of the ovaries or tube than the traditional bimanual examination, especially in patients with abdominal wall tenderness or trigger points. All ovaries are tender, so it is the degree of tenderness and the similarity to the chief pain complaint that are clinically useful.

Palpate the cecum on the right and the rectosigmoid on the left for masses, hard feces, and tenderness. Either or both may be abnormally tender in patients with IBS.

Perform traditional bimanual pelvic and rectal or rectovaginal examinations last. Marked discomfort with digital rectal examination often accompanies IBS or chronic constipation, as may hard feces in the rectum. Evaluate function of the internal and external anal sphincter by reflex wink and voluntary constriction. Carefully examine the rectovaginal septum for nodularity and tenderness, suggestive of endometriosis. Rectal examination should also include evaluation for rectal masses as many colorectal carcinomas are palpable this way. Tenderness of the anal canal may suggest abscess or fissures in the canal. Fecal occult blood test should be obtained.

Laboratory and imaging studies are not universally useful and should be done based on the clinical findings and differential diagnosis. Laparoscopy is commonly performed, especially by gynecologists, as a major part of the evaluation, but it also should be done based on the clinical findings and differential diagnosis.

A new approach to diagnostic laparoscopy, "conscious laparoscopic pain mapping," has been suggested as a way to improve the diagnostic capability of laparoscopy. Conscious laparoscopic pain mapping is a diagnostic laparoscopy under local anesthesia, with or without conscious sedation, directed at the identification of sources of pain. The technique used with conscious laparoscopic pain mapping is a gentle probing or tractioning of tissues, lesions, and organs with a blunt probe or forceps. Diagnosis of an etiologic lesion or organ is based on the severity of pain elicited and on replication of the pain that is the patient's presenting symptom. However, CPP is a multifaceted and complicated problem, and it is premature to assume that the findings with mechanically elicited tenderness at conscious pain mapping directly translate into cause and cure. For example, a study at the University of Rochester Medical Center evaluated laparoscopic diagnosis and treatment. A historical cohort of 65 patients treated before the introduction of conscious pain mapping was compared with 50 patients treated after introduction of conscious laparoscopic pain mapping. Data failed to show any improvement in outcomes.

Treatment

Clinically, there are two approaches to the treatment of CPP. The first is to treat chronic pain itself as a diagnosis, and the second is to treat diseases or disorders that might be a cause of or a contributor to CPP. These two approaches are not mutually exclusive, and in many patients, effective therapy is best achieved by using both.

Although several disorders may be associated with CPP (see Tables 17–1 through 17–5), the most frequent conditions seen in clinical practice include endometriosis, adhesions, IBS, and IC.

Cramer DW et al. The epidemiology of endometriosis. *Ann N Y Acad Sci.* 2002;955:11. [PMID: 11949940]

Howard FM et al. Conscious pain mapping by laparoscopy in women with chronic pelvic pain. *Obstet Gynecol.* 2000;96:934. [PMID: 11084181]

Lippman SA et al. Uterine fibroids and gynecologic pain symptoms in a population-based study. *Fertil Steril.* 2003;80:1488. [PMID: 14667888]

Tripp DA et al. Predictors of quality of life and pain in chronic prostatitis/chronic pelvic pain syndrome: findings from the National Institutes of Health Chronic Prostatitis Cohort Study. *BJU Int.* 2004;94:1279. [PMID: 15610105]

Zondervan K et al. Epidemiology of chronic pelvic pain. *Baillieres Best Pract Res Clin Obstet Gynaecol.* 2000;14:403. [PMID: 10962634]

Zubor P. Laparoscopy in chronic pelvic pain–a prospective clinical study. *Ceska Gynekol.* 2005;70:225. [PMID: 16047928]

American Pain Society http://www.ampainsoc.org

International Association for the Study of Pain http://www.iasp-pain.org

The Cochrane Collaboration http://www.cochrane.org/cochrane

The International Pelvic Pain Society http://www.pelvicpain.org

ADHESIONS

Pathogenesis

An adhesion is fibrous tissue by which anatomic structures abnormally adhere to one another. Adhesions may cause intestinal obstruction and infertility, but their role as a cause of CPP is controversial. Pelvic inflammatory disease, endometriosis, perforated appendix, prior abdominopelvic surgery, and inflammatory bowel disease are known causes of pelvic adhesions.

Prevention

At the time of surgery, adhesion barriers (biopolymers used at surgery to reduce adhesion formation), can be used and have been shown to have some, although not complete, efficacy in preventing surgical adhesions.

Clinical Findings

Pelvic pain due to adhesions is exacerbated by sudden movements, intercourse, or physical activities. The pain is often consistent in its location, although over time the area of involvement may expand. A history of one of the classic causes of adhesions is present in 50% of women with adhesions.

Complications

Surgical treatment of adhesions appears to have limited efficacy, yet may result in significant complications, especially intestinal injuries.

Treatment

Uncontrolled, observational studies suggest that laparoscopic adhesiolysis reduces pain in 60 to 90% of patients with CPP, but the only randomized trial (adhesiolysis by laparotomy, not laparoscopy) failed to show any significant improvement in pain symptoms. Only a subgroup of women with severe, stage IV adhesions showed any improvement in pain that could be attributed to adhesiolysis. A more recent randomized trial of laparoscopic adhesiolysis for chronic abdominal pain (not just pelvic pain) also failed to show significant improvement that could be attributed to adhesiolysis. Currently, no effective treatment has been confirmed with clinical trials.

Hammoud A et al. Adhesions in patients with chronic pelvic pain: a role for adhesiolysis? *Fertil Steril.* 2004;82:1483. [PMID: 15589847]

Swank DJ et al. Laparoscopic adhesiolysis in patients with chronic abdominal pain: a blinded randomised controlled multi-centre trial. *Lancet.* 2003;361:1247. [PMID: 12699951]

ENDOMETRIOSIS

Pathogenesis

Endometriosis is the presence of endometrial tissue in any location other than the uterine mucosa or muscularis. By definition, it requires histologic documentation of ectopic endometrial glands and stroma. Endometriosis is one of the most common gynecologic causes of CPP and is found in at least 33% of women who undergo a laparoscopy to evaluate CPP. The precise mechanisms by which it causes pain are not completely understood.

Prevention

At this time, there are no known ways to prevent the development of endometriosis. There is no evidence that early treatment with oral contraceptives prevents endometriosis.

Clinical Findings

Most women with endometriosis-associated pain are between 20 and 45 years of age. However, endometriosis can occur in adolescents and may be a more common cause of pain in teenagers than is generally recognized. It is rare in postmenopausal women but can occur if they are receiving estrogen replacement therapy.

Classically, the woman with endometriosis seeks medical attention complaining of one or more of the following triad: an adnexal mass (endometrioma), infertility, and pelvic pain. Endometriosis-associated pelvic pain often starts as dysmenorrhea, and about 75% of women with endometriosis-associated pelvic pain have dysmenorrhea as a component of their pain symptoms. Dyspareunia with deep vaginal penetration is also a frequent component of endometriosis-associated pain. Although CPP, dyspareunia, and dysmenorrhea are characteristic symptoms of endometriosis, they are not as specific or diagnostic as is commonly thought and by themselves do not justify a diagnosis of endometriosis.

In many women with endometriosis-associated pelvic pain, there is detectable tenderness only during menses. Therefore, it is sometimes helpful to do the examination during the first day or two of menstrual flow in women with suspected endometriosis. This may also increase the likelihood of finding tender endometriotic nodules in the pelvis or rectovaginal septum.

Complications

Complications of medical treatment include side effects of weight gain, edema, hot flushes, headaches, nausea, acne, hirsutism, abnormal uterine bleeding, decreased breast size, decreased libido, vaginal dryness, weakness, decreased bone density, and thromboembolic disease. Surgical complications vary with the severity of disease, but injury to pelvic viscera is a potential risk in women with endometriosis. Untreated endometriosis is rarely life-threatening, although there are cases of ureteral and bowel obstruction due to endometriosis as well as invasion of the urinary and gastrointestinal tracts.

Treatment

Treatment of endometriosis-associated pelvic pain is complex and none of the options for therapy are ideal for all patients (Table 17–6). The patient's age, reproductive plans, presence of infertility, pain severity, and attitude toward surgery or hormonal medications are a few of the factors that must be considered in designing a treatment plan. Plans may need to be modified based on the tolerance of drug therapies or persistence or worsening of symptoms.

Surgical treatment can be done at the time of laparoscopic diagnosis in symptomatic women. Conservative, laparoscopic surgical treatment has been shown to significantly improve pain in women with stage II, III, and IV endometriosis, with a number needed to treat to be effective being 2 to 2.5. Surgery for advanced-stage

Table 17–6. Some of the Treatment Options for Women with Endometriosis-Associated Pelvic Pain.

- Observation with palliative treatment
- Conservative surgery
    - Excision and ablation of endometriotic lesions
    - Presacral neurectomy
- Hormonal treatment
    - Combined oral contraceptives

    Low dose pills, continuously; double dose for 5 days if breakthrough bleeding occurs

    Low dose pills, cyclically

    - Medroxyprogesterone acetate, 10–100 mg/d
    - Norethindrone acetate, 10–40 mg/d
    - Danazol, 200–400 mg bid
    - Gonadotropin-releasing hormone analogues

    Nafarelin, 200–400 mcg bid

    Depot-leuprolide, 3.75–7.5 mg every 28 days

    Goserelin, 3.6 mg every 28 days

- Combined medical and surgical treatments
- Definitive extirpative surgery
    - Hysterectomy
    - Salpingo-oophorectomy

endometriosis can be challenging, tedious, frustrating, and prone to complications.

Presacral neurectomy (resection of the superior hypogastric plexus) and uterosacral neurectomy (uterine nerve resection or transection of the uterosacral ligament) have been recommended for relief of CPP associated with endometriosis. Data from clinical trials show that presacral neurectomy somewhat improves pain relief obtained with surgical treatment of endometriosis. However, presacral neurectomy may lead to intractable constipation in up to 5% of patients and bothersome urinary urgency in 5%. Data from clinical trials clearly show that uterosacral neurectomy does not improve pain relief when included in surgical treatment of endometriosis.

Medical treatment with gonadotropin-releasing hormone (GnRH) agonists, progestins, danazol, or combined oral contraceptives often relieves endometriosis-associated pelvic pain. The number needed to treat to be effective is 2 to 2.5.

GnRH agonists inhibit the production and release of luteinizing hormone and follicle-stimulating hormone, leading to a dramatic decline in estradiol levels, induction of amenorrhea, and improvement of pain levels. Examples of GnRH agonists available in the United States are depot leuprolide (3.75 mg intramuscularly every 28 days) and goserelin (3.6 mg subcutaneous implant every 28 days). When patients have a recurrence of pain within 1 year after treatment with GnRH analogues, retreatment appears to be reasonably effective, with about 67% of patients showing a significant reduction of pain levels during retreatment.

Loss of bone density with GnRH analogues is a serious concern. Clinical trials with GnRH agonists show that add-back therapy with conjugated equine estrogen or norethindrone acetate significantly decreases bone loss.

Danazol (200 to 400 mg orally twice a day), a 17-ethinyl-testosterone derivative, has efficacy similar to that of GnRH agonists. However, danazol is not as frequently used as GnRH agonists because of possible androgenic side effects, including significant weight gain, mood changes, and musculinizing symptoms.

Medroxyprogesterone acetate has been a recommended treatment for many years. Although a high dose of 100 mg/d was used in the only placebo-controlled trial of medroxyprogesterone acetate, lower doses are generally used in clinical practice.

Oral contraceptive treatment of endometriosis is a longstanding approach, using either cyclical or continuous dosing. Efficacy appears to be similar or somewhat less than the other hormonal treatments.

Combining medical and surgical treatments appear to result in the best relief of pain.

Prognosis

Endometriosis is often a progressive disease without treatment. Resolution of pain without treatment is uncommon. Surgical and medical treatments are efficacious, although only complete extirpation including hysterectomy and bilateral oophorectomy appears to have a high cure rate.

Abbott J et al. Laparoscopic excision of endometriosis: a randomized, placebo-controlled trial. *Fertil Steril.* 2004;82:878. [PMID: 15482763]

Busacca M et al. Post-operative GnRH analogue treatment after conservative surgery for symptomatic endometriosis stage III–IV: a randomized controlled trial. *Hum Reprod.* 2001;16:2399. [PMID: 11679528]

Gambone JC et al. Consensus statement for the management of chronic pelvic pain and endometriosis: proceedings of an expert-panel consensus process. *Fertil Steril.* 2002;78:961. [PMID: 12413979]

Howard FM. An evidence-based medicine approach to the treatment of endometriosis-associated chronic pelvic pain: placebo-controlled studies. *J Am Assoc Gynecol Laparosc.* 2000;7:477. [PMID: 11044498]

Jain KA. Sonographic spectrum of hemorrhagic ovarian cysts. *J Ultrasound Med.* 2002;21:879. [PMID: 12164573]

Jarrell J et al. Laparoscopy and reported pain among patients with endometriosis. *J Obstet Gynaecol Can.* 2005;27:477. [PMID: 16100643]

Lamvu G et al. The role of laparoscopy in the diagnosis and treatment of conditions associated with chronic pelvic pain. *Obstet Gynecol Clin North Am.* 2004;31:619. [PMID: 15450323]

Luciano AA. Leuprolide acetate in the management of endometriosis-associated pain: a multicenter, evaluator-blind, comparative clinical trial. *Glob Cong Gynecol Endo.* 2004;11(Suppl): S5.

Olive DL. Optimizing gonadotropin-releasing hormone agonist therapy in women with endometriosis. *Treat Endocrinol.* 2004;3:83. [PMID: 15743104]

Scarselli G et al. Diagnosis and treatment of endometriosis. A review. *Minerva Ginecol.* 2005;57:55. [PMID: 15758866]

Sutton C et al. A prospective, randomized, double-blind controlled trial of laparoscopic uterine nerve ablation in the treatment of pelvic pain associated with endometriosis. *Gynaecol Endoscopy.* 2001;10:217.

Tsai YL et al. Short-term postoperative GnRH analogue or danazol treatment after conservative surgery for stage III or IV endometriosis before ovarian stimulation: a prospective, randomized study. *J Reprod Med.* 2004;49:955. [PMID: 15656211]

Valle RF et al. Endometriosis: treatment strategies. *Ann N Y Acad Sci.* 2003;997:229. [PMID: 14644830]

Vercellini P et al. Laparoscopic uterosacral ligament resection for dysmenorrhea associated with endometriosis: results of a randomized, controlled trial. *Fertil Steril.* 2003;80:310. [PMID: 12909493]

Yap C et al. Pre- and postoperative medical therapy for endometriosis surgery. *Cochrane Database Syst Rev.* 2004;(3):CD003678. [PMID: 15266496]

Zullo F et al. Effectiveness of presacral neurectomy in women with severe dysmenorrhea caused by endometriosis who were treated with laparoscopic conservative surgery: a 1-year prospective randomized double-blind controlled trial. *Am J Obstet Gynecol.* 2003;189:5. [PMID: 12861130]

Zullo F et al. Long-term effectiveness of presacral neurectomy for the treatment of severe dysmenorrhea due to endometriosis. *J Am Assoc Gynecol Laparosc.* 2004;11:23. [PMID: 15104826]

Endometriosis Association http://www.endometriosisassn.org/

MedlinePlus: A service of the United States Library of Medicine and the National Institutes of Health http://www.nlm.nih.gov/medlineplus/endometriosis.html

IRRITABLE BOWEL SYNDROME

Pathogenesis

IBS is one of the most common disorders associated with CPP in women. Symptoms suggestive of IBS are present in 50 to 80% of women with CPP. Approximately 25 to 50% of all referrals to gastroenterologists are related to this diagnosis. In most Western countries, IBS is three times more common in women than in men.

IBS is a functional disorder, which means that, by definition, no structural or biochemical abnormalities are present that explain the symptoms. It is one of several functional digestive disorders. The pathophysiologic

mechanisms that cause IBS are not completely understood and likely are multifactorial. One alteration that may account for some symptoms of IBS is increased visceral sensitivity; patients with IBS have abnormal pain levels with intestinal distention.

Clinical Findings

IBS is defined by the presence of abdominal pain associated with bowel movements and changes of bowel function in the absence of other pathologies to explain the symptoms. The ROME II criteria are generally accepted as the clinical definition of this syndrome (Table 17–7).

A detailed history must be obtained about bowel function and the association with pain to discern whether the ROME II criteria are met and whether other diagnoses are likely. Abdominal pain must be present to have IBS. Pain is most often in the left lower quadrant but may be located in the middle or right lower abdomen as well. Many patients have two or more sites of pain. Eating commonly precipitates pain and defecation often relieves it. A complete history includes questions about anorexia, early satiety, nausea, vomiting, number of bowel movements per day, number of bowel movements per week, urgency to defecate, prolonged evacuation attempts, straining to defecate, stool color, weight loss without dieting, and increase of symptoms with sex or menses. A detailed dietary history is also important, particularly related to

Table 17–7. ROME II Criteria for Irritable Bowel Syndrome.

- At least 12 weeks, which need not be consecutive, in the preceding 12 months of abdominal discomfort or pain that has two of the following three features:

  - Relieved with defecation
  - Onset associated with a change in frequency of stool
  - Onset associated with a change in form (appearance) of stool

- Symptoms that support diagnosis:

  - < 3 bowel movements/week
  - > 3 bowel movements/day
  - Hard or lumpy stools
  - Loose or watery stools
  - Straining during a bowel movement
  - Urgency
  - Feeling of incomplete bowel movement
  - Passing mucus
  - Abdominal fullness, bloating, or swelling

lactose, sucrose, fructose, caffeinated products, and gas-producing foods.

A detailed medication history, including all current and past medications, both prescribed and over-the-counter, is necessary. Many medications alter bowel motility and may exacerbate symptoms of IBS. In particular, many patients take laxatives and do not realize that laxatives contribute to their symptoms. Antacids containing magnesium or aluminum can cause diarrhea or constipation, respectively.

Travel history, particularly overseas, is often important in the differential diagnostic evaluation of symptoms suggesting IBS. In addition, family history of gastrointestinal diseases, especially inflammatory bowel disease; colon cancer; or malabsorption states, such as sprue, is important in the differential diagnostic evaluation.

A history of rectal bleeding suggests a diagnosis other than IBS unless the bleeding is related to hemorrhoids or a fissure from straining. Similarly, a history of weight loss suggests the diagnosis is not IBS. Weight loss is unusual in a patient with IBS unless there is concomitant depression.

The symptoms of IBS are chronic, although variable in severity. Pain and bowel symptoms that are of a steadily progressive nature suggest a diagnosis other than IBS. Also, as a chronic disorder, IBS usually has an onset of symptoms that is gradual and vague, and it is unusual for the patient to be able to relate an exact date of onset of symptoms. If so, it is likely that she does not have IBS.

Either diarrhea or constipation, or alternating episodes of both, may be present. It is helpful to ask the patient to describe her bowel movements precisely. In particular, many patients complain of constipation if they do not have a bowel movement daily and do not realize that normal stool frequency is anywhere from 3 times a day to every 3 days. In patients with IBS and diarrhea, the volume of diarrhea is small (< 200 mL/d). Diarrheic stool volumes greater than 200 mL/d suggest the diagnosis is not IBS.

Characteristically, both pain and diarrhea resolve during sleep. Also, diarrhea associated with IBS usually resolves during a 24-hour fast. Awakening and noting pain is not the same as being awakened by pain, and it is important to try to have the patient make this distinction if possible.

IBS symptoms are often exacerbated during menses, so direct questions should be asked about a cyclic pattern corresponding with menses, but this correlation should not be assumed to mean the pain is of gynecologic origin. Even in women without IBS there is an increased occurrence of diarrhea, constipation, and increased gas at menses. Women with IBS also have an increased frequency of dyspareunia, compared with women without IBS.

The general physical examination is usually normal. Abdominal examination may reveal mild to moderate distention and mild to moderate tenderness, especially in the left lower quadrant. Rebound tenderness is not a common finding. Rectal and pelvic examinations are important to assess for masses or anal disease, such as hemorrhoids or fissures that could explain some of the symptoms.

In the patient with suspected IBS, a complete blood cell count with differential, chemistry profile, and sedimentation rate are suggested. With IBS, the chemistry profile should be normal, whereas in inflammatory bowel disease electrolyte abnormalities are more likely. To rule out infection with *Giardia,* amoeba, and other parasites, three stool specimens should be sent for ova-and-parasite testing.

Also, stool should be checked for occult blood; results should be negative in patients with IBS. Similarly, methylene blue stain of stool to look for white blood cells should be negative with IBS, as the presence of large numbers of white blood cells is diagnostic of inflammation. Stools should be checked for *Clostridium difficile* toxin if there is significant persistent diarrhea.

In women younger than 40 years of age, proctosigmoidoscopy with biopsy should be performed. Although the mucosa may appear grossly normal, biopsy may reveal microscopic or collagenous colitis. In patients older than 40 years of age, a barium enema and flexible sigmoidoscopy or a full colonoscopy may be indicated to rule out neoplasia. The insufflation during an air-contrast barium enema or colonoscopy often reproduces IBS symptoms.

Complications

Women with IBS have a disproportionately high predisposition to undergo hysterectomy. Of women with IBS, 21% of those 18 to 40 years of age have undergone hysterectomies; this is significantly higher than the national average of about 6%.

Clearly, it is important that accurate diagnosis and comprehensive treatment modalities be tried before hysterectomy is performed in women with pelvic pain and symptoms suggestive of IBS. Whether hysterectomy is capable of causing or worsening IBS symptoms is not clear.

Treatment

Dietary treatment is the mainstay of therapy, but most dietary interventions have not been experimentally validated. Elimination of dietary lactose, sorbitol, and fructose is advised. Lactose intolerance can mimic IBS and contribute to IBS symptoms; about 40% of patients with IBS also have lactose intolerance. Sorbitol, which is a common sweetening agent used in "sugar free" and other dietetic foods, may also contribute to symptoms.

Fructose, a major sugar component of fruit and an additive to a variety of processed foods, also can cause significant abdominal distress. Caffeinated products, including coffee, tea, and cola, carbonated products, and gas-producing foods may contribute to bloating. Smoking and chewing gum lead to more swallowed air and may increase gas and bloating. Excessive alcohol consumption may lead to increased rectal urgency.

Medical treatment of IBS is directed to symptomatic relief. Categorizing patients into one of three major sub-classifications can help in selecting medical therapy, depending on which symptoms are predominant:

1. Abdominal pain, gas, and bloating.
2. Constipation.
3. Diarrhea.

Unfortunately, many patients do not fall clearly into one of these three groups; rather, they have overlapping symptoms.

With predominantly abdominal pain, gas, and bloating, an antispasmodic may be useful. The commonly used antispasmodics are dicyclomine, hyoscyamine, atropine-hyoscyamine-phenobarbital-scopolamine formulation, and chlordiazepoxide with methscopolamine. Potential side effects of antispasmodic, anticholinergic medications include urinary retention, xerostomia, and mydriasis. It is helpful to discuss these side effects with the patient before initiating treatment. Because many patients have these symptoms postprandially, the timing of the dosing is crucial. Generally, it is best to give each of these medications 30 minutes before meals. However, if a sublingual preparation is prescribed, then it can be given at the time that the discomfort begins. Gas and bloating symptoms may be decreased by α-D-galactosidase (Beano) or a simethicone preparation. Peppermint oil may decrease abdominal distention and reduce flatulence.

With predominantly constipation, a trial of increased roughage and psyllium is often beneficial. However, many patients have increased gas with increased fiber, and about 15% cannot tolerate fiber therapy. In such cases, a stool softener or osmotic laxative can be tried. Long-term use of stimulant laxatives should be discouraged. The 5-HT$_4$ receptor agonist tegaserod maleate (6 mg PO twice daily) is effective and approved for short-term use in women.

With predominantly diarrhea, loperamide is the most commonly used agent. A particular advantage of loperamide is that it does not cross the blood-brain barrier, unlike other antidiarrheal agents. Tricyclic antidepressants may be another option for diarrhea-predominant patients.

Combining psychological treatment with medical therapies improves the clinical response in patients with IBS. Factors that predict a good response to psychotherapy include predominately diarrhea and pain symptoms, the association of overt psychiatric symptoms, intermittent pain exacerbated by stress, short durations of bowel complaints, and few sites of abdominal pain. Patients with constant abdominal pain do poorly with psychotherapy or hypnotherapy.

Kamm MA et al. Tegaserod for the treatment of chronic constipation: A randomized, double-blind, placebo-controlled multinational study. *Am J Gastroenterol.* 2005;100:362. [PMID: 15667494]

Kellow J et al. An Asia-Pacific, double blind, placebo controlled, randomised study to evaluate the efficacy, safety, and tolerability of tegaserod in patients with irritable bowel syndrome. *Gut.* 2003;52:671. [PMID: 12692051]

Lackner JM et al. Psychological treatments for irritable bowel syndrome: a systematic review and meta-analysis. *J Consult Clin Psychol.* 2004;72:1100. [PMID: 15612856]

Longstreth GF et al. Irritable bowel syndrome and surgery: a multivariable analysis. *Gastroenterology.* 2004;126:1665. [PMID: 15188159]

Novick J et al. A randomized, double-blind, placebo-controlled trial of tegaserod in female patients suffering from irritable bowel syndrome with constipation. *Aliment Pharmacol Ther.* 2002;16:1877. [PMID: 12390096]

Nyhlin H et al. A double-blind, placebo-controlled, randomized study to evaluate the efficacy, safety and tolerability of tegaserod in patients with irritable bowel syndrome. *Scand J Gastroenterol.* 2004;39:119. [PMID: 15000272]

Spiller RC. Irritable bowel syndrome. *Br Med Bull.* 2004;72:15. [PMID: 15767561]

Whitehead WE et al. The usual medical care for irritable bowel syndrome. *Aliment Pharmacol Ther.* 2004;20:1305. [PMID: 15606392]

Williams RE. Recognition and treatment of irritable bowel syndrome among women with chronic pelvic pain. *Am J Obstet Gynecol.* 2005;192:761. [PMID: 15746669]

Ziegenhagen DJ et al. Cisapride treatment of constipation-predominant irritable bowel syndrome is not superior to placebo. *J Gastroenterol Hepatol.* 2004;19:744. [PMID: 15209619]

American Gastroenterological Association http://www.gastro.org

International Foundation for Functional Gastrointestinal Disorders http://www.iffgd.org

Irritable Bowel Syndrome Association http://www.ibsassociation.org/

National Digestive Diseases Information Clearinghouse (NDDIC): A service of the National Institute of Diabetes and Digestive and Kidney Diseases http://digestive.niddk.nih.gov/ddiseases/pubs/ibs/

INTERSTITIAL CYSTITIS/PAINFUL BLADDER SYNDROME

Pathogenesis

Interstitial cystitis/painful bladder syndrome (IC/PBS) is a chronic inflammatory condition of the bladder characterized by CPP associated with bladder dysfunction. The disease appears to be unrelated to menopausal status, occurring both premenopausally and postmenopausally.

The etiology of IC/PBS is unknown. It is possible that more than one etiology and more than one disease are encompassed in the syndrome. Current thinking is that patients with IC/PBS have defects in the glycosaminoglycan layer of the bladder wall. The glycosaminoglycans of the bladder surface are extremely hydrophilic polysaccharides that form a layer of micelles of water on the bladder epithelium. This micellar layer acts as a barrier between the transitional epithelial cells and urine. It is hypothesized that a defect in this layer allows "leaking" of the epithelium, resulting in a dysfunctional epithelium with excessive permeability and exposure of the transitional epithelium and muscularis to noxious substances in the urine.

An autoimmune cause of this leakiness seems possible. Several researchers have demonstrated an increased number of mast cells in the bladder wall of patients with IC/PBS, potentially consistent with an autoimmune process. Detection of antinuclear antibodies and increased excretion of eosinophilic cationic protein in the urine also support an autoimmune mechanism. Other proposed mechanisms include viral infection, toxin exposure, or other inflammatory mediators. However, the failure to culture an organism and the failure of antibiotic therapy to alleviate symptoms argues against a bacterial infectious cause.

The physiologic causes of pain with IC are also not clear. The inflammatory reaction of the bladder wall may, via algesic substances released by this reaction, cause nociceptor stimulation of visceral neural pathways. This neuroinflammation may cause pain as well as urgency and frequency.

Clinical Findings

The definition and diagnostic criteria of IC/PBS are imprecise, but most commonly it is defined clinically by the following triad:

1. Irritative voiding symptoms.
2. Absence of objective evidence of another disease that could cause the symptoms.
3. A characteristic cystoscopic appearance of the bladder (glomerulations).

Dysuria or pain with voiding is not a characteristic symptom, but pain with the urge to void or after voiding is common. The urgency and frequency experienced is so severe that women with IC/PBS often have histories of recurrent treatment for urinary tract infections. This may be why there is typically a history of 3 to 7 years of symptoms before the diagnosis is established. Nocturia, with voiding at least two times per night, is also a characteristic and troublesome symptom. Incontinence is not a characteristic symptom of IC/PBS.

Pain is typically suprapubic and may radiate to the low back or the groin. Pain with intercourse is also common. Pain in the pelvic floor muscles, especially the levator ani, piriformis, and obturators is commonly associated with IC/PBS.

The physical examination in women with IC/PBS is usually normal. Many women may have anterior vaginal wall tenderness under the trigone and suprapubic pelvic tenderness, but this is variable. Tenderness of the pelvic floor muscles may be noted.

In patients with IC/PBS without infection, a urinalysis is generally normal. In the occasional patient with hematuria, urine cytology or cystoscopy is essential. Urine culture should be negative.

Cystoscopy with hydrodistention, with the finding of characteristic petechial, submucosal hemorrhages (termed "glomerulations") is the gold standard diagnostic criteria for IC/PBS, although clearly there are false-positives and false-negatives. Because the bladder needs to be significantly distended, which is painful in women with IC/PBS, general or spinal anesthesia is usually necessary. Occasionally, Hunner ulcer may also be noted, but it is not a consistent finding.

The potassium challenge also may be a useful diagnostic test for IC/PBS. With this test, the bladder is infused with 40 mL of sterile water, and the patient is asked to rate her pain level and sensation of urgency after the water is retained for 3 to 5 minutes. Patients with IC/PBS generally do not have a change of pain level with this volume of sterile water. The water is then drained, and 40 mL of a 400 mEq/L solution of potassium chloride is infused into the bladder. (This solution is easily made by mixing 40 mEq of potassium chloride with sterile water and bringing the volume to 100 mL.) The patient is again asked to rate her symptoms. A positive test is when the patient has a significantly greater increase of pain and urgency with the potassium chloride solution. Patients with radiation cystitis also have positive responses to the potassium challenge test.

Treatment

The treatments approved by the US Food and Drug Administration for IC/PBS are intravesical dimethylsulfoxide and oral pentosan polysulfate sodium. Dimethylsulfoxide is administered intravesically every 1 to 2 weeks for 2 to 3 months. Dimethylsulfoxide treatments result only in remission of disease, not cure. Other intravesical therapies for IC have been less extensively studied and efficacies are not established. Intravesical capsaicin, Bacillus Calmette-Guérin, clorpactin, heparin, and local anesthetics are examples of other medications used as intravesical treatments.

Pentosan polysulfate sodium is a polyanionic analogue of heparin. Reported results of its effectiveness have been mixed, but at least one placebo-controlled, double-blinded study showed a clinically significant response. Other nonsurgical treatments are often used, but evidence of their effectiveness is scant. Cyclosporine, L-arginine, nifedipine, antihistamines, and tricyclic antidepressants are some of the reported treatments.

Based on clinical observations, the mainstay of urologic treatment of IC for more than 50 years has been hydrodistention of the bladder. This procedure can be performed at the time of diagnostic cystoscopy if general or spinal anesthesia is used. It is too painful to be done without anesthesia.

Prognosis

In some patients, IC/PBS is a progressive disease with severe compromise of bladder function and incapacitating loss of bladder capacity. At times, this has led to the need for surgical treatments via augmentation cystoplasty and cystectomy-urethrectomy-continent diversion with a Kock or Indiana pouch.

Bernie JE et al. The intravesical potassium sensitivity test and urodynamics: implications in a large cohort of patients with lower urinary tract symptoms. *J Urol.* 2001;166:158. [PMID: 11435846]

Nordling J. Interstitial cystitis: how should we diagnose it and treat it in 2004? *Curr Opin Urol.* 2004;14:323. [PMID: 15626873]

Parsons CL et al. Gynecologic presentation of interstitial cystitis as detected by intravesical potassium sensitivity. *Obstet Gynecol.* 2001;98:127. [PMID: 11430970]

American Urological Association Foundation, Inc http://www.afud.org

American Urogynecologic Society http://www.augs.org

Interstitial Cystitis Association http://www.ichelp.org

National Kidney and Urologic Diseases Information Clearinghouse (NKUDIC): A service of the National Institute of Diabetes and Digestive and Kidney Diseases kidney.niddk.nih.gov/kudiseases/pubs/interstitialcystitis/

ADENOMYOSIS
Pathogenesis

Adenomyosis is growth of endometrial glands and stroma into the myometrium at least 2 to 3 mm below the endometrial surface. The reported incidence of adenomyosis ranges from 5 to 70%, varying with the scrutiny of histologic evaluation and the patient's symptoms, age, and parity.

Clinical Findings

Symptoms of adenomyosis are menorrhagia and dysmenorrhea, but many women with adenomyosis are asymptomatic. Many women with adenomyosis have tender uteri symmetrically enlarged up to 12 weeks' gestational size. Often, the uterus of a woman with adenomyosis is diffusely boggy to palpation, or it may have a nodular consistency, reminiscent of multiple small intramural fibroids.

Magnetic resonance imaging may be useful for the preoperative diagnosis of adenomyosis. On T_2 weighted images, diffuse adenomyosis distorts normal zonal anatomy of the uterus, causing enlargement of the functional zone, seen as a wide band with low signal intensity adjacent to the endometrium.

Diagnostic hysteroscopy may show small diverticula when there is a connection between the ectopic sites of adenomyosis in the endometrial cavity. In symptomatic patients with a normal appearing endometrial cavity, a hysteroscopic or laparoscopic myometrial biopsy may be helpful.

Treatment

Gonadotropin suppression with GnRH agonists, such as depot leuprolide or goserelin, may relieve symptoms, but they recur when suppression is discontinued. There may be a role for endometrial ablation or resection in some patients with adenomyosis. The principal method of diagnosis and therapy of adenomyosis is still hysterectomy.

Wang PH et al. Treatment of infertile women with adenomyosis with a conservative microsurgical technique and a gonadotropin-releasing hormone agonist. *Fertil Steril.* 2000;73:1061. [PMID: 10785242]

DYSMENORRHEA
Pathogenesis

Dysmenorrhea is severe, cramping pain in the lower abdomen, lower back, and upper thighs during menses. It is termed "primary dysmenorrhea" when it is not a symptom of another disorder. Secondary dysmenorrhea is the term used when dysmenorrhea is a symptom of pelvic pathology. Dysmenorrhea is not only a significant pain problem itself but is frequently a component of CPP.

Primary dysmenorrhea appears to be due principally to prostaglandins, in particular $F_{2\alpha}$ and E_2 released from the endometrium at menses. Both estradiol and progesterone levels influence the synthesis and levels of endometrial $PGF_{2\alpha}$.

Clinical Findings

Primary dysmenorrhea usually begins 6 to 12 months after menarche and coincides with the onset of ovulatory cycles. However, some patients complain of pain from the first cycle. Patients complain of spasmodic or cramping lower abdominal pain that may radiate suprapubically, to the low back, and to the anteromedial aspect of the thighs. The pain may also be described as continuous, dull, and aching. Other symptoms, such as headache, nausea, vomiting, diarrhea, and fatigue, often accompany the menstrual pain. Symptoms typically last 72 hours or less. They may also start 1 or 2 days before the onset of menses. Occasionally, the accompanying vasoconstriction in the acute phase may be so marked that the patient appears to be shocky.

The pelvic examination should be normal in women with primary dysmenorrhea and may be normal or abnormal in women with secondary dysmenorrhea. Sometimes a laparoscopy may have to be performed to rule out pelvic pathology, particularly endometriosis.

Treatment

Successful management of dysmenorrhea can be challenging. A healthy lifestyle (including nutritional supplements) and aerobic exercise (such as walking, swimming, and bicycling) may produce an overall benefit and decrease the impact of dysmenorrhea on the patient's daily activities. For appropriate selection of treatment, it is usually helpful to determine whether dysmenorrhea is primary or secondary.

Oral contraceptives provide significant relief of primary dysmenorrhea and are a good first-line therapy for many young women, especially if contraception is also needed.

Nonsteroidal anti-inflammatory drugs (NSAIDs) have had a pivotal role in treating primary dysmenorrhea. More than 70% of women obtain significant relief with NSAIDs. Unlike oral contraceptives, NSAIDs need to be taken only 2 to 5 days per month and do not suppress the hypothalamic-pituitary-ovarian axis. A trial of up to 3 to 6 months may be needed to demonstrate effective relief of symptoms. If a particular NSAID is ineffective, it is worth trying a different one, since there is significant variability of individual responsiveness to the NSAIDs (see Table 3–1).

Surgical interventions include hysterectomy, presacral neurectomy, uterosacral neurectomy, and cervical dilation but generally should be considered only if medical treatment has failed.

LEIOMYOMATA UTERI

Pathogenesis

A leiomyoma is a benign tumor of smooth muscle; other names are fibroid, fibromyoma, or myoma. Uterine leiomyomas are the most common tumors of the female pelvis and occur in one of four to five women, with the highest incidence in the fifth decade.

Clinical Findings

About 33% of women with uterine leiomyomas experience pain, but it is usually dysmenorrhea. CPP is more likely to be produced by associated pathology (eg, endometriosis or adhesions) than by a uterine fibroid. Occasionally, pressure-type symptoms, either directly from the leiomyoma or from pressure on the bladder or rectum, become severe and present as CPP. The onset of pain in such cases is usually gradual. Ureteral compression from very large myomas can produce hydronephrosis and back pain. Intermittent torsion of a pedunculated leiomyoma can cause sharp pelvic pain.

Leiomyomata can be diagnosed by finding an enlarged, firm, irregularly shaped uterus at the time of pelvic examination. With degeneration, the consistency of the myomas may become softer, or even cystic, to palpation. Rarely, the uterus may be tender. Sometimes, it is difficult to differentiate uterine myomata from an adnexal tumor.

Imaging studies, especially ultrasonography, can usually distinguish uterine from ovarian tumors. It also is valuable to document the number of fibroids, their location, degree of calcification, and rate of growth. Laparoscopy is helpful to discover associated pathology in patients with CPP.

Complications

Abnormal bleeding, including significant menorrhagia, is more common with leiomyomas than is pelvic pain. Such bleeding can at times become life-threatening and mandate intervention.

Treatment

Treatment of CPP associated with uterine fibroids includes expectant management, medical therapy, radiologic embolization, surgical removal or destruction of the myomas, and hysterectomy. Expectant management should include repeat examinations every 6 months to assure there is no rapid growth. NSAIDs can be used to treat dysmenorrhea and iron therapy may be necessary to treat anemia due to abnormal bleeding. GnRH agonists have been effective in reducing the size and symptoms of leiomyoma, but regrowth to pretreatment size occurs within 12 weeks after cessation of treatment. GnRH agonist therapy has been useful to reduce blood loss, treat iron deficiency anemia, and convert an abdominal to a vaginal hysterectomy.

Arterial embolization has been demonstrated to decrease the size of fibroids, but long-term results regarding pain relief are lacking.

Hysterectomy is usually the optimal way to ensure successful treatment with complete removal of all myomas and no recurrences. Myomectomy is an option for those patients wishing to retain their reproductive potential. Other medical and nonmedical therapies, including myolysis and mifepristone, are under investigation.

Prognosis

Uterine leiomyomas are almost always benign and rarely transform into malignancies, so the overall prognosis is good. Treatment improves quality of life.

OVARIAN RETENTION SYNDROME

Pathogenesis

Ovarian retention syndrome, also called residual ovary syndrome, is the presence of pelvic pain or dyspareunia (or both) after deliberate conservation of one or both ovaries at the time of hysterectomy. The reported incidence of ovarian retention syndrome ranges from 0.9% to 4.9%. Proposed mechanisms for pain from retained ovaries include the following:

1. Adhesions interfere with ovarian function and ovulation, leading to multiple cystic, atretic, or hemorrhagic follicles.
2. Adhesions hinder the ovary's ability to cyclically expand because of its encapsulation in dense adhesions.
3. Adhesions undergo distention with ovarian function and follicular development.

Prevention

Removal of the ovaries at the time of hysterectomy prevents ovarian retention syndrome, but obviously this is not clinically appropriate in many patients. Whether adhesion prevention barriers would decrease the likelihood of this syndrome is not known.

Clinical Findings

Patients with ovarian retention syndrome may complain of cyclic or continuous pain that may range from a bothersome ache to recurrent colicky pain to incapacitating cramps. Pain is often localized to the side of the retained ovary. The pain can also radiate to the lower back and into the legs. Deep dyspareunia occurs in at least 20% of patients.

On physical examination, most patients have a tender pelvic mass at the vaginal vault. Imaging studies may confirm the location and cystic status of the ovary or ovaries. Relief of pain with GnRH agonist suppression of ovarian function may confirm the retained ovary or ovaries as a source of pain. Laparoscopy may also be used as a diagnostic test and has the advantage of allowing simultaneous oophorectomy if indicated.

Treatment

Medical treatment with hormonal replacement therapy, continuous medroxyprogesterone, oral contraceptives, or GnRH agonists is often used, but studies confirming efficacy are lacking. Surgical treatment with salpingo-oophorectomy is the most common treatment but can be difficult due to extensive adhesions. Surgery can sometimes be performed laparoscopically but more often has been done by laparotomy due to the likelihood of severe adhesive disease.

Prognosis

Surgical removal of the retained ovary or ovaries has a high success rate, especially if the prior hysterectomy was not done for CPP.

Baxter N et al. The effect of gonadotropin-releasing hormone analogue as first-line management in cyclical pelvic pain. *J Obstet Gynecol.* 2004;24:64. [PMID: 14675984]

Howard FM. The role of laparoscopy as a diagnostic tool in chronic pelvic pain. *Baillieres Best Pract Res Clin Obstet Gynaecol.* 2000;14:467. [PMID: 10962637]

Mahdavi A et al. Laparoscopic management of ovarian remnant. *Obstet Gynecol Clin North Am.* 2004;31:593. [PMID: 15450320]

OVARIAN REMNANT SYNDROME

Pathogenesis

Ovarian remnant syndrome is the persistence of functional ovarian tissue inadvertently not removed at the time of intended extirpation of one or both ovaries, with or without hysterectomy. The incidence of ovarian remnant syndrome is not known, but it is probably more common than has previously been appreciated. The major predisposing factor to ovarian remnant syndrome is a difficult oophorectomy, usually due to adhesive disease, difficulty in hemostasis, or alteration of normal anatomy. It has been shown experimentally that incompletely excised, devascularized ovarian tissue can reimplant and function.

Prevention

Ensuring complete removal of all ovarian tissue at the time of oophorectomy is essential to prevent ovarian remnant syndrome. However, this may not always be achievable in particularly difficult cases.

Clinical Findings

Ovarian remnant syndrome should be considered in any woman with pelvic pain after hysterectomy and bilateral salpingo-oophorectomy. Too often, clinicians assume that it is impossible for these women to have a gynecologic disease. Ovarian remnant syndrome should also be considered in any woman with ipsilateral pelvic pain after a unilateral oophorectomy.

It usually presents as chronic pain of varying quality and severity in the abdominopelvic area, with or without a palpable pelvic mass. The absence of hot flushes in a woman not receiving hormonal replacement following bilateral oophorectomy should be a signal to investigate carefully for ovarian remnant.

Ovarian remnants are often too small to be palpated. Tenderness to palpation by pelvic examination is usually present on the same side as the remnant.

Without hormonal replacement therapy, women with ovarian remnant syndrome frequently have serum follicle stimulating hormone and estradiol concentrations at premenopausal levels. The diagnosis can also be confirmed using GnRH agonist stimulation. During the first week of administration, continuous GnRH agonist administration initially stimulates estrogen production. Thus, estradiol levels increase significantly 1 week after administration of a GnRH agonist, such as depot leuprolide, from their baseline levels in women with ovarian remnant syndrome.

Vaginal ultrasound shows a pelvic mass in 50 to 85% of cases. The diagnostic accuracy of ultrasound may be improved by stimulating follicular cyst formation with a 5- to 10-day course of clomiphene citrate.

Treatment

Ovarian remnant syndrome is most effectively diagnosed and treated surgically. Surgical extirpation is often difficult and complex, however, and has a postoperative recurrence rate of 8 to 15%. Alternatives include medical treatment via hormonal suppression of ovarian function and radioablative therapy. Sonographically directed aspiration of cysts has also been suggested.

Prognosis

Malignancies have rarely been reported in ovarian remnant syndrome.

Fleischer AC et al. Sonographic features of ovarian remnants. *J Ultrasound Med.* 1998;17:551. [PMID: 9733172]

Kaminski PF et al. Clomiphene citrate stimulation as an adjunct in locating ovarian tissue in ovarian remnant syndrome. *Obstet Gynecol.* 1990;76(5 Pt 2):924. [PMID: 2216258]

Narayansingh G et al. Ovarian cancer developing in the ovarian remnant syndrome. A case report and literature review. *Aust N Z J Obstet Gynaecol.* 2000;40:221. [PMID: 10925917]

Scott RT et al. Use of the GnRH agonist stimulation test in the diagnosis of ovarian remnant syndrome. A report of three cases. *J Reprod Med.* 1995;40:143. [PMID:7738926]

Vavilis D et al. Ovarian remnant syndrome: a case report and review of the literature. *Clin Exp Obstet Gynecol.* 2000;27:121. [PMID: 10968351]

PELVIC CONGESTION SYNDROME

Pathogenesis

Pelvic congestion syndrome is characterized by pelvic pain and dyspareunia associated with pelvic varicosities and pelvic venous congestion or stasis.

Clinical Findings

Women with pelvic congestion tend to have dull, aching, constant pain with premenstrual exacerbation. They also have episodes of severe, acute pelvic pain. The location of their pain tends to change or move, in contrast to the more consistent location of pain in women with CPP and other pelvic diseases. Women with pelvic congestion syndrome experience exacerbation of pain by walking, standing, lifting, bending, and stress. Deep dyspareunia and postcoital aching occurs in more than 50% of cases.

Deep abdominal palpation at the **ovarian point,** which lies at the junction of the upper and middle third of a line drawn from the anterior superior iliac spine to the umbilicus (Figure 17–3), reproduces the pelvic pain complained of by the patient. On pelvic examination, patients with pelvic congestion usually have bilateral ovarian tenderness.

Pelvic venography is performed to confirm the presence of pelvic varicosities and venous stasis and congestion. The two most common techniques used are selective retrograde ovarian venography and transuterine venography.

Treatment

Medical treatment with medroxyprogesterone acetate, 20 to 40 mg orally per day, or with GnRH agonists, such as goserelin at 3.6 mg subcutaneously implanted every 28 days, has been shown to significantly decrease pain. Adding psychotherapy to medical treatment may improve the clinical outcome. Radiologic transcatheter embolization of the ovarian or internal iliac veins has shown efficacy in observational studies.

Surgical treatment with hysterectomy and bilateral salpingo-oophorectomy has shown efficacy in women with venographically documented pelvic congestion syndrome who have not obtained long-term relief with medical therapy. Since most women with pelvic congestion syndrome are young, the benefits of extirpative surgery must be carefully weighed against the drawbacks of loss of fertility and the necessity of long-term hormone

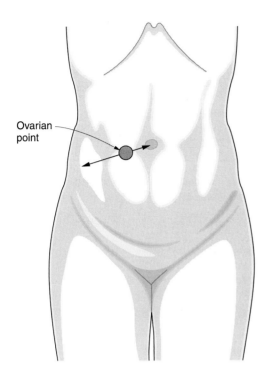

Figure 17–3. Location of the "ovarian point" a characteristic finding in pelvic congestion syndrome.

replacement therapies. Also, the use of objective diagnostic criteria is crucial.

Soysal ME et al. A randomized controlled trial of goserelin and medroxyprogesterone acetate in the treatment of pelvic congestion. *Hum Reprod.* 2001;16:931. [PMID: 11331640]

Venbrux AC et al. Pelvic congestion syndrome (pelvic venous incompetence): impact of ovarian and internal iliac vein embolotherapy on menstrual cycle and chronic pelvic pain. *J Vasc Interv Radiol.* 2002;13(2 Pt 1):171. [PMID: 11830623]

PELVIC FLOOR TENSION MYALGIA

Pathogenesis

Pelvic floor tension myalgia pain is caused by or associated with pain and tenderness of the levator ani, coccygeus, obturator, iliopsoas, or piriformis muscles or their associated fascia or insertions; pain is most often associated with the levator ani muscles. The pelvic floor muscles are major components of the musculoskeletal system of the pelvis and are frequently a source of CPP. The pain is often assumed to be analogous mechanistically to tension headaches. Many names (coccygodynia, pelvic floor myalgia, piriformis syndrome, levator ani spasm syndrome, and diaphragma pelvis spastica) have been used for pelvic floor pain, but it is not clear whether these multiple names contribute to further understanding of this syndrome.

Prevention

Abnormalities of posture are major contributors to the etiology of pelvic floor muscle pain. A marked kyphosis-lordosis, termed "typical pelvic pain posture," has been noted in most women with CPP. Occasionally, the abnormal posture is just a marked lordosis. Correct posture may prevent pelvic floor tension myalgia in some cases.

Clinical Findings

Most women with pelvic floor tension myalgia have been treated for numerous other problems, such as endometriosis, pelvic inflammatory disease, low back pain, lumbar disc disease, or degenerative joint disease, prior to the diagnosis of pelvic floor tension myalgia. Symptoms are usually vague and poorly localized. Pain may be diffuse within the pelvis, more localized about the rectum or the anterior pelvis, or unilateral. Low back pain and radiation to the sacrum at the area of insertion of the levator ani is not uncommon (>80% of patients). Radiation to the hip and down the back of the thigh, like sciatica, may also be noted and is particularly characteristic of piriformis spasm. Pain is most often described as aching, throbbing, or heaviness. Similar to patients with pelvic relaxation disorders, patients may describe the sensation as "everything falling out or dropping." Pain may be quite severe, and in some patients, has a characteristic of acute attacks that awaken the patient from sleep with rectal pain ("proctalgia fugax") or vaginal pain ("colpalgia fugax"). Characteristically, pain from spasm of the levator ani starts in the afternoon and becomes progressively worse. Pain is increased by prolonged sitting or standing in one position. The pain is not usually worsened by bowel movements. However, dyspareunia is a common symptom.

The most common physical finding with pelvic floor tension myalgia is tenderness and spasm of one or more of the levator ani muscles. Digital pressure on the involved muscle typically reproduces or intensifies the patient's pain. It is not unusual for the tenderness to be unilateral. In some patients with pelvic floor tension myalgia, there is also tenderness of the coccyx, lateral sacrum, or sacrococcygeal ligaments.

The diagnosis of pelvic floor tension myalgia is by clinical history and physical findings. No imaging or laboratory evaluations are useful in establishing the diagnosis. However, as pelvic floor tension myalgia may frequently occur secondary to other pelvic pathology, evaluations may be needed to rule out diagnoses such as endometriosis or adhesions. This is especially true if pelvic floor tension myalgia does not respond to appropriate physical therapy and medical treatment.

Treatment

The classic treatment for pelvic floor tension myalgia involves massaging the tender muscles with a firm sweeping motion. At each treatment session, 15 to 20 strokes are done, taking about 5 minutes. Treatments are repeated daily for 4 to 5 days, then every other day until improvement. About six sessions are usually needed. The initial sessions are usually quite uncomfortable, and most patients note an exacerbation of pain after the first one or two treatments. Many women find it less unpleasant if the technique is modified to transvaginal massage rather than transrectal.

Hot sitz baths may also be helpful. Vaginal and rectal diathermy, ultrasound, bed rest, relaxation exercises, biofeedback training, analgesics, skeletal muscle relaxants, Kegel exercises, transcutaneous electrical nerve stimulation, acupuncture, vaginal electrical stimulation, and infiltration with corticosteroid or local anesthetic (especially if trigger points are present) are all treatments for pelvic floor tension myalgia. There are no well-performed studies that allow a recommendation of any specific treatment modality or combination at this time. Coccygectomy is sometimes done for this syndrome but probably has little, if any, role in the modern management of the problem.

Tu FF et al. Musculoskeletal causes of chronic pelvic pain: a systematic review of diagnosis: part I. *Obstet Gynecol Surv.* 2005;60:379. [PMID: 15920438]

Chest Pain

18

Brad Stuart, MD

 ESSENTIALS OF DIAGNOSIS

- *Pain may be caused by cardiac, pulmonary, or gastrointestinal disease.*
- *Pain that results from cardiac disease may be due to stable angina pectoris, unstable angina, acute myocardial infarction, or aortic dissection.*
- *Pulmonary causes of chest pain include pulmonary embolism, pneumothorax, pulmonary hypertension, bacterial pneumonia, and cancer.*
- *Pain resulting from gastrointestinal causes may be due to esophageal rupture, gastroesophageal reflux disease, and abnormal esophageal motility.*

General Considerations

Approximately six million Americans seek medical attention each year complaining of chest pain. Of these cases, only about 40% can be attributed to cardiac, pulmonary, or gastrointestinal disease.

The prevalence of diseases resulting in chest pain varies with the population. For ischemic heart disease, the presence of cardiac risk factors and the age of the patient are important. For example, coronary disease is diagnosed in less than 10% of persons with chest pain who are younger than 35 years of age. However, the incidence of cardiac diagnoses may exceed 50% in persons over 40 years of age.

The first priority in assessing a patient with chest pain is to determine whether the chest pain is due to coronary disease. About 11% of chest pain presentations are due to stable angina pectoris and another 1.5% signal acute coronary syndrome (ACS), consisting of myocardial infarction (MI) or unstable angina pectoris. Despite the best efforts of medical providers, approximately 20,000 patients with chest pain are sent home after ACS has been incorrectly ruled out. These missed diagnoses result in as many as one in five medical malpractice suits in the United States.

Once coronary disease has been excluded, other life-threatening causes of acute chest pain (eg, pulmonary embolus, aortic dissection, esophageal rupture, or tension pneumothorax) must also be considered; then, a specific cause of the pain can usually be identified and treatment begun. A targeted history and physical examination, combined with selected tests such as electrocardiogram (ECG) or chest radiograph, will usually allow the physician to arrive at an accurate diagnosis, avoiding unhelpful terms such as "noncardiac" or "atypical" chest pain. In addition, the clinical evaluation helps estimate the pretest probability of organic causes of chest pain before ordering diagnostic tests. Determining pretest probability helps interpret test results and also avoid unnecessary and expensive procedures.

Pathogenesis

The mechanisms of most causes of chest pain are poorly understood. However, it is understood that angina pectoris results from myocardial oxygen demand exceeding oxygen supply, leading to ischemic episodes.

The neural pathways that transmit chest pain, however, are well defined. Deep retrosternal or precordial pain is not diagnostic of cardiac disease or any other specific disease process; rather, it indicates pain stimuli in a portion of the anatomic regions supplied by the dermatomes T1 to T6. These spinal neuroanatomic levels innervate the thoracic region from the mid-neck to beneath the xiphoid process and also extend down the anteromedial arms and forearms. The thoracic viscera, including the myocardium, pericardium, aorta, pulmonary artery, mediastinum, and esophagus are all supplied by sensory afferent fibers originating from T1 through T4. Lesions in any of these structures tend to produce poorly localized, deep, visceral pain that is felt maximally in the retrosternal region or the precordium. This pain often radiates into the neck, the left or right hemithorax or the anteromedial aspects of one or both arms and forearms.

Sensory fibers from T5 and T6 innervate the lower thoracic wall, the diaphragmatic muscles and their peritoneal surfaces, the gallbladder, the pancreas, the duodenum, and the stomach. Injury to any of these structures causes poorly localized, deep, visceral pain identical in character to that mentioned above but localized to the xiphoid region and the right subscapular area. However, this pain may extend to the T1 T4 dermatomes through posterior sympathetic connections, creating an anatomic pattern of pain indistinguishable from that originating from lesions above the diaphragm.

It has been said that pain from the umbilicus to the mandible is cardiac until proven otherwise. It is more accurate to state that visceral pain in the chest, like visceral pain elsewhere in the body, is not necessarily localized to the area of injury and its character is rarely specific for a particular lesion. However, a careful clinical evaluation and selected tests yield an accurate diagnosis in most cases.

Prevention

Knowledge of risk factors for the various etiologies of chest pain provides important information, both for prevention of underlying disease and regarding disease likelihood, which may help guide the clinical evaluation.

Retrospective studies of patients under 40 years of age with acute MI show that up to 98% of patients had at least one conventional coronary risk factor. Following are some coronary risk factors that increase the likelihood of other diseases causing chest pain:

1. The risk of myocardial ischemia is increased in the presence of hyperlipidemia, left ventricular hypertrophy, or a family history of premature coronary disease.
2. The presence of hypertension increases risks for both coronary disease and aortic dissection.
3. Cigarette smoking is a nonspecific risk factor associated with coronary disease, deep venous thrombosis and pulmonary embolism, aortic dissection, pneumothorax, and bacterial pneumonia.
4. A history of cocaine use (within the last 60 minutes) may increase the likelihood of MI.
5. A history of recent viral infection may indicate pericarditis or myocarditis.

Following are clinically identifiable risk factors for the development of venous thrombosis and pulmonary embolism:

1. Recent history of immobilization
2. History of surgery within 3 months
3. Stroke
4. Prior history of venous thromboembolism
5. Current malignancy

Clinical Findings

Clinicians must maintain diagnostic objectivity while evaluating a patient with chest pain. Studies have shown that patients were less likely to receive a cardiac workup if the physician viewed a histrionic portrayal of symptoms.

Furthermore, data suggest that women are not referred as often as men for appropriate diagnostic and therapeutic procedures for coronary disease, although this difference may be explained largely by the greater number of comorbidities in women with ACS, resulting in a greater burden of procedural complications related to coronary reperfusion.

A. HISTORY

1. Patient age—Acute, severe chest pain in men older than 60 years of age may be due to aortic dissection, whereas in younger men it may indicate spontaneous pneumothorax. A diagnosis of viral pleurisy is more common in younger adults of either sex.

2. Past history—Chest pain frequently recurs in such illnesses as peptic ulcer disease, gastroesophageal reflux, myocardial ischemia, cholecystitis and cholelithiasis that have not been treated surgically, cancer, and panic disorder. A diagnosis may be suggested if present pain is similar to that experienced in past exacerbations. A history of diabetes should raise the suspicion of an atypical presentation of myocardial ischemia. Recent blunt trauma to the chest may cause chest wall injury, pneumothorax, pulmonary or myocardial contusion, or a tear in the aorta, esophagus, or bronchus.

3. Description of chest pain

a. Quality—Patients with myocardial ischemia rarely complain of pain. Rather, they use such descriptors as squeezing, pressure, tightness, aching, constriction, burning, fullness, band-like sensation, lump in the throat, heavy weight ("elephant sitting on chest"), or toothache-like pain (with radiation to the mandible). In some cases, the patient places a closed fist over the sternum (the Levine sign). The quality of pain tends to be replicated in the same patient with repeated events of coronary ischemia. Coronary disease cannot be completely excluded in patients who describe the pain as sharp or stabbing, even though such qualities are not characteristic of myocardial ischemia.

The pain is less likely to be ischemic if it has a positional component, is reproducible by palpation, and if the patient has no history of angina or MI. The chest pain of myocarditis can be pleuritic in nature, but it can also be similar to pain typical of myocardial ischemia.

b. Location—Ischemic pain is often diffuse and may be difficult or impossible to localize. Pain that is localized to a small area on the chest (particularly when the patient can point to it with a finger) is more likely due to a lesion of the chest wall or pleura.

Pain due to myocardial ischemia may radiate to the lower jaw, teeth, neck, throat, upper extremity, or shoulder on either side. The pain of MI may radiate to many of these areas at once, and particularly to the right arm.

Radiation to both arms may be an even stronger indicator of acute MI.

Acute cholecystitis can cause pain in the right shoulder, although concurrent pain in the epigastrium or right upper quadrant is more common than chest discomfort. The pain of aortic dissection often radiates between the scapulae.

c. Time course—Temporal elements may be used to help distinguish between different causes of chest pain.

Myocardial ischemia is most often gradual in onset, and its intensity increases over time. Esophageal disease may also exhibit a crescendo pattern. On the other hand, aortic dissection and pneumothorax usually cause pain of abrupt onset that is immediately of maximal intensity. Musculoskeletal chest pain is often insidious in onset, sometimes taking hours or days to reach a peak.

The duration of pain may differ by etiology as well. Chest discomfort that lasts only for a few seconds or that is constant over days to weeks is almost certainly not secondary to myocardial ischemia. Pain that is unchanging over years is most likely functional. Chest discomfort due to myocardial ischemia generally lasts for minutes; it may be more prolonged when due to an MI. Myocardial ischemia, as well as MI, may demonstrate a circadian pattern, occurring more frequently from 6 A.M. to noon then later in the day due to changes in sympathetic tone.

d. Provoking factors—Pain on swallowing suggests an esophageal origin. Chest discomfort that occurs every time a patient eats is suggestive of upper gastrointestinal disease. However, it can also be seen in cases of severe coronary obstruction (eg, left main or three-vessel disease). Exertional chest pain is classic for angina, although occasionally esophageal spasm can present in a similar way. Myocardial ischemia can also be precipitated by exposure to cold, emotional stress, or sexual intercourse. Musculoskeletal chest pain can be exacerbated by movement or by adopting certain body positions, as well as by deep breathing. True pleuritic chest pain is worsened by inspiration and often by lying down; causes may be pulmonary embolism and infarction, pneumothorax, pleurisy, pneumonia, or pericarditis.

e. Relieving factors—Chest pain that is reliably palliated by eating food is probably caused by upper gastrointestinal disease. Neither nitroglycerin nor "GI cocktails" (eg, antacid plus a viscous lidocaine) reliably distinguish the pain of myocardial ischemia from noncardiac pain. However, chest pain that is relieved by physical rest strongly suggests a cardiac etiology.

f. Severity—The magnitude of the patient's pain does not reliably discriminate between cardiac and noncardiac pain. However, in the setting of confirmed coronary disease, the pain of MI may be more severe than the pain of stable or unstable angina.

B. Symptoms and Signs

Cardiac and gastrointestinal causes of chest pain may coexist in up to one-third of patients with chest pain. Associated symptoms may not reliably distinguish between these etiologies. Painful swallowing, belching, or a bad taste in the mouth are suggestive of esophageal disease, although these symptoms may occur in patients with myocardial ischemia as well. Similarly, vomiting may occur secondary to myocardial ischemia or upper gastrointestinal problems such as peptic ulcer disease, cholecystitis, acute pancreatitis, and also diabetic ketoacidosis, which in turn may be triggered by acute MI.

Other associated symptoms, such as diaphoresis, may occur more often in the setting of myocardial ischemia and may suggest that diagnosis. Dyspnea on exertion may precede chest pain due to myocardial ischemia and may also be seen in heart failure. Dyspnea concurrent with chest pain may occur in myocardial ischemia or such pulmonary disorders as pneumonia or pulmonary embolus. Presyncope may be seen in myocardial ischemia, but may also accompany aortic dissection, pulmonary embolus or critical aortic stenosis. Exertional dyspnea is common in aortic stenosis as well. Palpitations may occur with myocardial ischemia secondary to ventricular ectopy, although some patients may have a hypersensitive awareness of their own normal sinus rhythm. New-onset atrial fibrillation is uncommon in acute MI but is seen frequently in chronic coronary disease. Pulmonary embolism may cause chest pain and palpitations due to new atrial fibrillation as well. Cough is a nonspecific symptom that may be due to heart failure, lung cancer, pulmonary embolus, pneumonia, or occasionally gastroesophageal reflux disease. Severe fatigue may be a presenting symptom of MI in elderly patients.

C. Physical Examination

1. General appearance—Clinicians must be alert for signs of circulatory compromise, including pallor and diaphoresis; these are associated with high early mortality. Although panic disorder may be present in up to one-third of patients with chest pain without coronary ischemia, it may also coexist with coronary disease. In some patients, their level of alarm can be a more accurate reflection of the seriousness of their disease than is the severity of their symptoms.

2. Vital signs—Systolic blood pressure below 90 mm Hg, especially in conjunction with physical signs of circulatory compromise, indicate a need for emergent care. An elevation in heart rate and blood pressure may be seen in coronary ischemia secondary to sympathetic activation, but this is nonspecific. A marked difference in blood pressure between the two arms may suggest aortic dissection. A check for postural changes in heart rate and blood pressure is warranted, particularly in elderly patients with presyncope who may be volume depleted.

3. Chest wall palpation—Chest wall tenderness that exactly replicates the patient's pain is extremely suggestive of noncardiac disease, although occasionally chest wall tenderness may be present together with myocardial ischemia. Hyperesthesia in a dermatomal distribution, particularly when associated with a vesicular or patchy erythematous rash, may be due to herpes zoster.

4. Cardiac examination—Auscultation in sitting and supine positions can detect murmurs of acute aortic stenosis or insufficiency as well as the pericardial friction rub of acute pericarditis. A mitral insufficiency murmur due to papillary muscle dysfunction or an S_3 or S_4 gallop may be caused by myocardial ischemia. Palpation at the apex may also detect an abnormal left ventricular heave, which is sometimes felt during ischemic episodes due to an area of dyskinesis secondary to occlusion of the left anterior descending coronary artery.

5. Lung examination—Asymmetric or absent lung sounds may indicate pneumothorax. Basilar rales may be heard in cases of myocardial ischemia that is severe enough to raise end-diastolic pressure. Evidence of consolidation may indicate pneumonia or cancer; dullness at one of the lung bases may be seen with pleural effusion.

6. Abdominal examination—Tenderness in the epigastrium may be consistent with peptic ulcer disease or pancreatitis, whereas right upper quadrant tenderness may indicate cholecystitis. A pulsatile epigastric mass may be an extension of a thoracic aortic aneurysm presenting with chest pain.

D. Imaging Studies and Special Tests

Ancillary studies including chest radiography and electrocardiography may provide further information supporting or disproving initial diagnostic hypotheses as well as reducing the chance of missing serious etiologies of chest pain. Additional studies—including but not limited to exercise electrocardiography, myocardial perfusion scanning, echocardiographic stress testing, diagnostic acid suppression, ventilation-perfusion lung scanning, or chest computed tomography (CT)—may sometimes be required to narrow diagnostic possibilities.

1. Chest radiography—A chest radiograph aids in the diagnosis of chest pain due to cardiac or pulmonary causes, cancer, pneumothorax, or pneumomediastinum. The chest film may also be abnormal in aortic dissection, but other studies will usually be necessary for a definitive diagnosis. Up to one-quarter of chest radiographs done on patients with chest pain in an emergency setting yield information that influences therapy.

2. Electrocardiography—A 12-lead ECG provides critical information about the presence or absence of my-

ocardial ischemia. A normal ECG significantly reduces the probability that chest pain is due to acute MI. However, up to one-third of patients with unstable angina have a normal ECG, and up to 4% of patients with normal ECGs will have had an acute MI. On the other hand, an abnormal ECG with specific findings (eg, ST-segment elevation, ST-segment depression or new Q waves) is not only compatible with ACS (acute MI or unstable angina) but also is correlated with the need for invasive therapy, a complicated hospital course, or death. Nonspecific ST-T wave abnormalities are commonly seen and may indicate heart disease; more than two-thirds are associated with noncoronary diagnoses.

Chun AA et al. Bedside diagnosis of coronary artery disease: a systematic review. *Am J Med.* 2004;117:334. [PMID: 15336583]

Eslick GD. Usefulness of chest pain character and location as diagnostic indicators of an acute coronary syndrome. *Am J Cardiol.* 2005;95:1228. [PMID: 15877997]

Fox KF. Investigation and management of chest pain. *Heart.* 2005;91:105. [PMID: 15604354]

Freeston J et al. Can early diagnosis and management of costochondritis reduce acute chest pain admissions? *J Rheumatol.* 2004;31:2269. [PMID: 15517642]

Differential Diagnosis

In evaluating the patient with chest pain, the clinician must first exclude life-threatening diagnoses and then provide emergent care if indicated. Once this has been accomplished, the next step is to establish a reasonable diagnosis that explains the patient's complaints. The list of potential diagnoses presented below appear in approximate order of prevalence seen in primary care practice, except that life-threatening diagnoses are discussed first. Table 18–1 summarizes the major causes of chest pain.

A. Cardiac Causes

1. Coronary heart disease—The first step in the evaluation of any patient with chest pain is to exclude coronary ischemia as the cause. Chest pain due to myocardial ischemia secondary to varying degrees of coronary artery obstruction includes a continuum of diagnoses including transmural MI, non–Q wave infarction, unstable angina pectoris, and stable angina. A careful history and physical examination accompanied by an ECG at rest furnishes a clinical diagnosis with 90% predictive accuracy for the presence of coronary disease. Other tests are rarely necessary to establish a working diagnosis of acute myocardial ischemia. However, up to 8% of cases of myocardial ischemia will be missed when clinical and ECG data alone are used to establish the diagnosis. If patients are discharged without treatment, the annual mortality rate is 6 to 8%. These patients tend to be women under the age

Table 18–1. Major Causes of Chest Pain.

Cause	Key pain characteristics	Key history elements	Key physical findings	Diagnostic tests
Coronary heart disease	Diffuse, dull substernal heaviness, pressure Gradual in onset Occurs with exertion, relieved by nitroglycerin (except with infarction) Radiates to arms, neck, or jaw Duration 2–20 min; longer with infarction	Coronary risk factors Associated dyspnea, nausea, diaphoresis Atypical (non-pain) symptoms in women, elderly, diabetics	Nonspecific	Rest ECG Serial cardiac enzymes: troponin T & I, CK-MB, myoglobin
Aortic dissection	Catastrophic onset Sharp, ripping, tearing Migratory	Male, age 60–80 years Hypertension Syncope Shock Symptoms of coronary, gut ischemia	Unequal pulses or blood pressure in upper extremities Aortic insufficiency murmur Pulsatile epigastric mass Neurologic findings	Chest radiograph ECG (negative unless coronary ostia involved) Chest CT or MRI scan Transesophageal echocardiography
Aortic stenosis	Similar to myocardial ischemia	Dyspnea Syncope	Systolic murmur	Echocardiography
Acute pericarditis	Anterior, sharp, worse on inspiration	Viral illness AIDS	Pericardial friction rub	ECG: diffuse ST elevation
Myocarditis	Variable	Viral illness	Heart failure in severe cases	Echocardiography
Syndrome X	Similar to myocardial ischemia	Premenopausal female Panic attacks Rheumatologic disease	Nonspecific	Exercise ECG: ST depression Coronary angiogram: normal
Pulmonary embolus	Sharp, worse on inspiration	Immobilization Recent surgery Cancer Dyspnea, hemoptysis	Tachypnea Rales Tachycardia	Ventilation-perfusion lung scan Lower-extremity venous ultrasound D-dimer Helical CT scan Pulmonary angiography
Pneumothorax	Sharp, worse on inspiration	Young male smoker COPD *Pneumocystis* pneumonia Respiratory distress	Unilateral loss of breath sounds Hypertympany Jugulovenous distention	Chest radiograph: tracheal shift

(*Continued*)

Table 18–1. Major Causes of Chest Pain. (*Continued*)

Cause	Key pain characteristics	Key history elements	Key physical findings	Diagnostic tests
Pulmonary hypertension	Exertional	COPD Dyspnea Syncope Peripheral edema	Right heart failure in advanced cases	Chest radiograph: "pruning" of pulmonary vasculature
Bacterial pneumonia	Sharp, worse on inspiration	Fever, chills Cough	Rales	Chest radiograph
Lung cancer	Variable Neuropathic	Cough Dyspnea Hemoptysis Weight loss	Nonspecific	Depends on presentation
Sarcoidosis	Dull	Cough Dyspnea	Nonspecific	Chest radiograph ECG
Pleuritis	Sharp, worse on inspiration	Rheumatic disease Procainamide Hydralazine Isoniazid	Nonspecific	Chest radiograph: Rule out pneumonia
Esophageal rupture (Boerhaave syndrome)	Sudden, excruciating	Lye ingestion Esophageal dilatation	Tachypnea Fever	Chest radiograph: mediastinal gas
Gastroesophageal reflux	Heartburn Similar to myocardial ischemia Nonradiating	Postprandial Regurgitation of stomach acid, especially nocturnal Relieved by antacids	Nonspecific	Acid suppression Ambulatory pH monitoring
Esophageal hypersensitivity	Similar to myocardial ischemia Rarely exertional	Nonspecific	Nonspecific	Esophageal manometry
Esophageal spasm, achalasia	Similar to myocardial ischemia	Dysphagia	Nonspecific	Esophageal manometry
Pill esophagitis	Odynophagia	Doxycycline ASA, NSAIDs KCl $FeSO_4$	Nonspecific	Endoscopy
Musculoskeletal	Slow, insidious onset Lasts hours to days Worse with movement	Rheumatic disease CABG Fibromyalgia	Chest wall tenderness	Depends on presentation
Psychogenic	Nonspecific	Panic disorder Hyperventilation Münchausen syndrome	Nonspecific	Depends on presentation

ECG, electrocardiogram; CK-MB, creatine kinase MB band; CT, computed tomography; MRI, magnetic resonance imaging; COPD, chronic obstructive pulmonary disease; ASA, aspirin; NSAIDs, nonsteroidal anti-inflammatory drugs; CABG, coronary artery bypass grafting.

of 55, nonwhite, reporting dyspnea as the primary symptom, and with a normal or nondiagnostic ECG.

The classic presentation of pain caused by coronary disease, most frequently seen in middle-aged men with risk factors for atherosclerosis, includes complaints of chest heaviness, pressure, tightness, and burning; patients often deny having pain and may have difficulty describing their discomfort. Typical anginal pain has a gradual onset, usually over several minutes, and does not change with respiration or position. It is diffuse, difficult to localize, and often radiates to other parts of the body, including the lower jaw and teeth (not the upper jaw), neck and throat, shoulders, inner aspects of upper arms and forearms, wrists, fingers, epigastric area, and occasionally to the interscapular region of the back. Ischemic pain almost always lasts more than 2 but less than 20 minutes, unless an MI is in progress, in which case the pain may last longer. Associated symptoms include dyspnea, nausea and vomiting, diaphoresis, lightheadedness, or palpitations.

Up to one-third of patients, especially women over 65 years of age who are obese as well as diabetics and the elderly, may not have chest pain but rather complain of such atypical symptoms as abdominal pain (in 33%), paroxysmal dyspnea (in over 15%), shortness of breath as a primary symptom, or fatigue. Patients with variant angina due to coronary vasospasm may have classic anginal pain precipitated by hyperventilation and occasionally by exercise. These patients are usually younger than 60 years of age and do not necessarily have classic cardiovascular risk factors. The rest ECG in these cases often shows transient ST-segment elevation. Life-threatening arrhythmias may occur.

Among patients considered to have acute coronary ischemia, several aspects of the primary presentation suggest the possibility of unstable angina or MI:

1. Typical anginal pain at rest, more than 20 minutes in duration.
2. New onset of typical anginal pain, severe enough to limit physical activity.
3. Typical anginal pain that is more frequent, longer in duration, or occurs with less exertion than have previous episodes.

Chest pain that is more likely due to nonischemic problems is generally characterized as the following:

1. Sharp or knifelike pain made worse by respiration or cough.
2. Primarily located in the mid- to lower abdomen.
3. Pain that can be localized by pointing one finger.
4. Exactly reproduced by movement or by palpation by the examiner.
5. Constant pain lasting more than 1 day.

6. Fleeting pain that lasts for less than a few seconds.
7. Pain that radiates to the legs or the upper jaw or above.

The clinician should remember that up to 25% of patients with sharp or stabbing pain may have ischemia. Also, patients with noncardiac pain may still have other potentially lethal conditions.

Information gathered from a 10-minute history and physical examination should allow the clinician to place the patient with suspected myocardial ischemia into one of four categories:

1. **Definite acute ischemia:** substernal discomfort caused by physical exertion, with typical radiation to the jaw, shoulder or arm, relieved by rest or nitroglycerin in less than 10 minutes.
2. **Probable acute ischemia:** patient exhibits most of the features of definite ischemia but may not be entirely typical in some aspects.
3. **Probably not acute ischemia:** atypical chest pain that does not fit the description of definite ischemia.
4. **Definitely not acute ischemia:** questionable chest pain history, unrelated to activity, appears to be clearly noncardiac, not relieved by nitroglycerin.

For those patients with **definite** or **probable** acute ischemia, an ECG and sequential cardiac enzymes (troponin T and I, creatine kinase CK-MB, and myoglobin) should be obtained to establish the diagnosis. Other routine measures include using supplemental oxygen, establishing continuous ECG monitoring, obtaining intravenous access, and giving 160–325 mg of aspirin (chewable if possible) as well as sublingual nitroglycerin for pain. Hospital admission should be arranged under the following circumstances:

1. Presence of ST-segment elevation or depression or new Q wave (which may take time to evolve) or left bundle branch block on ECG.
2. If ST elevation is present in two or more leads or if left bundle branch block is new, the patient may be presumed to have suffered an MI and should be admitted to intensive care with consideration for reperfusion therapy if fewer than 12 hours have elapsed from the onset of symptoms.
3. If ST-segment depression is present in two or more contiguous leads, the patient has high-risk ischemia and may be referred for early angiography and revascularization. Thrombolytic therapy should not be administered unless persistent ST-segment elevations appear on subsequent ECGs.
4. Cardiac enzymes are elevated, which does not occur until 4 to 6 hours after the onset of pain and may not become elevated for as long as 12 hours. Although the

sensitivity and negative predictive value at 90 minutes after onset of symptoms for the combination of myoglobin and troponin I are both high, myoglobin is not specific for myocardial necrosis; serum myoglobin levels may be elevated after recent cocaine use and in patients with impaired renal function. Elevated troponin levels, however, are highly specific for myocardial necrosis.

5. Any evidence of hemodynamic instability.

6. Unstable angina without cardiac enzyme elevation is diagnosed clinically. These patients may need urgent cardiac catheterization with possible revascularization.

For patients who have persistent chest pain suggestive of acute myocardial ischemia but who have a nondiagnostic ECG and initially negative cardiac enzymes, rest imaging tests may help with the diagnosis. Acute rest myocardial perfusion imaging may be performed with one of several radiopharmaceutical agents that accumulate in the myocardium in concentrations proportional to blood flow. However, false-positive results may occur in patients with prior infarction, and false-negative results may be seen if chest pain has been resolved for more than 3 hours.

Echocardiography can detect regional left ventricular wall motion abnormalities within seconds of coronary artery occlusion; the sensitivity of this procedure is high but specificity is limited due to the large number of alternative causes of regional wall motion abnormalities. Thus, echocardiography may be used to exclude MI during or immediately after an episode of chest pain but not to diagnose it.

Patients with pain typical of ischemia in whom initial ECG and cardiac enzymes are normal or indeterminate can be monitored for 6–24 hours in a chest pain observation unit or in the emergency department. A repeat ECG and cardiac enzymes in 6 to 12 hours should be obtained; if either or both are positive, the patient should be admitted to the hospital.

Patients with typical anginal pain that resolves, and who are otherwise clinically stable, can undergo stress testing. Exercise testing has been shown to be both safe and predictive of good prognosis in patients who have a negative test result. Exercise ECG testing is not indicated in patients whose pain is probably noncardiac and who also have a nondiagnostic initial evaluation. There is a relatively low incidence of coronary disease in these patients.

The long-term outcome is more favorable for patients who are found not to have had an MI after being admitted for suspected MI than for those patients in whom MI is diagnosed. However, up to 15% of troponin-negative patients experience an adverse cardiac event at 1 year; in large series, 10-year mortality did not differ between the groups.

2. Aortic dissection—Chest pain caused by aortic dissection is often severe, bordering on catastrophic. Early diagnosis and treatment are critical for survival, particularly when hemodynamic compromise is present. Patients tend to be men ranging from 60 to 80 years of age; up to 75% have a prior history of hypertension. Less frequent predisposing factors include bicuspid aortic valve, Marfan or Turner syndrome, coarctation of the aorta, pregnancy, or prior coronary artery bypass surgery. Recently, high-intensity weight lifting and the abuse of crack cocaine have become more commonly associated with aortic dissection.

Pain is sudden in onset, often migratory, and often described as a ripping or tearing sensation. Pain is usually felt in the chest, anteriorly with dissections of the ascending aorta or posteriorly with dissections distal to the takeoff of the left subclavian artery. The pain may radiate anywhere in the thorax or abdomen. Painless dissection is uncommon.

Associated symptoms are usually caused by cerebral, spinal, coronary, or visceral ischemia due to occlusion of arterial branches at the site of dissection or propagation. Syncope heralds a worse prognosis because it is often due to cardiac tamponade from proximal dissection or stroke from occlusion of the subclavian artery. Other ischemic symptoms include neurologic deficits or ischemia of the myocardium, gut, kidneys, or lower extremities. Acute heart failure may occur as a result of aortic insufficiency. Shock, hemothorax, or sudden death may occur if the aorta ruptures into the pericardial or pleural space.

The initial evaluation should include a check of pulses and blood pressures to ensure that they are symmetric bilaterally and in upper and lower extremities. Pulse deficits occur more commonly in proximal dissections but are present in <30% of patients. The examiner should check for a murmur of aortic insufficiency as well as a pulsatile epigastric mass and focal neurologic defects. The chest radiograph may show an abnormal aortic contour; this can also be seen in "unwinding" of the aorta, which is a normal variant often seen in the elderly. The mediastinum may be widened and the trachea displaced laterally. The ECG may be helpful, particularly in cases where chest pain is similar to that usually seen with angina; lack of ECG findings mitigates against myocardial ischemia, unless proximal dissection has compromised coronary arterial blood flow.

Definitive diagnosis is made by CT scan, magnetic resonance imaging (MRI) scan, or transesophageal echocardiography after the patient has been medically stabilized. Transthoracic echocardiography is not indicated because of its inability to visualize the transverse and descending aorta in most patients. Aortography is now performed in <5% of cases. Routine blood tests are nondiagnostic.

3. Valvular heart disease—Abnormalities of the heart valves, including aortic stenosis, mitral stenosis, and mitral valve prolapse, may cause chest pain.

Aortic stenosis may present with anginal pain, dyspnea, and syncope. Cardiovascular examination in cases of critical aortic stenosis may show weakened and delayed peripheral arterial pulses, a sustained cardiac apical impulse, and a pronounced systolic murmur at the left sternal border that often radiates to the carotids. The pressure gradient across the valve as well as left ventricular function may be measured with an echocardiogram. Exercise stress testing may be contraindicated.

Mitral stenosis is an unusual cause of chest pain. The pain may be similar to angina, although it results from pulmonary hypertension and right ventricular hypertrophy. There may be associated coronary artery disease. Atrial tachyarrhythmias may be an additional cause of intermittent pain.

Mitral valve prolapse causes atypical chest pain, often fleeting and sharp in character, frequently in young women. It is often associated with a mid-systolic click and late systolic murmur. Hemodynamically significant mitral insufficiency rarely occurs.

4. Pericarditis—Acute inflammation of the pericardium, often viral, idiopathic, or associated with AIDS, induces pain that is often sharp, localized to the anterior chest, and usually made worse by inspiration. Less commonly, a dull pressure-like pain may occur that is sometimes difficult to distinguish from MI. Pain may radiate to the trapezius ridge, and it may decrease when the patient sits up. The pain is often accompanied by a pericardial friction rub that is heard best with the diaphragm of the stethoscope while the patient is sitting up, leaning forward, and holding his or her breath in full expiration.

Widespread ST-segment elevation may be seen on the ECG; these changes can be distinguished from those due to MI by experienced ECG interpreters. The chest radiograph is typically normal. The echocardiogram may show no pericardial effusion; this does not exclude acute pericarditis. Cardiac troponin I may be elevated in some cases, corresponding with the degree of myocardial inflammation and, coincidentally, with the degree of diffuse ST elevation, sometimes confounding the workup in patients with angina-like pain. Coronary angiograms have been negative in these patients, and the complication rate was not elevated at 1 year. Sustained arrhythmias are generally not seen in patients without coronary disease.

5. Myocarditis—Inflammation of the myocardium is, in the United States at least, predominantly a viral illness. There is no gold standard for diagnosis; endomyocardial biopsy is performed in very few cases and generally yields only a lymphocytic infiltrate. Chest pain, if it occurs, is often associated with concomitant pericarditis and is therefore similar in character and location to that

entity. Like pericarditis, myocarditis can produce substernal pain similar to that associated with angina pectoris. In some studies, the majority of patients with a clinical presentation consistent with MI but with normal coronary artery angiograms were found to have focal or generalized myocarditis.

Myocarditis may be responsible for up to 25% of sudden cardiac deaths in patients under 30 years of age, presumably due to lethal ventricular arrhythmias. However, premature atrial or ventricular extrasystoles are much more common than are any serious sustained arrhythmias. Myocarditis may be responsible for more cases of heart failure than of chest pain; up to 10% of patients with heart failure due to cardiomyopathy rather than ischemic causes have cardiomyopathy on endomyocardial biopsy.

In severe cases, physical examination shows signs of fluid overload as well as an S_3 or S_4 gallop if heart failure is present. Routine blood tests are usually normal, except for cardiac enzymes, which may be elevated if there is associated myocardial necrosis. Cardiac troponin I or T may be more elevated than is CK-MB. Troponin elevations tend to occur early in the course of illness, probably reflecting a peak in myocardial necrosis within the first month.

ECG findings are variable, sometimes simulating those seen in MI or pericarditis. Chest film findings are usually consistent with whatever degree of heart failure is present. Serial echocardiography may reveal a spherical left ventricle early in the course of disease but a reversion to a more elliptical geometry as healing occurs. Wall motion abnormalities are usually global but occasionally segmental. Occasionally, mural thrombi may be seen, requiring anticoagulation. Echocardiography is also indicated to rule out valvular abnormalities and hypertrophic and restrictive cardiomyopathies as potential causes of heart failure. Endomyocardial biopsy may be indicated for patients with a rapidly deteriorating course or in those in whom a potentially reversible cause (eg, hemochromatosis or amyloidosis) is suspected.

6. Syndrome X—This disorder has the following nonspecific characteristics:

1. Chest pain similar to that of angina pectoris, precipitated by exertion.
2. ST-depression on exercise ECG.
3. Normal coronary arteriogram, with no evidence of spasm on ergonovine provocation.

The chest pain these patients experience is thought to be due to either myocardial ischemia of occult etiology, possibly due to clot with rapid lysis or microvascular disease, or to "hypersensitive heart syndrome." Most patients are premenopausal women who are typically younger than those with coronary disease, and there is a strong correlation between Syndrome X and panic attacks. About one-half of the patients have atypical pain, and those with angina-like pain experience it for unusually prolonged periods. Poor response to nitroglycerin is common. A significantly small number of patients labeled with Syndrome X have been found to suffer from associated rheumatologic diagnoses, esophageal dysfunction, or amyloidosis.

The ECG at rest may show no changes or nonspecific ST-T depression, but the exercise ECG typically shows horizontal or downsloping ST depression. Although an abnormal response to vasomotor stimuli (eg, adenosine) has been seen, myocardial perfusion and wall motion abnormalities are variable on imaging studies, leading some to suggest that ischemia, if present, may be limited to the subendocardium. A normal coronary angiogram is a necessary component of the diagnosis of Syndrome X. A positive response to ergonovine during catheterization confirms the alternative diagnosis of variant angina.

Aziz S et al. Acute dissection of the thoracic aorta. *Hosp Med.* 2004;65:136. [PMID: 15052903]

Bugiardini R et al. Angina with "normal" coronary arteries: a changing philosophy. *JAMA.* 2005;293:477. [PMID: 15671433]

Cava JR et al. Chest pain in children and adolescents. *Pediatr Clin North Am.* 2004;51:1553. [PMID: 15561173]

Lange RA et al. Clinical practice. Acute pericarditis. *N Engl J Med.* 2004;351:2195. [PMID: 15548780]

B. PULMONARY CAUSES

1. Pulmonary embolus—Over half a million patients in the United States are diagnosed with pulmonary emboli each year; this probably understates the incidence of the disorder because it is an uncommon cause of chest pain in the primary care setting. Consequently, up to one-half of all cases go undiagnosed. Pulmonary emboli cause approximately 200,000 deaths in the United States each year. A high index of suspicion combined with rapid diagnosis and treatment are critical for survival. The mortality rate without treatment is approximately 30%; most deaths are due to recurrent emboli. However, with accurate diagnosis and effective anticoagulation, the mortality rate is reduced to 2 to 8%.

Up to 90% of pulmonary emboli arise from the deep veins of the lower extremities; the rest originate in pelvic, renal, or upper extremity veins, or from the right heart. Clinically significant pulmonary emboli usually result from ileofemoral thrombi. Calf vein thrombi resolve spontaneously in about 80% of cases; the remainder propagate to the popliteal, femoral, or iliac veins.

Clinical presentation depends on the size of the thrombus. Hemodynamic compromise results when large thrombi lodge at the bifurcation of the main pulmonary artery or the lobar branches. Pleuritic chest pain occurs when smaller thrombi travel distally and lodge in segmental veins, which presumably initiates an inflammatory response adjacent to the parietal pleura. Pulmonary infarction only occurs in about 10% of cases. Impairment of gas exchange results from the release of inflammatory mediators from platelets and other components of the thrombus and its surrounding vasculature, causing vascular permeability changes and intrapulmonary shunting.

Predisposing factors to pulmonary emboli include immobilization, recent surgery, or malignancy. Up to 17% of patients with idiopathic venous thromboembolism have occult malignancy, particularly of the pancreas or prostate, although late-stage breast, lung, uterine, or brain cancers may also be associated with a hypercoagulable state.

Although most pulmonary emboli originate in the lower extremities, <30% of patients have leg symptoms at the time of diagnosis. On the other hand, patients with symptomatic deep venous thrombosis may have asymptomatic pulmonary emboli in over 25% of cases. When symptoms are present, they commonly include dyspnea, pleuritic pain, cough, and hemoptysis, which is usually characterized by blood-tinged sputum and is rarely massive. Physical signs include tachypnea, rales, tachycardia, a fourth heart sound, and an accentuated pulmonic component of the second heart sound. The most commonly recognized symptom complex, seen in approximately 67% cases, is pleuritic pain and hemoptysis. Cardiovascular collapse occurs in <10%. Unfortunately, no particular clinical finding is sensitive or specific for the diagnosis of pulmonary embolus.

Routine laboratory results are nonspecific, although arterial blood gases usually show hypoxemia, hypocapnia, and respiratory alkalosis. However, because typical arterial blood gas findings are not always seen, they should not be given excess weight in excluding or establishing the diagnosis. Similarly, pulse oximetry does not establish the diagnosis, although P_{A2} >95% at the time of diagnosis may be seen in patients who are at increased risk for complications, including respiratory failure, cardiogenic shock, and death. Serum troponins I and T are elevated in up to 50% of patients with moderate to large pulmonary emboli, proportional to acute right heart overload; these findings are associated with poor outcomes. ECG changes are nonspecific, although T-wave inversions in the precordial leads may indicate severe right ventricular dysfunction. Chest film findings can include cardiomegaly, atelectasis, pulmonary parenchymal abnormality, or pleural effusion, but these findings are also nonspecific.

Clinical variables alone are not sufficient for the diagnosis of pulmonary embolism, although they do serve the important function of helping the clinician formulate pretest probabilities of the likelihood of pulmonary embolus. Of the additional tests available, ventilation-perfusion lung scan is used most frequently. If the perfusion scan is completely normal, the diagnosis of pulmonary embolus is virtually excluded. Conversely, a high probability lung scan, particularly in a patient with a high pretest probability of pulmonary emboli, indicates a high likelihood of thromboembolic disease. Unfortunately, however, over 50% of lung scan defects are interpreted as intermediate or low probability. In addition, the false-positive rate of high probability scans approaches 15%, although it is reduced below 10% if patients with prior pulmonary emboli are excluded. Up to 75% of patients have combinations of clinical and lung scan probabilities that cannot finally confirm or exclude the diagnosis of pulmonary emboli. These patients may require pulmonary angiography for definitive diagnosis, although many series report that the majority of patients are treated without undergoing the test.

In patients with intermediate clinical and lung scan probabilities for pulmonary embolism, particularly those with leg symptoms, a positive lower-extremity venous ultrasound provides adequate rationale for anticoagulation, although up to 3% of results can be false-positive. In addition, thromboembolic disease is not completely excluded if a single leg study is negative, because the entire detectable clot burden may have already embolized, or emboli may have originated from a source other than the legs or from calf vein thrombi.

The sensitivity and negative predictive value of D-dimer, a degradation product of cross-linked fibrin, are both high, especially when the enzyme-linked immunosorbent assay (ELISA) method is used. A negative quantitative rapid ELISA result rules out venous thromboembolism, although a positive test lacks specificity because high D-dimer levels are commonly seen in patients with malignancy or who have recently undergone surgery; levels also rise with increasing age.

Helical CT scanning is used increasingly to rule out pulmonary embolus. Specificity of the procedure has been high in most studies; however, to avoid false-positive results, the radiologist should be experienced in interpreting helical CT scans. Sensitivity has been more variable; most studies show a higher likelihood of detecting clots in large proximal pulmonary veins than at the segmental level or in smaller vessels. However, patients with normal spiral CT studies experience subsequent embolic events in <2% of cases. In centers where radiologists are experienced, where multidetector row CT scanners with thin collimation are available, and particularly where additional images of pulmonary arteries and leg veins can be obtained without additional venipuncture or contrast administration, helical CT scanning can provide significant benefits. A recent study showed that a combination of D-dimer and multidetector-row CT scanning may rule out pulmonary embolus without lower extremity ultrasonography.

Pulmonary angiography, using four injections with four views, is the gold standard for diagnosing pulmonary emboli. If the order of vessel injection is prioritized based upon ventilation-perfusion scanning results, the contrast burden can be limited. A normal pulmonary angiogram with magnification excludes clinically significant pulmonary embolism. Procedure mortality is <0.5%, and only about 5% of patients experience complications, which are usually related to catheter insertion or contrast reactions.

To summarize, clinical assessment, ventilation-perfusion lung scanning, D-dimer testing, and venous ultrasound can be used to confirm or exclude the diagnosis of pulmonary emboli in many but not all patients:

1. In patients with a high pretest probability and leg symptoms, a diagnostic venous ultrasound.

2. Pulmonary embolus is unlikely in patients with low pretest probability and a negative D-dimer assay.

3. Pulmonary embolus is unlikely in patients with low to moderate pretest probability, a non-high probability lung scan, and either a normal venous ultrasound or a negative D-dimer assay.

4. D-dimer measurements are difficult to use in excluding pulmonary emboli in patients with cancer, in those who have recently undergone surgery, or in the very elderly.

5. Helical CT is used increasingly in many centers, and can yield a relatively noninvasive diagnosis if leg veins are included. Multidetector-row CT combined with negative D-dimer may rule out pulmonary embolus without lower extremity studies.

6. Pulmonary angiography is the gold standard and is indicated in up to 20% of patients with possible pulmonary emboli whose noninvasive workup is not definitive.

2. Spontaneous pneumothorax—Similar to acute pulmonary embolus, a clinical presentation including acute onset of pleuritic pain and respiratory distress should trigger consideration of spontaneous pneumothorax. Primary spontaneous pneumothorax usually occurs in young, tall, adult male smokers without prior history of lung disease; recurrence is common. Secondary spontaneous pneumothorax is superimposed on underlying lung disease, such as chronic obstructive pulmonary disease or *Pneumocystis* pneumonia. Although rare, tension pneumothorax is life-threatening unless diagnosed promptly and treated emergently. A "one-way valve" is created by a tissue flap from the injured lung, trapping air in the intrapleural space progressively with each inspiration. Compression of healthy lung can cause respiratory failure in minutes. Physical examination discloses unilateral loss of breath sounds with hypertympany; the trachea is shifted away from the injured side and jugular venous distention can occur. The diagnosis must be based on history and physical examination; pneumothorax should be decompressed through the insertion of a large-bore needle into the second intercostal space in the midclavicular line on the affected side, prior to a confirmatory chest radiograph.

3. Pulmonary hypertension and cor pulmonale— Primary pulmonary hypertension is rare. Patients with this condition who have chest pain on exertion may also experience syncope and edema; these are indicators of severe disease and impaired right heart function. In general, exertional dyspnea precedes exertional chest pain. Secondary pulmonary hypertension can occur in chronic obstructive pulmonary disease, chronic or diffuse pulmonary embolization, and some rheumatic diseases. Chest pain may be due to the underlying disease. Occasionally, chest pain is directly attributable to secondary pulmonary hypertension, but again this usually occurs later than dyspnea on exertion and also after fatigue and syncope with exertion. Patients who have concurrent mitral stenosis or congenital heart disease with cor pulmonale may have typical exertional angina even with normal coronary arteries. Chest pain in these cases may be due to pulmonary artery stretching or ischemia of the right ventricle.

4. Bacterial pneumonia—Approximately 80% of patients with bacterial pneumonia complain of sudden onset of shaking chills followed by fever, pleuritic chest pain, and cough productive of purulent sputum. Chest pain, occurring in up to 33% of patients, is sharp or stabbing in character and worse on inspiration. For patients with severe pain, opioid analgesics may be necessary until antibiotics quell the vigorous anti-inflammatory response to bacterial infection.

5. Cancer—Of the primary cancers causing pain in the chest, lung cancer is the most common; 90% of patients are symptomatic when they seek medical attention. Chest pain in the absence of other symptoms is relatively rare in this disease. Up to 50% of patients with lung cancer have experienced chest pain in conjunction with cough, dyspnea, weight loss, and hemoptysis. Pain due to tumor involvement is usually dull and intermittent. More severe or persistent pain may indicate chest wall, bony, or mediastinal invasion. Neuropathic pain involving the shoulder or upper extremity in a C8 to T1 distribution can be a manifestation of Pancoast tumor, when a superior sulcus malignancy spreads upward into the brachial plexus; Horner syndrome can be an associated manifestation. Pleural or pericardial effusion, hoarseness, or superior vena cava syndrome can also be seen. Isolated pleural effusions present more often with dyspnea or vague chest discomfort than with typical pleuritic chest pain.

6. Sarcoidosis—Chest pain is commonly seen in sarcoidosis, although it more commonly causes cough and dyspnea. Cardiac involvement by the granulomatous process may also lead to arrhythmias including heart block and sometimes sudden death; this event may be preceded by chest pain, palpitations, syncope, or lightheadedness.

7. Pleuritis—The acute onset of pleuritic pain in otherwise healthy young adults is usually due to viral pleurisy. However, underlying autoimmune diseases such as systemic lupus erythematosus or rheumatoid arthritis, or occasionally drug-induced lupus, may be responsible. Potential offending agents include procainamide, hydralazine, isoniazid, and others.

Goyle KK et al. Diagnosing pericarditis. *Am Fam Physician.* 2002;66:1695. [PMID: 12449268]

Kruip MJ et al. Diagnostic strategies for excluding pulmonary embolism in clinical outcome studies. A systematic review. *Ann Intern Med.* 2003;138:941. [PMID: 12809450]

Laack TA et al. Pulmonary embolism: an unsuspected killer. *Emerg Med Clin North Am.* 2004;22:961. [PMID: 15474778]

Perrier A et al. Multidetector-row computed tomography in suspected pulmonary embolism. *N Engl J Med.* 2005;352:1760. [PMID: 15858185]

C. Gastrointestinal Causes

Esophageal disease can cause visceral pain identical to that caused by myocardial ischemia because the heart and the esophagus share similar neurologic innervation. Esophageal pain, like myocardial ischemia, may cause chest pressure, may be provoked by exercise or a motion, may be palliated by rest or nitrates, or may exhibit a crescendo pattern. A single response of chest pain to therapy with an antacid and viscous lidocaine does not reliably distinguish cardiac from esophageal pain. Up to one-third of patients referred for cardiology evaluation after emergency assessment for chest pain may have esophageal symptoms; even experienced clinicians may have difficulty making the diagnosis on clinical grounds. Features that may suggest an esophageal source of chest pain include the following:

1. Associated heartburn, dysphagia, regurgitation.
2. Pain typically occurs after meals.
3. Pain typically persists for more than 1 hour.
4. Pain typically relieved by antacid.
5. Pain never radiates.

1. Esophageal rupture and mediastinitis—Severe straining from repeated vomiting can cause spontaneous perforation of the esophagus (Boerhaave syndrome). The patient complains of excruciating retrosternal and

Table 18–3. "ABCDEF" Management of Non–ST Segment Elevation Acute Coronary Syndrome.

Intervention	Medication	Indication	Starting dose
Antiplatelet therapy	Aspirin		162–325 mg as soon as possible, then 75–160 mg/d
	Clopidogrel		75 mg/d
Anticoagulation	Glycoprotein IIb/IIIa inhibitors	Early invasive therapy	Varies
ACE inhibitor therapy	Multiple	CVD, DM, CHF	Varies
	Angiotensin-receptor blocker	ACE inhibitor intolerance	Varies
β-Blocker therapy	Atenolol		25 mg/d
	Metoprolol		50 mg bid
Blood pressure control	Amlodipine	Intolerance to ACE inhibitors or β-blockers	5 mg/d
Cholesterol control	Statins	Low-density lipoprotein levels >70 mg/dL	Varies
	Niacin	High-density lipoprotein levels <40 mg/dL	250 mg/d
Cigarette smoking cessation	Bupropion (sustained-release)		150 mg bid
Diabetic management	Varies	Hemoglobin A_{1c} > 7.0	Varies
Dietary management[a]			
Exercise[b]			
Follow-up[c]			

[a]Includes eating vegetables, fruit, whole grains, and fish.
[b]Includes aerobic plus weight-bearing 30 min/d.
[c]Should occur 1–6 weeks after discharge.
ACE, angiotensin-converting enzyme; CVD, cardiovascular disease; DM, diabetes mellitus; CHF, congestive heart failure.

with high-density lipoprotein levels <40 mg/dL (1.0 mmol/L). *Cigarette smoking cessation* greatly lowers the risk of future coronary events; behavioral support, as well as bupropion with or without nicotine replacement, should be provided.

d. Diabetes management—Treatment should bring glycosylated hemoglobin levels below 7.0%. *Diet* should be enriched with protein, complex carbohydrates, fruits, vegetables, nuts, and whole grains; saturated fat, cholesterol, and salt should be restricted.

e. Exercise—All patients should be encouraged to participate in moderate levels of aerobic and weight-bearing exercise for at least 30 minutes on most days of the week, preferably within a cardiac rehabilitation program.

f. Follow-up—Close follow-up with a physician is recommended for all patients within 1 to 6 weeks after discharge, with regular follow-up thereafter. Patients of advanced age as well as those with heart failure, persistent ST-segment depression, renal insufficiency, and elevated enzyme levels tend to have a higher incidence of recurrent cardiovascular events at 1 year. For all others, risk approaches that of similar patients with coronary disease, especially after 1 year. Coronary angiography is recommended for those in whom new or recurrent ischemic symptoms or heart failure develops or who survive a cardiac arrest.

2. Managing stable angina pectoris—Chest discomfort in angina pectoris is caused by transient myocardial ischemia whenever myocardial oxygen demand exceeds oxygen supply. Treatment of angina is aimed at reducing the former and increasing the latter.

   a. Nonpharmacologic management—Underlying medical conditions, particularly hypertension, febrile illnesses, tachyarrhythmias, anemia or polycythemia, conditions causing hypoxemia, valvular heart disease or thyrotoxicosis, should be treated. The patient should be encouraged to reduce exercise in cold weather or after eating. All patients should take one baby aspirin (81 mg/d) or clopidogrel if aspirin is contraindicated; dipyridamole is ineffective. Patients should be encouraged to undertake a regular aerobic exercise program as recommended by the American College of Cardiology and the American Heart Association. Risk factor reduction, especially including treatment of hypertension, smoking cessation, lipid lowering, weight reduction, and glycemic control in diabetics, should be undertaken. Stress reduction as well as treatment of any underlying depression and anxiety are beneficial. An exercise ECG should be considered. Noninvasive measurement of global left ventricular systolic function is important for patients with documented MI or Q waves on ECG.

   b. Medical management—Nitrates, β-blockers, and calcium channel blockers are standard therapy for angina. High-risk patients with stable angina should probably be treated with an ACE inhibitor as well. Opioids (eg, oral morphine) are used for refractory angina in late-stage disease.

   Nitrates decrease myocardial oxygen demand by producing both systemic arterial vasodilation that reduces left ventricular systolic wall stress, as well as coronary vasodilation to a lesser degree. No difference has been found among nitrate preparations. Sublingual nitroglycerin (0.3 mg [1/200 grains]) repeated every 5 minutes times two is standard therapy for acute anginal episodes as well as prophylaxis for activities known to precipitate angina. Onset of action is less than 5 minutes, and duration of action is 30 to 40 minutes. Oral or transdermal nitrate preparations can prevent or reduce the frequency of recurrent anginal episodes. However, nitrate tolerance dictates a 12- to 14-hour nitrate-free interval each day. A commonly used regimen uses isosorbide dinitrate 10 to 40 mg at 8 A.M., 1 P.M., and 6 P.M. Extended-release isosorbide mononitrate can be started at 30 mg once daily and titrated to 120 mg once daily if needed, but its effect

Table 18–4. Selected β-Blockers Used to Treat Angina.

Drug	Starting dose
Atenolol	50 mg/d
Metoprolol	50 mg bid

is reduced after 12 hours, so supplementary nitrates or additional antianginal therapy may be required if nocturnal or rebound angina develops.

   β-Blockers both inhibit sympathetic stimulation of the myocardium and reduce systemic sympathetic tone. Although all types of β-blockers are equally effective in exertional angina, long-acting cardioselective agents (eg, atenolol or metoprolol) are preferred for the treatment of stable angina, because their diminished inhibition of β_2-receptors minimizes side effects in patients with chronic obstructive pulmonary disease, asthma, peripheral vascular disease, diabetes, and depression (Table 18–4). Target resting heart rate is 50 to 60 beats per minute, not to exceed 100 beats per minute with ordinary activity. β-Blockers have the added advantage of preventing reinfarction and improving survival in patients who have had an MI, although they have not been shown to prevent first infarctions. They should be used with caution in patients with chronic obstructive pulmonary disease or peripheral vascular disease, and started in low doses in patients with heart failure who are well compensated. β-Blockers should be avoided in patients with variant angina.

   Calcium channel blockers prevent calcium entry into vascular smooth muscle cells, initiating coronary and peripheral vasodilation, which reduces coronary and systemic vascular resistance and increases blood flow. Several types of calcium channel blockers are available. The dihydropyridines (eg, nifedipine, nicardipine, felodipine and amlodipine) have greater selectivity for vascular smooth muscle than for myocardium; they are potent vasodilators and cause less reduction in contractility and atrioventricular conduction. Verapamil has greater myocardial selectivity; it is a negative inotrope and chronotrope but a less potent peripheral vasodilator than are the dihydropyridines. Diltiazem has intermediate effects between the two. Of the available agents, short-acting dihydropyridines, especially nifedipine, should be avoided because they have been shown to increase post-MI mortality and to increase the incidence of infarction in patients with hypertension. Long-acting diltiazem or verapamil or a second-generation dihydropyridine (eg, amlodipine or felodipine) may be used alone, in combination with β-blockers, or substituted for them (Table 18–5). Calcium channel blockers are the preferred therapy for variant angina. Potential side effects include bradycardia,

Table 18–5. Selected Calcium Channel Blockers Used to Treat Angina.

Drug (trade name)	Starting dose (mg/d)	Comments
Amlodipine (Norvasc)	5	Both amlodipine and felodipine are long-acting dihydropyridines, which increase coronary blood flow
Felodipine (Plendil)	2.5	
Diltiazem (Cardizem LA)	120	Drug of choice for variant angina
Verapamil (Isoptin SR)	120	Lowers heart rate and contractility; may worsen congestive heart failure

which may proceed to heart block, aggravation of heart failure, constipation, flushing, headache, dizziness, and pedal edema. Calcium channel blockers tend to be discontinued more frequently than are β-blockers because of adverse reactions, but this difference is most marked with nifedipine.

Opioids (eg, oral morphine sulfate) are used to manage refractory angina in two settings: (1) at the time of presentation with ACS, when opioids are given intravenously for acute, severe chest pain; and near the end of life, when relief of symptoms is the highest priority, even if life may be shortened somewhat. Morphine diminishes sympathetic tone, reducing blood pressure and heart rate; oxygen consumption is also reduced, resulting in a decrease in chest pain. In addition, morphine reduces chemoreceptor sensitivity to CO_2, thereby diminishing dyspnea. Although a large retrospective study has shown that administration of morphine for ACS was associated with an increase in mortality, patients who received morphine also were seen more often by a cardiologist, were more likely to receive evidence-based medicine, and were more likely to undergo invasive procedures; these patients might have had more severe underlying disease. Randomized trials of opioids in the setting of ACS are needed.

β-Blockers and calcium channel blockers are equally effective in the management of stable angina. If there is no contraindication, β-blockers should be given to all patients who have a history of prior MI or who have stable heart failure and are receiving optimal ACE inhibitor therapy. Nitrates, although universally used to relieve anginal symptoms, may have limited usefulness in their slow-release form as first-line therapy because tolerance to

their effect usually develops. Combination therapy with a β-blocker and a calcium channel blocker, with or without the addition of long-acting nitrates, is indicated for patients who do not respond well to monotherapy. Opioids, such as oral morphine, should be used for angina that is refractory to other agents, particularly in terminal patients.

3. Managing coronary disease in women—Cardiovascular diseases are the most common cause of death in women in the United States, accounting for 35% of all-cause mortality. Symptoms of some form of cardiovascular disease develop in one of three women over 65 years of age. Because women are underrepresented in clinical trials, data concerning the management of women with ACS are limited. Available data suggest that women are not referred as often as men for diagnostic and therapeutic procedures, although this is probably due to the fact that women present with more comorbidities than men and, therefore, experience predictably higher complication rates from revascularization procedures. Available evidence supports the use of the same standard medical therapy for women as for men. However, women are more likely to receive nitrates, calcium channel blockers, diuretics, and sedatives than are men, while some studies suggest that women are less likely to receive β-blockers and aspirin. Estrogen supplementation has not been shown to have a cardioprotective effect in women with coronary disease.

In ST-elevation MI, indications for thrombolysis or stenting are generally the same for women as for men. In most series, however, women are less likely than men to undergo both procedures and are likely to experience a greater delay in treatment as well. This finding has raised questions of gender bias. However, women are often older and have a greater burden of risk factors than men. After adjustment for clinical and coronary variables, evidence indicates that women probably have equivalent access to both catheterization and revascularization.

In non–ST elevation ACS, outcomes in high-risk men are improved with an invasive strategy of early catheterization and revascularization, but available data conflict as to whether this benefit extends to women for uncertain reasons.

4. Special considerations in the elderly—Available data indicate that both optimal medical therapy and revascularization produce similar outcomes in quality of life, improvement in angina and death or nonfatal MI compared with younger patients. An invasive approach appears to be associated with greater risk, while medical therapy is associated with an almost 50% chance of later hospitalization and revascularization. Patient preference is an important determinant, since some patients will prefer to assume the risk of early revascularization to achieve better short-term outcomes, while others will prefer the lower-risk approach and the avoidance of surgical morbidity.

Braunwald E et al. ACC/AHA guideline update for the management of patients with unstable angina and non-ST elevation myocardial infarction—2002: Summary article. *Circulation.* 2002;106:1893. [PMID: 12383588]

Gibbons RJ et al. ACC/AHA 2002 guideline update for the management of patients with chronic stable angina—Summary article. *Circulation.* 2003;107:149. [PMID: 12570960]

Gluckman TJ et al. A simplified approach to the management of non-ST-segment elevation acute coronary syndromes. *JAMA.* 2005;293:349. [PMID: 15657328]

Tresch DD et al. Diagnosis and management of myocardial ischemia (angina) in the elderly patient. *Am J Geriatr Cardiol.* 2001;10:337. [PMID: 11684918]

Yang EH et al. Current and future treatment strategies for refractory angina. *Mayo Clin Proc.* 2004;79:1284. [PMID: 15473411]

American College of Cardiology American Heart Association 2002 Guideline Update for the Management of Patients With Chronic Stable Angina–Summary Article http://acc.org/clinical/guidelines/stable/summary_article.pdf

American College of Cardiology/American Heart Association 2002 Guideline Update for the Management of Patients with Unstable Angina and Non-ST-Segment Elevation Myocardial Infarction–Summary Article http://www.acc.org/clinical/guidelines/unstable/summary_article.pdf

B. Managing Chest Pain due to Pulmonary Disease

1. Managing acute pulmonary embolism—Patients with severe pleuritic pain secondary to pulmonary embolus can be treated with morphine, either oral or intravenous, while definitive treatment is started. Thrombolytics are used if there is hemodynamic compromise from a large embolus; otherwise heparin, either unfractionated or low-molecular-weight, is started concurrently with warfarin. Heparin and oral anticoagulation therapy should overlap for at least 5 days, or until the international normalized ratio (INR) has been therapeutic for more than 48 hours. Heparin may be continued longer in cases of massive pulmonary embolus, or for large-burden iliofemoral thrombosis. Anticoagulation should be continued for at least 12 weeks, keeping INR in the range of 2.0 to 3.0. Some patients with recurrent or multisite thrombosis, including some with multicentric thromboembolic disease related to malignancy, may require low-molecular-weight heparin instead of warfarin. Patients without reversible risk factors for first thromboembolic event should be treated for 6 months. Inferior vena cava filter placement is recommended under the following clinical circumstances:

1. Anticoagulation is contraindicated.
2. Thromboembolic events recur despite anticoagulation.

3. Presence of chronic recurrent thromboembolism with pulmonary hypertension.
4. In conjunction with pulmonary embolectomy or endarterectomy.

2. Managing pain in lung cancer—Chest pain in lung cancer is almost always due to tumor growth. Therefore, it is best controlled by definitive antitumor treatment with surgery, chemotherapy, or radiation. However, pain should be treated as soon as it occurs, because pain left untreated recruits previously uninvolved central nervous system elements. As acute pain becomes chronic, anxiety, depression, and other nonpain phenomena can emerge to complicate treatment. In cases where antitumor therapy is not practical, or when patients place a higher priority on comfort than on disease treatment, symptom management becomes the highest priority, and it should be pursued aggressively, even if life may be shortened in the process. In these situations, issues such as informed consent and advanced directives should be discussed fully with the patient, family, and caregivers. Hospice care is frequently the best way to ensure that symptom management and family/caregiver support are provided effectively until the end of the patient's life.

The principles underlying rational and effective treatment of chest pain in lung cancer are identical to those outlined for the treatment of cancer pain in Chapter 8. The World Health Organization three-step approach to pain management should be followed for the management of chest pain secondary to cancer (see Figure 3–1). Pain assessment, including measurement of each location and type of pain on a 1 to 10 scale, should be performed on a regular basis. Nonopioid analgesics, particularly nonsteroidal anti-inflammatory drugs, should be used, but "strong" opioids (eg, morphine) should be added whenever pain is severe, which usually means once pain reaches 6 or higher on a 10-point scale. Clinicians should watch carefully for neuropathic pain, which may be partially refractive to opioids; methadone may provide particular benefit, and its low cost should be borne in mind as well.

Clinicians should not be deterred from providing adequate pain management in lung cancer because of irrational fears of respiratory depression. Available data indicates that morphine, started at low doses and increased until pain is controlled, does not depress respiration even in patients with coexistent chronic obstructive pulmonary disease. The key is to "start low and go slow" in patients with chronic obstructive pulmonary disease; although morphine reduces chemoreceptor sensitivity to CO_2, patients become tolerant quickly. Pco_2 returns to baseline within 24 hours, whereas relief of both pain and dyspnea persist.

Kyrle PA et al. Deep vein thrombosis. *Lancet.* 2005;365:1163. [PMID: 15794972]

Rainone F. Treating adult cancer pain in primary care. *J Am Board Fam Pract.* 2004;17(Suppl):S48. [PMID: 15575030]

Watts E. Managing DVT and pulmonary embolus. *Practitioner.* 2004; 248:446. [PMID: 15214274]

American College of Chest Physicians: Management of Spontaneous Pneumothorax http://www.chestnet.org/education/hsp/ statements/pneumothorax/qrg

American College of Emergency Physicians: Critical issues in the Evaluation and Management of Patients Presenting with Suspected Pulmonary Embolism http://www.acep.org/library/pdf/ cpPulEmbolism.pdf

C. MANAGING CHEST PAIN DUE TO GASTROINTESTINAL DISEASE

Most cases of chest pain referable to the gastrointestinal tract result from gastroesophageal reflux disease. Reflux symptoms, including chest pain, are a function of the severity of esophageal epithelial injury, which in turn is related to the quantity of esophageal acid exposure. Effective treatment must be titrated to disease severity. Mild symptoms may be managed empirically by elevating the head of the bed; this is particularly important for patients with nocturnal or laryngeal symptoms. Patients should be encouraged to avoid reflux-inducing foods, which included chocolate, peppermint, fatty foods, and excessive alcohol. In addition, cola drinks, orange juice, cranberry juice, and red wine all have a pH below 3.5. Patients should also be counseled to avoid lying down shortly after meals, and to avoid eating large meals within 1 hour of bedtime. Smoking cessation is also useful, in part because it diminishes salivation; saliva neutralizes refluxed acid and speeds its clearance from the esophagus.

Gastric acid secretion can be reduced with either H_2-blockers or proton pump inhibitors (PPIs). The latter are preferred, especially in severe cases, because they are much more effective in healing esophagitis (therapeutic gain of up to 75% relative to placebo, compared with approximately 60% therapeutic gain with H_2-blockers). PPIs have also been shown to produce more rapid healing and symptom relief than H_2-blockers. Most of the available PPIs appear to have similar efficacy when given in equivalent doses, although few large trials have directly compared them (Table 18–6). Both H_2-blockers and PPIs work by raising intragastric pH; they do not prevent reflux.

Table 18–6. Selected Proton Pump Inhibitors to Treat Esophageal Reflux Disease.

Drug (trade name)	Starting dose (mg/d)
Esomeprazole (Nexium)	20
Lansoprazole (Prevacid)	15
Omeprazole (Prilosec OTC)	20
Pantoprazole (Protonix)	40
Rabeprazole (Aciphex)	20

In general, patients should be treated with the least potent regimen that relieves symptoms. An alternative is to start with a dose of PPI that is likely to relieve symptoms in most cases (eg, 60 mg/d of omeprazole), then to step down treatment at 2 to 4 week intervals, maintaining antisecretory treatment for 8 weeks. Patients whose symptoms are relieved can be given a trial off medication. Relapses that occur in less than 3 months can be managed with continuous therapy, while relapses that occur after 3 months can be managed with intermittent therapy. Patients on continuous PPI therapy should undergo endoscopy at least once to rule out Barrett esophagus, an atrophic condition that predisposes to esophageal cancer. In addition, atrophic gastritis, with attendant risk of gastric cancer, as well as vitamin B_{12} deficiency, may occur in some patients receiving long-term PPI therapy.

Patients whose symptoms are refractory to PPIs may be considered for a 24-hour pH study on medication or esophageal manometry to rule out esophageal motility disorder. Calcium channel blockers may be effective in managing documented esophageal spasm. Antireflux surgery may be considered for those patients who do not respond to other measures.

Inadomi JM et al. Step-down management of gastroesophageal reflux disease. *Gastroenterology.* 2001;121:1095. [PMID: 11677201]

Metz DC. Managing gastroesophageal reflux disease for the lifetime of the patient: evaluating the long-term options. *Am J Med.* 2004;117 Suppl 5A:49S. [PMID: 15478853]

Wolfe MM. Managing gastroesophageal reflux disease: from pharmacology to the clinical arena. *Gastroenterol Clin North Am.* 2003;32(3 Suppl):S37. [PMID: 14556434]

American Gastroenterological Association: Gastroesophageal Reflux Disease Monograph http://www.gastro.org/edu/GERDmonograph.pdf

Temporomandibular Disorders & Orofacial Pain

19

James Fricton, DDS, MS

ESSENTIALS OF DIAGNOSIS

- *Jaw or facial pain, earache, or temple headache described as a dull steady pain that fluctuates over time.*
- *Associated with masticatory muscle or joint tenderness upon digital palpation in every case.*
- *Objective findings of limited or deviation of range of motion of the incisal jaw opening and sometimes joint clicking or crepitus.*
- *Primary joint diagnoses is confirmed by CT or MRI scan showing degenerative changes or disk displacement.*
- *Primary muscle diagnosis is confirmed by duplicating pain on palpation of responsible muscles.*
- *Electromyography and other objective tests are normal.*
- *Pain may be alleviated with anesthetic injection into responsible tender muscle point.*

General Considerations

Several surveys of persistent orofacial symptoms indicate that approximately 7% of Americans (or 13 million Americans) suffer from an orofacial disorder causing face or jaw pain. Clinical subpopulations comprising those whose problems are sufficiently severe to prompt them to seek care include more women than men.

Neuropathic pain and headache pain are discussed in Chapters 10 and 12, respectively. Other causes of chronic orofacial pain are discussed under the section on differential diagnosis. Typical signs of chronic orofacial pain include joint noise, tenderness of masticatory muscles and joints, pain, and limitation and deviation in the range of motion of the mandible; the most common symptoms include jaw pain, facial pain, headache, distressing or disturbing joint noises, and difficulty with jaw function.

Macfarlane TV et al. Oro-facial pain in the community: prevalence and associated impact. *Community Dent Oral Epidemiol.* 2002;30:52. [PMID: 11918576]

Magnusson T et al. A prospective investigation over two decades on signs and symptoms of temporomandibular disorders and associated variables. A final summary. *Acta Odontol Scand.* 2005;63:99. [PMID: 16134549]

Nilsson IM et al. Prevalence of temporomandibular pain and subsequent dental treatment in Swedish adolescents. *J Orofac Pain.* 2005;19:144. [PMID: 15895837]

Pathogenesis

Understanding the theories of the pathophysiology of temporomandibular joint (TMJ) disk displacements and masticatory myofascial pain are important to understanding the etiologic factors. These two disorders are the most common disorders of the temporomandibular structures.

TMJ disk displacements are classified by progressive stages of masticatory dysfunction involving anterior or medial displacement of the disk relative to the condyle (Figure 19–1). It is often characterized by TMJ clicking and pain in the early stages and jaw locking, limited range of motion, and degenerative joint changes in the later stages. The early stage TMJ disk displacement is the most common TMJ disorder and is characterized by reciprocal clicking of the joint on opening and closing from the impaired gliding function of the disk.

Although the exact etiology of TMJ disk displacement is unknown, one of the most common theories suggests that abnormal biomechanical forces on the condyle may cause the articular tissues to change in shape, form, and function. The friction created by malposition of the disk and jaw function may lead to further displacement and eventual morphologic changes to the form and function of the disk.

In addition, the pressure and strain from the condyle on the posterior attachment leads to inflammation, synovitis, and pain in the joint. Synovitis inhibits the synovial membrane's capacity to produce hyaluronic acid. With

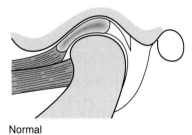

Normal

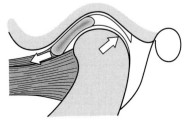

Slight displacement (clicking)

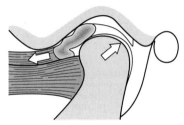

Advanced displacement (locked)

Figure 19–1. There are several stages of disk displacement relative to the temporomandibular joint. Each stage has different clinical characteristics.

time, the synovial fluid increases in viscosity, reducing its protective functioning. In a healthy joint, the side of the disk facing the condylar eminence is concave; during function, the condyle glides and expresses the synovial fluid out from this concavity, creating a negative relative pressure.

The healthy synovial fluid viscosity, allows a "hyaluronic fluid film" under the disk and enables the synovial fluid to flow back into this concavity as the condyle retrudes. If the synovial fluid is viscous, fluid may not be able to refill the concavity and the disk acts like a suction cup and maintains the anteriorly displaced position. If the disk maintains this position or is displaced farther forward, adhesions will form between the eminence and the disk, locking it in this forward position. With each translation, the head of the condyle rides over the disk's posterior band causing clicking and eventually causing the disk to fold forward. Adhesions may then form between the folded portions of the disk and prevent it from ever assuming its normal shape. In addition, abnormal mechanical loading may impair synthetic functions in affected tissues of the TMJ. Chondroblast failure with excessive loading may be associated with disruption of specific cytoskeletal elements, f-actin, and tubulin, affecting protein synthesis and repair potential.

Masticatory myofascial pain, on the other hand, is a regional muscle pain disorder characterized by localized muscle tenderness termed "trigger points" and is the most common cause of persistent regional pain (Figure 19–2). The affected muscles may also display an increased fatigability, stiffness, subjective weakness, pain in movement, and slight restricted range of motion that is unrelated to joint restriction. Masticatory myofascial pain is frequently overlooked as a diagnosis because it is often accompanied by other signs and symptoms in addition to pain, coincidental pathologic conditions, and numerous

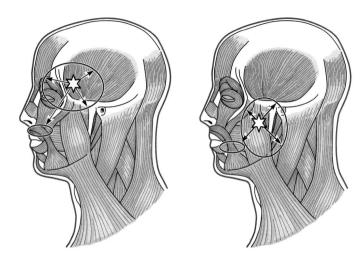

Figure 19–2. The most common muscles associated with masticatory muscle pain include the temporalis and masseters with associated pain referral patterns. Left: Temporalis refers pain to temples and frontal, retroorbital, and maxillary teeth. Right: Masseter refers pain to the jaw, ear, and retromandibular and mandibular teeth. ✴ = trigger point location; ◯ = referral patterns.

behavioral and psychosocial problems. As masticatory myofascial pain persists, chronic pain characteristics often precede or follow its development. Theories on the etiology of masticatory myofascial pain are based on a combination of peripheral and central theories.

The development of trigger points is hypothesized to be a progressive process with a stage of neuromuscular dysfunction of sustained muscle hyperactivity and irritability that is maintained by numerous perpetuating factors and then followed by a stage of neurobiologic changes in the muscle bands with the trigger points. The characteristics of masticatory myofascial pain often outlast the initiating events, setting up a self-generating pain cycle of central sensitization that is perpetuated through lack of proper treatment, sustained muscle tension, distorted muscle posture, pain-reinforcing behavior, and failure to reduce contributing factors such as clenching or sleep disturbances.

The initiating events, including macrotraumatic or microtraumatic events, may disturb the normal or weakened muscle through muscle injury (eg, whiplash, excess jaw opening) or sustained muscle contraction (eg, bruxism, muscle tension, postural habits). These traumas release free calcium within the muscle through disruption of the sarcoplasmic reticulum and, with adenosine triphosphate (ATP), stimulate actin and myosin interaction and local contractile and metabolic activity resulting in increases in noxious by-products. Substances such as serotonin, histamine, kinins, and prostaglandins sensitize and fire type III and IV muscle nociceptors, and a central sensitization is prolonged. These afferent inputs converge with other visceral and somatic inputs in the cells such as those of the lamina I or V of the dorsal horn on the way to the cortex, resulting in perception of local and referred pain.

These inputs may be facilitated or inhibited by multiple peripherally or centrally initiated alterations in neural input to this "central biasing mechanism" of the brainstem through various treatment modalities such as cold, heat, analgesic medications, massage, trigger point injections, and transcutaneous electrical stimulation. The cycle may be perpetuated by protective posturing of the painful muscle through distorted muscle posture and by avoiding painful stretching of the muscles. Any other perpetuating factors resulting in further sustained neural activity, such as continued muscle tension, poor postural habits, or inputs from pathologic viscera or dysfunctional joints, will support the reverberatory circuit.

With contractile activity sustained, local blood flow decreases, resulting in low oxygen tension, depleted ATP reserves, and diminished calcium pump. Free calcium continues to interact with ATP to trigger contractile activity, especially if actin and myosin are overlapping within the shortened muscle, and a self-perpetuating cycle is established. Sustained increases in local noxious by-products of oxidative metabolism then contribute to the beginning of the organic musculodystrophic stage with sensitization of nociceptors within the interstitial connective tissue at the trigger point and further disruption of the calcium pump. If normal muscle length is not restored and pain continues, functional, postural, and behavioral disturbances may further perpetuate the problem.

Borg-Stein J et al. Focused review: myofascial pain. *Arch Phys Med Rehabil.* 2002;83(3 Suppl 1):S40–7. [PMID: 11973695]

Emshoff R et al. Relative odds of temporomandibular joint pain as a function of magnetic resonance imaging findings of internal derangement, osteoarthrosis, effusion, and bone marrow edema. *Oral Surg Oral Med Oral Pathol Oral Radiol Endod.* 2003;95:437. [PMID: 12686927]

Giamberardino MA. Referred muscle pain/hyperalgesia and central sensitization. *J Rehabil Med.* 2003;(41 Suppl):85. [PMID: 12817663]

Graff-Radford SB. Myofascial pain: diagnosis and management. *Curr Pain Headache Rep.* 2004;8:463. [PMID: 15509460]

Haskin C et al. Physiological levels of hydrostatic pressure alter morphology and organization of cytoskeletal and adhesion proteins in MG-63 osteosarcoma cells. *Biochem Cell Biol.* 1993;71:27. [PMID: 8329174]

Katzberg RW et al. Normal and abnormal temporomandibular joint disc and posterior attachment as depicted by magnetic resonance imaging in symptomatic and asymptomatic subjects. *J Oral Maxillofac Surg.* 2005;63:1155. [PMID: 16094584]

Milam SB. Pathogenesis of degenerative temporomandibular joint arthritides. *Odontology.* 2005;93:7. [PMID: 16170470]

Nitzan DW et al. TMJ lubrication system: its effect on the joint function, dysfunction, and treatment approach. *Compend Contin Educ Dent.* 2004;25:437. [PMID: 15651234]

Prevention

Prevention of TMJ disk displacement and masticatory myofascial pain is based on reducing peripheral or central etiologic factors, or both. Peripheral factors that are most often cited as important in prevention of temporomandibular disorders includes oral parafunctional habits, occlusal dysharmony, and direct or indirect trauma to the jaw. These are among the numerous factors that drive the equilibrium of local tissues either toward normal or adaptive physiologic health and function or toward dysfunction and disease. However, peripherally based models of etiology do not address the issues of disparate findings in patients with similar objective findings or surgical treatments that fail.

Central factors that have been cited as important in the cause and progression of temporomandibular disorders include centrally mediated psychosocial factors (such as depression and poor coping strategies) and problems with abnormal central modulation of pain (such as somatization and fibromyalgia). Because of the multifactorial nature of chronic orofacial pain, most experts believe that it should be conceptualized and prevented from a broader biopsychosocial model rather than the traditional medical model commonly used for acute problems.

Clinical Findings & Differential Diagnosis

Diagnosis of temporomandibular disorders relies on measurement of range of motion, assessment of TMJ function, and palpation of the muscles and joints using standard and reliable procedures.

Range of motion of the jaw is measured from incisal edge to incisal edge of the central incisor with a millimeter rule. Minimum normal jaw opening is considered to be about two finger widths at the knuckles of the patient's dominant hand, or approximately 40 mm. Lateral motion should be 7 to 10 mm to both the right and left. Normal protrusive range is between 6 mm and 9 mm. **Limitation in range of motion** may indicate any of the following conditions: contracture of one or more of the jaw closing muscles, a nonreducing anterior displacement of the disk (closed lock), coronoid process interference, fibrous ankylosis of the joint, a hematoma, neoplasm, infection, or a systemic condition (such as scleroderma).

TMJ sounds may be detected by palpation of the joint during repetitive opening, closing, and lateral movements. They are common, and their presence does not imply the need for treatment. TMJ sounds may result from normal or pathologic mechanisms, including deviation in form or function of the disk, joint osteoarthritis, or anterior or medial TMJ disk displacement. Consider therapeutic intervention when limitation in movement or joint tenderness accompany joint pain.

Muscle and joint palpation is necessary to determine the presence of tenderness in the muscle, joint, and other soft tissue structures as the only sign found in masticatory pain disorders such as myofascial pain, myositis, TMJ synovitis, or capsulitis. Unfortunately, intra- and interexaminer reliability of muscle palpation is low and requires training and calibration to improve its consistency and replicability.

Imaging of the TMJ includes panoramic radiography; magnetic resonance imaging (MRI); and computed axial tomography (CT). Panoramic radiographic imaging of the jaw is convenient and inexpensive for TMJ screening. Although gross degenerative, traumatic, or dysplastic changes can be detected with panoramic radiographs, subtle condylar changes and abnormal disk/condylar/fossa relationships cannot be evaluated. Lateral open and closed mouth tomography or CT scans of the TMJ are usually recommended. MRI can provide a definitive diagnosis in most cases of suspected TMJ disk displacement. Patients with joint locking or restricted condylar motion, as demonstrated clinically or

with lateral tomography, can be evaluated with MRI to determine disk position and morphology. In addition, MRI scanning can be used to detect joint effusions or altered circulation due to inflammation using gadolinium-DTPA enhancement. Dynamic MRI can also be used to determine the functional relationships between the condyle and disk during rotatory and translatory movement of the condyle. Limitations of MRI include the relative lack of definition of bony surfaces of the joint and restriction to patients without magnetic metallic implants.

A. TEMPOROMANDIBULAR MUSCLE DISORDERS

Temporomandibular muscle pain disorders or masticatory myalgia are characterized by pain arising from pathologic or dysfunctional processes in the masticatory muscles. Pain is usually experienced over the involved muscle but is sometimes referred to distant structures, confusing the diagnostic process. There are several distinct types of masticatory muscle pain subtypes in the masticatory system.

Myofascial pain, the most common systemic muscle pain disorder, is characterized by regional pain associated with tender areas (trigger points) in taut bands of skeletal muscles, tendons, or ligaments. Although pain typically occurs over the trigger point, pain can be referred to distant areas (eg, the temporalis referring to the frontal area and the masseter referring into the ear). Reproducible pain upon palpation of the trigger point is diagnostic. Myofascial pain is the most common cause of masticatory pain, accounting for over 60% of all cases of temporomandibular disorders. Although the etiology of myofascial pain is unclear, current theories hypothesize that macrotrauma or microtrauma disturbs normal or weakened muscle through injury or sustained contraction (eg, bruxism or clenching). Such processes may induce peripheral and central changes that sensitize muscle nociceptors, resulting in tenderness and both local and referred pain.

Myositis is a less common acute condition involving inflammation of the muscle and connective tissue and associated pain and swelling. It may be septic or aseptic. Most areas of the muscle are tender, and there is pain within active range of motion. The inflammation is usually due to local causes such as acute overuse, local infection from an impacted third molar, pericoronitis, trauma, or cellulitis.

Muscle spasm is another acute disorder characterized by transient involuntary tonic contraction of a muscle. It can occur following overstretching of a previously weakened muscle, protective splinting of an injury, or acute overuse. A muscle in spasm is shortened and painful, producing limited range of jaw motion. Lateral pterygoid spasm on one side can also cause a shift of the occlusion to the contralateral side.

Muscle contracture is a chronic condition characterized by persistent shortening of the muscle. It can begin after trauma, infection, or prolonged hypomobility. If the muscle is maintained in a shortened state, muscular fibrosis and contracture may develop over several months. Pain is often decreased by voluntary or involuntary guarding or by avoiding use of the muscle.

B. TEMPOROMANDIBULAR JOINT DISORDERS

TMJ pain or arthralgia is usually due to capsulitis or synovitis, with associated joint inflammation, tenderness, pain, and fluid accumulation or effusion. The difficulty in diagnosing joint problems lies in determining whether pain in the area of the joint is due to muscle disorder, joint disorder, or a systemic disorder. Most TMJ arthralgias cause pain anterior to the ear, with occasional referral to surrounding (eg, temporal) regions; digital palpation and joint use are painful.

Several joint conditions can be associated with arthralgia. **Disk displacement with reduction** is characterized by clicking of the TMJ on opening and closing. The opening click reflects the condyle moving beneath the posterior band of the disk until it snaps into its normal relationship on the concave undersurface of the disk. The closing click reflects reversal of this process. The condyle moves under the posterior band of the disk until it snaps off the disk and on to the posterior attachment. The opening click occurs at a wider incisal opening than the closing click and at different points of incisal opening. Momentary dysfunction of the disk has been theorized to reflect articular surface irregularity, disk-articular surface adherence, synovial fluid degradation, disk-condyle incoordination as a result of abnormal muscle function, increased muscle activity around the joint, or disk deformation. As the disk becomes more dysfunctional, it begins to interfere with normal translation of the condyle and may even cause periodic jaw locking. An occasional patient has excessive opening due to ligament laxity and joint hypermobility and becomes at risk for open locking or subluxation of the joint.

Disk displacement without reduction is characterized by marked limited mouth opening due to interference with normal condylar sliding on the disk due to disk adhesion, deformation, or dystrophy. In this situation, the opening is usually restricted to 20 to 30 mm with a deviation of the jaw to the affected side on opening. Joint noise is minimal because little joint translation occurs. The masticatory muscles and joint frequently become tender and painful in response to the joint dysfunction. After the disk is permanently displaced, soft-tissue remodeling of the disk and associated ligaments in the joint occurs. After a permanent locking occurs, routine daily jaw function encourages the posterior attachment and collateral ligaments to accommodate to allow normal jaw opening and abatement of pain. Further adaptation

within the joint includes remodeling of the surfaces of the condyle, fossa, and articular eminence, with corresponding radiographic changes. Disk perforation may cause degenerative changes and coarse crepitus upon opening and closing. Successful remodeling allows patients to regain normal opening with minimal pain, but joint noise often persists. Sometimes, however, bony degenerative changes progress with severe erosion, loss of vertical dimension, occlusal changes, worsened joint and muscle pain, and greatly compromised jaw function.

The genesis of disk disorders and TMJ arthralgia has been at least partially attributed to abnormal biomechanical forces on the condyle, which alter the shape, form, and function of articular tissues. Friction due to abnormal jaw function and malposition of the disk may exacerbate both jaw displacement and changes to the form and function of the disk. In other cases, a blow to the jaw, inadvertent biting of a hard object, or abnormal chewing may be inciting factors. Occasionally, whiplash injury contributes to TMJ arthralgia and disk displacement.

Disk displacements are common in the general population, but those affected generally function adequately without treatment. When a patient seeks help for asymptomatic TMJ noises, continued observation, education about the condition, and self-care are sufficient (Table 19–1). Pain, intermittent locking, and difficulty using the jaw mandate closer observation and possible intervention.

TMJ subluxation or dislocation with or without a disk displacement is characterized by hypermobility of the joint due to laxity of the ligaments. It may be provoked in the dental office when the mouth is held open for an extended period, particularly in patients with systemic hypermobility. The condyle is anteriorly dislocated with respect to the disk and articular eminence, unable to return to the closed position because normal posterior translation is blocked. In most cases, the condyle can be moved laterally or medially by the patient or clinician to disengage the locking and allow normal closure. If the lock cannot be immediately disengaged, jaw manipulation inferiorly and anteriorly may be required before it can glide posteriorly.

Osteoarthritis of the TMJ involves degenerative changes of the articular surfaces of the joint that cause crepitus, jaw dysfunction, and radiographic changes. In osteoarthritis, pain, inflammation, and tenderness of the joint accompany the degenerative changes. Osteoarthritis can occur at any stage of a disk displacement as well as after trauma, infection, and other insults to the integrity of the joint, or with rheumatic or other conditions that cause polyarthritis. The latter include disorders such as systemic osteoarthritis, rheumatoid arthritis, psoriasis, lupus erythematosus, scleroderma, Sjögren syndrome, and hyperuricemia. A rheumatology consultation

Table 19–1. Self-Care for Masticatory Arthralgia and Myalgia.[a]

1. Apply moist heat or cold to the joint or muscles that are tender, whichever feels better. Either can reduce joint or muscle pain and relax the muscles. Apply heat for 20 minutes to the painful area several times daily. Microwave a wet towel until it is warm, and wrap it around a hot water bottle to keep it warm longer. For cold, use ice wrapped in a thin washcloth for 10 minutes several times each day (apply it to the painful area just before the onset of numbness).
2. Eat a softer diet. Avoid hard foods, such as hard bread or bagels. Avoid chewy food, such as steak or candy. Cut fruits and steam vegetables and cut them in small pieces. Chew with your back teeth rather than biting with your front teeth. Avoid chewing gum.
3. Chew your food on both sides at the same time or alternate sides to reduce strain on one side.
4. Keep your tongue up, teeth apart, and jaw relaxed. Place your tongue lightly on the palate behind your upper front teeth, allowing the teeth to come apart, and relax the jaw muscles. The upper and lower teeth should not touch at rest, except occasionally with swallowing. Monitor your jaw position during the day to keep it in a relaxed, comfortable position.
5. Avoid caffeine. Caffeine has effects in causing increased jaw tension and may disrupt sleep. This may contribute to jaw pain and headaches from overuse or withdrawal. Caffeine is present in coffee, tea, soda, and chocolate.
6. Avoid oral habits that strain the jaw muscles and joints. These include teeth clenching, teeth grinding (bruxism), teeth touching or resting together, biting the cheeks, pushing the tongue against the teeth, jaw tensing, and biting objects. Replace these habits with proper tongue position on the palate.
7. Avoid resting your jaw on your hand to reduce strain on the TMJ and maintain jaw muscles in a rest position.
8. Avoid activities that involve excessive or prolonged wide opening of the jaw (eg, yawning and prolonged dental treatments) for a period of time until the pain has been reduced.
9. Avoid stomach sleeping, which puts adverse forces on the jaw and neck muscles.
10. Use anti-inflammatory medications, such as ibuprofen and aspirin (without caffeine), to reduce TMJ and muscle pain.

[a]This program is typically provided to all patients with a temporomandibular disorder at their initial visit to encourage healing within the muscles and joints.
TMJ, temporomandibular joint.

is indicated if the joint, consistent with other joints, are painful and swollen, red, stiff, or crepitant.

Other temporomandibular joint disorders include ankylosis, traumatic injuries and fractures, neoplasms, and developmental abnormalities. Ankylosis or total lack of joint movement can be due to osseous or fibrous attachment of the condyle to the fossa. Extracapsular conditions, such as coronoid process interference or muscle contracture, can also cause significant jaw limitation. Traumatic injuries usually result in either a contusion with joint hemorrhage, a sprain with tearing of the joint capsule and ligaments, or a fracture of the condylar neck or head or of the external auditory canal. TMJ injuries are usually accompanied by pain and limited range of motion. Developmental abnormalities, primary benign and malignant tumors, myxoma, fibrous dysplasia, and metastasis or local extension of neighboring malignancies to the TMJ can also occur but are rare.

C. Other Causes of Orofacial Pain

Periodontal ligament pain is characteristic of deep somatic pain of the musculoskeletal type and is from repetitive strain to the periodontal ligaments through clenching, gross occlusal prematurities, or trauma to the teeth.

Periodontal ligament pain is generally a dull aching pain in and around the teeth and can affect multiple teeth. Inflammatory fluid accumulation may cause displacement of the tooth in its socket with a resulting acute malocclusion and pain. The most common sign is tenderness of the teeth to percussion in the absence of pulpitis or periapical or periodontal abscess. Treatment consists of placing a splint and reducing oral habits.

Neuropathic facial or dental pain is a continuous, daily pain often described as a burning or tingling that is limited to a specific nerve distribution. Historically, the pain usually begins following surgery or injury of the face, teeth, or gums but continues despite healing and the absence of a demonstrable etiology. Anesthetic nerve blocks can be used diagnostically to decrease the pain for the duration of the anesthetic. Anticonvulsants, tricyclic antidepressants, and other medications traditionally used for neuropathic pain can be of help.

Complete or incomplete tooth fractures can cause persistent tooth pain that is difficult to diagnose. Pain can result when the pulp is exposed from fractures to the enamel and dentin that become displaced when mechanical strain is placed on the tooth. Diagnosis is difficult, particularly if an incomplete fracture is present, but can be made by visual inspection, exploration of the tooth for loose fragments, tooth mobility tests, tooth discoloration, and tooth provocation tests that cause pain when the fractured segment is moved. The pulps of these teeth may or may not respond to an electric pulp test or to thermal testing. Fractures need to be treated with temporary banding, crowns, or endodontic treatment.

Pulpitis and periodontal pathology can present a diagnostic dilemma if it refers pain to areas that are distant from the involved tooth. Although not common, patients may complain of a toothache in a tooth that responds normally to all available tests. Further pulp testing or radiographs reveal that an adjacent tooth or other distant tooth or periodontal structure is inflamed. Subsequent treatment to the inflamed tooth resolves the referred pain.

Sympathetically maintained pain is often characterized by a constant burning sensation that is frequently associated with a prior history of tissue damage. The main clinical features include pain described as burning and continuous, exacerbated by movement, cutaneous stimulation, or stress, with onset usually weeks after injury. Confirmation and treatment of early cases of sympathetically maintained pain of the tooth or facial area is achieved by stellate ganglion blockade of the sympathetic nerve input to the painful region. Chronic cases are often considered permanent with pain relief achieved by pharmacologic medications, such as tricyclic antidepressants, clonidine, gabapentin, or carbamezapine.

Burning mouth syndrome is typically characterized by a burning sensation as if the mouth or tongue were scalded or on fire and can accompany other oral complaints, including xerostomia and dysgeusia. The oral tissue often appears normal. There are many factors that can cause burning mouth syndrome, including candidiasis, painful geographic or fissured tongue as well as parafunctional habits, allergies, xerostomia, and injury following dental treatment. Systemic disease and medication side effects have also been shown to cause burning mouth either directly or indirectly from the resultant xerostomia that may be present. Thus, it is not as difficult to diagnose a condition as burning mouth syndrome as it is to identify the underlying cause that will suggest a treatment.

Dionne RA. Pharmacologic advances in orofacial pain: from molecules to medicine. *J Dent Educ.* 2001;65:1393. [PMID: 11780658]

Dworkin SF et al. A randomized clinical trial of a tailored comprehensive care treatment program for temporomandibular disorders. *J Orofac Pain.* 2002;16:259. [PMID: 12455427]

Fricton J. Atypical orofacial pain disorders: a study of diagnostic subtypes. *Curr Rev Pain.* 2000;4:142. [PMID: 10998727]

Forssell H et al. Application of principles of evidence-based medicine to occlusal treatment of temporomandibular disorders: are

there lessons to be learned? *J Orofac Pain.* 2004;18:9. [PMID: 15022533]

Milam SB. Pathogenesis of degenerative temporomandibular joint arthritides. *Odontology.* 2005;93:7. [16170470]

Complications

The most significant complication associated with orofacial pain is the relationship between the development of chronic pain, depression, and related lifestyle problems. Recent studies show that some, but not all, patients with chronic pain are depressed, with over 30% having major depressive disorders. Thus, it appears that there is a subgroup of patients with chronic pain who are depressed and have severe pain and lifestyle limitations, such as difficulty using the jaw, home or work disability, task avoidance, and sleep disturbance. It is possible that depression may intensify pain and cause increased suffering, disturbances in lifestyle, and therefore be a risk factor for development of chronic pain.

Treatment

Management of all patients with orofacial pain from temporomandibular disorders aims to (1) reduce or eliminate pain, (2) restore normal jaw function, (3) reduce the need for future health care, and (4) restore normal lifestyle functioning. Specific interventions and their sequencing parallel treatment of musculoskeletal disorders in general. A key determinant of success in chronic pain management is the success in educating the patient about the disorder to enhance adherence to the self-care aspects of management, including jaw exercises, habit change, and proper use of the jaw. The treatments included here are supported by randomized controlled trials.

A. SELF-CARE

Most acute temporomandibular disorder symptoms are self-limited and resolve with minimal intervention. Therefore, initial treatment for masticatory myalgia and arthralgia should be a self-care program (Table 19–1) to reduce repetitive strain of the masticatory system and encourage relaxation and healing of the muscles and joints. Most patients respond well to self-care in 4 to 6 weeks; if not, further assessment and treatment are indicated.

B. ORTHOPEDIC INTRA-ORAL SPLINTS

The two most common splints include the anterior positioning splint and the stabilization splint and both have evidence to support their efficacy. The anterior repositioning splint places a patient's mandible and TMJ into an anterior position so as to reduce a TMJ click that occurs on opening and closing of the jaw. The anterior repositioning splint is typically placed on the maxillary arch with an anterior ramp that first engages mandibular teeth on initial closure and shifts the jaw forward into final closure, when all mandibular teeth contact the splint. The stabilization splint provides a flat passive occlusal surface that is adjusted with contact on all short-term posterior teeth to allow passive protection of the jaw and reduction of oral habits. Although both splints can reduce temporomandibular disorder symptoms, the indications for each differ somewhat.

Anterior repositioning splints can be efficacious for intermittent jaw locking with limited range of motion, especially upon awakening, or for persistent TMJ arthralgia not responsive to other therapy (including a stabilization splint). They are recommended only for short-term, part-time use, primarily during sleep, because they can cause occlusal changes if worn continuously or long term.

The stabilization splint is most efficacious for masticatory myalgia and TMJ arthralgia, especially if the pain is worse upon awakening. This type of splint can also be used during the day for oral habit management. Such splints are designed to provide postural stabilization and to protect the TMJ, muscles, and teeth.

Partial coverage splints may cause occlusal changes in some patients. All splints should cover all of the mandibular or maxillary teeth to prevent movement of uncovered teeth, with malocclusion. The splint's occlusal surface can be adjusted to provide a stable occlusal posture by creating single contacts in all posterior teeth in the habitual closure position.

C. Cognitive-Behavioral Therapy

Approaches to changing maladaptive habits and behaviors, such as jaw tensing and clenching and grinding of the teeth, are important in treating painful tissues. Cognitive-behavioral therapies, such as habit reversal, biofeedback, relaxation techniques, and stress management, can be effective alone or in conjunction with other treatments.

Behavior modification strategies, such as habit reversal, are the most common techniques used to change these habits. Although many simple habits are easily abandoned when the patient becomes aware of them, changing persistent habits requires a structured program that is facilitated by a clinician trained in behavioral strategies.

Habit correction can be accomplished by (1) becoming more aware of the habit, (2) knowing how to correct it (ie, what to do with the teeth and tongue), and (3) knowing why to correct it. When this knowledge is combined with a commitment to conscientious self-monitoring and a focus upon the goal, most habits will change. Supplemental behavioral strategies, such as biofeedback, may also be helpful.

Even when clenching is unconscious or nocturnal, correcting it during the day may help reduce it at night. Splints may also increase patients' awareness of oral habits. If muscle tensing is the inciting factor, biofeedback and relaxation techniques may be indicated. Another major issue to address is pacing or hurrying related to a busy day. For triggers such as depression and anxiety, psychological therapy can helpful. If the problem is a sleep disorder, sleep hygiene self-care can be instituted by the psychologist for nonpathologic sleep disturbances, or the patient can be referred to a sleep laboratory for more detailed evaluation.

D. Pharmacotherapy

Common medications used for temporomandibular disorder pain are classified as nonsteroidal anti-inflammatory drugs (NSAIDs), corticosteroids, opioids, muscle relaxants, anxiolytics, hypnotics, and antidepressants. Analgesics are used to allay pain; muscle relaxants and anxiolytics for anxiety, fear, and muscle tension; hypnotics for enhancing sleep; and antidepressants for pain, depression, and with certain agents, insomnia.

Randomized controlled trials of NSAIDs for temporomandibular disorder suggest adopting a low threshold for their use as a supplement to self-care. Long-term NSAID use is best approached with caution due to their systemic and gastrointestinal effects. For more severe joint inflammatory symptoms, corticosteroids are effective in TMJ synovitis, either as brief, tapering oral doses ("dose packs"), injected, or given via iontophoresis. Injection of hyaluronic acid is as effective as corticosteroid injections without being associated with higher risk of degenerative joint disease. Repeated injections of corticosteroids can lead to chondrocyte apoptosis and acceleration of the degenerative process.

For myalgia, especially with limited opening, NSAIDs and benzodiazepines are effective. Cyclobenzaprine has also been shown, in clinical trials of muscle pain, to be effective in reducing pain and improving sleep.

In patients with chronic pain due to a temporomandibular disorder, tricyclic antidepressants, such as 10 to 25 mg of amitriptyline or nortriptyline at night with gradual titration, significantly ameliorate insomnia, anxiety, and pain. These medications can be used long term. Selective serotonin reuptake inhibitors should be used with caution in patients with temporomandibular disorder since these agents may increase masticatory parafunctional muscle tension and aggravate muscle pain.

E. Physical Medicine

Physical medicine interventions can be efficacious for patients with temporomandibular disorder (TMD) pain and restricted motion. Jaw exercise is the primary and often the only physical medicine treatment required. Jaw exercises include relaxation, rotation, stretching (range of motion), isometric exercise, and postural exercise.

Stretching exercises, together with cold or heat, are effective in reducing pain and improving range of motion. Their benefit is enhanced when incorporated into the patient's daily routine in conjunction with relaxation techniques and a relaxed posture to reduce strain from sustained jaw contraction.

If exercises are ineffective or worsen pain, other physical modalities can be considered: ultrasonography, shortwave diathermy, low-intensity laser, pulsed diathermy, iontophoresis, phonophoresis, superficial heat, cryotherapy (cold), and massage have all demonstrated efficacy. In the short term, such modalities can reduce jaw pain and increase range of motion, thereby allowing jaw exercises to proceed. When range of motion of the jaw is restricted by a TMJ disk displacement without reduction, short-term manipulation of the jaw by a physical therapist or self-mobilization by the patient can help in remodeling the disk to improve joint translation, range of motion, and pain.

F. Surgery

If persistent pain is localized to the TMJ and is associated with specific structural changes in the joint, surgical intervention can be considered if comprehensive non-surgical care is unsuccessful. Muscle pain and associated contributing factors should be addressed and controlled prior to TMJ surgery. In general, the less invasive surgeries are as effective as those that are more invasive, so the health care provider should consider an arthrocentesis or arthroscopic procedure before more invasive interventions, such as diskectomy or disk repair. Postoperative management includes appropriate medications, physical therapy, splint therapy when indicated, and continued behavioral treatment as appropriate.

G. Dental Treatment

There is no consistent evidence from randomized controlled trials with persistent TMD that altering the occlusion through occlusal adjustment will benefit temporo-mandibular disorders. Likewise, other dental treatments, such as prosthodontic and orthodontic treatments, are not recommended as a primary treatment for the management or prevention of TMD. However, patients with TMD may require these procedures as part of normal dental care. In these cases, care should be exercised to minimize additional strain to the muscles and joints and aggravation of an existing TMD during these procedures.

Prognosis

As treatment approaches are better defined and validated through clinical trials, triaging patients to appropriate treatment strategies will most likely result in improved, more predictable outcomes. However, patients with similar diagnoses may have quite different histories, contributing factors, and outcomes. In some cases, the causative web of persistent pain is complex, and unraveling it may require a team that includes a dentist, physician, physical therapist, health psychologist, or other health professionals. Factors such as depression, fibromyalgia, and secondary gain may play a role in delaying recovery leading to chronic pain. Patients with chronic temporomandibular disorder, like others with chronic pain, bear witness to the fact that chronic pain is a disease whose remission depends on timely and appropriate application of drug and nondrug therapies.

Al-Ani MZ et al. Stabilisation splint therapy for temporomandibular pain dysfunction syndrome. *Cochrane Database Syst Rev.* 2004;(1):CD002778. [PMID: 14973990]

Crider AB et al. A meta-analysis of EMG biofeedback treatment of temporomandibular disorders. *J Orofacial Pain.* 1999;13:29.

Forssell H et al. Application of principles of evidence-based medicine to occlusal treatment of temporomandibular disorders: are there lessons to be learned? *J Orofacial Pain.* 2004;18:9. [PMID: 15022533]

Koh H et al. Occlusal adjustment for treating and preventing temporomandibular joint disorders. *Cochrane Database Syst Rev.* 2003;(1):CD003812. [PMID: 12535488]

Pain in HIV & AIDS

 20

Gaurav Mathur, MD & Peter A. Selwyn, MD, MPH

ESSENTIALS OF DIAGNOSIS

- *HIV-related pain can be as severe as cancer pain, and treatment should be aggressive.*
- *HIV-related pain is often underdiagnosed and undertreated.*
- *Pain can be a result of opportunistic illness, HIV therapy, or the HIV virus itself.*
- *Pain management should be accompanied with primary therapy for the causative illness whenever possible.*

■ REVIEW OF HIV/AIDS

General Considerations

A. EPIDEMIOLOGY

An estimated 38 million people are infected with HIV worldwide. More than 20 million people have died of HIV or AIDS since it was first identified in 1981. The rate of infection continues to climb at a staggering pace. In 2003, five million people were newly infected. Public health workers struggle to control the epidemic while clinicians struggle to manage its devastating consequences for patients and their families: preventing and treating opportunistic infections, maintaining quality of life through increasingly sophisticated but complicated medications, and ensuring adequate social support. The task is even more daunting in HIV-infected patients who suffer from substance abuse, psychiatric illness, and marginalization due to race, gender, and poverty.

B. ETIOLOGY

Pain is one of the most common symptoms in persons with HIV and AIDS. Pain affects up to 90% of all HIV-infected patients and is often severe. It is disappointingly undertreated, and many patients never receive effective pain management. There are many obstacles to the ef-

fective assessment and treatment of HIV pain. Unlike illnesses that cause pain in a single identifiable pattern, HIV produces a multitude of pain syndromes from a variety of causes. Patients with HIV experience pain caused directly by opportunistic infections, by the virus itself, and by antiretroviral treatment.

HIV-infected patients are susceptible to a variety of **opportunistic infections and malignancies,** and many of these illnesses are painful. Most of these illnesses are uncommon in the general population; moreover, opportunistic illnesses may present in different ways in different patients, fooling even the most skilled of clinicians.

Even in the absence of opportunistic infection, **the HIV virus itself can cause pain and painful sequelae**. HIV can cause painful arthritis and avascular necrosis of certain joints. HIV also directly infects the nervous system and causes painful neuropathies. Neurologic findings can be subtle; repeated assessments may be necessary to pinpoint the cause.

Unfortunately, **antiretroviral treatments** for HIV can also induce pain. Specifically, stavudine, didanosine, and zalcitabine (the latter now rarely used) have all been found to cause a painful distal symmetric polyneuropathy. Many of the antiretrovirals can induce potentially painful syndromes such as hepatitis and pancreatitis, making the treatment of HIV even more difficult.

Pain in HIV-Infected Women

HIV-infected women are at greater risk for gynecologic illnesses than nonHIV-infected women. Human papillomavirus can cause cervical dysplasia and cervical cancer, and HIV-infected women are more at risk for human papillomavirus infection and its sequelae. Pelvic inflammatory disease and many sexually transmitted diseases are also more common in HIV-infected women. Many of these illnesses are very painful. The clinician should make every effort to evaluate the patient for gynecologic illness in the pain assessment.

HIV Pain & Substance Abuse

Injection drug use has become one of the highest exposure risk categories for HIV transmission in recent years.

Patients who have a history of substance abuse are often the most challenging patients to treat. The clinician must balance the critical need for effective pain management against the consequences of substance abuse, especially when deciding whether to prescribe opioids. There are numerous issues that cause concern, such as the risk of drug diversion by the patient, the fear that patients will use prescribed opioids to get high, and the fear that patients are lying about their pain to obtain opioids simply to feed their addiction. In addition, patients who are tolerant to large doses of opioids generally require much higher doses than opioid-naive patients.

Furthermore, clinicians may be concerned about law enforcement agencies targeting well-intentioned clinicians for prescribing opioids that were eventually diverted without the knowledge of the prescriber. It is not surprising, therefore, that pain in HIV-infected patients with current or past substance abuse is woefully undertreated. In order to effectively treat these patients, clinicians should use a variety of strategies (Table 20–1), keeping in mind the principles of sound prescribing, knowledge of legal issues in prescribing, and a commitment to reduce suffering in all patients.

Table 20–1. Approach to Pain Management in Substance Abusers with HIV Disease.

- Substance abusers with HIV disease deserve pain control; clinicians have an obligation to treat pain and suffering in all patients.
- Accept and respect the report of pain.
- Be careful about the label "substance abuse"; distinguish between tolerance, physical dependence, and addiction (psychological dependence or drug abuse).
- Not all substance abusers are the same; distinguish between active users, individuals in methadone maintenance, and those in recovery.
- Individualize pain treatment.
- Use the principles of pain management outlined in analgesic ladder established by the World Health Organization (see Figure 3–1).
- Establish clear goals and conditions for opioid therapy: Set limits, recognize drug abuse behaviors, make consequences clear, use written contracts, and establish a single prescriber.
- Use a multidimensional strategy, including pharmacologic and nonpharmacologic interventions, attention to psychosocial issues, and a team approach.

Reprinted with permission from Breitbart W et al. *Oncology.* 2002;16:964.

Palliative Care for AIDS

Patients with AIDS can benefit greatly from palliative care. The recognition that the illness is beyond cure allows clinicians to focus on quality of life and thereby ease suffering. Relief of pain, dyspnea, nausea, diarrhea, and depression are examples of ways in which suffering can be improved. Antiretroviral therapy can have a great impact on health early in the course of the illness; however, as HIV infection progresses to AIDS, the side effects of highly active antiretroviral therapy (eg, diarrhea or pancreatitis), can become very troublesome. In many cases, discussing whether to discontinue antiretroviral therapy may be worthwhile, especially if a multidrug-resistant virus is suspected. Other medications can also be discontinued if burdens of treatment outweigh the benefits. At the very end of life, patients with AIDS may resemble those with cancer. Cachexia and wasting are common, and patients become severely debilitated. Oral intake is limited, consciousness declines, and breathing becomes labored and distressed. Patients may experience great pain and agitation. Just as in patients with cancer, clinicians should make every effort to keep patients with AIDS as comfortable as possible while making sure that dignity is preserved.

Clinicians should discuss goals of care with their patients, including such issues as whether or not to resuscitate in the event of death, who the patient's health care agent should be in case the patient is incapacitated, and whether or not the patient would desire artificial nutrition and hydration. It is not possible to prepare for every medical scenario, but with some clear guidelines and communication, most patients can make their wishes known. A clear and honest description of prognosis is essential to this discussion. It is also important to have these discussions early; do not wait until the patient is seriously ill to discuss how to treat serious illness.

Principles of Pain Management in HIV

The principles of pain management in HIV/AIDS are similar to those of every patient. Often, the most difficult task is simply the recognition of how severe HIV-related pain can be. Evidence demonstrates that clinicians usually underestimate and, consequently, undertreat pain.

Many patients whose pain is initially mild experience worsening of pain with disease progression. Clinicians must be empathic to their illness and use a multimodality strategy, including pharmacotherapy, interventional procedures, psychological treatment, and complementary/alternative treatment when appropriate. Most importantly, clinicians should advise patients that pain in HIV is common, but effective pain control is possible in the vast majority of cases.

The treatment of HIV-related pain must include **primary therapy** as well as direct pain management. Primary therapy refers to treatment of HIV disease and HIV-related complications, notably painful opportunistic infections and malignancies (eg, amphotericin B for cryptococcal infection, radiotherapy for Kaposi sarcoma.) Many opportunistic illnesses improve and pain management may be temporary; other illnesses, such as peripheral neuropathy, generally persist and pain management will be ongoing. Effective primary therapy usually substantially reduces the accompanying pain. Clinicians should be mindful that antiretrovirals—the primary therapy for HIV disease—may cause painful conditions.

In addition, **direct pain management** with opioids and other therapies should be thoughtfully applied to treat the pain that accompanies the primary illness. An "analgesic ladder" has been developed by the World Health Organization for the treatment of pain (see Figure 3–1). This set of guidelines suggests the initial use of nonsteroidal anti-inflammatory drugs (NSAIDs) or acetaminophen for mild pain and strongly supports the role of opioids in the treatment of moderate to severe pain (see Chapter 3).

For both pain and other symptoms commonly seen in palliative care, it is also important to recognize the unique possibilities for drug-drug interactions between medications used for pain and palliative care and those used for HIV-specific and related anti-infective therapy. For example, several of the nonnucleoside reverse transcriptase inhibitors (eg, nevirapine, efavirenz) as well as the rifamycins, which are used to treat mycobacterial infections, are potent inhibitors of the cytochrome P-450 enzyme system in the liver. Several of the protease inhibitors (eg, ritonavir, indivanir, saquinavir) are inhibitors of the P-450 enzyme system or its subunits to varying degrees. These pharmacologic properties may affect the metabolism of certain opioids (eg, methadone), antidepressants (eg, tricyclic antidepressants), anticonvulsants (eg, phenytoin), or other drugs when these are used together with the HIV-related medications. It is not possible to keep track of all the individual interactions, but it is important to be aware that these must be considered when providing both palliative and disease-specific care to patients with HIV/AIDS. Clinicians are strongly urged to use available print and Internet-based resources to check for drug-drug interactions in this setting (see below).

Montessori V et al. Adverse effects of antiretroviral therapy for HIV infection. *CMAJ.* 2004;170:229. [PMID: 14734438]

O'Neill JF, Selwyn PA, Schietinger H, eds. *A Clinical Guide to Palliative and Supportive Care for HIV/AIDS.* Rockville, MD: Health Resources and Services Administration, 2003.

Piscitelli SC et al. Interactions among drugs for HIV and opportunistic infections. *N Engl J Med.* 2001;344:984. [PMID: 11274626]

Yeni PG et al. Treatment for adult HIV infection: 2004 recommendations of the International AIDS Society-USA Panel. *JAMA.* 2004;292:251. [PMID: 15249575]

World Health Organization. *Cancer Pain Relief.* Geneva: WHO, 1986. AIDS *info* http://www.aidsinfo.nih.gov Web-based resource for up-to-date HIV treatment consensus guidelines as well as information about drug-drug interactions and links to other resources.

■ PAIN SYNDROMES IN HIV

Organ systems that are often affected by pain syndromes include neurologic, musculoskeletal, gastrointestinal, and dermatologic. Often several painful processes may coexist, making assessment more complex. Clinicians who make a skillful and comprehensive assessment can relieve much of the pain associated with HIV.

NEUROLOGICALLY RELATED PAIN SYNDROMES

Virtually all HIV-infected patients have some degree of involvement of the central nervous system or peripheral nervous system, or both, and most will have some neurologic illness during the course of the disease. Patients may be affected by pain caused directly by the effects of the virus or pain due to opportunistic infections and malignancies that affect the nervous system. Medications and treatments can also cause neurologic pain.

1. Headache

Headache is commonly seen in patients with HIV/AIDS (Table 20–2). Headache can signify a wide spectrum of illnesses, from benign causes, such as tension headache, to severe and life-threatening illness, such as toxoplasmosis. The clinician must include a wide differential diagnosis. It is important to recognize that several etiologies may coexist to cause headache. Some causes of headache in immunocompetent persons may present more frequently in HIV-infected persons.

Diagnosing the cause of headache can be challenging. Benign illness, such as migraine, can present with severe headache, while the headache from a dangerous illness, such as cryptococcal infection, may be mild. The quality and characteristics of the pain can sometimes be helpful, but they cannot be consistently relied upon for accurate diagnosis.

Diagnostic studies that are likely to be helpful include lumbar puncture, computed tomography (CT) scanning,

Table 20–2. Selected Causes of Headache in HIV Disease.

Illness	Clinical features	Diagnostic findings	Comments
Caused by HIV Disease			
Subacute encephalitis	Headache, confusion, memory loss, seizures, and progressive dementia weeks to months preceding death	CT and MRI scans show cortical atrophy. Elevated protein and pleocytosis on cerebrospinal fluid examination	May also be caused by cytomegalovirus
Atypical aseptic meningitis	Occurs early in illness, possibly immune mediated Fever Headache Photophobia Nuchal rigidity	Lymphocytic pleocytosis on cerebrospinal fluid examination	Does not occur in late stages of HIV illness
Caused by Opportunistic Cancer			
Primary central nervous system lymphoma	Headache, vomiting, mental status changes caused by increased intracranial pressure	MRI/CT with pathologic confirmation	Tends to develop in brain parenchyma
Metastatic central nervous system lymphoma	Headache, vomiting, mental status changes caused by increased intracranial pressure	MRI/CT with pathologic confirmation	Tends to be spinal epidural or meningeal in location Radiation may improve pain and other neurologic symptoms
Caused by Opportunistic Disease			
Toxoplasmosis	Headache Visual disturbance Cranial nerve palsies Motor or sensory disturbance. Seizures. Altered mental status progressing to coma and death	Ring-enhancing lesions on contrast CT or MRI Serology not helpful in AIDS patients	
Cryptococcal meningitis	Meningitic symptoms including headache, photophobia, nuchal rigidity Fever is often absent	Culture of cerebrospinal fluid, blood, or urine Cerebrospinal fluid latex agglutination generally positive	Pulmonary and systemic involvement may occur
Mycobacterium tuberculosis	Fever, headache, nausea, progressing to stupor, coma, and death	Low cerebrospinal fluid glucose, elevated cerebrospinal fluid protein, and lymphocytosis Polymerase chain reaction examination of cerebrospinal fluid	Abscesses may form in the brain parenchyma
Caused by Diagnosis and Treatment			
Medication induced	Usually self-limited, but sometimes persistent	Headache associated with medication initiation	Most common with zidovudine
Post lumbar puncture headache	Dull occipital pain beginning hours to days after lumbar puncture Nausea and dizziness may occur	Rule out more severe causes	Supine position may help Epidural blood patch in severe cases

CT, computed tomography; MRI, magnetic resonance imaging.

and magnetic resonance imaging (MRI). Clinical judgment is crucial in assessing which of these tests are necessary, keeping in mind that headache in the immunocompromised may need etiologic investigation even when mild.

Clinical Findings

HIV and cytomegalovirus can cause a **subacute encephalitis** that may progress over months. Headache, confusion, memory loss, seizures, and progressive dementia may develop in patients weeks to months preceding death. Cerebrospinal fluid examination findings are nonspecific but may include pleocytosis and elevated protein. CT or MRI may reveal cortical atrophy.

Aseptic meningitis is a common illness that may present in any but the late stages of HIV, suggesting that it may be an immune-mediated disease. It commonly presents during primary HIV infection. Symptoms include headache, photophobia, and lymphocytic pleocytosis on cerebrospinal fluid examination.

Opportunistic cancers include primary B-cell (non-Hodgkins) lymphoma and systemic lymphoma with central nervous system involvement. Primary central nervous system lymphomas are much more commonly seen in HIV patients than in immunocompetent persons. The lymphoma causes a mass effect and consequent increased intracranial pressure. Presenting symptoms include focal neurologic deficits, including cranial nerve findings, headache, and seizure; papilledema may also be seen. In severe cases, herniation may occur with devastating consequences. Corticosteroids are helpful to reduce the mass effect. Radiation and chemotherapy can also be helpful. Systemic lymphoma may involve the central nervous system, most commonly, the leptomeninges, in about 20% of patients. Pain and other focal neurologic deficits may be alleviated by radiation. Rarely, Kaposi sarcoma involves the central nervous system.

Opportunistic infections are a common cause of headache and can be life threatening. **Toxoplasmosis** and **cryptococcal meningitis** are the two most common opportunistic causes of headache in the HIV-infected patient. *Toxoplasmosis gondii* accounts for 38% of all secondary central nervous system infections in AIDS patients and 28% of first seizures. The organism is a protozoan parasite, and infection occurs through ingestion of cat feces or undercooked meat, which should be avoided by immunocompromised patients and pregnant women because the illness is also dangerous to the fetus. Disease in HIV/AIDS patients is more often due to reactivation of a preexisting latent infection than to newly acquired infection. Generalized CNS symptoms, including headache, visual disturbance, cranial nerve palsies, motor or sensory disturbance, and seizures may develop. Mental status may be altered, with progression to coma and, if untreated, death. Serology is used in immunocompetent persons but is not helpful in AIDS patients. Instead, the cerebrospinal fluid may demonstrate lymphocytic pleocytosis and elevated protein levels. Contrast CT or MRI scans will demonstrate dense rounded lesions with characteristic ring enhancement.

Cryptococcus neoformans is a yeast-like fungus and is the leading cause of **meningitis** in HIV patients. Fever, nausea, vomiting, headache, altered mental status, and meningeal signs are common; seizures and focal neurologic deficits are not. Symptoms are thought to be due to generalized brain edema. Patients may have subacute disease for weeks or months before diagnosis. Culturing the cerebrospinal fluid, blood, or urine can help make the diagnosis; a cerebrospinal fluid latex agglutination test can provide a more rapid diagnosis. Pulmonary manifestations and systemic illness can also be present.

Syphilis is caused by *Treponema pallidum,* a spirochete bacteria with primary, secondary, and tertiary stages of infection. There are diverse clinical manifestations and the course may be accelerated in the presence of HIV. Neurosyphilis is generally diagnosed during the second or third stage of infection; presenting symptoms and signs include acute meningitis, deafness, stroke, or retinitis. Acute syphilitic meningitis may present with headache, neck stiffness, and cranial nerve lesions with occasional papilledema.

Tuberculosis is caused by *Mycobacterium tuberculosis;* transmission generally occurs through inhalation of aerosolized droplets. Although tuberculosis most commonly causes pneumonia, extrapulmonary manifestations are also common in HIV, including tuberculosis meningitis and brain abscesses. Like other forms of meningitis, tuberculosis meningitis is characterized by fever, stiff neck, and stupor that if untreated progresses to coma and death. Tubercle bacilli can form an abscess in the brain parenchyma that can also be very dangerous. Diagnosis is made by cerebrospinal fluid examination, but organisms may not be seen on smear or even culture. A low cerebrospinal fluid glucose, elevated cerebrospinal fluid protein, and lymphocytosis is suggestive. Polymerase chain reaction examination of cerebrospinal fluid is most helpful.

Antiretroviral therapy for HIV and AIDS, most notably zidovudine, can also cause headache. A history of headache that coincides with medication initiation may help guide the diagnosis. Headache is usually temporary and resolves with time, but some patients may have persistent pain. Other benign causes of headache include migraine, tension-type headache, and sinusitis; evidence suggests that migraine frequency may decrease and tension headache frequency may increase as HIV infection progresses.

Post lumbar puncture headache is typically described as a dull occipital discomfort that may radiate to the frontal head or to the shoulders. Nausea and dizziness are common, and in severe cases may be accompanied by vomiting and diaphoresis. In some patients, supine position may help alleviate the pain. Pain usually develops hours to several days after the procedure, and is believed to be related to a reduction in cerebrospinal fluid volume due to leakage through the dura. This complication can be reduced by using a small gauge spinal needle with a non cutting rounded tip and a lateral opening. If headache is persistent, an epidural "blood patch" may be used; several milliliters of autologous blood are obtained and sterilely injected into the epidural space at the site of the lumbar puncture.

Treatment

Treatment of headache should include primary therapy of the underlying illness as well as effective pain management. As in most illnesses, opioids are the mainstay of treatment, and patient-controlled analgesia is optimal in allowing the patient to participate in effective pain relief. In chronic headache, many adjuvants are available, including antidepressants, anticonvulsants, migraine-specific medications, and others (see Chapter 12). If HIV therapy is the cause of pain, the clinician should consider the benefits of changing therapies versus continuing the pain-producing medication and treating the headache.

2. Neuropathic Pain

Pain can be described as nociceptive or neuropathic. Nociceptive pain is thought to be maintained by ongoing tissue injury. In contrast, neuropathic pain is sustained by abnormal somatosensory processing due to damage to nerve tissue. It is typically characterized by the descriptions of burning and electric-type pain and is often accompanied by paresthesias and dysesthesias. On physical examination, the presence of allodynia (pain induced by nonpainful stimuli) and hyperalgesia (increased perception of painful stimuli) further suggests this diagnosis. Electrophysiologic nerve studies may reveal decreased conduction velocity, which is suggestive of demyelination, or decreased conduction amplitude, which is suggestive of axonopathy.

Clinical Findings

In HIV, neuropathic pain can be caused by a variety of illnesses (Table 20–3). In general, several different neuropathic syndromes tend to present at various times during the progression of HIV to AIDS. The syndromes can be polyneuropathies that affect many nerves in generally symmetric distributions (eg, stocking-glove pattern) or mononeuropathies that affect many nerves in patchy distributions, such as radiculopathies, plexopathies, and

Table 20–3. Causes of Neuropathic Illness in HIV and AIDS.

- Immune-mediated
- Infectious
  - HIV
  - Cytomegalovirus
  - Varicella-zoster virus
  - Hepatitis C virus
  - *Mycobacterium avium* complex
- Other illnesses
  - Diabetes mellitus
  - Alcoholism
  - Vitamin B_6 or B_{12} deficiency
- Antiretrovirals
  - Didanosine
  - Stavudine
  - Zalcitabine
- Other antimicrobials
  - Foscarnet
  - Dapsone
  - Metronidazole
  - Isoniazid
  - Rifampin
  - Ethionamide
  - Ethambutol
- Antineoplastics
  - Vincristine
  - Vinblastine
  - Paclitaxel

specific mononeuropathies. Depending on the type of nerve injury, patients may experience sensory changes, motor disturbances, or both. Pain is common in the distribution of the affected nerve(s); muscle tenderness and swelling may also be present.

In the acute seroconversion stage of HIV infection, some patients acquire an **acute inflammatory demyelinating polyneuropathy,** which is characterized by progressive distal weakness extending proximally in a pattern similar to Guillain-Barré syndrome (Table 20–4). Patients become areflexic, but there are minimal sensory changes. This illness is thought to be autoimmune mediated and is generally self-limited; however, in severe cases, treatment with plasmapheresis, intravenous immunoglobulin, and even corticosteroids may be required. Acute and chronic demyelinating polyneuropathies may continue to occur during the clinically latent phase of infection.

As the patient enters the transition phase to immunodeficiency, susceptibility develops to **zoster (shingles),** a painful sensory neuritis caused by reactivation of latent herpes zoster virus, often in the distribution of a

Table 20–4. Overview of Neuropathic Pain Syndromes in HIV and AIDS.

Type of neuropathy	Phase of HIV encountered	Mechanism	Clinical features	Comments
Acute inflammatory demyelinating polyneuropathy	Early (seroconversion)	Thought to be autoimmune mediated	Weakness extending proximally (similar to Guillain-Barré syndrome)	May require plasmapheresis, intravenous immunoglobulin, and cortico-steroids
Mononeuropathy multiplex	Early, immuno-competent	Autoimmune-mediated demyelination Vasculitis of vasa vasorum	Asymmetric, patchy sensory or motor deficits	
Zoster	Transition to immunodeficiency	Varicella-zoster virus reactivation	Burning pain in dermatomal distribution followed by vesicular rash	Postherpetic neuralgia may persist long after infection
Cytomegalovirus polyradiculopathy	Late	Cytomegalovirus	Pain in lumbosacral nerve root distributions	Ganciclovir may be helpful
Distal sensory polyneuropathy	Late	Axonal destruction by HIV	Ascending dysesthesias in stocking-glove pattern	Ventilatory impairment in severe cases

single dermatome. A vesicular eruption develops in a dermatomal pattern several days after the onset of pain. Although the infection is self-limited, treatment with antivirals can shorten the duration of pain. Postherpetic neuralgia is a feared complication of the neuritis and is often described as an intense burning pain that may persist long after the acute infection has healed. Opioids, tricyclic antidepressants, gabapentin, and topical lidocaine have been shown to be beneficial. Topical capsaicin may be of benefit but its side effect of burning limits its tolerability.

Mononeuropathy multiplex occurs in a patchy multifocal pattern, affecting the peripheral nervous tissue apparently in a random pattern. Demyelination is the underlying disorder in a subset of patients with mononeuropathy multiplex and is thought to be autoimmune mediated, (like the demyelinating neuropathies described above), and treatment is similar. A vasculitis of the vasa vasorum is responsible for the neuropathy in many of the remainder of patients with mononeuropathy multiplex; the underlying disorder may be polyarteritis nodosa or one of the connective tissue diseases.

The late phase of HIV is characterized by immunodeficiency and the progression to AIDS. Cytomegalovirus infection of the nerve roots may develop and result in **cytomegalovirus polyradiculopathy,** which can cause severe pain in lumbar and sacral nerve root distributions. The illness may progress to involve the cauda equina. Ganciclovir can help arrest the disorder.

Distal sensory polyneuropathy is the most commonly seen neuropathic pain syndrome in patients with HIV or AIDS. It usually occurs relatively late in the course of the illness. Patients generally report onset of a tingling, prickly sensation on the soles of the feet or the tips of the toes. As illness progresses, sensation is lost in an ascending fashion, first throughout the foot, and motor deficits may follow. Ankle jerk reflex is generally lost, and by the time sensory disturbances reach the upper shin, similar dysesthesias may be noted in the fingertips. This distribution is a result of axonal destruction and is directly related to the length of the axon. In severe cases, disease may progress so proximally that ventilatory function may be impaired.

Treatment

The treatment of neuropathic pain in HIV is similar to treatment of neuropathic pain in immunocompetent patients. Many adjuvant medications exist for the treatment of neuropathic pain in conjunction with opioids (see Chapter 10). An anticonvulsant (such as lamotrigine, gabapentin, carbamazepine) or, less commonly, one of the tricyclic antidepressants can usually be used with moderate to good results. Selective serotonin reuptake inhibitors (SSRIs), serotonin-norepinephrine reuptake inhibitors (SNRIs), corticosteroids, and N-methyl-D-aspartate (NMDA) receptor agonists can also be used in the treatment of neuropathic pain (see Chapter 10). Experimental studies with recombinant nerve growth factor suggested possible efficacy, but this product is not in commercial development at this time. Recent preliminary studies have suggested possible benefit from a transdermal capsaicin patch in the treatment of chronic neuropathic pain in AIDS.

Primary therapy with antiretrovirals may halt the progression of neurologic damage and arrest the worsening neuropathic pain. However, in some cases, antiretrovirals may be the cause of the neuropathy and may need to be discontinued. In the case of neuropathy caused by viral or other infectious illness, primary treatment of the infection will often help improve the pain.

Belman AL. HIV-1 infection and AIDS. *Neurol Clin.* 2002;20:983. [PMID: 12616678]

Keswani SC et al. Incidence of and risk factors for HIV-associated distal sensory polyneuropathy. *Neurology.* 2003;61:279. [PMID: 12874429]

MUSCULOSKELETAL PAIN SYNDROMES

Patients with HIV infection are at risk for painful illnesses arising in the musculoskeletal system (Tables 20–5 and 20–6). Presentations vary according to risk factors and stage of HIV infection. Pain may arise due to direct injury from HIV virus, from opportunistic illness, or from primary antiretroviral therapy. Familiarity with these pain syndromes can allow a skilled clinician to treat the underlying source of pain effectively. Note that while NSAIDs are often used to treat the inflammatory component of illness, they may not be efficacious for pain management. Opioids should be used whenever necessary to treat moderate to severe pain.

1. Muscular Pain Syndromes

Polymyositis, also known as idiopathic inflammatory myositis, is characterized by weakness in the proximal muscles, usually in the shoulder girdle and hips. It generally occurs in the early stages of HIV disease. Insidious

Table 20–5. Painful HIV-Related Muscular Illnesses.

Illness	Etiology	HIV stage	Clinical features	Diagnostic findings	Treatment
Polymyositis (idiopathic inflammatory myositis)	Unclear	Occurs early in HIV illness	Insidious onset Muscle weakness and aching in shoulder girdle and hips Muscle tenderness and wasting	ESR and CPK may be elevated MRI, EMG, and muscle biopsy may be helpful	Anti-inflammatories or corticosteroids or both
Zidovudine-induced myopathy	Zidovudine-induced mitochondrial effects	Occurs early in HIV illness	Similar to polymyositis	Similar to polymyositis (muscle biopsy can distinguish between the two)	Cessation of zidovudine
Pyomyositis	Bacterial, commonly *Staphylococcus aureus*	Occurs late in HIV illness	Fevers and cramp-like pain, progression to abscess, septic shock, and death	MRI and CT scanning	Antibiotics Surgical drainage

ESR, erythrocyte sedimentation rate; CPK, creatine phosphokinase; MRI, magnetic resonance imaging; CT, computed tomography.

Table 20–6. Painful HIV-Related Skeletal Illness.

Illness	Clinical features	Diagnostic findings	Treatment
HIV arthralgia	Acute joint pain, commonly in the knee Often occurs at time of primary HIV infection	Physical examination, aspiration, and radiography are normal	Self-limited
HIV arthritis	Acute onset, persists for 1 week to 6 months Generally in the knees and ankles	Synovial biopsy demonstrates chronic mononuclear cell infiltrate	Intra-articular corticosteroid injection or NSAIDs
Acute symmetric polyarthritis	Ulnar deviation and swan neck deformities in the hands Acute onset	Radiography shows joint space narrowing and periarticular osteopenia Rheumatoid factor negative	NSAIDs are primary therapy
Reactive arthritis and psoriatic arthritis	Moderate to severe arthralgias in feet and ankles de Quervain, Achilles, and rotator cuff tendinitis "AIDS foot"	Clinical diagnosis Psoriatic skin rashes distinguish psoriatic arthritis	NSAIDs are primary therapy
Hypertrophic osteoarthropathy	Lower extremity pain, nonpitting edema, clubbing Warm edematous shiny skin Commonly associated with *Pneumocystis jiroveci* pneumonia	Radiography: periosteal changes in the long bones	Treatment of underlying pulmonary infection
Septic arthritis and bursitis	Monoarticular pain and fever, often hips and knees Usually caused by *Staphylococcus aureus* Bursitis commonly in the olecranon and prepatellar bursae	Plain films MRI Joint aspirate	Antibiotics Surgical debridement Drainage
Osteomyelitis	Fever, chills, pain, and bony tenderness Many different causative bacteria	Blood cultures, bone aspirate, elevated ESR MRI is the best test	Antibiotics Surgical drainage
Osteonecrosis (avascular necrosis)	Intermittent deep throbbing pain, progressively worsening Possible association with protease inhibitors	MRI is the most sensitive test	Physical therapy Reduced weight bearing Surgical intervention in advanced cases

NSAIDs, nonsteroidal anti-inflammatory drugs; MRI, magnetic resonance imaging; ESR, erythrocyte sedimentation rate.

muscle weakness, fatigue, and aching pain in the affected muscles develop first, although pain is commonly absent. Muscle tenderness and wasting can be found on physical examination, and erythrocyte sedimentation rate and creatine phosphokinase may be elevated. Presently, the etiology is unclear; however, evidence suggests that the illness may be due to either direct infection of muscle cells by HIV and subsequent cell death or by an autoimmune response to muscle cells harboring HIV; further studies are needed. MRI, electromyography, and muscle biopsy are generally helpful in making the diagnosis. Treatment usually includes anti-inflammatories or corticosteroids, or both. Zidovudine commonly causes a similar myopathy, possibly due to mitochondrial effects, and it may be difficult to distinguish zidovudine-induced myopathy from polymyositis; laboratory test results may also be similar. If suspected, a muscle biopsy can be helpful in distinguishing the illness. Cessation of zidovudine generally reverses the clinical findings.

Pyomyositis is an infection of skeletal muscle tissue. Until recently, it was only commonly found in sub-Saharan Africa but is now emerging in incidence in HIV-infected persons in the United States. It tends to occur relatively late in HIV illness, often after the development of AIDS, and is usually caused by *Staphylococcus aureus,* although other bacteria and mycobacteria have been implicated. Large muscle groups in the lower extremities are more commonly infected, especially the quadriceps. Usually, a cramp-like muscle pain, muscle stiffness, and low-grade fevers develop first. As infection progresses, high-grade fever develops and an abscess may develop within the muscle. The muscle then begins to necrose and sepsis ensues; septic shock and death may occur if left untreated. Early diagnosis is crucial; MRI and CT scanning can be helpful. Treatment consists of antibiotics and surgical drainage.

2. Skeletal Pain Syndromes

HIV arthralgia is a very common manifestation of HIV and can occur at almost any stage of the disease, commonly occurring at the time of primary infection. Most patients experience mild to moderate pain in one or several joints that can be persistent or migratory. The etiology is unclear but is believed not to be truly inflammatory in nature. Some patients may have an acute painful arthralgia that lasts less than 24 hours, most commonly in the knee. Although symptoms may mimic septic arthritis, examination, aspiration, and radiography of the knee are generally normal. The illness is generally self-limited.

HIV arthritis has been described as a self-limited subacute oligoarthritis that may persist from 1 week up to 6 months. Patients experience acute onset of joint pain, generally in the knees or the ankles. Synovial biopsy demonstrates a chronic mononuclear cell infiltrate; there

is debate as to whether the illness is caused by direct HIV infection of the synovial tissue or by reactive immune complexes within the synovium. Primary therapy may consist of intra-articular corticosteroid injection or NSAIDs; opioids may be needed for pain control.

Acute symmetric polyarthritis bears resemblance to rheumatoid arthritis. Physical examination reveals ulnar deviation and swan neck deformities of the hands, and radiography demonstrates joint space narrowing and periarticular osteopenia. However, unlike rheumatoid arthritis, onset is generally acute and radiologic findings are seen rapidly; rheumatoid factor is generally negative.

Reactive arthritis, or Reiter syndrome, is much more common in HIV-infected persons than in immunocompetent persons, with a prevalence of 5 to 10% of the HIV-infected population. Although the etiology is not well understood, there appears to be an association with the HLA-B27 antigen, while additional evidence points to a link to some bacterial infections such as *Yersinia, Campylobacter,* and *Shigella.*

Reiter syndrome consists of a triad of arthritis, conjunctivitis, and urethritis, but the full triad is not often seen. Most patients have involvement of the feet and ankles, but the hands and other large joints can also be involved. Some patients have a mild course that resolves on its own; in others, severe arthritis may develop at multiple sites and fever may also be present. Other connective tissue sites may be involved as well, including tendons and fascia. Patients may experience tendinitis of the Achilles, rotator cuff tendinitis, and de Quervain tenosynovitis. A symptom termed "AIDS foot" may develop in some patients and is a particularly severe consequence consisting of involvement of the Achilles tendon, the anterior and posterior tibial tendons, extensor tendons, and plantar fascia. These patients may have a wide gait and ankle stiffness in order to reduce painful load on the heel. Other patients may have uveitis, oral ulcers, involvement of the glans penis, and scattered hyperkeratotic skin lesions. NSAIDs are generally helpful for primary therapy; opioids may be necessary for pain control.

It may be difficult to distinguish reactive arthritis from **psoriatic arthritis,** a clinically similar illness found in 2 to 3% of HIV-infected patients. Psoriatic arthritis often, but not always, presents with skin manifestations of psoriasis, including confluent circumscribed, discrete reddish, silvery-scaled maculopapules, predominantly on the elbows, knees, scalp, and trunk. Pitting of the nails is often present as well. Treatment is similar to that of reactive arthritis.

Hypertrophic osteoarthropathy is characterized by severe pain in the lower extremity, often with clubbing of the digits, nonpitting edema, and joint pain. Skin over affected areas may demonstrate edema, warmth, and a shiny appearance. Radiography reveals periosteal and subperiosteal changes in the long bones of the affected areas. It appears to be associated with pulmonary infections, most commonly *Pneumocystis jiroveci* pneumonia. The condition usually resolves with treatment of the opportunistic illness.

Septic arthritis refers to the acute bacterial infection of a joint space and is very common in HIV-infected patients. Risk factors include hemophilia, injection drug use, and male homosexual sex. Patients generally complain of monoarticular pain and fever; physical examination findings are consistent with septic arthritis, and joint aspirate is helpful in diagnosis. The most common pathogen is *S aureus,* but many others have been implicated. The hip and knees are most commonly affected; however, HIV-infected patients can be affected in unusual locations, such as the sternoclavicular joint. **Septic bursitis** refers to the infection of the bursa surrounding the joint space, and commonly involved sites include the olecranon and prepatellar bursae. Plain films and MRI are helpful in making the diagnosis. Treatment of these conditions is with antibiotics, surgical debridement, and drainage.

Osteomyelitis refers to the progressive infection of bone and is commonly seen in HIV-infected patients, usually late in the disease course. Patients usually seek medical attention complaining of sudden onset of high fever, chills, and pain and tenderness of the involved bony area. Commonly involved bones include the spine and long bones. Additional risk factors include injection drug use and vascular insufficiency. Erythrocyte sedimentation rate is elevated. Blood cultures are essential, and bone aspirate can help reveal the causative organism. Plain films are generally normal in early disease, but early findings may include periarticular demineralization of bone; bony erosion and periosteal reaction may be seen 2 weeks later. MRI is the most sensitive test, especially when soft-tissue involvement is a concern. Nuclear medicine studies may detect multifocal sites of infection. The most common pathogen is *S. aureus,* but many organisms have been found to cause osteomyelitis, including *M. tuberculosis* infection. Tuberculosis osteomyelitis can be particularly dangerous and this diagnosis should be considered in all HIV-infected patients with osteomyelitis. Treatment for osteomyelitis is very difficult, consisting of appropriate long-term antibiotic therapy (often parenteral) and surgical drainage.

Osteonecrosis, also called avascular necrosis, is the pathologic destruction of bone tissue as a result of vascular compromise. Osteonecrosis appears to be more common in the HIV-infected population, with an estimated prevalence of 4 to 5%. The precise etiology of the vascular compromise resulting in HIV osteonecrosis is unclear. In recent years, the use of protease inhibitors has been associated with an increased risk for osteonecrosis of the femoral head, through a mechanism that is not yet clear. Patients with osteonecrosis most commonly have an intermittent deep throbbing pain. The pain may begin suddenly or insidiously and is often associated with weight bearing and physical activity. However, pain can occur at rest in advance disease, while some patients with osteonecrosis never experience pain until much later in the illness. It occurs most commonly in the hip, and other sites may include the knee, shoulder, ankle, and wrists; multiple joints are frequently involved in the same patient. Radiographs, CT, and nuclear medicine studies can all be helpful, but MRI is the most sensitive test. In its early stages, management consists of reducing weight bearing on the affected joint in order to slow progression. As illness progresses, surgical intervention may be needed to revascularize, stabilize, or replace the joint. Pain may greatly intensify as the illness progresses; aggressive pain control is invaluable.

Plate AM et al. Musculoskeletal manifestations of HIV infection. *AIDS Read.* 2003;13:62. [PMID: 12645490]

Tehranzadeh J et al. Musculoskeletal disorders associated with HIV infection and AIDS. Part I: infectious musculoskeletal conditions. *Skeletal Radiol.* 2004;33:249. [PMID: 15034682]

Tehranzadeh J et al. Musculoskeletal disorders associated with HIV infection and AIDS. Part II: non-infectious musculoskeletal conditions. *Skeletal Radiol.* 2004;33:311. [PMID: 15127244]

GASTROINTESTINAL PAIN SYNDROMES

HIV-infected patients are susceptible to a wide range of illnesses involving the entire gastrointestinal tract, including the oral mucosa, esophagus, stomach, pancreas, hepatobiliary tract, small and large bowel, and anorectum (Table 20–7). As with other pain manifestations in HIV, clinicians should pay heed to the diagnosis and treatment of the pain-producing illness as well as the management of the pain itself. Painful opportunistic illnesses are frequent in the gastrointestinal tract. Pain may also be caused by illnesses that are found in the non–HIV-infected persons, such as peptic ulcer disease. Antiretroviral therapy for HIV can cause painful illness as well. In addition, patients may experience pain caused by more than one etiology.

Diagnosis of gastrointestinal disorders in HIV-infected persons, such as candidiasis, may occasionally be apparent by accurate history taking and findings on physical examination. Laboratory data is usually helpful, and the skilled use of radiologic tests is generally of great value. However, additional diagnostic data is often required and may necessitate consultation with a gastroenterologist for such procedures as endoscopy and biopsy.

Disturbances in motility, absorption, and oral intolerance can result in the patient being unable to take oral medications. This is a challenge to effective pain management. The clinician should be astute to these needs and be prepared to prescribe medications that can be taken

Table 20–7. Selected Painful Gastrointestinal Disorders in HIV.

Site	Illness	Etiology	Clinical features	Diagnostic findings	Treatment
Esophagus	Candidiasis	*Candida albicans*	Odynophagia Dysphagia Oral thrush may not be present	Endoscopy reveals white plaques on esophageal mucosa	Antifungals
	CMV or herpes simplex virus esophagitis	CMV Herpes simplex virus	Odynophagia, concurrent systemic infection. Occurs in profound immunodeficiency	Endoscopy reveals large characteristic ulcerations	Antivirals
	Idiopathic esophageal ulceration	HIV	Odynophagia Dysphagia	Endoscopic biopsy demonstrates only HIV virus	Corticosteroids and preventive antifungals
Stomach	CMV gastritis	CMV	Severe epigastric pain but commonly asymptomatic	Endoscopy shows inflamed ulcerated gastric mucosa	Antivirals
Pancreas	Drug-induced pancreatitis Infectious: cryptosporidiosis, CMV, MAC, tuberculosis Gallstones, alcohol, and other causes common to general population	Drug induced: didanosine, zalcitabine, stavudine, lamivudine, ritonavir, pentamidine	Deep epigastric pain with radiation to the back, accompanied by nausea and vomiting	CT scanning shows fluid collection and abscess Elevated amylase/lipase Ultrasonography or ERCP reveals gallstones	Cessation of offending drug ERCP for gallstones Supportive care
Liver	Infectious hepatitis	Various—see text	Fever Abdominal pain Nausea Vomiting Jaundice Encephalopathy	Transaminase and other liver enzyme abnormalities Imaging as appropriate	Treatment of underlying infection
Gallbladder and biliary tree	Acalculous cholecystitis AIDS associated cholangiopathy	CMV *Cryptosporidium* Microsporidians	Fever Abdominal pain Right upper quadrant tenderness Jaundice	Ultrasonography Radionuclide hepatobiliary scintigraphy CT scanning	ERCP
Anorectum	Hemorrhoids Fistulas Anal fissures	Various	Severe pain in anorectum Visualized lesions on examination	Clinical history and examination	Dietary modification Stool softeners Antimotility agents Topical therapies
	Condyloma lesions Abscesses Proctitis	STDs (syphilis, gonorrhea, chlamydia, herpes simplex virus, human papillomavirus)	Painful lesions Occasionally constitutional symptoms	Clinical history and examination	Antibiotics Incision and drainage Surgical intervention as needed

CMV, cytomegalovirus; MAC, *Mycobacterium avium* complex; CT, computed tomography; ERCP, endoscopic retrograde cholangiopancreatography; STDs, sexually transmitted diseases.

via the transmucosal, transdermal, rectal, and parenteral routes.

Treatment of the underlying illness can be complex and is essential for relief of suffering. Many illnesses respond to treatment, and the need for pain management will diminish. In addition, as HIV illness progresses, other gastrointestinal symptoms, such as nausea, vomiting, diarrhea, and constipation, may cause suffering that is no less intense. These symptoms may coexist with pain; indeed, patients may have difficulty distinguishing the cause of the intense discomfort. As illness progresses, palliative management of these symptoms must intensify as well. Fortunately, therapy is often successful even when the underlying etiology is not identified.

1. Esophagus

Odynophagia is often described as a sharp substernal pain that occurs predominantly on swallowing and can be distinguished from *pyrosis,* or "heartburn," which is retrosternal wavelike pain associated with gastroesophageal reflux. Such pain deserves investigation, especially in immunocompromised persons. Causes of esophageal pain include viral, bacterial, fungal, or parasitic infection; pill esophagitis; and opportunistic malignances. In general, endoscopy is the procedure of choice for diagnosis, and endoscopic brush biopsy can be very helpful. Other radiologic studies, such as barium swallows, are less helpful.

There are numerous infectious causes of esophagitis. **Candidiasis** is one of the most common causes; characteristic white plaques on the esophageal mucosa can be visualized by endoscopy. Dysphagia (difficulty in swallowing) is common, and odynophagia, while less common, can still occur. The presence or absence of oral thrush is not a reliable indicator of esophageal candidiasis. If candidiasis is suspected in an otherwise stable patient, the clinician may decide to empirically start antifungal therapy. However, if there has been no response for several days, the patient should be reassessed.

Viral etiologies of esophagitis include cytomegalovirus, herpes simplex virus, varicella-zoster virus, and a self-limited HIV esophagitis. **Cytomegalovirus,** the most common viral esophagitis, causes odynophagia more commonly than dysphagia. It occurs in patients who are profoundly immunodeficient and often manifests concurrently with symptomatic infection at other sites in the body, such as the retina. Cytomegalovirus esophageal ulcers are often very large and can be visualized on endoscopy, which is the procedure of choice. Primary therapy with antivirals is crucial for treatment.

Herpes simplex virus uncommonly causes a viral esophagitis with a similar presentation. Endoscopic biopsies reveal diffuse erosive esophagitis or multiple shallow ulcerations. Treatment is with antivirals.

Idiopathic esophageal ulceration can also cause odynophagia and dysphagia and is usually associated with severe immunodeficiency. Endoscopy reveals multiple ulcerations of varying depth. While the appearance may mimic other types of viral esophagitis, biopsy will demonstrate only HIV virus. Treatment includes corticosteroids, which is generally accompanied by antifungal therapy to decrease the likelihood of infection with candidiasis. Other infections that have been reported to involve the esophagus include *Cryptosporidia, Pneumocystis jiroveci, Mycobacterium* sp., *Nocardia,* and *Actinomyces* sp..

Opportunistic malignances that cause esophagitis include **Kaposi sarcoma** and **Non-Hodgkin's lymphoma.** These should also be included in the differential diagnosis. In some cases, swallowed pills can cause **pill esophagitis;** zidovudine, zalcitabine, doxycycline, tetracycline, and clindamycin have been reported as causative agents. Pill esophagitis can be prevented by swallowing while in the upright position and following with plenty of water.

2. Stomach

In HIV-infected patients, gastric disorders are frequently not related to HIV disease and may, in fact, be illnesses found in the general population, such as *Helicobacter pylori* infection. However, opportunistic disorders can cause gastric illness, especially in advanced HIV disease. Gastrointestinal illnesses can manifest with abdominal pain, nausea, vomiting, anorexia, early satiety, or hematemesis.

Cytomegalovirus can cause inflammation or ulceration of the gastric mucosa, which is best evaluated by endoscopy. Epigastric pain may be severe, but infections are often asymptomatic. Other infectious etiologies of gastritis have been reported but are less common. **Kaposi sarcoma** is the most common opportunistic malignancy to involve the stomach, and cutaneous illness is usually present. Patients may be asymptomatic, but pain can be severe, and hemorrhage may be present. Diagnosis is confirmed with endoscopy.

3. Small & Large Intestines

HIV-infected patients are at risk for numerous intestinal infections as well as several opportunistic malignances. Small bowel disease may produce cramplike pain associated with nausea, vomiting, and diarrhea, which may be explosive and occur in large volumes. Malabsorption and weight loss may be present. Colitis often produces lower abdominal pain and cramping associated with urgency and tenesmus. However, there is considerable overlap in disease presentation, and it may be quite difficult to distinguish between small and large bowel illness.

Table 20–8. Common Infectious Illness in the Small and Large Intestines in HIV-Infected Patients.

- Bacterial
  - *Campylobacter* sp.
  - *Clostridium difficile*
  - *Escherichia coli*
  - *Mycobacterium* sp.
  - *Salmonella* sp.
  - *Shigella flexneri*
- Viral
  - Adenovirus
  - Cytomegalovirus
  - Norwalk virus
  - Rotavirus
- Parasitic
  - *Cryptosporidium parvum*
  - *Cyclospora cayetanensis*
  - *Entamoeba histolytica*
  - *Giardia lamblia*
  - *Isospora belli*
  - *Microsporidia*

Numerous bacterial, viral, and parasitic organisms can infect the small and large bowel, often causing significant pain in the process (Table 20–8). Typically, the workup begins with an extensive history and physical examination, including assessment of risk factors for exposure to enteric pathogens (eg, recent travel). This is followed by culture of the stool for enteric pathogens as well as stool examination for leukocytes, ova and parasites, and *Clostridium difficile* toxin. If the cause remains unclear, upper endoscopy or colonoscopy should be considered, depending on the nature of the patient's symptoms and the presumed location of illness. In as many as 50% of cases, no cause is found. Some of these patients have **AIDS enteropathy,** the pathology of which is still not fully understood but thought to be caused by the HIV virus itself.

Kaposi sarcoma can involve multiple areas of the gastrointestinal tract including the colon. Patients often have cutaneous manifestations of the illness. Although colonic lesions are often clinically silent, patients may present with bleeding or abdominal pain. The lesions can become quite large and can obstruct and even perforate the bowel. **NonHodgkins lymphoma** and colonic adenocarcinoma can also involve the bowel. Diagnosis can usually be made by colonoscopic biopsy.

4. Pancreas

In addition to the causes of pancreatitis in the general population (eg, trauma, alcohol, gallstones), HIV-infected patients are susceptible to pancreatitis caused by **opportunistic infections,** including cryptosporidiosis, cytomegalovirus, *Mycobacterium avium* complex, and tuberculosis. Patients may also be at risk for **drug-induced pancreatitis;** some predisposing medications include didanosine, zalcitabine, stavudine, lamivudine, ritonavir, and pentamidine. Typically, patients feel a deep boring pain in the epigastrium that radiates to the back, accompanied by nausea and vomiting. CT scanning of the abdomen and pelvis is the best imaging technique to visualize the pancreas and differentiate fluid collections, abscesses, and other infectious etiologies. If necessary, CT-guided biopsy can be performed. Gallstones can be best visualized or excluded by ultrasonography. Endoscopic retrograde cholangiopancreatography (ERCP) can be both diagnostic and therapeutic in visualizing gallstones and removing them. Treatment of pancreatitis consists of aggressive pain control and primary therapy, including treatment of infection. Any offending drug should be discontinued.

5. Liver

Many opportunistic infections can cause **hepatitis** and patients may experience fever, abdominal pain, nausea, and vomiting, in addition to other symptoms. Jaundice may also be present. Fungal infections such as cryptococcosis, coccidiosis, histoplasmosis, and candidiasis can cause hepatocellular damage and consequent inflammatory response. Extrapulmonary tuberculosis can cause abscesses in the liver, and *M avium* is the most common pathogen to infect the liver, often at the later stages of the disease. Parasitic infections can also occur.

Viral infections include cytomegalovirus, Epstein-Barr virus, herpes simplex virus, and adenovirus. While not technically opportunistic infections, hepatitis B and hepatitis C viruses may coinfect many HIV-infected injection drug users. The coexistence of HIV may increase the likelihood of hepatitis B virus infection to become chronic and may accelerate the course of hepatitis C virus disease.

Opportunistic malignancies include **Kaposi sarcoma,** which can cause hepatomegaly and abdominal pain, and less commonly **non-Hodgkins lymphoma. Hepatocellular carcinoma** may be present in patients with cirrhosis.

Many **medications** are toxic to the liver and must be carefully assessed. Acetaminophen produces fulminant hepatic necrosis if taken in large quantities through the depletion of glutathione, which normally detoxifies the drug. Clinicians must be very careful with antiretrovirals; many of them can cause elevated transaminase levels, hepatic steatosis, and lactic acidosis, which can be very dangerous. Zidovudine, nevirapine and ritonavir have been shown to be particularly hepatotoxic. Periodic monitoring of transaminase levels may be prudent. Other drugs can cause hepatocellular necrosis through different mechanisms, including isoniazid, methyldopa, monoamine oxidase inhibitors, indomethacin, propylthiouracil, phenytoin, diclofenac, and halothane. Isoniazid toxicity is enhanced by coadministration of rifampin. Some of these medications can cause a persistent hepatitis that may appear clinically similar to viral hepatitis. Pain is not always present; indeed liver toxicity may remain subclinical. If medication toxicity is suspected, stopping the offending medication is the first step in pain control.

6. Biliary Tree & Gallbladder

HIV-infected patients are at risk for opportunistic infections of the biliary tree and gallbladder. Fever, abdominal pain, and tenderness in the right upper quadrant are typically the presenting symptoms. Laboratory studies show elevated alkaline phosphatase levels. Gallstones lead to cholecystitis in many patients, but a substantial number have an infectious **acalculous cholecystitis.** Cytomegalovirus, *Cryptosporidium,* and microsporidians account for many of these cases, and other pathogens are not uncommon. These pathogens also commonly cause **AIDS-associated cholangiopathy,** or infection of the biliary tree, and symptoms may be similar. Ultrasonography, radionuclide hepatobiliary scintigraphy, and CT scanning are all diagnostic tests that can be helpful. ERCP can be diagnostic and therapeutic.

7. Anorectum

Hemorrhoidal disease is the most common anorectal disorder in both the general and HIV-infected populations, and pain can be severe. Fistulas and anal fissures can also be quite painful. Dietary modifications and stool softeners can be used to reduce hard painful stools. Patients with diarrhea may experience painful irritation of lesions, and antimotility agents may be helpful. Topical therapies may be helpful for hemorrhoids.

Homosexual men who engage in receptive anal intercourse are at risk for **sexually transmitted diseases** in the anorectum, including syphilis, gonorrhea, chlamydia, herpes simplex virus, and human papillomavirus. Manifestations include condyloma lesions, proctitis, and abscesses. Many of these can be very painful, and primary therapy should be directed at the infection, including antibiotics, drainage and, if necessary, surgical intervention.

Slaven EM et al. The AIDS patient with abdominal pain: a new challenge for the emergency physician. *Emerg Med Clin North Am.* 2003;21:987. [PMID: 14708816]

Wallace MR et al. Gastrointestinal manifestations of HIV infection. *Curr Gastroenterol Rep.* 2000;2:283. [PMID: 10981025]

DERMATOLOGIC PAIN SYNDROMES

Kaposi sarcoma is caused by disregulation of vascular cell growth, and evidence points to a causative role in human herpesvirus 8. Due to transmission of the virus, the lesion has typically been seen most in homosexual men; however, Kaposi sarcoma can also develop in women who have sex with bisexual men. Lesions may occur in virtually any organ, and commonly occur on the skin, oropharyngeal mucosa, lymphatic tissue, lungs, and gastrointestinal tract. Cutaneous lesions generally present as firm macular reddish or purple colored rashes, often resembling a bruise. This is due to the vascular nature of the lesion. Cutaneous lesions are generally not painful, but lesions involving the oropharyngeal mucosa are more likely to cause pain and bleeding. Lesions involving lymphatic structures can cause painful distal lymphedema. Gastrointestinal Kaposi sarcoma can cause severe bleeding but is rarely painful. Treatments include radiation therapy, cryotherapy, and chemotherapy. Kaposi sarcoma is rarely the cause of death in AIDS patients; however, it remains a considerable source of morbidity.

HIV-infected patients are at risk for **bacterial skin infections,** such as *S aureus* as well as others. Infections can progress from localized folliculitis to frank cellulitis, furuncles, carbuncles, and abscess (Table 20–9). Secondary impetigo can superinfect other lesions, such as eczema, scabies, herpetic lesions, and Kaposi sarcoma. Bacterial infections can become very painful and, if severe, life-threatening. Treatment generally consists of topical or systemic antibiotics (or both) and when appropriate, surgical drainage.

Aphthous stomatitis are generally small (<1 cm) white circular lesions surrounded by an erythematous margin and are often disproportionately painful. They occur on soft mucosal surfaces like the inner lips, bucca, tongue, soft palate, and pharynx. The pain usually persists for 4 to 5 days, after which the ulcer heals. Though there is no clear infectious etiology, HIV patients are at risk for the progression of these lesions, and they frequently enlarge and become chronic, causing great pain, often limiting oral intake and increasing suffering. Laser ablation or intralesional corticosteroids can be used to treat the ulcers. Pain can be controlled with topical corticosteroids, topical tetracycline, and viscous topical lidocaine.

Herpes simplex virus (types 1 and 2) causes **genital and oral herpes.** Lesions are highly painful and are more troublesome in immunocompromised persons than in immunocompetent persons. Primary infection consists of fever and the distinctive vesicles, which burst and

Table 20–9. Selected Painful Dermatologic Conditions in HIV and AIDS.

Illness	Clinical features	Treatment	Comments
Kaposi sarcoma	Firm cutaneous reddish or purple macules	Radiotherapy Cryotherapy Chemotherapy	May involve gastrointestinal tract, lungs, lymphatics
Bacterial skin infections	Folliculitis Cellulitis Furuncles Carbuncles Abscesses	Topical or systemic antibiotics Surgical drainage	Can be life threatening Superinfection of preexisting lesions is common
Aphthous stomatitis	Small white circular lesions, erythematous margins Occurs on soft mucosal oropharyngeal surfaces	Laser ablation Intralesional corticosteroids Topical: lidocaine, corticosteroids, tetracycline	May become chronic and cause great suffering in HIV-infected patients
Oral and genital herpes	Primary infection: fever, distinctive vesicles Secondary infection: prodromal tingling/burning followed by vesicles	Systemic and topical antiherpetics, as soon as prodromal symptoms manifest	Treatment reduces duration of illness
Herpes zoster	Prodromal pain Characteristic vesicles Dermatomal distribution	IV acyclovir, famciclovir, or valacyclovir	Primary infection is chickenpox (varicella) Consult ophthalmologist immediately if ophthalmic involvement is suspected
Toxic epidermal necrolysis	Localized painful erythema and blisters that may peel off Fevers and malaise	Discontinue offending agent and hospitalize Supportive care	Continuum of symptoms includes erythema multiforme and Stevens-Johnson syndrome

form painful ulcerations; these then crust and usually heal completely. Like aphthous stomatitis, pain may greatly limit oral intake. Pain typically lasts 10 to 14 days, and the virus then recedes to the sensory ganglion where it remains latent. It can, however, be reactivated by stress or immunodeficiency, resulting in secondary infection or reactivation. Patients typically feel a prodromal tingling or burning in the affected area, followed by the development of the lesions, which last 4 to 5 days. Both systemic and topical antiherpetic therapies are available and should be used as soon as the patient feels the prodromal sensation, as duration of symptoms can be modestly reduced.

Herpes zoster (shingles) is caused by varicella-zoster virus. The primary manifestation of this virus is chickenpox, an illness that usually occurs in childhood. Like herpes simplex virus, the virus remains latent in sensory nerve ganglia and may be reactivated by immunodeficiency. Patients usually experience pain at the involved site 2 to 3 days before the onset of the characteristic rash; vesicles develop on an erythematous base in the distribution of a sensory dermatome. Pain may be severe. If ophthalmic involvement is suspected, an ophthalmologist should be consulted immediately in order to prevent eye involvement and vision loss. Topical remedies such as wet compresses may be helpful, and systemic treatment may consist of intravenous acyclovir, famciclovir, or valacyclovir.

Postherpetic neuralgia occurs after some cases of zoster; see the section on Neurologically Related Pain Syndromes.

Drug Reactions

Sulfonamide drugs, such as sulfamethoxazole and sulfadiazine, can cause a severe skin reaction called **toxic epidermal necrolysis,** which is believed to exist on a continuum of symptoms from erythema multiforme to

Stevens-Johnson syndrome. Localized painful erythema and blisters that may peel off develop; this may be accompanied by fevers, malaise, and chills. The illness can be life-threatening, and patients must be hospitalized for treatment. Some other medications that have been associated with painful rash include nevirapine, delavirdine, efavirenz, amprenavir, and fosamprenavir. Any suspected offending agent should be discontinued, and the patient should be treated immediately.

Garman ME et al. The cutaneous manifestations of HIV infection. *Dermatol Clin.* 2002;20:193. [PMID: 12120434]

Pain in the Elderly

Joshua M. Hauser, MD

ESSENTIAL CRITERIA

- *Elderly persons have a less predictable pain reaction to a specific disease or injury than do younger persons.*
- *Obtain an accurate medication history by asking patients to bring their medication to the appointment.*
- *Unidimensional pain assessment scales (eg, Visual Analogue Scale or Numeric Rating Scales) are particularly helpful in elderly patients, especially those who have cognitive impairment.*

General Considerations

Pain in the elderly can be a challenging diagnostic and therapeutic problem for clinicians of many disciplines. The majority of elderly patients in pain will not be seen by geriatricians but rather by internists, family practitioners, oncologists, surgeons, and palliative care physicians. It is critical, therefore, that physicians within these specialties be able to recognize, treat, and consider the special circumstances of the elderly with pain.

A. EPIDEMIOLOGY

In the Assessing Care of Vulnerable Elders (ACOVE) project, which began in 2000, an expert panel of geriatricians, epidemiologists and health services researchers convened to identify geriatric conditions as optimal targets for quality improvement. After the panel members initially identified 78 common conditions among the elderly, they reduced the list to 35 on the basis of prevalence, impact on health, effectiveness of interventions, and disparities in the quality of care for these conditions among providers. Of these 35 conditions affecting the elderly, pain management ranked fifteenth in importance, ahead of pneumonia, influenza, malnutrition, and osteoarthritis.

The prevalence of pain in the elderly varies according to the setting. Consider whether the elderly person lives in the community or in a long-term care facility, or whether he or she is hospitalized with an acute illness. The studies reviewed below generally include any type of pain (eg, neuropathic or nociceptive) occurring at any anatomic site. The general goal is to give a sense of the overall burden of pain in the elderly, not to characterize specific diagnoses or management strategies.

1. In the community—The prevalence of pain in the elderly who live in the community has been shown to range from 25 to 56%. The sources of pain include back pain (21 to 49.5%), joint pain, and headaches. A study of community-dwelling elderly using the Minimum Data Set (MDS) for Home Care (3046 patients) found that between 39 of age and 41% of patients older than 65 years reported daily pain. Of those who reported daily pain, 25% received nonopioid therapy for mild pain, 6% received opioids plus nonopioids for moderate pain, and 3% received opioids plus nonopioids for severe pain (see Figure 3–1). Two specific groups within the elderly appeared to confer added vulnerability to pain: Both the oldest old and those with diminished cognitive ability were at increased risk for not receiving analgesia. In a separate study of over 300 elderly patients in California, undertaken as part of the ACOVE project, the prevalence of pain was documented to be 33%. Even more alarming, 40% of these patients reported being screened for pain.

2. In the nursing home setting—Since significant numbers of elderly persons live in nursing homes, the problem of pain prevalence and control in this setting is crucial to consider. In an examination of data from the MDS, Teno and colleagues found that almost 15% of nursing home residents had persistent pain on two separate assessments and 41.2% of residents in pain at first assessment were in severe pain 60 to 180 days later. This rate was fairly uniform across the country, varying from 37.7 to 49.5% in different states and suggests that even when pain is recognized, it is frequently not addressed. A more recent study, which also used the MDS to analyze 21,380 nursing home residents, found that 49% of residents had persistent pain. The differences may be due to differing standards for "persistent pain."

A more recent study of a national sample of nursing home patients showed a relatively small subset of patients (4%) reported "daily pain that was excruciating at some time in the previous week"; nearly half of these patients had a similar report in a follow-up assessment a week later. All of these studies suggest significant problems not only in the recognition of pain but also in its treatment once recognized. Clearly, pain in nursing homes is frequently underrecognized, undertreated, and the source of significant morbidity.

There are multiple quality improvement projects that have attempted to address this issue through both educational and systems interventions. For example, Miller and colleagues compared pain management of nursing home patients receiving hospice with pain management of those not receiving hospice in over 800 nursing homes. They found that hospice patients had more favorable pain treatment by a number of measures:

1. 15% of hospice residents and 23% of nonhospice residents in daily pain received no analgesics.

2. A lower proportion of hospice residents (21%) than of nonhospice residents (29%) received analgesics not recommended by the American Medical Directors Association.

3. Controlling for clinical confounders, hospice residents were twice as likely as nonhospice residents to receive regular treatment for daily pain.

Studies such as these suggest that a concerted clinical or educational effort can impact pain assessment and treatment in the nursing home setting.

However, there is one important caveat in these studies: the source of the data (the MDS) has been shown to significantly underestimate pain in the elderly. In a recent study, Cadogan and colleagues interviewed patients concerning pain and compared their findings with the patients' scores on the MDS, which is filled in by health care providers. They found that the MDS reported prevalence was between 15 and 30% in the nursing homes sampled, but 27 to 47% of residents reported pain when interviewed. Another study compared MDS scores to reports of clinical nursing assistants caring for residents. Similar problems with the MDS were found: Clinical nursing assistants who used a standard measurement of pain for patients with dementia found a prevalence of 48%, compared with a prevalence of 20% found using the MDS.

The implications of this measurement mismatch is that even the relatively high levels of pain among the elderly reported in the MDS may be underestimating the burden of pain in elderly nursing home residents. Therefore, the information obtained from MDS data must be treated as a fairly crude estimate.

3. In the hospital setting—In a comprehensive study of pain in hospitalized patients in a tertiary care hospital, Whelan and colleagues found an overall prevalence of 49.3% in elderly patients reporting moderate or severe pain. A larger study of elderly hospitalized patients over 80 years of age, a part of the SUPPORT (Study to Understand Patient Preferences for Outcomes and Treatment) study, showed a prevalence of pain ranging from 43% in patients with congestive heart failure to 60% in patients with colon cancer.

These aforementioned studies focused on elderly patients hospitalized on medical services. A parallel group of studies has looked at patients on surgical services and found that postoperative pain has also been shown to be inadequately managed in the elderly. Sauaia and colleagues evaluated patient satisfaction with postoperative pain management in elderly persons who underwent a variety of procedures. They found that 62% reported severe pain and documented inconsistent strategies to address it in eight hospitals. Interestingly, 87% of patients reported being "satisfied" with treatment, suggesting that patients may have low expectations of pain treatment. A recent review of pain management for the elderly in the orthopedic setting suggests that the weight of multiple studies in this area show between 50 and 75% of older adults do not have pain adequately managed. A failure to assess pain, low knowledge about assessment and management, a view that pain is a natural consequence of aging, and concerns about the use of analgesics in patients with cognitive dysfunction or other comorbid illnesses all play a role in the undertreatment of pain in the elderly.

B. ETIOLOGY AND CLASSIFICATION

The elderly are vulnerable to both acute and chronic pain. Acute pain is defined as distinct in onset, with a clear cause, and often a limited duration. This type of pain is associated with an injury, an acute illness, or an acute exacerbation of a chronic illness. Very frequently, it has a much clearer underlying cause than chronic pain.

In contrast to acute pain, chronic pain (also called persistent pain) has a duration of at least 3 months, a less predictable pattern of beginning and ending, and a less clear etiology than acute pain.

The etiology of pain in the elderly may be classified by pathophysiology (eg, nociceptive pain caused by inflammation, trauma, or tumor; or neuropathic, caused by diabetic neuropathy, postherpetic neuropathy, or medication-induced neuropathy). It may also be classified by the condition that is causing the pain (eg, cancer, diabetes mellitus, musculoskeletal disorders). In general, the prevalence of chronic diseases is higher in the elderly and the prevalence of musculoskeletal disorders, such as osteoarthritis and chronic low back pain, rises significantly in the elderly (Table 21–1).

Table 21–1. Pain Syndromes in the Elderly.

Cause	Example
Musculoskeletal	Fibromyalgia Polymyalgia rheumatica Osteoarthritis Rheumatoid arthritis Temporal arteritis
Neurologic	Diabetic neuralgia and neuropathy Trigeminal neuralgia Postherpetic neuralgia
Oncologic	Pain secondary to cancerous involvement of bowel, liver, bones
Vascular	Angina Peripheral arterial disease
Trauma	Pain secondary to fracture or fall

Reproduced, with permission, from Ferrell BA. Acute and Chronic Pain. In: Cassel CK et al (editors). *Geriatric Medicine.* 4th ed. New York: Springer; 2003.

Cadogan MP et al. A minimum data set prevalence of pain quality indicator: is it accurate and does it reflect differences in care processes? *J Gerontol A Biol Sci Med Sci.* 2004;59:281. [PMID: 15031314]

Chodosh J et al. The quality of medical care provided to vulnerable older patients with chronic pain. *J Am Geriatr Soc.* 2004;52:756. [PMID: 15086657]

Desbiens NA et al. Pain and suffering in seriously ill hospitalized patients. *J Am Geriatr Soc.* 2000;48:S183. [PMID: 10809473]

Ferrell BA. The management of pain in long-term care. *Clin J Pain.* 2004;20:240. [PMID: 15218408]

Fisher SE et al. Pain assessment and management in cognitively impaired nursing home residents: association of certified nursing assistant pain report, Minimum Data Set pain report, and analgesic medication use. *J Am Geriatr Soc.* 2002;50:152. [PMID: 12028260]

Karani R et al. Systemic pharmacologic postoperative pain management in the geriatric orthopaedic patient. *Clin Orthop Rel Res.* 2004;(425):26. [PMID: 15292784]

Landi F et al. Pain management in frail, community-living elderly patients. *Arch Intern Med.* 2001;161:2721. [PMID: 11732938]

Miller SC et al. Does receipt of hospice care in nursing homes improve the management of pain at the end of life? *J Am Geriatr Soc.* 2002;50:507. [PMID: 11943048]

Sauaia A et al. Postoperative pain management in elderly patients: correlation between adherence to treatment guidelines and patient satisfaction. *J Am Geriatr Soc.* 2005;53:274. [PMID: 15673352]

Sloss EM et al. Selecting target conditions for quality of care improvements in vulnerable older adults. *J Am Geriatr Soc.* 2000;48:363. [PMID: 10798460]

Teno JM et al. Daily pain that was excruciating at some time in the previous week: prevalence, characteristics, and outcomes in nursing home residents. *J Am Geriatr Soc.* 2004;52:762. [PMID: 15086658]

Teno JM et al. Persistent pain in nursing home residents. *JAMA.* 2001;285:2081. [PMID: 11311096]

Whelan CT et al. Pain and satisfaction with pain control in hospitalized medical patients: no such thing as low risk. *Arch Intern Med.* 2004;164:175. [PMID: 14744841]

Won AB et al. Persistent nonmalignant pain and analgesic prescribing patterns in elderly nursing home residents. *J Am Geriatr Soc.* 2004;52:867. [PMID: 15161448]

Assessment & Diagnosis

The assessment and diagnosis of pain in the elderly should begin with a thorough history and physical examination. Information from family caregivers may be particularly helpful, especially when the patient has co-existing cognitive deficits. Because of the complexities of patient and family reporting of pain, clinicians should assess patients both in the presence of family members and, if possible, alone. Family members often provide key information about a patient's condition, but the phenomenon of clinicians deferring to family members and ignoring the patient is well documented.

During the assessment of elderly patients with pain, five key issues need to be addressed: changes in pain perception, polypharmacy, functional status, pain measurement scales, and assessment of pain in persons who are cognitively impaired.

A. CHANGES IN PAIN PERCEPTION

In general, age-related changes in the elderly alter their perception of pain. Although many studies of neurologic decline have not been specific to pain perception, the neurologic changes that have been documented include decreases in pain receptors in the skin, decreased density and conduction of both myelinated and nonmyelinated neurons, and loss of neurons in the dorsal horn of the spinal cord. Clinically, investigators have observed that myocardial infarction or abdominal illness presents with less pain in the elderly than in younger patients. Furthermore, a study that directly measured pain perception by inserting an intravenous line in elderly and younger persons showed that elderly persons reported significantly less pain in response to this procedure than younger patients. Therefore, evidence suggests that a patient who is elderly has a less predictable pain reaction to a specific disease or injury than a younger patient.

B. POLYPHARMACY

Many elderly persons take multiple medications that put them at risk for adverse drug events as well as missing medications and doses. It is not clear that polypharmacy in itself is a cause of pain, but it is clear that the more medications a patient takes, the higher his or her likelihood is of missing doses. Therefore, a "treatment failure" may be that the person is not taking the medication that the physician thinks he or she is taking. There may have been no change in a patient's underlying pathophysiology to explain the pain; the only change may be in the missing of medication. A thorough medication history is vital in all patients and even more so in this population. One technique that is encouraged is the so-called "brown bag" test in which a patient is asked to bring all of his or her medication to an appointment in a brown bag; examining the contents of the medicine bottles is often more accurate than the list of medications in a patient's medical record that he or she is "supposed to be taking."

C. FUNCTIONAL STATUS

Comprehensive assessment of the elderly is the cornerstone of geriatrics and stems from the realization of the close correlation between functional status and quality of life. The elderly are at higher risk than younger patients for having both diminished and diminishing functional status, and pain has been shown to be correlated with worsened functional status. Its relief, therefore, has the potential to result in improved functional status.

D. MEASUREMENT SCALES

In addition to the usual tools of history taking, physical examination, laboratory tests, and radiologic studies, a variety of pain scales are available to assess pain in the elderly. Since pain is, by definition, a subjective symptom, efforts to measure it have been widespread. There are multiple pain assessment scales used in clinical care and research. The sheer number of these is less important than how they have been applied clinically and which are specific to the elderly. Some of these have been validated in multiple populations with multiple types of pain (eg, the McGill Pain Questionnaire) while others are more specific to cancer pain (eg, Wisconsin Brief Pain Inventory, the Memorial Sloan-Kettering Cancer Center Pain Scale). Ferrell and colleagues have developed a validated scale for use in the elderly that consists of 22 yes or no items and two 0 to 10 scales.

In the elderly and especially in the cognitively impaired, it may be more feasible to use a unidimensional scale. These include a Visual Analogue Scale, which is a 10-cm line that is either horizontal or vertical and has clear end points where a patient can indicate the level of pain; scales with pictures, such as the Memorial Sloan-Kettering Pain Assessment Card; or a verbal 0 to 10 scale. For patients with visual difficulties, a spoken 0 to 10 scale may be most effective at assessing their pain. For patients with hearing difficulties, a visual scale is most appropriate.

E. PAIN IN THE SETTING OF COGNITIVE IMPAIRMENT

Although standardized pain scales are useful in multiple populations of patients in pain, it is in patients with cognitive impairment that they are probably most valuable. In patients with cognitive impairment, assessment is a particular challenge. The challenge is one of accurate measurement and assessment in patients whose ability to interact has been compromised. A recent review of available assessment tools identified 39 instruments used to assess pain in the setting of cognitive impairment. Of 30 that met minimum standards, 18 were self-reported and 12 were staff reported. Of particular note, no instruments met all major tests of validity and reliability. In general, the simpler instruments had more extensive testing.

In one study that compared multiple assessment scales among cognitively impaired patients, Krulewitch and colleagues assessed cognitively impaired patients using a Visual Analogue Scale; a FACES Pain Scale; and the Philadelphia Pain Intensity Scale, a six-item self-report scale. They found that the Philadelphia Pain Intensity Scale was most likely to be filled out by patients and their caregivers. There was, importantly, relatively high correlation between the FACES and Visual Analogue Scale in their study.

The need for scales is compounded by recent findings that there is some evidence that the accuracy of physician assessment decreases as cognitive status worsens. A study that compared the pain assessments of patients' personal geriatricians with those of experts found that although assessments for patients with moderate impairment were accurate, the assessment in the most cognitively impaired group (average Mini-Mental Status Examination score of 1.91 out of a possible 30) was poor.

In severely cognitively impaired patients, scales of pain assessment consist of observed behaviors of the patient. One example that is fairly widely used is the Hurley Discomfort Scale. This scale consists of a trained examiner observing the breathing, vocalizations, facial expressions, and body movements in patients with dementia (Table 21–2). It has been reported to have moderate reliability. Even in cases where the full scale cannot be used, nonverbal cues to pain (eg, furrowing of the brow, moaning, calling out, restlessness, increased agitation) are critical to a thorough assessment. Physicians, nurses, and other health care professionals should routinely note such observations in the assessments. The presence of any of these nonverbal cues should prompt a therapeutic trial of analgesic medications. Family caregivers can also be asked about these signs of pain and also about positions, manipulations, or other actions that they have seen relieve or exacerbate pain.

Another example of a tool used to assess patients with cognitive impairment uses a mnemonic called BODIES. This tool was recently developed by Snow and colleagues

Table 21–2. Pain Assessment in Advanced Dementia—PAINAD.

	0	1	2	Score[a]
Breathing independent of vocalization	Normal	Occasional labored breathing Short period of hyperventilation	Noisy labored breathing Long period of hyperventilation Cheyne-Stokes respirations	
Negative vocalization	None	Occasional moan or groan Low-level speech with a negative or disapproving quality	Repeated troubled calling out Loud moaning or groaning Crying	
Facial expression	Smiling or inexpressive	Sad Frightened Frown	Grimacing	
Body language	Relaxed	Tense Distressed pacing Fidgeting	Rigid Fists clenched Knees pulled up Pulling or pushing away Striking out	
Consolability	No need to console	Distracted or reassured by voice or touch	Unable to console, distract, or reassure	
				Total

[a]Pain score of 4 or greater requires intervention. Pain score of 3 or less requires careful monitoring (screening with vital signs).

Reproduced, with permission, from Warden V et al. Development and psychometric evaluation of the Pain Assessment in Advanced Dementia (PAINAD) scale. *J Am Med Dir Assoc.* 2003;4:9–15.

for nursing assistants to help in the assessment of pain in nursing home residents with dementia. This mnemonic consists of the following fields:

B—What **behaviors** did you see?
O—How **often** did the behaviors occur?
D—What was the **duration** of the behaviors?
I—How **intense** were the behaviors?
E—How **effective** was treatment, if given?
S—What made the behaviors **start** and **stop**?

Although it uses relatively nonspecific items for caregivers to assess, this highlights important areas for further development of valid scales.

Cohen-Mansfield J et al. Pain in cognitively impaired nursing home residents: how well are physicians diagnosing it? *J Am Geriatr Soc.* 2000;48:1607. [PMID: 12110063]

Ferrell BA et al. The Geriatric Pain Measure: validity, reliability and factor analysis. *J Am Geriatr Soc.* 2000;48:1669. [PMID: 11129760]

Gibson SJ et al. Age-related differences in pain perception and report. *Clin Geriatr Med.* 2001;17:433. [PMID: 11459714]

Goulding MR. Inappropriate medication prescribing for elderly ambulatory care patients. *Arch Intern Med.* 2004;164:305. [PMID: 14769626]

Krulewitch H et al. Assessment of pain in cognitively impaired older adults: a comparison of pain assessment tools and their use by nonprofessional caregivers. *J Am Geriatr Soc.* 2000;48:1607. [PMID: 11129750]

Li SF et al. Effect of age on acute pain perception of a standardized stimulus in the emergency department. *Ann Emerg Med.* 2001;38:644. [PMID: 11719743]

Snow L et al. Pain management in persons with dementia. BODIES mnemonic helps caregivers relay pain-related signs, symptoms to physicians and nursing staff. *Geriatrics.* 2005;60:22. [PMID: 15877481]

Stolee P et al. Instruments for the assessment of pain in older persons with cognitive impairment. *J Am Geriatr Soc.* 2005;53:319. [PMID: 15673359]

Treatment

A. ANALGESIC THERAPY

The principles of analgesic treatment in the elderly parallel the principles for all patients. A thorough history and physical examination as well as the appropriate use of laboratory and radiologic testing are critical to identify the cause of pain. In some cases, such as lower back pain, a specific cause will be elusive. In other cases, a specific anatomic cause or injury can be identified. In all cases, it is crucial to define the extent of diagnostic workup by the goals of the patient and his or her family. In the elderly, especially those who may be close to the end of life, issues of goals of care can help determine the level of diagnostic testing that is desired, which means that clinicians may not always be able to discover a clear cause to help guide treatment. For example, for a patient who has dementia and is severely debilitated, contracted, and bedbound, a simple x-ray film of the lumbar spine may be a significant burden—far greater than it might be for a 60-year old. This does not mean that clinicians should hesitate to treat pain until an etiology can be found; quite the contrary, clinicians should feel comfortable treating pain even if a clear etiology is not known.

Both the American Geriatrics Society (AGS), the main professional society for geriatricians, and the American Medical Directors Association, the main professional society for physicians in long-term care, have position statements and clinical guidelines concerning geriatric pain. These guidelines stress a step-wise approach to pain treatment that is consistent with the original pain ladder established by the World Health Organization (see Figure 3–1). This approach is applicable to the setting of acute and chronic pain. It consists of beginning with a nonsteroidal anti-inflammatory drug (NSAID) or acetaminophen and then moving to different strength opioids if the pain is not relieved. Adjuvant medications, especially for neuropathic pain, are efficacious in the elderly. Their side effects should be carefully monitored: tricyclic antidepressants have more significant anticholinergic effects in the elderly than in younger patients and the elderly are at increased risk for glycemic changes and mood changes from corticosteroids. While this does not mean that these medications should be withheld, it does mean that their risk-benefit profile needs careful consideration.

1. Nonsteroidal anti-inflammatory drugs—These have been shown to be effective in a variety of conditions, particularly osteoarthritis. NSAIDs may be combined with opioids or used as single agents. Acetaminophen can be given in doses up to 4000 mg/d but should be reduced in patients with concurrent alcohol use or liver dysfunction. NSAIDs, such as ibuprofen, have a higher incidence of bleeding complications in the elderly compared with the nonelderly. Although gastroprotective drugs offer some protection, this is not complete. They also do not change the known renal toxicity of long-term NSAID use in the elderly.

2. Opioids—Opioids have been found in repeated trials to be safe and effective for the elderly in both chronic and acute pain. The issue of opioid use is one of slow and careful titration of dosage rather than avoidance. For example, Roth and colleagues found around-the-clock, controlled-release oxycodone therapy to be safe and effective treatment for patients with moderate to severe pain due to osteoarthritis. The most common opioids for use in the elderly include morphine, oxycodone, and hydrocodone. In patients with renal dysfunction, hydromorphone is a preferred opioid. Starting doses are shown in Table 21–3.

3. Opioids to be avoided—The AGS makes a specific recommendation against the use of several opioid medications, including methadone (whose variable half-life is especially problematic in the elderly) and tramadol (which can lower seizure threshold). Although not specifically mentioned in the AGS guidelines, the use of meperidine is not recommended in the elderly because of the neuroexcitatory effects of its metabolite normeperidine. In response to adverse events concerning meperidine, some hospitals have taken it off their formulary. In addition, propoxyphene is not recommended in any person because of its poor analgesia, high acetaminophen content and, of particular concern in the elderly, the neurotoxic effects of the metabolite norpropoxyphene.

B. NONPHARMACOLOGIC APPROACHES

Given the presence of increased vulnerability to side effects, many clinicians in the geriatrics community have called for the integrating of nonpharmacologic approaches to pain. These are most commonly used in conjunction with pharmacologic approaches and can be appropriate both in the setting of acute and chronic pain.

One approach has been to use exercise as an adjunctive pain relief technique. Ettinger and colleagues conducted a randomized trial comparing aerobic exercise and resistance exercise in the treatment of pain in older adults with osteoarthritis. They found that both types of exercises improved pain and disability scores, with pain scores showing more improvement in the resistance exercise model. Iversen and colleagues found improvements in pain and quality of life in a small sample of elderly patients with chronic low back pain who underwent a bicycle exercise program three times a week for 12 weeks. In their clinical practice guidelines, the American Geriatrics Society recommends an exercise prescription for adults with osteoarthritis. Although it is tempting to extrapolate that all elderly persons with pain will benefit from exercise, some caution is warranted. For example, it is likely only those with a functional status to allow appropriate participation will benefit from exercise. There is some suggestion that these benefits from exercise may be isolated to elderly with relatively preserved functional

Table 21–3. Selected Opioid Analgesic Medications for Pain.

Drug	Starting dose (oral)	Description	Comments
Morphine	15 mg q4h	Short-intermediate half-life Older people are more sensitive than younger people to side effects	Titrate to comfort; continuous use for continuous pain; intermittent use for episodic pain; anticipate and prevent side effects
Codeine	30–60 mg q4–6h	Acetaminophen or NSAIDs limit dose Constipation is a major issue	Begin bowel program early; do not exceed maximum dose for acetaminophen or NSAIDs.
Hydrocodone	5–10 mg q3–4h	Toxicity similar to morphine, acetaminophen, or NSAID combinations Limit maximum dose	Same as above
Oxycodone	20–30 mg q3–4h	Toxicity similar to morphine, acetaminophen, or NSAID combinations Limit maximum dose Oxycodone is available generically as a single agent	Same as above
Hydromorphone	2 mg q3–4h	Half-life may be shorter than morphine Toxicity similar to morphine	Similar to morphine
Sustained-release morphine (MS Contin, Oramorph, Kadian)	MS Contin 15–30 mg q12h Oramorph 15–30 mg q12h Kadian 15–30 mg q24h	Morphine sulfate in a wax matrix tablet or sprinkles MS Contin and Oramorph should not be broken or crushed Kadian capsules can be opened and sprinkled on food but should not be crushed	Titrate dose slowly because of drug accumulation Immediate-release opioid analgesic often necessary for breakthrough pain
Sustained-release oxycodone	15–30 mg q12h	Similar to sustained-release morphine	Similar to sustained-release morphine
Transderm fentanyl	25–mcg patch q72h	Reservoir for drug is in the skin, not in the patch Equivalent dose compared with other opioids is not very predictable (see package insert) Effective activity may exceed 72 h in older patients	Titrate slowly using immediate-release analgesics for breakthrough pain Peak effect of first dose may take 18–24 h Not recommended for opioid-naïve patients
Fentanyl lozenge on an applicator stick	Rub on buccal mucosa until analgesia occurs, then discard	Short half-life Useful for acute and breakthrough pain when oral route is not possible	Absorbed via buccal mucosa Not effective orally

Ferrell BA. Acute and Chronic Pain. In: Cassel CK et al (editors). *Geriatric Medicine.* 4th ed. New York: Springer; 2003.

status. In a small trial among elderly persons with dementia and incontinence, a controlled exercise program failed to show improvement in pain scores.

Another nonpharmacologic approach that has shown some promise is acupuncture. In a recent trial of acupuncture for patients with chronic low back pain, Meng and colleagues demonstrated significant improvements in disability measured by the Roland Disability Questionnaire, which includes pain. A larger study by Berman and colleagues compared true acupuncture with sham acupuncture in 570 patients. Although they had some limitations in follow-up in both groups, they found significant improvements in pain scores among the patients who received true acupuncture compared with the sham group.

AGS Panel on Persistent Pain in Older Persons. The management of persistent pain in older persons. *J Am Geriatr Soc.* 2002;50(6 Suppl):S205. [PMID: 12067390]

American Geriatrics Society Panel on Exercise and Osteoarthritis. Exercise prescription for older adults with osteoarthritis pain: consensus practice recommendations. A supplement to the AGS Clinical Practice Guidelines on the management of chronic pain in older adults. *J Am Geriatr Soc.* 2001;49:808. [PMID: 11480416]

Berman BM et al. Effectiveness of acupuncture as adjunctive therapy in osteoarthritis of the knee: a randomized controlled trial. *Ann Intern Med.* 2004;141:901. [PMID: 15611487]

Ettinger WH Jr et al. A randomized trial comparing aerobic exercise and resistance exercise with a health education program in older adults with knee osteoarthritis. The Fitness Arthritis and Seniors Trial (FAST). *JAMA.* 1997;277:25. [PMID: 8980206]

Iversen MD et al. Enhancing function in older adults with chronic low back pain: a pilot study of endurance training. *Arch Phys Med Rehabil.* 2003;84:1324. [PMID: 13680569]

Meng CF et al. Acupuncture for chronic low back pain in older patients: a randomized, controlled trial. *Rheumatology (Oxford).* 2003;42:1508. [PMID: 12890859]

Roth SH et al. Around-the-clock, controlled-release oxycodone therapy for osteoarthritis-related pain: placebo-controlled trial and long-term evaluation. *Arch Intern Med.* 2000;160:853. [PMID: 10737286]

Simmons SF et al. Effects of a controlled exercise trial on pain in nursing home residents. *Clin J Pain.* 2002;18:380. [PMID: 12441832]

Special Issues

A. DEPRESSION AND PAIN

Depression has been shown to influence pain in both elderly and nonelderly populations. In a prospective random sample of more than 18,000 persons, which included elderly and nonelderly, chronic pain was shown to be strongly associated with major depression. The message is clear that patients with pain should be evaluated for depression and vice versa. The coexistence of these two diagnoses can make both assessment and treatment of pain more complex for the elderly.

A recent study reviewed the effect of two different depression care interventions on pain reports in a large sample of elderly with arthritis. The findings showed that an intervention consisting of antidepressants and problem-solving psychotherapy not only improved patients' depression but also improved the patients' pain reporting. Unutzer and colleagues examined the prevalence of pain and functional decline in a sample 1801 patients with depression. They found that 79% of patients reported functional impairment from pain in the previous month, and 57% reported a diagnosis of treatment for chronic pain in the previous 3 years. Yet, only 51% reported any analgesic use.

What might be the mechanism by which depression and chronic pain influence each other? In a prospective cohort study, investigators monitored 226 patients with disabling musculoskeletal pain and examined levels of depressive symptoms and self-efficacy. Both depression and a measure of low self-efficacy were correlated with higher pain scores.

B. PAIN AND QUALITY OF LIFE

Depression is a relatively specific clinical diagnosis. Its correlation with pain has naturally led investigators and clinicians to wonder how pain more generally influences quality of life and self-reported health. The intuitive concern that pain always decreases quality of life is often but not always borne out in the literature. In a small study at one center, Kong and colleagues recently studied the impact of pain on health-related quality of life for stroke survivors. Using one of the most widely accepted quality of life measures, the SF-36 (Short Form-36), they found that although pain was common in poststroke patients (42% prevalence), there was no difference in scores (with the exception of the subscale of the SF-36 that concerns pain) between patients with persistent poststroke pain and those without persistent pain.

Mantyselka and colleagues examined the relationship between chronic pain and self-rated health in more than 6500 patients in Finland. Their study included adults 15 to 74 years of age, and found the prevalence of chronic pain increased consistently with age, with 30% of those in the oldest group (70 to 74 years) reporting daily pain and 15% reporting pain several times a week. There was a similar consistent increase in the numbers of patients who reported poor perceived health.

The correlation is not just between self-reported health and pain but to a variety of objective measures of poor health. Leveille and colleagues, for example, have shown that pain is associated with increased falls in the elderly. In a prospective cohort study of over 1000 patients in Baltimore, Maryland, they found that women with pain were 1.66 times more likely to have reported falls. However, they found that those treated for pain were less likely to have experienced falls. Since falls themselves are associated with significant, morbidity and mortality in the elderly, the role of pain in contributing to their increased incidence is crucial to understand.

Finally, Won and colleagues assessed more than 49,000 nursing home residents and examined the associations between the presence of pain and activities of daily living, mood, and activity involvement. In addition to a high prevalence of daily pain (26%), they found that pain was correlated with decreased ability to perform activities of daily living, low mood, and less involvement in activity.

None of these studies are able to elucidate a mechanism by which pain is related to quality of life, activities of daily living, and depression. However, they do illustrate a clear correlation. The lesson for clinicians is that pain does not occur as an isolated phenomenon but has myriad connections with other parts of patients and families lives.

C. Family Caregivers

The elderly are more likely to have family members involved in assessing and treating their pain than are younger patients. Therefore, it is vital to understand how family caregivers assess pain among patients. Studies in this area have shown that family caregivers have extensive involvement and confidence in their ability to judge patients' pain yet also find this role distressing.

Focus groups of caregivers and patients suggest that improvements in communication between clinicians and family members, increasing participation of family members by clinicians in care, and addressing fears of using pain medications are key interventions that health systems need to consider. More recently, a group has developed instruments such as the Caregiver Pain Medicine Questionnaire to measure concerns about reporting pain and administering medications. In an initial study of this 22-item instrument, investigators found that although very few caregivers had concern about overall communication, more than 25% had concerns about addiction to pain medications and about their ability as a caregiver to decide how much medication to administer.

When caregiver and patient reports are compared, caregivers have been shown to overestimate pain prevalence in the elderly. Redinbaugh and colleagues explored this phenomenon of noncongruence between patients and their family caregivers. They examined 31 patient-caregiver pairs and found that caregiver knowledge of cancer pain management was not significantly associated with accuracy of ratings. However, the caregivers' experience of pain was significantly associated with the accuracy of their ratings. For example, caregivers who reported their loved one to be in distress secondary to his or her pain more accurately reported the pain, and caregivers who themselves were more distressed more accurately reported the pain.

Kimberlin C et al. Cancer patient and caregiver experiences: communication and pain management issues. *J Pain Symptom Manage.* 2004;28:566. [PMID: 15589081]

Kong KH et al. Prevalence of chronic pain and its impact on health-related quality of life in stroke survivors. *Arch Phys Med Rehabil.* 2004;85:35. [PMID: 14970965]

Letizia M et al. Barriers to caregiver administration of pain medication in hospice care. *J Pain Symptom Manage.* 2004;27:114. [PMID: 15157035]

Leveille SG et al. Musculoskeletal pain and risk for falls in older disabled women living in the community. *J Am Geriatr Soc.* 2002;50:671. [PMID: 11982667]

Lin EH et al; IMPACT investigators. Effect of improving depression care on pain and functional outcomes among older adults with arthritis: a randomized controlled trial. *JAMA.* 2003;290:2428. [PMID: 14612479]

Mantyselka PT et al. Chronic pain and poor self-rated health. *JAMA.* 2003;290:2435. [PMID: 14612480]

Ohayson MM et al. Using chronic pain to predict depressive morbidity in the general population. *Arch Gen Psychiatry.* 2003;60:39. [PMID: 12511171]

Redinbaugh EM et al. Factors associated with the accuracy of family caregiver estimates of pain. *J Pain Symptom Manage.* 2002;23:31. [PMID: 11779666]

Reid MC et al. The relationship between psychological factors and disabling musculoskeletal pain in community-dwelling older persons. *J Am Geriatr Soc.* 2003;51:1092. [PMID: 12890071]

Shega JW et al. Pain in community-dwelling persons with dementia: frequency, intensity, and congruence between patient and caregiver report. *J Pain Symptom Manage.* 2004;28:585. [PMID: 15589083]

Unutzer J et al. Pharmacotherapy of pain in depressed older adults. *J Am Geriatr Soc.* 2004;52:1916. [PMID: 15507072]

Won A et al. Correlates and management of nonmalignant pain in the nursing home. SAGE Study Group. Systematic Assessment of Geriatric drug use via Epidemiology. *J Am Geriatr Soc.* 1999;47:936. [PMID: 10443853]

Yates P et al. Family caregivers' experiences and involvement with cancer pain management. *J Palliat Care.* 2004;20:287. [PMID: 15690831]

Barriers to Pain Control

Barriers that may explain the overall low level of recognition and treatment of pain in the elderly include deficiency of knowledge, inadequate systems to assess and monitor pain relief, and attitudinal barriers. A study of six community-based and one Veterans Affairs long-term care facilities, explored the barriers among both residents and staff to pain treatment. The study compared residents, nurses, and clinical nursing assistants and found that among residents, attitudes that interfered with adequate pain control included the belief that chronic pain does not change, a fear of addiction, and fear of dependence. The major attitude that nurses identified was that complaints from residents to staff frequently went unheard. Clinical nursing assistants believed lack of time and complaints being unheard were the major barriers.

Other investigators have identified barriers that are clinician based: a failure to assess for pain, inadequate knowledge about management principles, a perception that pain is an inevitable part of growing old, and concerns about the use of pain medications in patients with cognitive difficulties or multiple comorbidities. Many of these barriers are amenable to education. Other barriers, such as the lack of availability of opioids in pharmacies that serve lower income patients, have economic and cultural causes and will require policy, legislative, and economic solutions.

Karani R et al. Systemic pharmacologic postoperative pain management in the geriatric orthopaedic patient. *Clin Orthop Rel Res.* 2004;(425):26. [PMID: 15292784]

Morrison RS et al. "We Don't Carry That"—failure of pharmacies in predominantly nonwhite neighborhoods to stock opioid analgesics. *N Engl J Med.* 2000;342:1023. [PMID: 10749965]

Weiner DK et al. Attitudinal barriers to effective treatment of persistent pain in nursing home residents. *J Am Geriatr Soc.* 2002;50:2035. [PMID: 12473018]

Legal & Regulatory Issues in Pain Management

22

Perry G. Fine, MD & Scott Fishman, MD

Clinicians worry about appropriate use and iatrogenic consequences of long-term opioid therapy in patients with persistent pain syndromes. Legal and regulatory concerns often focus on indications for, and legitimate use of, opioid analgesics for pain syndromes that are poorly responsive to other pain-relieving modalities. Uncertainty arises because principles of practice, clinical consequences, standards of monitoring, and outcomes for long-term opioid therapy are still evolving. Meanwhile, in day-to-day clinical practice, great tension exists between traditional ethical duties—and more recently, legal imperatives—to relieve suffering and optimize health status, and real or perceived legal and regulatory constraints. The situations that confront most clinicians are not easily reduced to "black and white," even when there is apparent clarity or consensus around some of the associated ethical and legal issues.

Recognizing that there are innumerable variations on the many clinical themes and scenarios that confront practitioners, and countless case examples involving possible legal and ethical issues pursuant to opioid prescribing, the intent of this chapter is to outline and clarify the contemporary legal, regulatory, and related ethical issues that pertain to this class of drugs in commonly encountered medical contexts. Prescribing clinicians must understand the regulations and laws that govern the use of controlled prescription drugs and must be able to structure a prescription regimen that is consistent with the perceived risk of abuse or addiction and includes the monitoring necessary to identify problems early if they occur.

Armed with this information, clinicians should be better prepared to address the issues that arise in their practices, protecting themselves and their patients in a world where no equally efficacious alternatives to the opioid analgesics for many pain conditions yet exist. To set the stage for this discussion, several cases are presented that typify the types of quandaries experienced in typical practice.

COMMON ISSUES CLINICIANS FACE

The ambiguities and difficulties encountered in practice can be illustrated in the following five cases. We invite you to compare your thoughts with the notes the authors provide to address the issues raised by each case.

Case 1: Long-Term Prescribing of a Controlled Substance

An otherwise healthy young man underwent lumbosacral spine fusion surgery for a work-related injury. He has completed an intensive rehabilitation program focused on "work hardening" and pain control, due to persistent postinjury and postoperative pain. He has returned to work and he is referred back to his primary care physician for long-term management. His discharge disposition included recommendations for continuing use of sustained-release morphine for ongoing pain control. His physician feels wary about his obligation to write monthly prescriptions for controlled substances for, perhaps, many years to come.

Discussion

Persistent debilitating pain is too prevalent, indications for opioid analgesic therapy too common, and pain specialists are too few for primary care physicians to defer these cases. When no other therapies exist that provide similar efficacy and positive therapeutic outcomes, physicians need to overcome their reluctance and learn how to manage these case skillfully and with confidence. Using the analogy of other chronic conditions and the importance of having structured disease management strategies (eg, diabetes, heart failure, obstructive airways disease), expertise is gained both through formal and self-directed continuing education and practice. Associating informally with a physician who has expertise in long-term opioid therapy, in order to discuss issues when they arise, may be a helpful strategy. However, the primary care physician should also recognize when referral to a pain treatment center, mental health professional, or chemical dependency program is indicated—knowledge and skill developed through continuing education.

Case 2: Balancing Therapeutic & Potentially Adverse Outcomes

A middle-aged man with chronic daily headaches has undergone thorough evaluation as well as multiple non-pharmacologic and nonopioid pharmacologic treatment approaches in several specialty headache clinics for his debilitating pain syndrome. After an exhaustive array of treatments, he reports that he can only maintain a functional life with several doses of a short-acting opioid each week. He has acknowledged suicidal ideation due to the severity of his headaches, but when his pain is controlled, he has no signs or symptoms of depression. He has no prior history of chemical dependency. However, he has demonstrated a tendency to dose-escalate over time, re-quiring opioid rotation every few months and "drug holidays" every year or so. He requires testosterone supplementation due to opioid-induced hormone suppression. His physician feels "caught between a rock and a hard place." She asks herself, "In the long run, by continuing to prescribe opioids, am I helping him or causing harm? If there is a bad outcome such as a suicide attempt, in what ways am I most—or least—culpable"?

Discussion

The ongoing evaluation and reevaluation of benefit versus burden of potentially harmful therapies attends most medical decisions when treating chronic conditions, including cancer, heart disease, and psychiatric conditions. This should be an iterative process. A well-structured plan of care that includes regularly scheduled follow-up visits, a treatment agreement (eg, one prescribing clinician, one pharmacy, no early refills, keeping appointments, and urine drug screens), and ongoing evidence of therapeutic benefit that is well documented will satisfy the physician's ethical obligations to her patient while protecting herself.

Case 3: Possible Drug Diversion

A young woman with multiple sclerosis is being treated with a sustained-release opioid analgesic for control of pain that is refractory to other therapies. She also requires one or two doses of an immediate-release opioid formulation every few days for severe, debilitating pain exacerbations that are unpredictable (breakthrough pain). Her physician receives a note from the patient's mother, with whom she lives, stating that she is worried that her daughter is "hoarding" her medications and that she is "running with a crowd" that may be taking advantage of her, using her medications for "recreational purposes." The doctor does not know what to do.

Discussion

The receipt of information from third parties must be handled with great care, both from ethical and legal standpoints. Since this patient is a competent adult, her permission is required to communicate with her mother about her medical condition and related matters. This is probably a good idea since her mother is (and likely will increasingly be) an important ally in her ongoing care. This is an important opportunity to deepen the therapeutic alliance with the patient, not weaken it, by compassionate but direct and clear communication about her responsibilities. An appointment needs to be scheduled wherein there is unhurried and ample time to let her know the serious legal risks and consequences to her and you as her physician if there is ever any diversion of her prescriptions. As in the previous cases, a structured treatment plan needs to be implemented and documented. These types of cases present a timely opportunity to initiate counseling as part of the renegotiated treatment plan since there is no criminal intent but rather maladaptive psychosocial issues.

Case 4: Rekindling Substance Abuse

A young man with HIV-related pain is not responding adequately to nonopioid therapies. His pain is unrelenting, severe, and contributing to sleep deprivation, anorexia, anxiety, and depression. The patient's physician suspects that the pain can be appreciably reduced with around-the-clock opioid analgesia. However, both the patient and his physician are afraid to initiate a trial of opioid therapy because the patient is an acknowledged opioid addict in drug-free recovery.

Discussion

There is no right answer in these cases. The patient's fears are quite justified, and they need to be fully heard and appreciated (validated). In the absence of other effective pain-mitigating therapies, and in collaboration with both an addiction disorder and pain management specialist, it is feasible to have successful therapeutic intervention with opioids in patients with a history of substance abuse. With little empiric evidence to rely upon, anecdotal experience suggests that successful outcomes require agreement on distinct goals (eg, sleep, mood, functional improvement) and contingencies (treatment agreement), coupled to a time-limited trial of medication (ie, an "exit strategy" if the plan is not working).

Daily prescription of methadone, or every-third-day prescription of a fentanyl patch, seems to be most effective, allowing for close monitoring of medication use and effects, and direct contact with the patient to provide psychological support. With adherence and positive therapeutic outcomes, duration between visits can increase. However, because this is a very time-intensive process, few practices may be able to sustain such attention.

Case 5: Hastening Death

A widowed older woman with metastatic colon cancer and severe abdominal pain has been well managed on oral opioid therapy for several months. She has become quite frail and was recently admitted to a nursing home. A hospice program has been called in to help manage terminal care. Her abdominal pain and nausea have dramatically increased, requiring change to a continuous subcutaneous infusion of opioids. Her mental status has declined, making patient self-report difficult. Some of the nurses express concern that the patient is exhibiting distress that they think is due to unrelieved pain. The medical director at the long-term care facility is hesitant to increase her opioid dose, fearing that this will be interpreted as intentionally hastening her death.

Discussion

Clinicians who care for patients at the end of life have an ethical obligation to become adept at evaluating and treating pain in cognitively impaired patients, or to be able to make timely and appropriate referrals. Pain is such a common concomitant symptom of life-limiting illnesses, and its adverse effects on well-being are so clear, that it is not tenable to actively or passively allow undertreatment. In all institutional settings, patients should be assessed frequently, and conferences between family members and clinical care providers should be held to review the morbid effects of pain, behaviors that signal pain, the indications for analgesics, and the ethical principles involved, so that everyone understands the plan of care.

HISTORY OF OPIOIDS AS A REGULATED CLASS OF DRUGS

Creation of a Regulatory Environment

Early in the twentieth century, increasingly common use of opioids and other drugs with abuse potential led to public clamor for legislative action. The Pure Food and Drug Act was passed in 1906, giving the federal government authority and responsibility to regulate drugs, including the obligation to establish safety and efficacy for drugs being sold in the United States. Shortly thereafter, the most enduring and influential law affecting opioid prescribing was passed: the Harrison Narcotics Act of 1914. It applied strict controls to opioid analgesics and included prohibitions against prescribing this class

of drugs to known addicts. Importantly, and problematically, "addiction" was not clearly defined as a psychophysiologic condition distinct from pharmacologic properties such as dependence upon or tolerance to opioids for medical indications related to pain control. This absence of clarity has led to a century of confusion and conflict.

In 1919, the Supreme Court upheld the Harrison Act, with opinions stating that physicians could not legally provide *narcotics* (opioids) for maintenance of an addict. As a result, opioid maintenance centers were closed, driving procurement underground. Addicts—and all those who required daily dosing of opioids, lest they experience abstinence—were considered to be criminals, since their ability to obtain opioids became dependent on illegal means. Drug use subsequently became the purview of the criminal justice system, rather than a health care–related issue. The Marijuana Tax Act of 1937, outlawing cannabis and heroin (diacetyl morphine), added to the criminal code and further blurred distinctions among pharmacologic classes of drugs, lumping them under the legal/regulatory rubric of *narcotics*.

Efforts to curb opioid use mounted over the proceeding decades with little differentiation between illicit use and medical need. In 1970, the Federal Controlled Substances Act (CSA) increased governmental oversight of manufacturing, prescribing, and dispensing of opioids. Currently, the framework of laws and regulations governing the use of opioids and other controlled substances has three tiers: (1) international laws and treaties, (2) federal laws and regulations, and (3) state laws and regulations.

National governments are encouraged to ensure the availability of opioid drugs for legitimate medical and scientific purposes. International treaties have been designed to achieve a balance between ensuring the availability of controlled substances for medical purposes and preventing illegal diversion. The International Narcotics Control Board was established in 1968 as an independent and quasi-judicial body empowered to implement the United Nations drug conventions. It attempts to ensure that adequate supplies are available for medical and scientific uses, and that diversion from licit sources to illicit traffic does not occur. To accomplish this, it administers an "estimates system" for opioid drugs and monitors international trade in drugs. It also monitors government control over chemicals used in the illicit manufacture of drugs, and assists governments in preventing diversion of these chemicals into illicit traffic. Finally, the Board also attempts to identify where weaknesses in the national and international control systems exist.

At the federal level, the Food and Drug Administration (FDA) and the Drug Enforcement Agency (DEA) work together to regulate drugs and thereby prevent drug diversion and abuse. The DEA enforces the CSA and laws regulating the manufacture, distribution, dispensing, and record-keeping requirements for controlled substances. The DEA also sets production quotas for controlled drugs, which are intended to accommodate all legitimate medical and scientific uses of scheduled drugs. Each state works with the federal government to oversee the movement of controlled prescription drugs and minimize abuse and diversion. Individual states also have sole responsibility for maintaining standards of health care practice through licensure of professionals. Medical practice and licensure is governed through state medical boards, whose members are appointed by the executive branch. Law enforcement occurs at the local and the state level through numerous agencies.

Before a pain medication can reach patients, the FDA must determine its efficacy and safety, including its potential for abuse. If a product does not receive marketing approval (or an exemption) from the agency, then it cannot be legally produced or prescribed. The CSA empowers the DEA to classify drugs into different groups, called schedules, based on the risk of abuse and diversion, medical use, and safety. It requires registration of all prescribers of controlled substances and categorizes potentially abusable drugs into one of five schedules, each with progressively more stringent regulatory mandates, from schedule V (low abuse potential) up to schedule I (for which there are no approved medical indications in the United States; heroin resides in this group).

Schedule II opioids include morphine, methadone, fentanyl, oxycodone, hydromorphone, levorphanol, and oxymorphone. The law stipulates that drugs in schedule II cannot be prescribed by telephone nor can they be refilled without a new, written prescription. Schedule III includes those opioids that are either combined with other dose-limiting coanalgesic agents (ie, hydrocodone with acetaminophen) or considered to be less subject to abuse, such as tramadol. Whereas federal regulations apply throughout all states, individual states have created an array of their own complex laws and regulations that vary from one jurisdiction to another.

The "Law" of Unintended Effects

A consequence of the unique regulatory milieu surrounding this aspect of medical practice has led clinicians to fear investigation, stigmatization, sanctions, and criminal prosecution. In particular, under-utilization of opioids in situations where their use is medically indicated, and especially where no other sufficient means of pain control is possible, has been attributed to the emotionally charged regulatory environment. In recognition of this, and the increasingly evident need to manage debilitating pain in a demographically and medically very different world than that of prior generations (eg, a rapidly growing population of aging individuals living for many years with multiple, and very often pain-producing, chronic, progressive conditions), significant changes among regulatory agencies—both in knowledge and attitude—are evolving.

Specifically, indications for long-term opioid analgesic therapy are openly acknowledged and increasingly accepted. In parallel, though, increased therapeutic use comes with greater demands for vigilance and monitoring for the ever-present risk of medication misuse and abuse, adverse effects, and iatrogenic addiction: conditions that are fundamentally medical rather than legal.

Toward Improved Public Policy

The ethics and laws applying to pain management have greatly evolved over the past few decades, especially with regard to the use of opioid analgesics. Before this rather dramatic shift in social thought and policy, neither the ethical imperatives of the health profession (formalized in normative bioethics) nor health care jurisprudence (formalized in statutes and codes) played a positive role in pain management. In many cases, their influences created barriers to adequate pain relief for many patients. Historically, definitive statements on pain management centered on the admonition to avoid fostering addiction in patients by overprescribing opioid analgesics. Disciplinary actions were taken against physicians who were perceived as having failed to follow this injunction.

Only recently has there been due attention paid to the positive duty to relieve pain and mitigate the suffering caused by it, and a convergence of this ethical imperative with regulatory policies and the law. Legal precedents are being set in court cases at both ends of the pain management spectrum. In rare cases, physicians have been convicted of criminal charges for opioid prescribing that is believed to be excessive and outside the scope of medical practice. At the opposite extreme, there have been two cases where physicians have been found guilty of elder abuse for insufficient pain control. This creates a pressing need for clinicians to attend to pain as a humanistic, medical, and forensic issue. Clinicians must become sufficiently knowledgeable to recognize the indications for opioid therapy without erring on one side (undertreatment) or the other (iatrogenic harm from opioids).

Current policy redirection is founded upon the view that adverse public health and criminal consequences of drug abuse, addiction, drug diversion, and trafficking of prescription opioids can be anticipated, recognized, and prevented by prescribers. Presumably, these policies are implemented to the extent that licit practice is not significantly curtailed. However, there is growing debate over the unintended but highly consequential role of law enforcement in the practice of medicine, particularly in relation to use of opioids. The "principle of balance" has been invoked as an appropriate response to competing needs and challenges surrounding prescription opioids (Table 22–1). Representatives from public policy,

Table 22–1. The Principle of Balance.

Medical Availability
- While opioid analgesics are controlled drugs, they are also essential drugs and are absolutely necessary for the relief of pain.
- Opioid analgesics should be accessible to all patients who need them for relief of pain.
- Governments must take steps to ensure the adequate availability of opioids for medical and scientific purposes, including:

   – Empowering medical practitioners to provide opioids in the course of professional practice.

   – Allowing them to prescribe, dispense, and administer according to the individual medical needs of patients.

   – Ensuring that a sufficient supply of opioids is available to meet medical demand.

Drug Control
- When misused, opioids pose a threat to society.
- Clinicians must recognize that a system of controls is necessary to prevent abuse and diversion. Although the system of controls is not intended to interfere with legitimate medical uses, they are necessary to protect the public health and should be understood and supported by the clinical community.
- Minimizing risk of abuse and diversion during the treatment of individual patients is part of the essential skill set needed for the safe and effective clinical use of opioid drugs.

Adapted from http://www.medsch.wisc.edu/-painpolicy/index.htm Pain and Policy Studies Group at the University of Wisconsin Comprehensive Cancer Center. Accessed October 13, 2005.

regulatory, and scientific and clinical bodies have joined to address the need to ensure sufficient access to appropriate therapeutic use of opioids while addressing the potential for harm. Exactly where this balance point sits remains in question, particularly in light of ongoing serious disagreements between the DEA and many pain experts around interpretation of the CSA. Among several points of contention, there is heated debate around the therapeutic value versus putative harm of high-dose opioid therapy in nonterminally ill chronic pain patients.

Notwithstanding these unresolved issues, the compelling need to implement the principle of balance motivated the Federation of State Medical Boards of the United States to create *Model Policy for the Use of Controlled Substances for the Treatment of Pain (2004)*. This model policy is meant to serve as a guideline for states and has been endorsed by several federal and state regulatory bodies, professional organizations, and patient advocacy groups. A report card on how each of the states is faring with regard to policies that positively and negatively impact pain management is available through the University of Wisconsin's Pain and Policy Studies Group (*Achieving Balance in State Policy: A Progress Report Card*) at http://www.medsch.wisc.edu/painpolicy. It is recommended that clinicians access this information so that they can understand what is occurring within their own practice jurisdictions.

Opioid Analgesics & State Licensing Boards

Only within the last decade have state medical boards offered policy statements or guidelines on pain relief, including aggressive symptom control in the treatment of dying patients. Typically, disciplinary actions admonished or sanctioned physicians for excessive use of opioids, in contrast to minimal attention to undertreatment of pain, signaling that "abuse of prescribing privileges" was a one-way street. In retrospect (and still today in too many cases), medical board members lack sufficient knowledge about pain medicine, opioid pharmacology, and addiction medicine to make informed decisions.

In response to what has been acknowledged as an epidemic of uncontrolled pain, several states have enacted "intractable pain" (or similarly titled) statutes. Such statutes are a response to the perceptions of many clinicians that their licensing boards are hostile to the use of opioids for the management of chronic noncancer pain, and uncomfortable about the high doses of opioids that may be required to mitigate against unnecessary pain in patients with progressive, fatal diseases, such as cancer—especially during the terminal phase of the disease. Intractable pain statutes are well intentioned, but they may also have some limitations. In many cases, they single out physicians, leaving out other clinicians (eg, nurse practitioners) with prescribing authority who may be involved in patient care.

Legal protections are not necessarily guaranteed for clinicians who adhere to the statutes. To date, there has been no all-inclusive remedy to these limitations that include ambiguities of language. For instance, New York law defines an addict as "a person who uses a controlled substance for nonlegitimate or unlawful use; and who by reason of such use is dependent thereon." That would seem reasonable were it not for the fact that it goes on to strictly limit the clinical conditions for which controlled substances can be administered or dispensed to "addicts" or "habitual users," precluding patients with severe noncancer chronic pain or cancer pain prior to the determination that it is "incurable and fatal".[1] Similarly, Texas law governing the prescribing of controlled substances uses the maltropisms "narcotic drugs" and "dangerous drugs" instead of pharmacologic classifications of FDA-approved medications. These examples point to the necessity for prescribing clinicians to be knowledgeable about the regulations and statutes that govern controlled substances in the states in which they hold licensure.

Fine PG, Portenoy RK. *A Clinical Guide to Opioid Analgesia.* Minneapolis: McGraw Hill; 2004:1–8.

Fishman SM. The debate on elder abuse for undertreatment of pain. *Pain Med.* 2004;5:212.

Fishman SM et al. Regulating opioid prescribing through balanced prescription monitoring programs. *Pain Med.* 2004;5:255. [PMID: 15367312]

Gilson AM et al. A reassessment of trends in the medical use and abuse of opioid analgesics and implications for diversion control: 1997–2002. *J Pain Symptom Manage.* 2004;28:176. [PMID: 15276196]

Mendelson D. Aspects of legal liability in pain management involving opioid medications. *J Law Med.* 2001;9:145. [PMID: 12375494]

Pain and Policy Studies Group: Achieving balance in federal and state pain policy: a guide to evaluation. 2nd ed. Madison, WI: University of Wisconsin Comprehensive Cancer Center, 2003. Available at www.mesch.wisc.edu/painpolicy/2003_balance/.

RISKS OF OPIOID MISUSE, ABUSE, & ADDICTION

Treatment of severe pain in cancer patients over the course of many years has suggested that long-term opioid therapy in populations with no prior history of substance abuse is rarely associated with de novo development of abuse or addiction. Similarly, very large surveys of patients who receive opioids to treat acute pain indicate that this therapy has a very low risk of precipitating addiction. In persons with acute pain or pain due to cancer, there are considerable challenges in treating persons with a known history of drug abuse, but the risk of iatrogenic addiction among those without this history appears to be very low.

Notwithstanding the reassuring data concerning the de novo development of addiction in the nonabusing cancer pain and acute pain populations, the incidence and prevalence, or impact, of various aberrant drug-related behaviors are not known in the oncologic setting, no less noncancer chronic pain patients. The reasons for, and rates of, all types of aberrant drug-related behavior

within these diverse populations remain an important topic of current and future research.

The patient with severe pain who is no longer actively abusing drugs raises a special challenge that is similar to other dual diagnoses where a needed treatment for one disease may worsen the other. Since pain relief is a fundamental human right as well as good clinical and ethical practice, the disease of addiction does not eliminate this right or relinquish the physician's responsibility to respond to suffering. In these cases, physicians are therefore required to become risk managers (not dissimilar to the judicious use of treatments that are known to cause metaplasia in cancer treatment or disimmune effects in transplant medicine). Unfortunately, when it comes to treating pain, physicians may feel they accept excessive risk whether they treat or not. This inconsistent attribution of blame for "iatrogenic" harm in pain treatment is only beginning to be openly recognized, evaluated, and discussed.

Questionable Drug-Related Behaviors

Surveys have shown that the occurrence of aberrant drug-related behavior during opioid therapy is common among those patients referred to pain specialists. For example, studies of urine drug screens suggest that as many as 1 of every 3 patients referred to specialized multidisciplinary pain clinics who are prescribed opioid drugs and are not subsequently suspected of abuse may be using other drugs without clinician knowledge. Because patients referred to pain specialists are far more likely than the general population with chronic pain to have comorbid psychiatric disease, including prior substance abuse, it is reasonable to maintain heightened vigilance for the possibility of addiction.

It must be recognized that the base rate of addictive disease in the general population is relatively high (estimated at about 15% for alcoholism and about 5% for cocaine or heroin addiction). On this basis, it has been estimated that at least 10% of adults (and probably higher) have a genetic susceptibility to addiction. With this level of genetic vulnerability, and with other factors (psychological and social) also potentially driving aberrant drug-related behavior, it is prudent to acknowledge the risk of problematic behavior, and even addiction, whenever opioids (or other abusable drugs) are prescribed. Although the risk may be small in some subpopulations, it can never be considered to be zero, and clinicians who prescribe opioids must incorporate risk assessment (and management if needed) at the start of therapy and repeatedly during its course.

It is not surprising that patients with a past history of substance abuse or addiction are at higher risk for a similar problem developing with prescribed opioids. These

---

[1] New York Consolidate Law Laws, Public Health § 3302(1);3350–3351.

Table 22–2. Strategies to Minimize Risk of Abuse and Enhance Monitoring.

- Written agreement following detailed consent discussion.
- Prescribe long-acting drug without rescue dose.
- Frequent visits and small quantities prescribed.
- Urine drug screen at baseline and expressed intention to request occasional screens in the future.
- Requirement that only one pharmacy be used (with permission to contact).
- Instruction to bring pill bottle to appointment (for count).
- Instruction that there will be no early refills and no replacement of lost prescription without police report documenting loss.
- Requirement for nonopioid therapies, including psychotherapy.
- Requirement for all prior records and permission to contact all other health care providers.
- Required referral to addiction medicine specialist.
- Requirement that others (eg, spouse) be allowed to give feedback to the physician.
- In states with electronic prescription reporting and tracking, intention to query the database on a regular basis.

obvious cases establish the need for close monitoring, vigilance, well-established rules and, perhaps, specialist consultation at the outset when opioids may be indicated for pain control. Recent studies have attempted to go beyond this characterization and identify other patient characteristics that can be useful in predicting aberrant drug-related behavior or addiction during opioid therapy for chronic pain. Several screening tools have recently been developed, but they all require additional validation in large prospective studies before they can be relied upon in routine practice.

Although there is no standard approach yet to the prediction of risk, clinicians should ensure that the assessment of the patient receiving long-term opioid therapy for pain include a variety of items related to the risk of abuse and addiction (Table 22–2). In this way, patients may be classified as relatively low risk versus high risk for future problems, and this classification, in turn, can determine the approach used to administer and monitor therapy over time. Risk assessment that supplements comprehensive evaluation, timely and regular follow-up, and documentation of salient clinical issues serve as the best protection for the patient and prescriber alike (Figure 22–1).

High-Risk Patients

Physicians are ethically bound to act in the best interest of the patient and within the law. In many cases, the risk that a patient may deteriorate due to pain may grossly outweigh the risk of relapse into addiction. In such a situation, the physician is confronted with a common dilemma over whether to use a treatment that has risk of adverse effects. For example, in the treatment of serious infectious disease, drugs that are potentially harmful to normal tissues and organs are routinely administered. Clinicians accept these risks and monitor for adverse outcomes, since the risk of not using such a treatment is even more grim. The common application of this principle, known as "double effect," in all areas of medical practice provides the ethical foundation for almost all modern medical and surgical interventions. This is the perspective that must be considered in patients with severe pain who also have a history of opioid addiction that is in remission.

Based on the severity of problematic behavior, past history, and the findings of the reassessment, the clinician must decide about continuation of treatment and referral. Pain treatment may be continued with opioids (using a different structure for prescribing) or continued without opioids, or the patient may be discharged from the practice. The decision to continue treatment with the opioid is based on the severity of the problematic behavior and evidence of functional improvement with opioid treatment from structured reassessment. Treatment should not be continued unless favorable outcomes (ie, pain relief and maintained or improved function) are manifest, ample resources are available and implemented for detecting any further signs or symptoms of addiction, there is a high likelihood that control over the therapy can be reacquired, and restructuring will allow better monitoring of drug-related behavior.

Since the manifestation of drug addiction focuses on the dysfunction or harm derived from compulsive use of a drug, and the objective outcome of effective analgesia (pain relief) is improved function, the safe use of opioids in a patient with a history of opioid addiction relies on distinguishing these opposing potential outcomes. Physicians are often confronted with helping a patient manage one risk against another. Patients often have more than one illness where treating one disease may harm another. Patients who have chronic pain as well as addiction in remission are in this situation, and physicians must manage the relative risks associated with each. To ignore one problem out of fear of protecting the other may not be in the best interest of either one as the patient must be viewed and treated as a whole person. Similarly, the social context within which the patient lives, with the relative

Patient Identifiers: Name   Medical Record No.

PROGRESS NOTE

Current Analgesic Regimen

Drug name	Strength	Frequency	Max Total Daily Dose
_____	_____	_____	_____
_____	_____	_____	_____
_____	_____	_____	_____
_____	_____	_____	_____

The PADT is a clinician-directed interview; that is, the clinician asks the questions, and the clinician records the responses. The Analgesia, Activities of Daily Living, and Adverse Events sections may be completed by the physician, nurse practitioner, physician assistant, or nurse. The Potential Aberrant Drug-Related Behavior and Assessment sections must be completed by the physician. Ask the patient the questions below, except as noted.

Analgesia

If zero indicates "no pain" and ten indicates "pain as bad as it can be," on a scale of 0 to 10, what is your level of pain for the following questions?

1. What was your pain level on average during the past week?
No Pain 0 1 2 3 4 5 6 7 8 9 10 **Pain as bad as it can be**

2. What was your pain level at its worst during the past week?
No Pain 0 1 2 3 4 5 6 7 8 9 10 **Pain as bad as it can be**

3. What percentage of your pain has been relieved during the past week? (Write in a percentage between 0% and 100%.) _____

4. Is the amount of pain relief you are now obtaining from your current pain reliever(s) enough to make a real difference in your life?
☐Yes ☐No

5. *Query to clinician:* Is the patient's pain relief clinically significant?
☐Yes ☐No ☐Unsure

Activities of Daily Living

Please indicate whether the patient's functioning with the current pain reliever(s) is Better, the Same, or Worse since the patient's last assessment with the PADT.*

	Better	Same	Worse
1. Physical functioning	☐	☐	☐
2. Family relationships	☐	☐	☐
3. Social relationships	☐	☐	☐
4. Mood	☐	☐	☐
5. Sleep patterns	☐	☐	☐
6. Overall functioning	☐	☐	☐

 If the patient is receiving his or her first PADT assessment, the clinician should compare the patients functional status with other reports from the last office visit.

Adverse Events

1. Is patient experiencing any side effects from current pain reliever(s)? ☐Yes ☐No
Ask patient about potential side effects:

	None	Mild	Moderate	Severe
a. Nausea	☐	☐	☐	☐
b. Vomiting	☐	☐	☐	☐
c. Constipation	☐	☐	☐	☐
d. Itching	☐	☐	☐	☐
e. Mental clouding	☐	☐	☐	☐

Figure 22–1. Pain Assessment and Documentation Tool (PADT™). (Copyright Janssen Pharmaceutica, 2003. Used with permission.)

f. Sweating	☐	☐	☐	☐
g. Fatigue	☐	☐	☐	☐
h. Drowsiness	☐	☐	☐	☐
i. Other ———	☐	☐	☐	☐
j. Other ———	☐	☐	☐	☐

2. Patient's overall severity of side effects?
☐None ☐Mild ☐Moderate ☐Severe

Activities of Daily Living

*Please **check** any of the following items that you discovered during your interactions with the patient.* Please note that some of these are directly observable (eg, appears intoxicated), while others may require more active listening and/or probing. Use the "Assessment" section below to note additional details.

☐ Purposeful over-sedation
☐ Negative mood change
☐ Appears intoxicated
☐ Increasingly unkempt or impaired
☐ Involvement in car or other accident
☐ Requests frequent early renewals
☐ Increased dose without authorization
☐ Reports lost or stolen prescriptions
☐ Attempts to obtain prescriptions from other doctors
☐ Changes route of administration
☐ Uses pain medication in response to situational stressor
☐ Insists on certain medications by name
☐ Contact with street drug culture
☐ Abusing alcohol or illicit drugs
☐ Hoarding (ie, stockpiling) of medication
☐ Arrested by police
☐ Victim of abuse
Other:_____

PROGRESS NOTE

Assessment: (This section must be completed by the physican.)
Is your overall impression that this patient is benefiting (eg, benefits, such as pain relief, outweigh side effects) from opioid therapy? ☐Yes ☐No ☐Unsure
Comments:_____

Specific Analgesic Plan:
☐ Continue present regimen Comments:_____

☐ Adjust dose of present analgesic Comments:_____

☐ Switch analgesics Comments:_____

☐ Add/Adjust concomitant therapy Comments:_____

☐ Discontinue/taper off opioid therapy Comments:_____

Date: _____
Physician's signature:_____

Figure 22–1. *(Continued)*

support or risks that are there, may determine the course and choices of treatment.

Should the decision to discontinue opioids be indicated, a plan should have already been put in place, and agreed upon, in order to manage expectations and smooth the transition. Discharge from the practice may be warranted if the possibility of therapeutic progress has been severely undermined by mistrust or the assessment reveals that the patient lacks interest in any nonopioid treatments. Ethical and legal protection is gained by clear documentation that the patient was provided with reasonable and available alternative options for care.

When aberrant drug-related behavior occurs, the clinician must also decide about the need for referral for consultation beyond the clinician's expertise. If a diagnosis of addiction is tenable, referral to a specialist in addiction medicine or an addiction program should be strongly considered, although this may be highly problematic in areas where there are insufficient referral centers. Addiction is a serious illness; once it is suspected, it is ill-advised to neglect treatment, as with any other complex, potentially life-threatening disease.

If the decision is made to continue prescribing, strategies should be implemented to reduce the risk of further problems and enhance the opportunity to monitor therapy. For patients who have a proclivity toward substance abuse or addiction, a more rigid structure for therapy, such as frequent visits, small quantities prescribed, the use of urine drug screens, single designated pharmacy use, and collateral information from individuals in daily close contact with the patient who can comment on function and dysfunction, may be helpful in maintaining control. This structure also provides the clinician with the reassurance necessary to continue to act in the patient's best interest. Patients who are taught that a new structure for prescribing is not punitive, but rather, fundamentally therapeutic, are more likely to accept the new restrictions without difficulty. Indeed, patients may express gratitude that the clinician is willing to continue a helpful therapy and assist them in maintaining control. When therapy is restructured, it is important that documentation be comprehensive and complete. The medical record should reflect all aspects of the thoughtful reassessment and the written plan should be explicit. It may be useful to provide the patient with a letter that clarifies the next steps, the patient's obligations, and consequences should problems recur.

Role of Opioid Agreements

A formal written agreement between the patient and physician at the start of opioid therapy is becoming a common tool for defining expectations and documenting informed consent. These agreements are often called "contracts" and are probably enforceable against clinicians who break their own terms irrespective of the title given (eg, contract, agreement, or consent) (Figure 22–2).

There may be good reasons either to implement or not implement an agreement. On the "pro" side, these agreements outline the clinician's policy for providing controlled prescription drugs, and describe the consequences of problematic drug-related behavior. They can reinforce that these medications must be used responsibly and also assure patients that medication will be prescribed, as long as there is adherence to the plan of care. Lastly, they can be used as educational tools.

On the "con" side, these agreements can contribute to the stigmatization of opioid therapy and possibly reduce the likelihood of success. If they are framed in a manner that the patient perceives as threatening, they may contribute to assessment difficulties as the patient withholds or skews information in an effort to meet expectations. If they make insupportable demands (like no driving, even after dose equilibration and habituation to sedating effects) that are inconsistent with the literature and compromise function and quality of life, they could undermine the goals of therapy or encourage the patient to lie. If they give a clinician a false sense of security, and thereby reduce the vigilance, monitoring, and use of appropriate ongoing strategies that are essential to risk management, they could paradoxically increase risk. Finally, if they implicitly hold a clinician to a certain level of clinical performance, they could ultimately be used adversely in a medicolegal dispute. Given these potential negatives, and the lack of consensus about the role of this approach, each clinician must decide whether the use of an agreement is appropriate and likely to be beneficial.

Adams LL et al. Development of a self-report screening instrument for assessing potential opioid medication misuse in chronic pain patients. *J Pain Symptom Manage.* 2004;27:440. [PMID: 15120773]

Fishman SM et al. The opioid contract. *Clin J Pain.* 2002;18:S70. [PMID: 12479256]

Friedman R et al. Treating pain patients at risk: evaluation of a screening tool in opioid-treated pain patients with and without addiction. *Pain Med.* 2003;4:182. [PMID: 12873264]

Michna E et al. Predicting aberrant drug behavior in patients treated for chronic pain: Importance of abuse history. *J Pain Symptom Manage.* 2004;28:250. [PMID: 15336337]

OPIOIDS & TERMINAL ILLNESS

The obligation to relieve suffering is an ethical imperative of the medical profession and is especially important

Patient name:_____

Medical Record: _____

Doctor: _____

Goals for taking opioid medications:

Medication and proposed duration of use:

Agreements:

- Only your pain doctor will prescribe opioid medications for you.
- You agree not to ask for opioid medications from any other doctor without the knowledge and assent of your pain doctor.
- You agree to keep all scheduled appointments, not just with your physician but also with recommended therapists and psychological counselors. Three or more missed appointments or same day cancellations will lead to patient dismissal.
- You agree to provide regular samples for drug screens. Positive tests for any illegal substances, or opioids not prescribed by your pain doctor, will result in your dismissal and referral elsewhere for substance abuse evaluation and management.
- No prescriptions will be refilled early.
- No prescriptions will be refilled if you lose, destroy, or have any of your medication stolen.
- Prescription refills will be authorized only during regular office hours. If you want the prescription mailed to you, contact our office 7 working days prior to the refill date. If you want to pick up the prescription in person, call 2 working days in advance of renewal date. You may be required to provide postage-paid self- addressed envelopes in advance for mailed prescriptions.
- You agree to comply fully with all aspects of your treatment program including behavioral medicine (psychology/psychiatry) and physical therapy, if recommended. Failure to do so may lead to discontinuation of your medication and referral to another provider or treatment center.
- Successful pain management entails using multiple interventions, including active participation in regular physical exercise and the use of psychological coping strategies. A pattern of passive reliance on medications, resistance to more active physical treatments, and repeated failure to demonstrate the implementation of psychologically based coping strategies that have been taught to you may lead to discontinuation of medications and/or referral to another provider or treatment center.

It is understood that emergencies can occur and under some circumstances, exceptions to these guidelines may be made. Emergencies will be considered on an individual basis.

Opioids may cause drowsiness that can be worsened with alcohol, benzodiazepines, and other sedating medications. Use care when driving or operating machinery. An overdose can cause severe side effects, even death.

Other common, usually temporary, side effects include nausea, itching, and sweating. Psychological depression and altered testosterone levels, and other hormones, may also occur. Sleep apnea, if present, may be worsened by opioids. Constipation commonly occurs, and often does not improve with time. It is impossible to predict opioid side effects in any individual patient. Having side effects on one opioid does not necessarily mean there will be side effects on another opioid.

You must take opioids only as directed. Federal law prohibits giving this medication to anyone else. Physical dependence will develop with regular use but does not by itself indicate addiction; this means that a withdrawal syndrome will probably develop if you stop your medication abruptly. Tolerance can develop to the pain relieving effects of opioids; this means that the pain relief may decrease over time, but it usually occurs slowly, if at all.

Not all pain conditions respond to opioids. Some pain may only be partially responsive to opioid therapy. Total elimination of pain is an unrealistic goal. Escalating dosages may indicate that opioids are not effective or that there is an underlying problem with addiction or psychological dependence. Discontinuation of opioid medications may need to be done under these circumstances: not enough pain relief, persistent side effects, not achieving goals of opioid treatment (such as improvement in funtion), problematic dose escalation, or inability to comply with the treatment agreement.

I, the undersigned, agree to follow these guidelines that have been fully explained to me. All of my questions and concerns regarding treatment have been adequately answered.

I give permission to my pain doctor to contact my other healthcare providers, or prescription databases, for the purposes of sharing information concerning my situation, as is deemed necessary for coordinated, high-quality care.

If I do not follow these guidelines fully, my doctor may taper and stop opioid treatment and refer me elsewhere for care.

A copy of this document has been given to me.

Patient signature: _____

Date:_____

Witness signature:_____

Figure 22–2. Sample Medication Management Agreement.

in the care of persons who are dying. Among the greatest harm to dying patients, and their loved ones, is to abandon them in their need for comfort, of which relief

Table 22–3. Principles of Prescribing Opioids in Terminally Ill Patients.

- Choose the least invasive, most readily available and acceptable route. Provide around-the-clock analgesic coverage and a plan for breakthrough pain if the pain pattern warrants it.
- Be prepared for an alternative route if the patient loses the ability to swallow or absorb medications via the oral route.
- Educate caregivers about the approach to pain management and ensure that professional and nonprofessional caregivers and family members understand the principles involved (eg, recognition of nonverbal signs of pain; titration to comfort).
- Distinguish pain from anxiety, delirium, or "terminal restlessness," if possible. This may require an opioid trial in the nonverbal or cognitively impaired patient. Distressed behaviors that do not respond to anxiolytics or antipsychotics suggest a pain etiology.
- Pain crises that respond poorly to basic analgesic approaches merit consultation with a specialist as soon as possible. More aggressive therapeutic methods may be warranted. Interventional techniques, such as epidural or intrathecal catheterization, certain types of nerve blocks or neurolytic procedures, or use of drugs such as ketamine, may be appropriate in selected patients.
- Escalating doses of opioids in patients who are not demonstrating pain behaviors may be interpreted as hastening death. Physician assisted suicide is only permissible under state law (and highly circumscribed conditions) in Oregon.

from pain is paramount. Patients and family members expect that physicians will honor this need by effectively treating pain.

When providing opioid therapy to patients near death, the ethical principle of double effect must be understood and clearly communicated. This principle is particularly important in addressing the fear that aggressive opioid therapy at the end of life could potentially hasten death. According to the principle of double effect, a foreseeable "bad" outcome of an action (such as a potentially hastened death) is ethically acceptable if the intention is beneficent (the relief of suffering), and the need to accomplish the good is more important than the need to avoid potentially negative consequences. At the end of life, this principle guides the aggressive use of opioids and other interventions. Physicians must defend the ethical nature of aggressive pain control and clearly distinguish pain treatment from euthanasia.

Although clinicians should understand and invoke the principle of double effect when using opioids in dying patients, it is nonetheless reassuring to know that there is no convincing scientific evidence that demonstrates a significant risk of hastened death if the opioid dose is appropriately titrated at the end of life. Indeed, there is more anecdotal evidence to the contrary. Given these reassuring observations, and the well-recognized adverse physiologic and psychological effects from unrelieved pain, aggressive titration of the opioid dose to maintain relief of pain is warranted until the very end of life (Table 22–3).

Bercovitch M et al. Patterns of high-dose morphine use in a home-care hospice service: should we be afraid of it? *Cancer.* 2004;101:1473. [PMID: 15368335]

Fine PG. The ethical imperative to relieve pain at life's end. *J Pain Symptom Manage.* 2002;23:273. [PMID: 11997196]

Fine PG. The evolving and important role of anesthesiology in palliative care. *Anesth Analg.* 2005;100:183. [PMID: 15616075]

Index

Note: Page numbers followed by a *t* indicate tables; numbers followed by an *f* indicate figures.